Mycobacterial Skin Infections

Domenico Bonamonte • Gianni Angelini
Editors

Mycobacterial Skin Infections

Springer

Editors
Domenico Bonamonte
University of Bari "Aldo Moro"
Department of Biomedical Science and Human Oncology
Bari
Italy

Gianni Angelini
University of Bari "Aldo Moro"
Dermatology
Bari
Italy

English editing by Mary VC. Pragnell, B.A. (HONS).

ISBN 978-3-319-48537-9 ISBN 978-3-319-48538-6 (eBook)
DOI 10.1007/978-3-319-48538-6

Library of Congress Control Number: 2017951315

Printed on acid-free paper

This Springer imprint is published by Springer Nature
The registered company is Springer International Publishing AG
The registered company address is: Gewerbestrasse 11, 6330 Cham, Switzerland

To Davide
Elizabeth
Gianmarco

Preface

The overview of mycobacterial skin infections presented in this work is justified by the current worldwide increase in diseases induced by both old and new mycobacteria. Until the late 1980s, such diseases had been notably declining, but after that period, the trend reversed, and an exponential increase began to be observed. There are various reasons for this rise not only in developing countries but even in urban areas in the most developed nations.

Being the cause of tuberculosis and leprosy, the *Mycobacterium* genus has probably caused mankind more suffering than all the other bacterial genera combined. Moreover, in addition to the obligate pathogens, namely, the *Mycobacterium tuberculosis* complex and *M. leprae*, this genus is continually being enriched by the addition of many other species. Although usually encountered as environmental saprophytes, in some conditions that depend on the host immune status, they can induce extremely severe, sometimes fatal, clinical pictures.

It is well known that tuberculosis (TB) is one of the oldest diseases ever to affect mankind, but nowadays, it is emerging once more as an enormous and growing global health problem.

According to the World Health Organization (WHO) (Global Tuberculosis Report 2016, World Health Organization), in 2015 there were an estimated 10.4 million new (incident) TB cases worldwide, of which 5.9 million (56%) were among men, 3.5 million (34%) among women, and 1.0 million (10%) among children. HIV-infected people accounted for 11% of all new TB cases. Six countries accounted for 60% of the new cases: in descending order, India, Indonesia, China, Nigeria, Pakistan, and South Africa.

The rate of decline in TB incidence remained worldwide at only 1.5% from 2014 to 2015. This need to accelerate to a 4–5% annual decline by 2020 to reach the first milestones of the End TB Strategy. The WHO End TB Strategy (approved by the World Health Assembly in 2014), in fact, calls for a 90% reduction in TB deaths and an 80% reduction in the TB incidence rate by 2030, compared with 2015.

According to many authors, the high present TB incidence is attributable to increased levels of poverty in our overpopulated world, to the breakdown of healthcare systems and to the impact of the HIV/AIDS pandemic. Further complicating the situation, there has been a worrying rise in multidrug-resistant TB (MDR-TB) (defined as resistance to isoniazid and rifampicin), and now we also face the recent emergence of extensively drug-resistant TB (defined as resistance to many other drugs). In 2015, there were an estimated 580,000 new cases of MDR-TB. India, China, and the Russian Federation accounted for 45% of the combined total of 580,000 cases. The WHO estimated that in 2015 there has been 1.4 million TB deaths and an additional 0.4 million deaths resulting from TB infection among HIV-infected people. Although the number of TB deaths fell by 22% between 2000 and 2015, TB remained one of the top 10 causes of death worldwide in 2015.

Extrapulmonary TB manifests only in 8.4–13.7% of cases, while cutaneous TB comprises only a small proportion (<1–2%) of all cases of TB. All the same, in view of the current high prevalence of TB worldwide, these numbers become significant. Assuming that 1% of all cases of TB will have cutaneous involvement, dermatologists in countries such as India, where 1,847,000 new cases of TB were reported in 1999, must expect to see an annual incidence of about 18,000 cases of cutaneous TB. In any event, factors such as HIV infection and migration are ensuring that cutaneous TB will necessarily have to be included in differential diagnosis made by dermatologists all over the world.

Apart from *M. tuberculosis*, TB in man is induced also by *M. bovis*, which has a greater number of potential hosts than the tubercle bacillus. Various studies have shown that 0.3–1.5% of TB in humans is due to *M. bovis* in developed countries. Due to inappropriate methods for identifying the pathogen, in developing countries the incidence is unknown, but is most likely higher than in industrialized countries. In 1992, the European Union declared infection by *M. bovis* one of the four most important zoonoses (European Union. Council Directive 29/117/EEC, 1992. Off J Eur Comm 1993; L62:38), and in 1995, the WHO labeled the infection a global emergency (Guidelines for speciation within the *Mycobacterium tuberculosis* complex. Geneva: World Health Organization, 1995). Among the various modes of transmission of this organism to man (respiratory, gastrointestinal), we must include direct skin contact that occurs mainly in some occupational fields.

Meanwhile, the modes of transmission of *M. leprae* are still not fully understood. There is solid evidence of transmission among contacts, as well as of zoonotic leprosy in southern states in the USA. Current findings suggest that aerosols/droplets and shedding of bacteria in the environment, as well as skin-to-skin contact, are possible culprits. Globally, the number of leprosy cases is now below the elimination threshold of 1 case/10,000 people, as defined by the WHO. In various countries and subnational regions, however, the number of leprosy patients is still above this threshold. Moreover, despite the near-universal use and efficacy of multidrug therapy, the annual number of newly detected cases has remained fairly constant at around 200,000–300,000 cases in the last years. This demonstrates that the current control measures are insufficient to arrest the process of leprosy transmission.

The experience we gained over several years of assiduous attendance of the Hansenian Colony in Gioia del Colle (Bari, Italy), one of the largest in Europe, validated by clinical-therapeutic studies of the disease, has been of inestimable aid in writing the relative chapter about leprosy.

To compound the issue, nontuberculous mycobacteria (NTM) are common in nature, and, except perhaps in extreme environments such as deserts and polar regions, humans are regularly exposed to them. Unlike the obligate pathogens,

NTM may occur as transient commensals on the skin and in various other organs (the pharynx, lower urethra, gastrointestinal tract), so their isolation does not necessarily indicate the presence of disease. The pathogenicity of NTM is directly correlated to the host immune system, and in fact since the 1930s, many species have been strongly associated with some human diseases. The development of new diagnostic tools has resulted in a huge increase in the number of infections associated with specific species, as well as the number of new species identified as causal agents. NTM can cause a vast spectrum of diseases that are often quite difficult to diagnose. A high suspicion index is important, and the diagnostic conclusions must be based on a number of microbiological and radiological investigations. It must also be borne in mind that the search for bacilli in various clinical specimens may not always be positive. Even histopathology is not definitive because granulomatous tubercle findings are rare, whereas nonspecific inflammatory aspects are common.

The aim of this work is, therefore, to offer dermatologists a tool to help them recognize the different clinical mycobacterial manifestations, make a prompt diagnosis, and institute effective treatment. Unfortunately, older dermatologists tend to have become less familiar with these very important diseases in recent decades, while younger dermatologists have perhaps never encountered them before. By contrast, the current globalization process, and all its accompanying implications as regards infectious diseases that may be more or less widespread in the different countries, "demands" as wide as possible a knowledge of these among clinicians.

Bari, Italy
May 2017

Gianni Angelini, MD
Domenico Bonamonte, MD, PhD

Acknowledgments

This book has been produced thanks also to the valuable contributions of various colleagues, to whom go our most grateful thanks.

Professor Roger Pradinaud, chairman of the Dermatology Service of the Andrée Rosemon Hospital, Cayenne (French Guyana), a great expert on tropical dermatology, offered valuable information about *Mycobacterium ulcerans* infection: his wise suggestions and in-depth knowledge of the subject, illustrated in numerous publications, provided us with inestimable guidance. We are also grateful to Professor Roger Pradinaud for clinical images of this disease.

Professor Giorgio Leigheb, former chairman of the Dermatological Clinic of the University of Novara (Italy), famous entomological dermatologist and great friend, kindly provided us with various clinical images of *Mycobacterium ulcerans* infection, a topic that he has studied widely in the nations with the highest incidence of this infection.

Doctors Angela Filoni, Paolo Romita, Pietro Verni, and Michelangelo Vestita, of the Dermatological Clinic of Bari University Hospital (Italy), contributed enormously with their enthusiasm and skill to the completion of this work.

We would like to thank the publishers Springer-Verlag (Berlin), Cambridge University Press (Cambridge, UK), and Piccin (Padova, Italy) and John Libbey Eurotest, editor of the *European Journal of Dermatology* (Montrouge, France), for having kindly authorized the reproduction of various figures.

Finally, we are very grateful to Springer-Verlag for their assiduous commitment to producing this volume.

Gianni Angelini
Domenico Bonamonte

Contents

Contributors

Gianni Angelini, MD Professor of Dermatology, Former Professor and Chairman, University of Bari "Aldo Moro", Bari, Italy

Domenico Bonamonte, MD, PhD Associate Professor of Dermatology, Department of Biomedical Science and Human Oncology, University of Bari "Aldo Moro", Bari, Italy

Angela Filoni, MD University of Bari "Aldo Moro", Bari, Italy

Paolo Romita, MD University of Bary "Aldo Moro", Bari, Italy

Pietro Verni, MD University of Bari "Aldo Moro", Bari, Italy

Michelangelo Vestita, MD University of Bari "Aldo Moro", Bari, Italy

Mycobacteria

1

Domenico Bonamonte, Paolo Romita,
Pietro Verni, and Gianni Angelini

As compared to other Schizomycetes, mycobacteria (from the Greek muxes:mycetes and bacterion: rod) present some atypical characteristics that cause them to resemble mycetes. Nevertheless, there is no doubt as to their status as bacteria: they belong to the order of the *Actinomycetaceae*, and the family of *Mycobacteriaceae*. This family includes only the *Mycobacterium* genus, that accounts for more than 170 species, many of which are of no clinical interest [1, 2].

Despite a few peculiar differences observed in some species, the morphology of mycobacteria tends to be homogeneous. They are long, slender bacilli ranging from 1 to 5 μm in length and 0.2–0.6 μm in diameter. Coccobacillary forms, although rarely found in pathological samples, are common in colony-forming preparations. Mycobacteria have no locomotor organules and are strictly aerobic or microaerophylic, as well as being Gram-positive and pleomorphic. Their pleomorphism is due to the fact that they normally grow in filaments, sometimes branched (hence the name of this genus, to indicate their resemblance to mycetes, that being moulds, have a filament-like branched morphology), that fragment into bacilli or coccobacilli.

Mycobacteria are not mobile nor sporogenic, and except for a few species, show fairly slow reproductive rhythms. In fact, while mean duplication time is about 20 min in *Enterobacteriaceae*, in the case of mycobacteria it exceeds 15 h. Except

D. Bonamonte, MD, PhD (✉)
Department of Biomedical Science and Human Oncology,
University of Bary "Aldo Moro", Bari, Italy
e-mail: domenico.bonamonte@uniba.it

P. Romita, MD • P. Verni, MD
University of Bary "Aldo Moro", Bari, Italy

G. Angelini, MD
Professor of Dermatology, Former Professor and Chairman, University of Bary "Aldo Moro",
Bari, Italy

D. Bonamonte, G. Angelini (eds.), *Mycobacterial Skin Infections*,
DOI 10.1007/978-3-319-48538-6_1

for *M. leprae*, all the species can be cultured, even if most of them require very complex culture media. The colonies show morphological differences among the species but generally feature a rough surface.

1.1 Habitat and Diffusion

Mycobacteria are widespread in the environment; apart from in man, they are present in all types of water (including domestic), in the soil, air, plants, foods and in various hot- and cold-blooded animals. Mycobacteria have the same degree of resistance to heat and ultraviolet rays as other bacteria, but are more resistant to drying and chemical disinfectants, probably due to their high lipid content.

1.2 Cellular Structure

Under the electronic microscope, mycobacteria are seen to have a very thick cell wall, inwards from which extend the first sprouts of the transverse septa, that will lead to cell division (mesosomes). The components of the cell wall include peptidoglycan and diaminopimelate, as well as polysaccharides (glucan, mannitol, arabinogalactan, arabino-mannitol). There is a wealth of cytoplasmic inclusions, especially lipids, glycogen and polymetaphosphates.

Most of the properties of mycobacteria are directly or indirectly owed to the structure of the cell wall. The lipid content, that is already very high overall in mycobacteria cells (25%, that is 10–15 times higher than that of other bacteria) reaches extremely high values at the level of the cell wall (more than 60% of the dry weight). Another important characteristic of mycobacteria, that is unusual among Schizomycetes, is the presence of some large compounds with associated sugars and glycoproteins, that therefore give rise to the formation of glycolipids and glycopeptidolipids called mycosides.

The basic constituents of mycosides are mycolic acids, that are often esterified in lipid molecules. These are beta-hydroxylated fatty acids, characterized by a long saturated chain (ramified in the alpha position) of carbon atoms (from 83 to 93). These mycolic acids are not present in other bacteria species. At the level of the external surface of the cell wall, mycolic acids have the function of phagic receptors. The proportion of different types of mycosides remains constant within each single species, and is therefore also a valid aid for taxonomic purposes.

Another very important class of lipids, that is also present in corynebacteria, is that of waxes, fatty acid esters (including mycolic acids) and alcohols. One mycoside that has undergone close study is dimycolil-trehalose, known as the cord factor because when tubercular mycobacteria lack this substance, they lose the ability to develop as tortuous bands on particular culture media. This characteristic is likely due to the virulence of these bacteria. In fact, the greater the cord factor content the more virulent the species. Moreover, this factor is lethal in mouse, inhibiting the migration of polymorphonuclear cells [3]. However, the virulence seems to be also correlated to a sulfonate glycolipid that is present in high quantities in those species featuring this property.

Mycobacteria waxes are subdivided into four classes (A, B, C, D): the most important is wax D, that has an immunological adjuvant action, boosting the production of antibodies against other antigens that may be present (in particular of proteinaceous type).

1.3 Antigenic Structure

Various antigens have been identified in mycobacteria, many of which are common to several species. Some antigens crossreact with the Nocardia and Corynebacterium genuses, whose cell wall has some affinities with that of mycobacteria.

As stated above, the most abundant substances in the chemical composition of mycobacteria are lipids, that determine many of their peculiar properties. These are not important from the antigenic standpoint because they are non immunogenic, but it seems that they may act as haptens.

Polysaccharide antigens consist largely of arabino-galactan; from the immunological standpoint they are haptens, that can stimulate the production of antibodies only if inoculated together with the entire bacterial cell.

Proteic antigens are complex and quite difficult to purify. They are weakly immunogenic, although their activity is reinforced by class D waxes, that act as adjuvants. These antigens are responsible for delayed hypersensitivity reactions, as induced by the tuberculin test.

1.4 Sensitivity to Antibiotics

Mycobacteria behave rather differently toward antibiotics as compared to other microorganisms. For example, *M. tuberculosis* is resistant to all the antibiotics normally used to treat Gram-positive and Gram-negative infections, but it is sensitive to a small number of drugs that are therefore denominated antitubercular; sensitivity to these drugs is generally fairly constant, at least as regards those strains isolated from untreated subjects. By contrast, resistance may arise during treatment, related to various factors. It should also be borne in mind that in vitro susceptibility results are not always correlated with the same drug results in vivo.

Most of the clinical pictures induced by mycobacteria are treated with one or two active drugs. The association of drugs is necessary to reduce the likelihood of onset of resistant mutants. It is estimated, for example, that in a tubercle bacilli culture the frequency of isoniazide resistant mutants is 1 in 10^5, of streptomycin mutants 1 in 10^6, while the frequency of mutants resistant to both drugs is lower, being 1 in 10^{11} [2].

It is not necessary to test the drug sensitivity of most of the strains isolated if the patient has never previously taken antitubercular drugs. In any case, there is no need to wait for the results of susceptibility tests before starting treatment, that can be begun with drugs known to be more active against the strain isolated. Instead, it is important to determine the sensitivity of the isolated strain when the patient has already undergone antitubercular treatment (owing to the common onset of resistance), or shows worsening during the treatment, or else when the culture does not become negative within 4–6 months from the start of treatment or if a nontubercular species is isolated.

1.5 Nontubercular Bacteria

The existence of mycobacteria other than *M. tuberculosis* complex and *M. leprae* has been known since the time of the discovery of the tubercle bacillus in the late 1800s. They are ubiquitous in the environment and have been variously denominated "atypical", "anonymous", "opportunistic", or "non classified". These terminologies have since been abandoned and these mycobacteria are now denominated "nontubercular mycobacteria" (NTM). This denomination can be considered to correspond to the acronym MOTT (Mycobacteria Other Than Tubercle bacilli) used by Anglo-Saxon writers. Some authors prefer to use the denomination "environmental mycobacteria" in view of their ubiquity in the environment [4, 5].

Today, more than 170 species have been identified (www.bacterio.net/mycobacterium.html), thanks to the advent of molecular techniques and 16s rRNA gene sequencing for defining new species [6–9]. There is no evidence of human-to-human or animal-to-human transmission of infections due to NTM. The source of infection in man is always the environment, even if the precise source is not always identified [10].

1.6 Classification

In 1959 Runyon proposed a classification of mycobacteria in four groups, based on the speed of growth and the pigmentation of the colonies (Table 1.1) [11]. It was later seen that there were several strains within each group, and also that the different strains could elicit different reaction patterns from those considered as typical. Certain species may therefore belong to more than one group; for example, *M. szulgai*, that features slow growth, is scotochromogenic if incubated at 37°C and photochromogenic when incubated at 22–25°C. Many species may be lightly pigmented and so misinterpreted, causing classification errors.

Table 1.1 Classification of nontubercular mycobacteria according to Runyon

Group I: photochromogens	*M. asiaticum, M. kansasii, M. marinum, M. simiae*
Group II: scotochromogens	*M. flavescens, M. gordonae, M. scrofulaceum, M. szulgai, M. xenopi*
Group III: non chromogens	*M. avium, M. intracellulare, M. haemophilum, M. malmoense, M. terrae, M. nonchromogenicum, M. triviale, M. gastri*
Group IV: rapidly growing mycobacteria	*M. chelonae, M. fortuitum, M. phlei, M. smegmatis, M. vaccae*

Moreover, *M. tuberculosis, M. africanum, M. bovis, M. leprae* and *M. ulcerans* are not included in the Runyon classification. It is now therefore largely of historical interest and has been replaced by more precise methods for determining the different species [12, 13].

In the Runyon classification the first group includes slow growth photochromogenic species, i.e. those that are able to produce pigment only after exposure to light. The second group is that of slow growth scotochromogenic (or true chromogenic) species that can produce pigment even in the dark (but the *M. xenopi* species is assigned by some authors to the third group). The third group includes slow growth nonchromogenic species, and the fourth, rapidly growing species.

1.7 Complexes

Depending on their bio-physiological appearance, the different mycobacteria species are generally grouped in "complexes" named after the most representative species. However, some species, that show no resemblance to any of these groups, or whose characteristics are poorly delineated, are not included in any of the complexes.

Table 1.2 reports only some of the complexes, in particular those species that most commonly cause disease in man.

Table 1.2 The most common complexes and most representative species isolated in man

1- Mycobacterium tuberculosis complex
a. M. tuberculosis
b. M. bovis
c. M. africanum
2- Mycobacterium avium complex
a. M. avium
b. M. intracellulare
c. M. xenopi
3- Mycobacterium scrofulaceum complex
a. M. scrofulaceum
b. M. simiae
4- Mycobacterium gordonae complex
a. M. gordonae
b. M. szulgai
5- Mycobacterium kansasii complex
a. M. kansasii
b. M. gastri
6- Mycobacterium terrae complex
a. M. terrae
b. M. nonchromogenicum
c. M. triviale
7- Mycobacterium fortuitum complex
a. M. fortuitum
b. M. chelonae
8- Mycobacterium parafortuitum complex
a. M. parafortuitum
b. M. vaccae

1.8 Microscopic Examination

This examination has a major diagnostic importance owing to the peculiar property of mycobacteria, namely that they are acid-fast. This property seems to be linked to the lipid component of the cell wall: the mycolic acids form a complex with fuchsin, impeding its release despite alcohol and acid treatment.

The most commonly employed staining method is Ziehl–Neelsen, that involves the use of fuchsin and heat. Preparations are observed in immersion (1000×) and the bacilli stain red against a blue background.

Fluorescent microscopy is also based on acid-fastness: in this case after the fluorochrome has stained the mycobacteria they do not release it despite alcohol and acid treatment [14]. The reagent is fluorochrome (0.1 g auramine-O in 10 ml of 95% ethanol; 3 ml of liquid phenol in 87 ml of H_2O). Preparations must be observed under a blue light fluorescence microscope (mean excitation wave length 460 nm). There are some advantages of this method as compared to Ziehl–Neelsen staining, namely faster reading thanks to the greater width of the microscope observation field and the lesser importance of observer chromatic discrimination.

A slide treated with auramine can be counterstained with Ziehl–Neelsen if it may help to interpret any fluorescent bodies with an untypical morphology.

Kinyoun staining, that also employs fuchsin, is similar to Ziehl–Neelsen staining but has the advantage of not requiring the use of heat. Preparations are observed using a 100× oil immersion objective.

The preparation findings are generally reported as semiquantitative assessments, indicating the presence of bacilli as + (sporadic bacilli), ++ (bacilli in several microscope fields), and +++ (numerous bacilli in all the fields observed). This assessment provides the clinician with useful indications as regards the effects of therapy, and can also help to identify the onset of resistance (observation of a high bacterial load after microscope monitoring had demonstrated the reduction or absence of bacilli).

However, we wish to underline once more here that a negative result of a bacterioscopic examination is not a certain indication of negative results; in fact, the limit of detection of the current microscope observation method is calculated to be about 5×10^4 bacilli per ml of sample material [15]. Similarly, a positive result is not equivalent to an etiological diagnosis of the species and hence a specific disease, since examination at the microscope only reveals the presence of acid-fast bacilli, that may or may not be pathogenic.

1.9 Culture Media

All mycobacteria are obligate parasites, saprophytic or intermediate forms, that differ as regards nutrient requirements and hence culture methods. Some species grow on fairly simple culture media while others need media enriched by particular substances (potato flour, egg, albumin, glycerine, casein hydroxylate, oleic acid, various salts, vitamins), and others can only be cultured in living cells. In general they show a fairly slow growth, ranging from about 3 days to 8 weeks or more, depending on the cell division time, that ranges from 2 to more than 20 h.

Mycobacteria culture media are generally fairly complex because they are particularly demanding microorganisms. Liquid media are normally unsuited to the isolation of mycobacteria from biological samples. Exceptionally, they may be used for seeding sterile matter (CSF, blood, cavitary fluids), while they are largely used to enrich pure culture media and to prepare bacterial suspensions for sensitivity or typing tests [15]. The most common liquid media are the Dubos, Middlebrook 7H9 and Middlebrook 7H12 broths (the latter being used only for radiometric culture methods). Solid media, in practice the only ones employed for primary isolation, have an egg or synthetic base. The former contain, together with egg, natural substances (potato flour, glycerol, milk, mineral salts); the addition of malachite green has the function of inhibiting the development of any associated flora that have survived the decontamination process. Among the various natural solid media those most commonly employed are Jehnsen modified Löwenstein (Löwenstein-Jehnsen, certainly the one in most widespread use), Petragnani medium, the American Thoracic Society medium, and the International Union Tuberculosis Medium. Some species of mycobacteria require specific substances to foster growth: for example, *M. bovis* needs pyruvate, instead of glycerol, as carbon source [15]. The basic ingredients of synthetic media are agar and oleic acid; Middlebrook 7H10 and 7H11 are among the best known. Added with the single antimicrobial agents, these media are used to perform sensitivity testing.

The pathological material used for seeding to isolate mycobacteria is often contaminated by other microbial flora and so needs to be adequately decontaminated to eliminate concomitant flora. These have a faster growth and so could impede mycobacterial development by invading the entire medium. When reading and reporting the results, a positive response to a culture medium is always preceded by ascertainment that the colony-forming bacilli are acid-fast. In general, the results of microscopy and culture coincide but positive results to one and negative to the other may occur. Unless gross errors have been made, positive results to microscopy and negative to culture may be due to the presence of non vital bacilli (this is not infrequent in patients undergoing treatment) or the use of a harmful decontaminant, and the reverse result, to a minor mycobacterial load in the sample.

1.10 Biological Testing

Biological testing in guineapigs, by subcutaneous inoculation of test matter in the inguinal region, is no longer performed because the animals have a reduced receptivity to some mycobacterial strains. In fact, they are refractory not only to NTM, but also to isoniazide- and rifampicin-resistant strains of *M. tuberculosis*.

1.11 Identification

In itself, a positive culture provides some information about the species, according to the type of material from which the strain was isolated, the temperature and the growth speed of the primary culture, the morphology and pigmentation of the

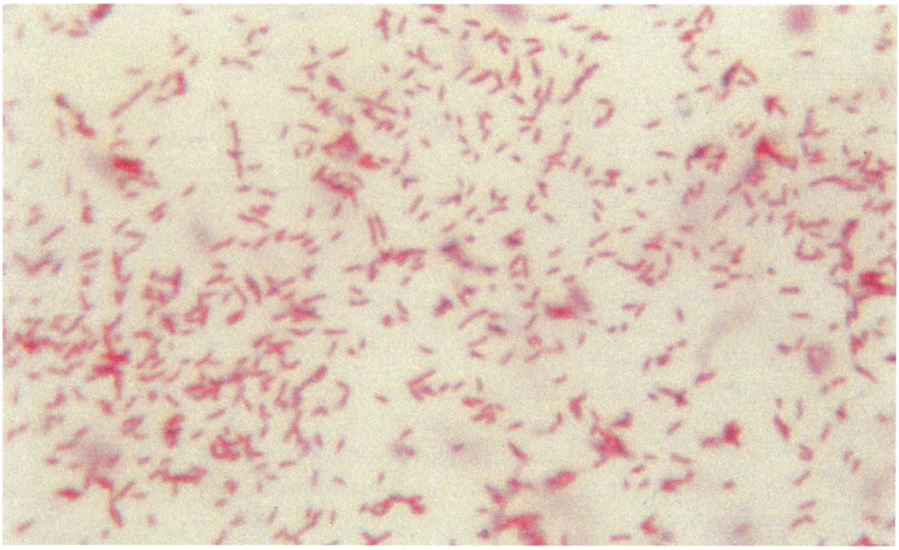

Fig. 1.1 *Mycobacterium fortuitum*

colonies obtained (that may range from yellow to a deep orange, due to the production of carotene crystals).

A series of tests is then employed to make a definitive identification of the species and subspecies. For *M. tuberculosis* tests of niacin, nitrates and catalase heat inactivation are generally sufficient. In the case of NTM, as well as different culture tests (media incubated at different growth temperatures, one of which will be wrapped in aluminum foil to protect it from light; media containing specific nutrient substances), biochemical tests and some other complementary tests are necessary (e.g. sensitivity to ciprofloxacin to discriminate *M. fortuitum*, sensitive, from *M. chelonae*, resistant), and must all be performed in a single session (Fig. 1.1).

1.12 Rapid Methods

Compared to conventional tests, so-called rapid tests allow faster positive results to be obtained. The radiometric method is based on the discrimination of radiolabeled CO_2 released by the metabolic activity of the microorganism on a substrate containing C^{14} [16]. A beta-counter removes culture medium (7H12 broth) daily from the flask, and from a gas sample, measures the radioactivity, transforming the resulting value into a growth index. Use of this method speeds positivization time by 30% [15].

The molecular probes technique is based on the following principle: as well as nucleotide sequences that may be more or less homologous to those of other species (the homology varies according to the philogenetic distance), living organisms possess some entirely species-specific sequences in their genome. These specific genome fractions can be used as probes once they have been identified, cloned and made available in single helix form. The genomic material of a species to be identified is added with a probe of known specificity: if there are complementary nucleic acid filaments in the reaction mix (this condition will occur only if the unknown microorganism belongs to the same species as the probe) they will unite to form a double helix. The probe target can be denatured nuclear DNA or ribosomal RNA; in the latter case the sensitivity of the method is enormously increased because there are about 10,000 ribosomes per cell. This technology is widely employed in the mycobacteriological field thanks to the availability of specific probes for clinically important mycobacteria.

Chromatography is based on analysis of the lipids making up the bacterial wall: the different mycobacterial species can be identified on the basis of the differences in lipid content. The various chromatography techniques separate and identify the single lipid components of the cell wall of the species under study and the species can then be identified on the basis of analysis of the lipid pattern [15].

References

1. Esposito R (1985) Parassitologia clinica e medicina tropicale. Masson Italia Editori, Milano
2. Nicoletti G, Nicolosi VM (1993) Dizionario di batteriologia umana. Normale e patologica, 2nd edn. Mediserve, Milano
3. Noll H (1956) The chemistry of cord factor, a toxic glycolipid of *Mycobacterium tuberculosis*. Adv Tuberc Res 7:149
4. Mandler F, Peona V (1987) Micobatteriosi e micobatteri non tubercolari. Masson Italia Editori, Milano, p 126
5. Griffith DE, Aksamit T, Brown-Elliott BA et al (2007) An official ATS/IDSA statement: diagnosis, treatment, and prevention of nontuberculous mycobacterial diseases. Am J Respir Crit Care Med 175:367
6. Tortoli E (2003) Impact of genotypic studies on mycobacterial taxonomy: the new mycobacterial of the 1900s. Clin Microbiol Rev 2:319
7. Mc Nabb AD, Eisler K, Adlie M et al (2004) Assessment of partial sequencing of the 65-kilodalton heat shock protein gene (hsp65) for routine identification of mycobacterium species isolated from clinical sources. J Clin Microbiol 42:3000
8. Yeager H (2011) Nontuberculous mycobacteria. Introduction. In: Schlossberg D (ed) Tuberculosis and nontuberculous mycobacterial infections, 6th edn. ASM Press, Washington, DC, p 525
9. Van Ingen J (2013) Diagnosis of nontuberculous mycobacterial infections. Semin Resp Crit Care Med 34:103
10. Von Reyn CF, Arbeit RD, Horsburgh CR et al (2002) Sources of disseminated *Mycobacterium avium* infection in AIDS. J Infect 44:156
11. Runyon EH (1959) Anonymous mycobacteria in pulmonary disease. Med Clin North Am 43:273
12. Marks J (1972) Classification of mycobacteria in relation to clinical significance. Tubercle 53:210
13. Kubica GP (1973) Differential identification of mycobacteria. VII: key features for identification of clinically significant mycobacteria. Am Rev Respir Dis 107:9
14. Richards OW, Miller DK (1941) An efficient method for the identification of tuberculosis bacteria with a single fluorescence microscope. Am J Clin Pathol Tech 5:1
15. Tortoli E, Simonetti MI (1990) I micobatteri. Caleidoscopio, vol 51. Medical Systems S.P.A., Genova
16. Middlebrook C, Reggiardo Z, Tigert WD (1977) Automatable radiometric detection of growth of *Mycobacterium tuberculosis* in selective media. Am Rev Respir Dis 115:1066

Cutaneous Tuberculosis

2

Domenico Bonamonte, Angela Filoni, Pietro Verni, and Gianni Angelini

2.1 History

Tuberculosis (TB) is one of the most ancient diseases of humankind; it spread around the globe together with human migration as people moved to populate the earth [1–3]. The disease manifestation has always been characterized by great epidemics followed by periods of quiescence: in total, *Mycobacterium tuberculosis* may have killed more people on earth than any other microbial pathogen [1].

The modern molecular biology techniques and genome sequencing of several strains of *M. tuberculosis,* together with the low mutation rate of the germ, have made it possible to estimate the time of origin of TB. An early progenitor of *M. tuberculosis* was present in East Africa about 3 million years ago, and presumably infected early hominids [4]. However, the various members of the *M. tuberculosis* complex (*M. tuberculosis*, *M. africanum*, *M. canettii*, *M. microti, M. caprae, M. pinnipedii, M. bovis*) likely date back to a common African ancestor about 35,000–15,000 years ago [4–6]. The current strains of *M. tuberculosis* seem to have originated from a common ancestor about 20,000–15,000 years ago [7]. The current circulating strains fall into six major lineages, all present in East Africa, and with a variable global circulation [8]; they diversified between 250 and 1000 years ago [9].

D. Bonamonte, MD, PhD (✉)
Department of Biomedical Science and Human Oncology, University of Bary "Aldo Moro", Bari, Italy
e-mail: domenico.bonamonte@uniba.it

A. Filoni, MD • P. Verni, MD
University of Bary "Aldo Moro", Bari, Italy

G. Angelini, MD
Professor of Dermatology, Former Professor and Chairman, University of Bary "Aldo Moro", Bari, Italy

D. Bonamonte, G. Angelini (eds.), *Mycobacterial Skin Infections*,
DOI 10.1007/978-3-319-48538-6_2

Skeletal abnormalities due to TB have been observed in ancient Egyptian mummies dating back 5000 years [10, 11], and their cause has been ascertained thanks to studies of DNA amplified from tissues of the mummies [12, 13]. In India, texts dating back 3300 years speak of TB, as do 2300 year old texts from China [14]. TB is also mentioned in the Biblical books Deuteronomy and Leviticus [15]. In classical Greece, TB was well known, and named phthisis (consumption, wasting disease) [16]. Hippocrates described the clinical picture and claimed that the disease has a predilection for young adults and that "consumption" is the main symptom. Also the Greek physician Galen wrote about TB in the second century AD; he recommended treatment with fresh air, milk, and sea voyages [1]. Bony tuberculosis has been demonstrated in Peruvian mummies, and it is certain that the disease was present in America prior to the arrival of European explorers [17–20]. In various sites scattered all over Europe, TB epidemics occurred during the millennium that followed the fall of Rome in the fifth century [21].

It was the Frenchman René Théophile Hyacinthe Laënnec, the inventor of the stethoscope, who first elucidated the pathogenesis of TB [22]; in 1819, in his book "D'Auscultation Mediate" he described the physical signs of the pulmonary disease and introduced the terminology that is still in use today [23]. By the Laënnec era, TB was diffuse in Europe and deadly epidemics struck down thousands every year. This was why John Bunyan gave it the famous definition by which it is still known in Anglo-Saxon countries today, "the Captain of all these men of death" [2]. In 1865, the French military surgeon Jean-Antoine Villemin (1827–1892) demonstrated the infectious nature of TB by inoculating a rabbit with a small quantity of purulent matter extracted from a tuberculous cavity in a man who died of TB: 3 months later, extensive TB was revealed at autopsy [1].

On March 24, 1882, Hermann Heinrich Robert Koch made his presentation, "Die Aetiologic der Tuberculose", to the Berlin Physiological Society, where he illustrated the tubercle bacillus that he had identified. He was awarded the Noble Prize in Medicine in 1905 for this discovery [24]. In 1907, Clemens von Pirquet, a pediatrician in Vienna, used a vaccination lancet to introduce a small amount of tuberculin intracutaneously [25, 26]. In 1908 Charles Mantoux introduced the use of a cannulated needle and syringe to inject tuberculin intracutaneously, and during the 1930s Florence Seibert developed a purified protein derivative (PPD); this is the form that is still currently used [1].

A more direct aid to public health arrived with Albert Calmette and his associate Camille Guérin, who set up a TB vaccine with attenuated *M. bovis*. The BCG (Bacille Calmette-Guérin) vaccine was experimented in 1921: the first recipient was a child born of a mother who died of pulmonary tuberculosis; the child survived and did not develop TB. In the following 7 years, more than 100,000 children were immunized, including Calmette's children, and from France the use of the vaccine spread all over Europe [27–29].

The history of TB changed radically after the introduction of chemotherapy. The first drugs to be used, both bacteriostatic, were para-amino salicylic acid (PAS), discovered by Jorgen Lehmann in 1943, and thiosemicarbazone, discovered by Gerhard Domagk [1]. In 1944, streptomycin, the first both antibiotic and bactericidal agent effective against *M. tuberculosis* was isolated [16, 30]. Isoniazide, the first oral mycobactericidal drug, followed in 1952 and rifampicins in 1957, triggering a new era in the treatment of the infection, that finally led to the closure of the sanatoriums.

2.2 Epidemiology

TB is ranked among the leading 10 causes of death worldwide, and is one of the worst kinds of epidemics that humankind has ever had to face; it is a reflection of our incapacity to alleviate poverty [31]. More than 20 years after the World Health Organization (WHO) declared TB a global emergency [32], the disease is still a major cause of human suffering and death, and is a pandemic of devastating proportions [31]. The progress made in combating the disease and the renewed efforts made recently are aimed at eradicating TB as a public health problem by 2050, the target adopted by the international community [33]. However, new challenges such as the persistent adverse social conditions, high rates of migration of infected people from areas of relatively high prevalence to low endemic areas, the co-existent human immunodeficiency virus (HIV) epidemic, and the appearance of extensively drug-resistant TB have all contributed to worsen the pandemic and offset the efforts made in the last years.

In 2008, the WHO estimated that there were 9.4 million incident cases (139 cases per 100,000 population) worldwide, 3.6 million of which were women. There were also 11 million prevalent cases of TB (164 cases per 100,000 population) [34]. South-East Asia and African regions accounted for 3.2 million and 2.8 million new cases, respectively, while 80% of the 9.4 million new cases were recorded in India (1.9 million), China (1.3 million), and 20 other countries. In 2008, there were an estimated 1.3 million deaths (20/100,000 population) among HIV-negative incident cases, 0.5 million of which were women. An additional 0.5 million deaths occurred among HIV-positive subjects with incident TB. Thus, in 2008 the total number of deaths worldwide attributable to TB amounted to 1.8 million [31].

2.2.1 Impact of the HIV Epidemic

In recent years, the epidemiology of TB has been adversely affected by the HIV pandemic: in fact, HIV infection is now the most important predisposing factor to the development of active TB. Moreover, TB and HIV infection pose the two greatest global public health threats owing to their high morbidity and mortality rates [35, 36]. This is particularly evident in Sub-Saharan Africa, where more than 20 million of the globally estimated 33 million patients with HIV type 1 infection live [37].

TB is an opportunistic infection in subjects infected by HIV. While the risk of developing post-primary TB later in life is about 10% in a non-immunocompromised patient infected by *M. tuberculosis* who has overcome the primary infection, the risk is multiplied 20–37 times in an HIV-positive patient [38, 39]. Patients with both HIV and TB infection have a 10% risk per year of developing TB [40]. The association between the two infections is due to a synergic interaction of HIV and *M. tuberculosis*: HIV induces immunosuppression and so is an important risk factor for the progression of infection by the tubercle bacillus; meanwhile, the tubercle bacillus accelerates the progression of HIV infection.

In patients with HIV infection, a defective *M. tuberculosis*-mediated alveolar macrophage apoptosis (a critical mechanism for the elimination of the tubercle bacillus) has recently been identified [41]. This defect reduces the killing of *M. tuberculosis* and increases the susceptibility to active TB, even among HIV-infected patients with relatively well preserved CD4+ T cells [42].

TB is observed in all stages of HIV infection. If more than 350 CD4+ T cells/ mm^3 are present, the clinical and histopathologic features of TB are similar to those in subjects without HIV infection, featuring granuloma, with or without central caseation [43]. As the immunosuppression condition progresses, however, granulomas are unformed or absent but there are abundant tubercle bacilli and abscess formation in soft tissues, and disseminated TB is more frequent [44]. Despite antiretroviral therapy, that should reduce the risk of TB in most populations, the risk remains on average 5–10-fold higher than in the HIV-unaffected population, even if the therapy is shown to be active [45]. This may be partly explained by an incomplete restoration of the tuberculosis-specific immune response [46, 47].

TB induces the progression of HIV immunosuppression by means of several mechanisms [48]: the increase of HIV RNA (due to HIV replication in monocytes and macrophages through tumor necrosis factor-alpha and chemoattractant protein-1) [49–51], and transcriptional activation of latent HIV in alveolar macrophages [48].

Because the clinical severity of TB varies according to the host immune response to the infection, there is inevitably a wide range of TB symptoms, depending on the level of HIV-induced immunosuppression. In cases with modest immunosuppression, TB is similar to the condition in HIV-unaffected subjects. But as the immunosuppression progresses, the TB picture becomes "atypical", showing unusual radiological manifestations, non-reactive skin tests, and disseminated and extrapulmonary forms (Table 2.1) [52, 53].

Table 2.1 Clinical features of tuberculosis in patients with HIV infection (modified, by [35])

A. In early HIV infection:
Pulmonary disease with upper lobes involvement and cavitation
Positive PPD in >50% of cases
Good response to treatment
B. In advanced HIV infection:
Involvement of any organ
Common extrapulmonary involvement (bones, joints, lymphatics, meningi, pleura, liver, kidneys, spleen, skin) and miliary dissemination, with manifestations similar to those in patients without HIV infection
Unusual radiographic manifestations
PPD positive in <40% of cases
Good response to therapy but possible high early mortality

In view of the high frequency of coinfection, all patients infected by HIV must undergo screening for a latent TB infection or active TB, and conversely, subjects with TB must be tested for HIV infection [54]. The diagnostic tools employed to identify the two infections are well known but great care must be taken in interpreting the results due to the risk of false-negative results and the lack of specific symptoms [35]. To treat HIV/AIDS infection, the interested reader should consult the standard texts; therapy for TB, also in cases with coexisting HIV infection, will be considered in a later section. For preventive purposes, the *M. bovis* BCG vaccination is not recommended in patients with HIV [55, 56], because a study conducted in South Africa demonstrated that about 992 per 100,000 BCG-vaccinated HIV-infected children then developed disseminated BCG disease [57], compared to the estimated 5 per million in the general population [58]. It has also been demonstrated that in children with HIV infection the CD4+ and CD8+ T cell response to BCG was severely impaired, and hence little or no benefit was gained from the vaccination [59].

In any case, it should be borne in mind that TB is both preventable and treatable even in subjects with HIV infection.

2.2.2 Impact of Drug and Multidrug Resistance

Effective control of TB is threatened by the emergence of *M. tuberculosis* strains that are resistant to one or more of the standard anti-tuberculosis drugs [31, 60]. Such resistance is attributable to bacterial mutation in patients treated with inadequate or inappropriate drug regimens or poorly formulated combination drugs, and in patients receiving suboptimal therapy. This type of resistance is termed secondary or acquired resistance, whereas in a person infected by an already resistant strain, the resistance is denominated initial or primary resistance. Multidrug-resistant TB (MDR-TB) is defined as TB resistant to at least two of the most potent first-line drugs, namely isoniazid and rifampicin, while extensively drug-resistant TB (XDR-TB) is defined as MDR-TB plus additional resistance to second-line drugs, such as any of the fluoroquinolones and any of the three injectables (amikacin, kamamycin, and capreomycin) [31].

The factors contributing to acquired resistance are reported in Table 2.2 [60]. It should be noted that in cases of MDR-TB, patients must be treated with more costly, less effective and more toxic drugs for extended periods: as a consequence, many patients in developing countries are not treated and so spread the infection to other people. The WHO has carried out surveys of the prevalence of drug resistance in the world [61]. The prevalence of MDR among new cases of TB ranged from 0 to 28% across different settings over 15 years of surveillance [62]. A high prevalence of MDR-TB has been identified in some areas of the world (including Mexico, India, Peru, Mozambique, Sierra Leone, South Africa, Botswana, Guinea), and in particular in countries of the former Soviet Union and some provinces of China [31]. In addition to MDR-TB, combined data from 50 countries and territories suggest that 5.4% of all

Table 2.2 Factors contributing to acquired drug and multidrug resistance

Inadequate or inappropriate drug regimens
Poorly formulated combination drugs
Suboptimal therapy
Poor compliance in taking drugs
Irregular supplies of drugs
Unacceptably high cost of drugs for the patient and hence intermittent medication
Irregular intake of drugs due to various reasons
Use of time-expired or mishandled drugs
Unregulated over-the-counter sale of drugs

MDR-TB cases have already evolved toward XDR-TB [62]. The extensive resistance to second-line drugs is obviously a very serious challenge, since there are currently only a few promising new compounds in the research pipeline.

2.2.3 Impact of Solid Organ Transplantation

M. tuberculosis is a significant opportunistic pathogen in solid organ transplant (SOT) recipients [63–65]. The frequency of TB in SOT recipients ranges from 1.2 to 15% [63, 64], being 20 to 74-fold higher than in the general population in a given geographic area. However, the true incidence of TB in SOT recipients is not known.

In any case, SOT recipients must be regarded as a high risk group for TB, even if the risk differs according to the transplanted organ type. The TB incidence is particularly high in lung transplant cases, for instance [66, 67], being 5.6 times higher than in other transplant patients, and 73.3 times higher than in the general population [68].

Most cases of TB in SOT recipients are caused by the reactivation of a latent infection after immunosuppressive therapy has been started. Other risk factors include a history of previous exposure to *M. tuberculosis* (positive PPD and/or residual TB lesions seen on pre-transplant chest X-rays). Yet other factors are any pre-transplant diseases and the intensity of the immune suppression (Table 2.3). It is known that some SOT recipients are over-immunosuppressed after an initial rejection episode [63, 68, 69]. Bearing in mind that the use of some new immunosuppressive drugs does not seem to increase the risk of TB, it is reasonable to suppose that in transplant recipients there are also other contributing risk factors.

The time of onset of the symptoms of TB after the transplant varies: some recipients develop the infection already in the first year after the transplant (mean time 9 months), and others after the first year. More than to the type of immunosuppression, the early onset of TB seems to be due to a possible preexisting history of TB, and hence to a reactivation [65].

Most SOT patients develop pulmonary forms of TB. However, the percentage of patients who develop disseminated or extrapulmonary forms of TB is higher than in the general population (with an incidence ranging from 38 to 64%) [70]. The most common symptoms are fever, coughing, dyspnea, musculoskeletal pain, night sweats, weight loss, and lymphadenopathy [71]. Unlike in the general population, however, TB

Table 2.3 Risk factors for tuberculosis in solid organ transplant recipients (modified, by [65])

History of previous exposure to *Mycobacterium tuberculosis*
Positive PPD
Radiological evidence of previous untreated tuberculosis
Pretransplant diseases
Chronic renal failure
Hepatitis C virus
Diabetes mellitus
Chronic liver disease
Deep mycoses
Cytomegalovirus
Immunosuppressive therapy
Anti-T-cell antibodies
Intensification of immunosuppression due to graft rejection

in SOT recipients is often asymptomatic, and diagnosed only at routine surveillance cultures. Pulmonary TB manifests with fever, coughing, hemoptysis, and radiological involvement in the upper lobes, often diffuse involvement or miliary dissemination. Unlike in AIDS-positive patients, cavitation images are rare. Gastrointestinal TB presents with fever, gastrointestinal bleeding, and abdominal pain, while patients with urological TB develop fever, urinary symptoms, back pain, and sterile pyuria [65].

2.3 Risk Factors

Apart from HIV infection and transplantation, there are many other risk factors for TB (Table 2.4). Some infections like measles, whooping cough, and chronic malaria, and causes of lung damage, in particular smoking and exposure to silicon and other industrial dusts, are included among these risk factors. Other predisposing conditions are malnutrition, diabetes, renal failure (especially in cases requiring hemodialysis), liver failure, cancers (particularly hematological malignancies), as well as immunosuppressive drugs and corticosteroids [60]. Transmission of the infection is favored by overcrowding and poor ventilation conditions, and so is often linked to poverty.

Tuberculin reactivity is a risk factor: usually, it is indicative of a previous infection by *M. tuberculosis*; however, the link between this reactivity and the risk of development of TB is not a close one. In general, minor reactions imply a degree of protection and do not pose an increased risk, whereas major reactions do increase the risk, even if there are regional variations in this regard [60].

2.3.1 Immunosuppressive Drugs and Corticosteroids

Patients in treatment with immunosuppressive drugs after transplantation or for other reasons are particularly susceptible to TB, that often has an insidious onset, and may be of disseminated type. Anti-TB prophylaxis must be considered, above all in tuberculin-negative patients who receive organs from tuberculin-positive donors [72].

Table 2.4 Risk factors for tuberculosis

Age (in particular, under 5 years and older age)
Geographic area (in particular, Asians and Africans)
Immune suppression
HIV infection
Malnutrition
Congenital immunodeficiencies
Immunosuppressive drugs
Corticosteroids
Vitamin D deficiency
Various diseases
Liver failure
Renal failure
Diabetes mellitus
Cancers (in particular, hematological malignancies)
Industrial dusts (pulmonary diseases due to silicosis, asbestosis)
Measles
Alcoholism and other substance abuse
Pulmonary damage due to smoking
Gastrectomy
Jejuno-ileal bypass
Organ transplants
Genetic factors
Environmental mycobacteria

TNF-α inhibitors are an effective treatment in some immune-mediated inflammatory diseases (rheumatoid arthritis, Crohn's disease, ankylosing spondylitis, and psoriasis). Nevertheless, TNF is a protective cytokine for the host defenses against *M. tuberculosis.* In fact, together with other cytokines it plays an important role in the development and maintenance of granulomas that localize bacilli. Although the increased incidence is documented only for rheumatoid arthritis, TNF inhibition with anti-TNF treatment using infliximab can cause a 4 to 5-fold higher incidence of TB in patients with latent infection [73, 74]. The onset of TB rapidly follows the start of treatment, after a mean of 12 weeks and in 98% of cases within 6 months. Disseminated extrapulmonary forms can also be observed [75]. An increased incidence of TB has also been reported with the use of the TNF receptor antagonist etanercept, and the monoclonal antibody adalimumab. Before starting treatment with infliximab it is necessary to exclude a latent or active TB infection. The skin test is often a false negative but in association with QuantiFERON-TB Gold it can help to detect a latent infection.

It is commonly believed that treatment with steroids predisposes to TB, even if the evidence for this is weak. However, the American Thoracic Society recommends that patients on long-term corticosteroid treatment and with healed pulmonary TB should receive isionazid chemoprophylaxis for 1 year [75]. Others have claimed that in patients on long-term steroid therapy, prophylaxis must also be administered in other circumstances, such as a history of inadequate anti-tubercular treatment, an abnormal chest radiograph, a tuberculin reaction of 10 mm or more in diameter, and recent exposure to a tuberculosis patient [70].

The joint statement of the American Thoracic Society and the Centers for Disease Control and Prevention (CDC) acknowledges that ≥15 mg/day of prednisone (or its equivalent) administered for ≥1 month is a risk factor for TB [76], in particular because this dosage has been shown to suppress tuberculin reactivity [75, 76]. However, specific dose and duration thresholds that could increase the risk for TB are still unknown [77, 78]. To examine this issue, a case-control study of TB cases identified during 1990–2001 was conducted in the United Kingdom using the General Practice Research Database [79]. The study encompassed 497 new cases of TB and 1,966 controls at risk for developing incident TB in the study base population. This study showed that patients concurrently exposed to a glucocorticoid had an approximately 5-fold increased risk for developing new TB. The association was independent of other risk factors, such as smoking, diabetes, a lower body mass index, and pulmonary disorders [80]. It is well known that systemic corticosteroids have profound effects on the cellular immune response required to control TB. The study also demonstrated that a minor adiposity (low body mass index) was associated with a 3-fold increased risk of TB as compared with subjects with a normal body mass.

2.3.2 Age and Sex

Children up to the age of 3 years are highly prone to TB, in particular miliary TB and tuberculous meningitis, while those aged 3–15 seem relatively resistant. In developing countries most cases of TB are observed in people aged between 15 and 59 years.

Various studies have shown that men are more affected than women. The effect of pregnancy on TB is not clear: according to some authors it is protective, others claim that it can worsen the disease, while a third group believes it has no effect [81].

2.3.3 Contact Tracing

Most cases of TB are spread within households; small epidemics can also be observed in schools, prison, hospitals, and in other crowded places. Procedures for contact tracing are therefore essential.

2.3.4 Occupational Tuberculosis

TB has long been recognized as an important occupational disease for health care workers (HCWs) [82, 83]. In the pre-antibiotic era, TB caused severe morbidity and mortality among medical and nursing students [84]. With the advent of antibiotics, as well as thanks to the reduced incidence of TB in high-income countries, the risk of nosocomial transmission has declined. Instead, in low- and middle-income countries the risk of TB among HCWs remains high.

An important review of the literature demonstrated that TB remains a very important occupational risk for HCWs in low- and middle-income countries and for workers in some institutions in high-income countries. The median prevalence of latent TB infection in HCWs was 63% (range 33–79%) in developing countries and 24% (range 4–46%) in developed countries. The median annual incidence of TB infection was 5.8% (range 0–11%) in low- and middle-income countries and 1.1% (range 0.2–12%) in high-income countries. Rates of active TB in HCWs were much higher than in the general population in all countries [83].

These data underline the fact that TB infection and disease continue to be an important occupational hazard for HCWs all over the world.

2.3.5 Tuberculosis and Air Travel

A low risk of transmission of TB infection during air travel has been documented [85, 86], and also emerged in studies conducted between 1993 and 1995 by the Centers for Disease Control and Prevention [87].

Most of the subjects who did become infected were passengers seated beside infected patients; exposure must be prolonged, on flights lasting more than 8 hours. On shorter flights the risk is still lower.

2.3.6 Genetic Factors

A genetic predisposition to TB is known, as demonstrated in studies among monozygotic and dizygotic twins [88].

It seems that race can also play a part; in the same conditions, blacks were twice as likely to become infected as whites; in vitro studies have demonstrated that monocytes from black donors are relatively permissive of mycobacterial growth [89–91]. Associations between TB and some HLA alleles have also been shown [92–94].

2.3.7 Other Factors

Substance abuse is a risk factor in patients with TB [95], as also drug injection abuse [39, 96]. In urban areas, alcoholics have a 10-fold risk of TB, especially among those with an alcohol intake of more than 40 g of alcohol per day [97]. Cigarette smoking increases the TB risk 1.5–2-fold, and also influences the risk of recurrence [98].

Industrialization and urban sprawl are the optimal transmission conditions, owing to the crowded living conditions and lack of health care and proper housing. Most of the increases in TB incidence have been observed in cities with a population of more than 500,000 inhabitants [99]. Among the urban poor, the homeless have been shown to be a risk group [100].

2.4 Etiology

M. tuberculosis is the etiological agent of tuberculosis (from the Latin "tuberculum": small protuberance, and the Greek suffix "osis": state, condition) in man, in other primates, in the dog and in many other animals that come in contact with man. Discovered by Robert Koch (hence its other name, the "Koch bacillus") in 1882 in the sputum of patients affected by pulmonary TB, he identified it 2 years later also in cases of lupus vulgaris. *M. tuberculosis* is the most widespread species of the *Mycobacterium* genus in the world, as well as being the most virulent of the mycobacteria. It is also one of the most sensitive to the currently available anti-tubercular drugs.

Tubercle bacilli are necessarily aerobic (the predilection for the lung tissue is correlated to their need for molecular oxygen for growth), non-motile, non-sporing, often slightly curved rods 2–5 μm in length and 0.3–0.5 μm in diameter. In tissues they are found isolated, in pairs or in clusters. In common with other mycobacteria, they stain deep-red with the Zihel-Neelsen method, since they retain the red carbol-fuchsin color even after bleaching with strong mineral acids (H_2SO_4) and alcohol. This acid-alcohol-fast staining property is due to some constituents of the cell body, in particular to mycolic acid, and depends on the structure of the cell body.

M. tuberculosis is not inserted in the Runyon classification and belongs to the mycobacteria class to which it gives the name. It can be isolated using solid or liquid media containing minerals, proteins, amino acids, carbohydrates, and water-soluble fatty acid esters (tweens) that foster the growth of bacilli-rich colonies. The Petragnani and Löwenstein-Jensen media are generally used. In culture media, at an optimal temperature of 37°C, the colonies grow slowly and develop only after 3–4 weeks of incubation.

A protein known as the old Koch's tuberculin is extracted from bacillary cultures; this protein was used for many years to test for tuberculin sensitivity in the skin. Subsequently, the old tuberculin was purified by precipitation with trichloroacetic acid and semi-saturated ammonium sulphate and then by filtration, obtaining a purified protein derivative (PPD) of tuberculin. PPD consists of immunologically active tubercle proteins with a constant potency and composition. It is a mixture of proteins, carbohydrates and some lipids, obtained from cultures of *M. tuberculosis* through precipitation after boiling. PPD is used for testing and standardized tuberculin units (IU) have been established by the WHO.

The virulence of *M. tuberculosis*, which is an elective intracellular parasite, seems to be strictly correlated with its ability to survive and multiply inside macrophages. Since the mycobacterium has a very thick cell wall (lipids account for over 50% of its dry weight), once phagocytized it can resist intracellular lysis and multiply. It seems to cause inhibition of the fusion of lysosomes with phagosomes within the histiocytes.

2.4.1 *Mycobacterium tuberculosis* Complex

A few years after Koch's discovery of the tuberculous bacillus, Theobald Smith noted that there were constant phenotypical differences between tuberculous bacilli of human origin and those isolated from cattle. He therefore subdivided the species into human and bovine tubercle bacilli [101, 102]. The two species share some common characteristics but there are differences, the most important of which is probably the low pathogenicity of human strains for animals, while the bovine bacillus can infect both animals and humans, and is also an important cause of extrapulmonary TB in humans [103].

Since then, new species of tuberculous bacilli have been described, some of which can cause disease in humans [104, 105]. All these species, together with the species *M. tuberculosis*, form the *M. tuberculosis* complex, but there are important differences among them in terms of epidemiology, microbiology, and even therapy (Table 2.5).

2.4.1.1 *Mycobacterium africanum*

This species includes strains which share phenotypic characteristics with *M. tuberculosis* and *M. bovis* [102]. Strains of this species have been isolated in Sub-Saharan African countries, where they cause variable percentages of human TB. In developed countries, instead, the isolation of *M. africanum* is uncommon, and associated with immigrants from Africa; obviously, they can infect natives of the new country of residence.

The species was previously subdivided into two groups, from East and West Africa, but taxonomic studies have recently demonstrated that the East strains are *M. bovis* and the West strains are true *M. africanum* [106]. The latter has peculiar phenotypic and genetic characteristics. Nowadays, it can be identified with a genetic test available on the market.

The disease caused by *M. africanum* is identical to the one caused by *M. tuberculosis*. The only differences are that *M. africanum* induces less clustering cases, and less frequently involves the lower lung lobe than *M. tuberculosis* [107]. Subjects affected by *M. africanum* are generally older than *M. tuberculosis* patients and are more frequently HIV-infected; they also show more severe disease on the chest X ray [108]. Therapy for *M. africanum* disease is the same as for *M. tuberculosis*; there do not seem to have been multidrug resistance outbreaks up to now.

Table 2.5 Species included in *Mycobacterium tuberculosis* complex

Species	Human pathogen
Mycobacterium tuberculosis	Frequent
Mycobacterium bovis	Frequent
Mycobacterium bovis BCG	Rare
Mycobacterium africanum	Frequent
Mycobacterium canettii[a]	Rare
Mycobacterium microti	Rare
Mycobacterium caprae	Occasional
Mycobacterium pinnipedii	No

[a]Not considered a separate species or subspecies

2.4.1.2 *Mycobacterium caprae*

Strains isolated from goats in Spain were initially described as *M. tuberculosis* subspecies *caprae*. The isolates were then classified as *M. bovis* subspecies *caprae,* and finally as a new species, *M. caprae* [104, 109]. This species has also been isolated in other mammals in various European countries [110].

M. caprae has also been reported to cause human disease, and retrospective studies have demonstrated that it consists of a variable percentage of strains previously identified as *M. bovis* [111, 112]. The two species have similar epidemiologic characteristics. Therapy is also the same as for *M. bovis*, even if *M. caprae* is susceptible to pyrazinamide.

2.4.1.3 *Mycobacterium microti*

This strain has been reported to cause disease in voles and other animals [113, 114], but is considered non pathogenic in man. Nevertheless, recent molecular studies have shown that *M. microti* can actually cause human infection, especially in immune suppressed cases [113–115]. The disease is clinically similar to classic TB and the treatment is the same.

2.4.1.4 *Mycobacterium pinnipedii*

This is the most recently described member of the complex. It causes disease in seals and some other animals. In a recent study, the possibility of human infection was suggested, even if there have been no reports of the disease to date [105, 116].

2.4.1.5 *Mycobacterium canettii*

Some *M. tuberculosis* strains that produce glossy, smooth colonies (a rare finding among this species) have been given the name of *M. canettii*. Although some cases of human TB from these strains have been reported, they are not considered as a separate species or subspecies in the *M. tuberculosis* complex [117, 118].

2.5 Transmission

Although they can affect all the organs, the entry routes of the bacilli are virtually always the lungs. The bacilli are commonly discharged into the atmosphere by aerosolization of pulmonary secretions when a diseased pulmonary patient coughs, sneezes, speaks, and sings [73]. Aerosol droplets dry rapidly, leaving tiny droplet nuclei, some of which contain a few bacilli [119]. Large droplets fall to the ground, while droplet nuclei in the range of 1–10 μm can be inhaled. The larger ones are blocked at nasal level or expelled into the pharynx by the mucociliary mechanism of the lower respiratory tract and then swallowed and digested without causing damage. Instead, the smaller droplets can reach the alveoli and cause infection [73]. Droplet nuclei of patients with a productive cough and positive sputum smears have a rich bacillary content [120]. The number of bacilli in airborne aerosols depends on the expulsion force of the cough and on the presence of lung cavitation [119, 120].

Other possible transmission routes are rare. In the past the transmission of *M. bovis* commonly occurred through the consumption of infected cows milk but nowadays this means of infection no longer exists in developed countries, thanks to the elimination of diseased cattle and the pasteurization of milk. However, this transmission route is still prevalent in developing countries due to the consumption of unpasteurized milk, to direct contact with infected animals and to eating insufficiently cooked meat [121]. A recent genetic study showed the possibility of inter-human transmission of *M. bovis* among HIV-infected subjects. Albeit less frequently, *M. bovis* has also been identified as a cause of human TB in developed countries; about 7% of cases of TB in San Diego, California, are caused by *M. bovis* [122]. In the United States, from 1995 to 2005 *M. bovis* was isolated in 1.4% of 11,860 linked cases. Most of the cases were extrapulmonary disease in young US-born Hispanics, and likely related to food-borne exposure [123].

Extrapulmonary TB has rarely been considered contagious, but in the literature some new cases of infection of hospital personnel handling tuberculosis lesions have been reported [124, 125]. It is also possible for transmission to occur via inoculation of the bacilli through the skin. This source of infection is an occupational hazard among pathologists and laboratory workers who handle infected issues and tuberculosis cultures.

Fomites, like books, clothes, bedding, and eating utensils, do not pose a risk of infection [73].

In the great majority of cases, airborne transmission of TB occurs. Close contacts of smear-positive patients are at highest risk of infection, even if TB is actually less contagious than some viral diseases. Some studies have shown that among close contacts, the risk of infection ranges from 25 to 50% [126, 127]. It would also seem that prolonged contact with smear-negative culture-positive patients can be dangerous. In short, epidemiologic data demonstrate that to contract the disease, there must be close, prolonged contact, and the environment must be heavily laden with droplet nuclei; in addition, there must be a defect of the protective inborn defenses [73].

2.6 Pathophysiology

The pathogenesis of TB can be seen as a battle between the host and *M. tuberculosis* [128]. The host defense relies on activated macrophages that can kill the bacilli by phagocytosis, as well as on their ability to stop intracellular bacillary growth in non-activated macrophages by killing these macrophages, and creating an inhibitory environment of solid caseous tissue. On the other hand, tubercle bacilli have the capacity to multiply logarithmically within non-activated macrophages and extracellularly in liquefied caseous material. Therefore, it is the non-activated macrophages (that permit intracellular growth of the bacilli) and the liquefied caseous material (the only host environment where extracellular bacilli growth can occur) that make the host vulnerable. Instead, the bacilli are vulnerable in the presence of activated macrophages and solid caseous tissue [128].

Table 2.6 Preventive measures for contagion (modified, by [128])

1. During a cough or sneeze patients must turn their heads away from others, and cover their mouth and nose with a hand, or preferably a cloth or tissue
2. The attending staff must wear tight-fitting, effective masks
3. Tuberculin-negative people exposed to tubercle bacilli must be vaccinated with an effective bacillus Calmette-Guérin (BCG) strain
4. Air exchange must be achieved in rooms where patients reside using an exhaust fan, HEPA filter, UV light, or all of these together

Table 2.6 shows the prophylactic measures to be adopted to prevent or reduce the risk of contagion; these are particularly important in subjects exposed to antimicrobial-resistant bacilli [128–130].

2.6.1 Human Pulmonary Tuberculosis

As stated above, only the inhaled droplet nuclei, that contain 1–3 bacilli, are capable of transmitting the infection when they enter the alveolar spaces. Heavier droplets, containing more bacilli and/or bits of caseous material, instead, are blocked at the bronchial mucosa level or are ingested by the gastrointestinal mucosa. In such circumstances, very large numbers of bacilli are needed to achieve the infection [128].

The virulence of the tubercle bacilli varies according to genetic and phenotypic factors. Over the years, the *M. tuberculosis* genome has changed relatively little [7, 131]. However, there have been evolutionary changes in members of the *M. tuberculosis* complex: *M. microti*, for example, despite its 99% genomic identity, is naturally attenuated in man [132, 133]. BCG is attenuated from the virulent *M. bovis*, through a series of passages in media with an ox bile base [134, 135]. Even the virulence of human-type tubercle bacilli H37Rv can be reduced by culture series, dessication or by exposure to sunlight [136, 137].

In the same way as bacilli can be more or less virulent, the microbicidal power of alveolar macrophages can vary: some have a rich content of lysosomal and oxidative enzymes and microbicides, others a lower content [138], depending on the native genetic resistance of each person and on phenotypic factors. The mean number of inhaled bacillary particles needed to induce primary pulmonary tubercle in man is not known but the range is probably between 5 and 200 for virulent human type tubercle bacilli [139].

2.6.2 Stages of Pulmonary Tuberculosis

There are five stages of pulmonary TB [128, 140]. In stage 1, the stage of no bacillary growth, there are mature activated resident alveolar macrophages that destroy or inhibit the bacilli they have ingested. Most of the alveolar macrophages are non-specifically activated by many stimulating factors, including the ingestion and digestion of inhaled particles and occasional extravasated erythrocytes.

Stage 2 is the initial primary tubercle, in which the bacilli multiply logarithmically inside the vacuoles of immature non-activated macrophages that have emigrated from the bloodstream to the new lesion. This stage is known as the symbiosis stage, because the bacilli multiply without damaging the host, and the macrophages multiply without damaging the bacilli.

In stage 3, after 3 weeks the tubercle has a caseous necrotic center, surrounded by partly activated macrophages and lymphocytes. The caseation is due to the immune response, mainly a tissue-damaging delayed-type hypersensitivity (DTH) reaction. In response to the tuberculin like products of the bacilli, DTH kills the non-activated macrophages in which the bacilli are multiplying. As well as in the macrophages, intact or fragmented bacilli are present also within the caseum. In the solid caseous center of the tubercle the bacilli, being extracellular, do not multiply. Around them there are non-activated macrophages (with multiplying bacilli inside), and partly activated macrophages (immature epithelioid cells) produced through the intervention of cell-mediated immunity (CMI).

The caseous necrosis seen in TB is a DTH reaction produced by the T cells, including cytotoxic T cells and NK cells, that induces apoptosis of the macrophages. The reaction also relies on anoxia (by thrombosis: macrophages produce clotting factors), cytokines (TNF), reactive oxygen and nitrogen intermediates, complement, and toxic products released from dead bacilli [128].

In stage 4, the decisive stage for the development of the disease, CMI is activated. If the CMI is weak, the bacilli move from the caseous center of the tubercle back to the surrounding non activated macrophages. Cytotoxic DTH acts on the latter, killing them and thus causing a further enlargement of the caseous center, and hence progression of the disease. Instead, if the CMI is strong, a mantle of activated macrophages will surround the caseous necrosis and kill the bacilli. In this case the development of the lesion is arrested at a subclinical stage.

In stage 5, the liquefaction stage, the bacilli evade the host defenses. In the presence of liquid caseous necrosis, the extracellular bacilli multiply very rapidly. The resulting very high local concentration of tuberculin-like products that they release activates the DTH cytotoxic response; this erodes the bronchial wall, forming a cavity. Then the bacilli enter the bronchial airways and invade other portions of the lung. They are also spread to the environment when the subject coughs. The ability to prevent the disease at this stage depends on the host control of the bacilli and their products [128].

2.6.3 Susceptibility to Tuberculosis

The mean number of infectious 1–3 bacilli particles that man must inhale for the tuberculin skin test to be positive is unknown but estimated to be about 5–200. However, only 10% of subjects with a positive tuberculin skin test will develop active TB during their lifetime. Most individuals are able to arrest the infection thanks to an adequate CMI response [128].

HIV-coinfected subjects or those with immunosuppression due to other causes are more susceptible to the disease after inhaling exogenous bacilli or due to endogenous (latent) bacilli inhaled years before. Among these subjects with latent bacilli,

5–10% of tuberculin-positive HIV-infected subjects will suffer a disease reactivation in a given year, whereas 5–10% of tuberculin-positive non-HIV-infected subjects will undergo a disease reactivation in their lifetime [128].

The susceptibility to TB also depends on various genetic polymorphisms, such as the genes for natural-resistance-associated macrophage protein 1 (NRAMP-1), and the vitamin D receptor [93, 141–143].

2.6.4 Primary and Post-Primary Tuberculosis

Traditionally, TB is subdivided into two forms: (1) primary and (2) post-primary. Post-primary TB refers to the endogenous reactivation of latent or dormant primary lesions, even if an exogenous reinfection is possible, especially in immunosuppressed subjects.

As pointed out above, most infected subjects never develop clinical disease, and the primary infection goes unnoticed. An effective immune response encapsulates the organism and contains it throughout life. Only about 2–5% of infected individuals will develop clinically evident primary TB, and a further 2–5% then develop post-primary disease [60].

In cases with pulmonary infection, some bacilli will move from the primary focus to the regional lymph nodes (mediastinal, paratracheal, and rarely supraclavear nodes), where secondary lesions will develop. The set of primary focus lesions, lymphangitis and lymphadenitis is termed the "primary complex". In most cases, thanks to an effective immune response, the lesions become fibrotic and then calcified, while the bacilli can persist inside the dormant lesions for years or decades.

After about 3–8 weeks from the initial infection, a conversion to dermal reactivity and to tuberculin occurs. The dermal induration of the positive tuberculin reaction is due to tissue edema linked to immunological and other processes. Thus, a positive test indicates a recent or past infection by the tubercle bacillus or a BCG vaccination, but not the immune status of the infected host [60].

Post-primary TB develops directly from a primary lesion, or more commonly, from the latent phase that has been dormant for many years. Post-primary lesions develop in other parts of the same lung and often in the other lung, through the bronchial tree. Then the bacilli infect other organs through the bloodstream; they can also be ingested and cause ulceration of bowel tracts, or through the bronchial secretions, can cause tuberculous laryngitis. Unlike primary TB lesions, post-primary lesions are generally walled-in by fibrosis, so lymphatic or hematogenous dissemination of the disease is rare [60].

2.7 Immunology

There is considerable controversy about the immunological mechanism underlying the development of TB, because it is known to be highly complex and variable, and to depend on the interaction of myriad factors that are often difficult to control [128, 144–148].

One of the most debated problems is *M. tuberculosis'* ability to prevent or evade effective host responses [144]. For thousands of years *M. tuberculosis* has co-evolved with humans, and this constant relationship has enabled the mycobacteria genome to encode mechanisms that allow the bacilli to resist attacks by man's immune system. *M. tuberculosis* can establish latent or progressive infection and persist even in the presence of a fully functional immune system. This ability reflects the highly evolved immune evasion strategies it has developed to interfere with human innate and adaptive immunity [144].

2.7.1 Cell-Mediated Immunity

CMI and DTH, both mediated by Th1 lymphocytes, play a key role in the immunopathogenesis of TB. In response to tuberculin-like antigens, DTH kills non activated macrophages in which the bacilli are proliferating exponentially, inducing toxic levels of tuberculin-like antigens, while CMI prevents the multiplication of the bacilli by activating the macrophages [128]. The bacillary antigens that trigger DTH are active already at low concentrations, while those producing CMI are active when they reach high concentrations. In general, the tuberculoproteins, peptides and carbohydrates in tuberculin promote DTH, while other proteins, with carbohydrates and lipids, favor CMI [149, 150].

CMI is brought about by antigen-specific T lymphocytes that produce cytokines (IFN-γ and TNF- α), attracted from the bloodstream to the lesion, where they activate lymphocytes, monocytes/macrophages and dendritic cells (DCs). IFN-γ also stimulates the monocytes/macrophages production of IL-2, an additional phagocytes activating cytokine [151, 152]. Activated macrophages produce reactive-oxygen and reactive-nitrogen intermediates, lysosomal enzymes and other factors that kill the bacilli [153, 154].

Acquired cellular resistance therefore relies on the macrophages, that enter the tubercle lesion in a non-immune, non-activated state, and are activated and develop a microbicidal ability only when they reach the bacillary antigens.

DTH occurs in the same cells and cytokines. However, its cytotoxic activity is not sufficient to block the progression of the disease, because viable bacilli escape from the necrotic area and move to the peripheral zone of the tubercle, where they must then be ingested and destroyed by activated macrophages.

2.7.2 Innate Immune Response

The phagocytosis of bacilli by the macrophages occurs thanks to recognition receptors, including the mannose receptor, complement receptor, fibronectin receptor, nuclear oligomerization domain (NOD) receptors, and Toll-like receptors, that are all involved in the host innate immune response [144–148, 155]. Close study has been made in particular of the Toll-like receptors (TLRs) family, of which some members recognize various mycobacterial cell wall components [155–157].

These receptors bind *M. tuberculosis* to the macrophages and internalize them in phagosomes. Normally, these phagosomes fuse with lysosomes, undergo acidification, and receive lysosomal enzymes that degrade the ingested microorganisms. However, *M. tuberculosis* can subvert phagosome-lysosome fusion and the resulting maturation of the phagosome in the microbicidal compartment [158] and also resist the degrading action of the lysosomal enzymes. In addition, it can inhibit the entry of many microbicidal factors into the phagosome [158–161].

As well as blocking the phagosome-lysosomes fusion, *M. tuberculosis* evades the various innate immune recognition pathways and can limit the development of potentially more potent adaptive immune responses [162]. In this way, thanks to the intervention of myriad powerful mechanisms (see 128, 144–147) for evading antimicrobial responses and subverting the innate immune crosstalk with adaptive immunity, *M. tuberculosis* can tilt the balance towards pathological rather than protective immune responses [145].

The major innate immune cell types in humans are macrophages, neutrophils, dendritic cells and NK cells. Recently, some other, non classic immune cells, such as airway epithelial cells, have been shown to contribute to the immune response to *M. tuberculosis* in animal models [163] and in vivo studies with human cell lines [164].

In response to *M. tuberculosis* infection, the macrophages upregulate effectors and signaling pathways in order to prevent bacterial replication, and recruit other immune cells to the site of the infection. Various components of *M. tuberculosis*, like lipoarabinomannans, lipomannans, phosphatidylinositol mannosides, and heat shock proteins, are recognized by various cell receptors. Following the recognition of *M. tuberculosis*, host effectors, such as NF-κB and peroxisome proliferator activated receptor γ, are activated in order to upregulate antimicrobial factors. The latter have effector and signaling functions that can interfere with bacterial replication and recruit activated neutrophils, dendritic cells and T cells. On the other hand, *M. tuberculosis* interferes with macrophage effector and signaling pathways, downregulating MCH II expression on macrophages to prevent the interaction with antigen specific T-cells. Moreover, *M. tuberculosis* interferes with IFN-γ signaling; this T cell cytokine mediator serves to upregulate the inherent antimicrobial capacity of macrophages during infection [145].

During infection, neutrophilis secrete various antimicrobial enzymes that are necessary to restrict bacterial growth inside the macrophages. These neutrophil effectors promote apoptosis of the infected macrophages, thereby limiting survival of the bacilli. However, these enzymes also mediate pulmonary tissue damage and the inflammatory response [145].

Dendritic cells, that are involved in innate and adaptive immunity, are the primary antigen-presenting cells in the immune system, and play a central role in the activation and differentiation of T cells by presenting antigenic peptides. But *M. tuberculosis* subverts the dendritic cells functions, thereby impairing T cell responses during infection [145].

Natural killer cells are innate granular lymphocytes with a potent cytolytic activity. They intervene at an early stage during infection and can restrict bacillary replication through the production of soluble mediators such as GM-CSF, IL-12, IL-22,

INF-α, and IFN-γ. These mediators upregulate the antimicrobial function of the infected macrophages and activate antigen-specific T cell responses during the infection [145].

In short, the success of *M. tuberculosis* infection likely relies on an early interaction with the cells of the innate immune system. Macrophages and neutrophils can engulf and kill the bacteria, but may be subverted by *M. tuberculosis* to promote chronic lung inflammation. Dendritic cells can generate *M. tuberculosis* specific T cells that can bolster immunity, but are manipulated to reduce the T cell responses. Finally, even the functional capacity of the NK cells, that directly and indirectly bring about killing of the bacilli, can be hampered in some way. All these cells, that play a role in the host defense against *M. tuberculosis*, are therefore coopted into helping bacilli to establish a long term infection [145].

Various immunogenetics studies have demonstrated the importance of the innate immunity in the control of mycobacterial infections. Patients with mutations in two innate immune autosomal genes (IL12B and IL12Rβ1) suffer widespread and recurrent mycobacterial infections early in life [164–167]. In these subjects with polymorphisms in the IL-12 locus, treatment with exogenous IL-12 makes them less susceptible to fatal infections, underlining the role of macrophage and/or dendritic cells-derived IL-12 in the generation of INF-γ responses that control infection [168]. Other innate pathways implicated in the immune response to mycobacterial infection are the TLRs. Polymorphisms in TLR2, TLR9 [169], TLR1 [170], and TLR8 [171] have been associated with susceptibility to mycobacterial infections. Yet other studies have shown that mutations in the inflammasome pathway, and IL-1 in particular, may be critical in promoting an enhanced immunity against *M. tuberculosis* [172, 173]. Subjects with low serum levels of vitamin D3 metabolites also show an increased susceptibility to active TB [174]; as we know, vitamin D boosts the responsiveness of macrophages to INF-γ [175, 176], and acts synergistically with IFN-γ to increase antimycobacterial activity in human monocytes [177]. These data illustrate how human immunogenetic studies can contribute to the knowledge of the various mechanisms underlying resistance to *M. tuberculosis* [145].

2.8 Laboratory Diagnosis

The success of TB control programs depends to a large extent on the quality of the diagnostic services. Nowadays, in clinical microbiology laboratories a number of accurate, rapid diagnostic tests are available, including molecular biology techniques, that have greatly reduced the waiting times for results. However, the sensitivity of all these methods is dependent on appropriate selection and collection of those clinical specimens most likely to contain *M. tuberculosis,* and these must be considered only in cases of suspected active TB [60, 178]. The tests below serve to confirm the diagnosis and monitor the results of treatment:

1. Bacteriology: identification of *M. tuberculosis* by microscopic tests and culture of various clinical samples (sputum, blood, lymph node aspirate, skin, caseous exudates, pleural fluid, bone marrow).
2. Imaging techniques: radiology, ultrasound, computed axial tomography scanning, magnetic resonance imaging, and radioisotope scans.
3. Tissue biopsy: for histopathology (to reveal granulomas and identify acid-fast bacilli), bacteriology (culture), and identify mycobacterial DNA.
4. Molecular techniques: nucleic acid amplification systems (polymerase chain reaction: PCR, ligase chain reaction: LCR), applied to the various clinical specimens to identify mycobacterial DNA.
5. Hematology and biochemistry: hemoglobin, erythrocyte sedimentation rate (ESR), C-reactive protein, liver function tests, urea, and electrolytes.
6. Tuberculin skin test.
7. Serology.

Naturally, in cases when none of these tests are available, the diagnosis will be based on clinical acumen and simple microscopic tests.

2.8.1 Bacteriological Identification

2.8.1.1 Specimen Collection

Various body fluids and tissue biopsies are employed for mycobacterial culture. In cases of suspected pulmonary TB the specimen most commonly employed in culture is sputum, collected in the early morning. The patient must be instructed to expectorate a specimen with no nasal secretion or saliva after taking a deep breath. Sputum (sample volumes of 5–10 ml) must be collected for three consecutive days. Sample collection with swabs is not useful because little material is collected and so there is a risk of a false negative result of culture. In cases of subjects who are unable to produce sputum, hypertonic saline (5–15%) can be nebulized to induce matter. If this procedure is ineffective, too, the test of choice is bronchoscopy with bronchoalveolar lavage.

In cases of children or adults who are completely unable to expectorate sputum, gastric lavage is an alternative. The resulting specimens must be processed within 4 h because gastric acid is potentially harmful to the mycobacteria. If rapid processing is impossible, the gastric specimens must be neutralized with sodium carbonate or another buffer salt to a pH of 7.0.

In cases of suspected extrapulmonary TB, appropriate specimens from the specific organs must be collected. All specimens, collected and transported in sterile conditions, must reach the laboratory as soon as possible. If this is not possible, then specimens must be refrigerated.

Obviously, specimen collection must be done before any treatment, since even a few days of therapy can induce negative results. Some specimens, such as sputum, urine, and bronchial and gastric aspirate, need to be decontaminated using various useful alkaline solutions, the most common of which is benzalkonium chloride with trisodium phosphate or 4% NaOH [178].

2.8.1.2 Culture

Isolation of *M. tuberculosis* in culture provides a definite diagnosis. The disadvantage of culture is the delay, usually 3–6 weeks, between receiving the specimen and the emergence of visible growth. Although mycobacteria are strictly aerobic, a CO_2 concentration between 5 and 10% is necessary for the primary recovery of solid media. The incubation must be done in high humidity conditions at a temperature of 35–37°C for non-cutaneous sources.

Solid Media

Mycobacterial culture media include egg-based, agar-based, liquid, and selective media. Löwenstein-Jensen, Petragnani and American Thoracic Society media are examples of egg-based media. Petragnani medium is the most inhibitory of contaminant bacteria thanks to its high content of malachite green, an antibacterial agent. They all contain whole eggs, potato flour, salts, glycerol, and malachite green [178]. Löwenstein-Jensen is the medium most commonly used for primary culture. Middlenbrook 7H10 and 7H11 are other common complex media. Selective media also contain antimicrobials to inhibit contaminating bacteria.

All media must be incubated for up to 8 weeks at 35°C to 37°C. In cases of positive acid-fast smears and negative culture for mycobacteria after 8 weeks of incubation on solid media, specimens must be incubated for a further 8 weeks. Cultures must be examined twice a week for visible evidence of growth. In the presence of colony growth, the next steps are acid-fast smears, subcultures for identification, susceptibility tests, and nucleic acid probe tests or other comparable molecular methods.

Broth Media

The MGIT tube system (Becton Dickinson, Sparks, MD) contains a 7H9-based medium with enrichment, antibiotics, and an oxygen-labile fluorescent indicator at the bottom of the tube. As the mycobacteria grow and use up oxygen, the indicator compound is excited, and the resulting fluorescence can be visually examined using an UV source. This medium was designed to replace the BACTEC 460 TB system, which was the previous gold standard but is no longer available. Various other commercial systems are available and all appear to be suitable alternatives to the BACTEC 460 TB system [178].

2.8.1.3 Staining Procedure

The same procedure is valid both for smears prepared directly from patients specimens and for culture-grown organisms. It must be borne in mind that in the same patient there can be smear-negative but culture-positive specimens, and that anyway smear specimens provide no indications as to the identity or the viability of the organisms, since all species of mycobacteria are acid-fast.

Two procedures are commonly employed: carbol fuchsin methods, including the Ziehl-Neelsen and Kinyoun procedure, and a fluorochrome method using auramine O or auramine-rhodamine dye. The Ziehl-Neelsen and Kinyoun methods stain the mycobacterial cells red against a methylene blue counterstain, while mycobacteria stained with auramine O are bright yellow against a dark background and are easily visualized using a 25× lens, whereas for the previous two methods a 100× oil immersion lens is necessary. Fluorochrome staining is more sensitive than carbol fuchsin techniques. All these methods also stain non-viable organisms. Obviously, a negative smear does not exclude the diagnosis of a possible infection by a *Mycobacterium* species, while the presence of mycobacteria at direct examination does not confirm the diagnosis of TB. Finally, it should be remembered that some non mycobacterial organisms can appear acid-fast, like *Rhodococcus*, *Nocardia*, *Legionella micdadei*, cysts of *Cryptosporidium*, *Cystoisospora*, and *Cyclospora* [178].

Apart from on acid-fastness, the identification of the *M. tuberculosis* complex relies on niacin production, nitrate reduction, and the inactivation of catalase at 68°C. The recovery time on solid media ranges from 12 days to 4–6 weeks, with an average of about 3–4 weeks. The colonies are rough, cauliflower-like, and colorless.

2.8.2 Radiological Imaging

Radiology is very sensitive, although exceptionally the radiograph may appear normal in patients with smear-positive pulmonary TB. However, it is not specific because a wide spectrum of radiological changes is possible, and all the changes associated with TB occur in other respiratory conditions. Chest X-ray is highly suggestive of post primary pulmonary TB if there are unilateral or bilateral patchy shadows in the upper zone, single or multiple cavities and calcification. The differential diagnosis must include atypical pneumonia, carcinoma, sarcoidosis, Kaposi's sarcoma, and unresolved pneumonia. High-resolution CT scanning may be required to distinguish these conditions. Radioisotope scans are useful to detect the extent of the disease especially in cryptic areas, such as bones and lymph nodes.

2.8.3 Hematological Examination

Hematological changes are fairly non-specific in TB. Blood examination may reveal a raised lymphocyte count, a raised ESR, elevated C-reactive protein levels, and a mild anemia. All these changes resolve with treatment. Elevated enzymes levels in various body fluids have been reported.

2.8.4 Molecular Methods

Nucleic Acid Probe Since the early 1990s, nucleic acid probes have been used to identify mycobacteria. The commercially available probes (AccuProbe, Gen-Probe) can identify the *M. tuberculosis* complex, *M. kansasii*, *M. avium-M. intracellulare* and *M. gordonae.*

The *M. tuberculosis* complex non isotopic probe has demonstrated a sensitivity and specificity of 100%, compared with its isotopic predecessor [179]. This test is used to confirm cultures of organisms on broth culture, such as BACTEC 12B medium and the MGIT system [180].

Nucleic Acid Amplification Molecular diagnostics are a good solution for a prompt detection and identification of mycobacteria. These methods include *M. tuberculosis* complex-specific nucleic acid amplification systems, as well as broad-range mycobacterial amplification assays followed by postamplification analyses, such as DNA sequencing or microarray hybridization. Genes that encode rRNA or RNA polymerase are used as genetic targets. The newer rapid-cycle PCR systems have less risk of contamination and provide very high specificity [181, 182].

The FDA-approved assays are the Amplified *Mycobacterium tuberculosis* Direct (AMTD) test by Gen-Probe and the Amplicor *M. tuberculosis* test by Roche Diagnostic Systems. The AMTD test has been approved for both acid-fast smear-positive and smear-negative respiratory tract specimens, and the Amplicor assay only for smear-positive respiratory specimens.

The AMTD test, whose target is 16S RNA, has various advantages: it detects rRNA, that in theory may exist in concentrations several thousand-fold higher than those found in genomic DNA of the organism, is highly sensitive, easy to perform and undergoes little or no contamination. Specimens for testing must be collected from untreated patients. The test may remain positive even after culture has become negative as a result of treatment [183]. It can also be used on non-respiratory tract specimens (urine, feces, tissue, bone marrow, cerebrospinal fluids, pleural exudates) [184]. The Amplicor *M. tuberculosis* test is a PCR-based assay: instead of detecting rRNA, it detects the rRNA gene in the genome (DNA) [184, 185].

Although these nucleic acid amplification methods provide rapid results, mycobacterial cultures are still required: these are essential to exclude the rare possibility of mixed infections, for further characterization or identification, and, most importantly, for complete antimicrobial susceptibility testing. The possible variations in test results from the same laboratory and in particular among different laboratories must also be stressed, as well as the importance of good laboratory practice [178].

In general, amplified tests must be used as well as culture. These tests, that are rarely used if specimen volume is an issue, or to detect *M. tuberculosis* in paraffin block sections, are expensive. The American Thoracic Society issued a statement in 1997 on the use for these tests [186] and the Centers for Disease Control and Prevention provided updated guidelines for their use in 2009 [187].

Broad-range PCR assays differ from the species-specific PCR assays in that they amplify nucleic acid from entire groups of organisms: in the case of mycobacteria, they will amplify DNA from all members of the genus. The amplified product can then be differentiated by post-amplification analysis methods, such as probe hybridization, reverse hybridization, traditional sequencing, and microarray analysis [182, 188].

2.8.5 Antimicrobial Susceptibility Testing

The reemergence of *M. tuberculosis* complex as a cause of disease and the increasing percentage of cases of drug resistance have further strengthened the importance of antimicrobial susceptibility tests [189]. These must be performed in untreated patients and in those undergoing therapy who yield positive acid-fast smears or cultures after 2 months of treatment; they must also be performed in patients with a history of treatment failure for TB, in contacts of patients with resistant TB, and in residents in high prevalence areas [178].

The traditional susceptibility test method is a 1% agar proportion method. Organisms are inoculated onto 7H10 or 7H11 agar plates containing the various antibiotic concentrations and incubated for 14–21 days. The BATEC 460 TB system is preferably used when much earlier results are needed, after 4–7 days [189]. There are also broth-based automated systems available on the market, that are valid alternatives to the now infrequently used BACTEC 460 TB system [178].

Molecular mechanisms of drug resistance for many of the more important antimycobacterial agents have now been elucidated [178, 190, 191]. One of the more thoroughly studied targets for drug resistance to rifampicin is *rpoB*, which encodes the β-subunit of RNA polymerase; the *katG*, *inhA*, *imabA* and *ahpC* genes are associated with isoniazid resistance. A real-time PCR assay has been developed to detect important mutations in the *inhA* and r*poA* genes associated with resistance [192]. The markers of resistance to other drugs, such as streptomycin (*rpsL* and *rrs*), ethambutol (*embCAB*), and fluoroquinolones (*gyrA*), have also been studied [178].

2.8.6 The Tuberculin Skin Test

The tuberculin skin test (TST), also known as the intradermal Mantoux test since 1910, is the classic diagnostic tool for latent tuberculosis infection (LTBI). It is the oldest diagnostic test in use in modern medical practice, and because of its limitations, it is the weakest element in the strategy of targeted testing of LTBI [193].

The TST is based on the development of delayed hypersensitivity to mycobacterial antigens, following an intradermal injection of a purified protein derivative (PPD). The PPD is a culture filtrate of tubercle bacilli [194] containing over 200 antigens shared with the bacille Calmette-Guérin (BCG) vaccine and most nontuberculous mycobacteria [195]. This lack of specificity is the main cause of false positive tests in individuals vaccinated with BCG. BCG is the most widely used vaccine in the world, and more than 3 billion people have received it [196]. A meta-analysis showed that BCG administration increases the false positive TST results for a period of up to 15 years after vaccination [197]. Thus, a positive test can result from clinical or latent TB, from BCG vaccination or from contact with environmental mycobacteria.

Apart from its low specificity, the TST is characterized by a poor sensitivity. In fact, as TST depends on a lymphocyte-induced delayed hypersensitivity reaction, it has low sensitivity in immunosuppressed patients. In addition, severely ill patients, including those with some forms of active TB, with HIV infection and those on immunosuppressant drugs including corticosteroids, may have false-negative responses.

2.8.6.1 Mantoux Test

The TST should be done by the Mantoux method, the only standardized and well validated technique. The PPD (0.1 ml = 5 tuberculin units) is injected intradermally into the volar aspect of the forearm using a 27-gauge needle to raise a small wheal.

The diameter of the induration is read after 48–72 h. In normal conditions, a cut-off of 5 mm induration targets individuals at high risk of TB infection, such as close contacts of active cases, subjects with radiographic abnormalities consistent with TB, subjects with HIV infection and individuals taking immunosuppressants, corticosteroids or other agents. A cut-off of 10 mm is observed in residents of endemic areas, health care workers, the homeless, patients with diabetes, renal disease, silicosis and other conditions associated with an increased risk of latent tuberculous infection. A cut-off of 15 mm, finally, targets subjects with no risk factors [198].

Regardless of the above parameters, the size of the dermal tuberculin reaction has little or no prognostic significance, either during the disease or after recovery. A wide reaction during the disease may mean that the host has a high native and acquired resistance to TB, with high numbers of lymphocytes and macrophages in tuberculous lesions and at the site of the tuberculin reaction. A wide reaction can also be observed in subjects with a low native and acquired resistance and numerous bacilli that provide high doses of antigen for sensitization. If the wide reaction persists for years after recovery, it is possible that few dormant bacilli are still present in hidden caseous foci. From these, bacilli are released from time to time and then destroyed, thus boosting the whole immune system, including the level of tuberculin sensitivity [128].

Subjects with a recent infection can later become tuberculin negative, with or without antimicrobial treatment. In most of these subjects a tuberculin sensitivity recall is produced by the antigens in the tuberculin injected for skin testing. Therefore, when retested with intermediate-strength PPD, a subject with negative results a few weeks before becomes positive due to the booster effect of the tuberculin itself [199, 200]. The previous PPD injection can expand the tuberculin-sensitive T-cell population (memory T cells) to such an extent that the number of these cells is enough to induce a positive TST when the test is repeated [201]. Thus, in view of this booster effect, conversion of the TST must not necessarily be regarded as a sign of a recently acquired active infection.

By contrast, in subjects with active TB, the TST may be negative. This may be due to the fact that the pulmonary lesions collect most of the antigen specific circulating T cells, so few are left to contribute to the dermal tuberculin reaction. This possibility is supported by the fact that lymphocytes from diseased tissues obtained by bronchoalveolar lavage or from pleural exudates, contain a large population of antigen-specific T cells, secrete higher quantities of cytokines and showed a greater tendency to proliferate than T lymphocytes in peripheral blood [202, 203]. Moreover, TST negative subjects with active TB have a greater number of suppressor monocytes and lymphocytes in peripheral blood, producing transforming growth factor beta (TGF-β) and IL-10 [204].

Table 2.7 Heaf test: grades of reactions (modified, by [198])

Grade	Reaction
0	No reaction
I	At least 4 discrete papules
II	Confluent papules in a ring
III	Induration disc
IV	Induration disc >10 mm or vesiculation of the disc

Apart from the Mantoux test, other TST test forms are the Heaf and tine tests. The Heaf test (used in the UK) employs a spring-loaded "gun" which drives six needles into the skin of the volar aspect of the forearm through a drop of undiluted PPD. The method is easy but the gun needs to be autoclaved. The test result is read after 48–72 h; the reaction score is illustrated in Table 2.7. Grades III and IV correspond to a Mantoux reaction of 15 mm or more and are considered as evidence of infection; grade II corresponds to a Mantoux reaction of 10–14 mm and indicates a probable infection [198].

In the tine test the PPD is dried onto four spikes (tines) on a small, single use, disposable unit. The device is pressed firmly onto the skin so that the tines penetrate the cutis and is held in place for 10 s, while the dried PPD dissolves in the tissue fluids. The results are more variable than with the other tests [198].

2.8.7 Interferon-Gamma Assays

One third of the world population bears a latent tuberculosis infection (LTBI): this condition is characterized by a positive TST in a clinically asymptomatic subject, and 5–10% of these subjects will develop active disease. This is a major world health problem bearing mind that every year 2 million people die from TB [205]. Diagnosing LTBI is therefore imperative in order to be able to control the disease, but the TST is far from being the "gold" standard. A new generation of immune-based rapid blood tests for the diagnosis of LTBI seems to offer a significant upgrade of the century-old TST [193, 206–209].

Advances in mycobacterial genomics have revealed an *M. tuberculosis* genomic segment, termed "region of difference-1", deleted from all strains of the BCG vaccine and most nontuberculous mycobacteria [210]. Two proteins encoded by this stretch of DNA, early secretory antigen target protein 6 (ESAT-6) and culture filtrate protein 10 (CFP-10), are strong targets of T-helper type 1 T cells in subjects with TB infection [209, 211, 212]. A T-cell response to these antigens is thus, at least in theory, a specific marker of *M. tuberculosis* infection. An antigenic cross-reactivity of PPD is theoretically avoided in these new tests. There are now two methods for the rapid measurement of antigen-specific T-cell responses, the QuantiFERON-TB Gold Test (Cellestis, Carnegie, Australia) and the T-SPOT.TB test (Oxford Immunotec, Oxford, UK) [193, 209]. They are based on the fact that the predominant host response to the tubercle infection is by antigen-specific memory T cells, that release IFN-γ in response to the previously encountered mycobacterial antigens. The QuantiFERON-TB Gold Test, based on a whole-blood ELISA developed in the late

1980s, has recently been approved by the FDA for in vitro diagnostics, and the Centers for Disease Control and Prevention have published guidelines for its use [213]. The T-SPOT.TB test is based on the *ex vivo* overnight enzyme-linked immunospot (ELISpot) assay developed by Prof. Lalvani and Coworkers in the late 1990s [211]. It is approved for in vitro diagnostic use in Europe.

These two new blood tests have some common features but differ in various ways, also compared to their predecessor TST test (Table 2.8) [193, 208, 209]. The interferon-gamma tests have several advantages over the TST. They are based on a blood test taken at a single visit, and a return visit may not be necessary; automated testing has the advantage of offering an objective interpretation of the results. The booster phenomenon does not occur and so repeated screening of subjects at risk, exposed to TB (e.g. health care workers), is feasible. These tests are a better marker of LTBI. However, the interferon-gamma tests have some limitations: they require at least a basic laboratory and so are not currently in widespread use.

Various studies have shown that the two interferon-gamma tests are more specific than the TST for the diagnosis of LTBI in BCG-vaccinated populations. In fact, the T-SPOT.TB is more sensitive than the TST in immunocompetent subjects with LTBI and in patients with active TB, including those with an impaired cellular immunity, at high risk of false-negative TST results. The QuantiFERON-TB Gold

Table 2.8 Characteristics of the new blood tests and of the tuberculin skin test (TST) (modified, by [209])

Variables	QuantiFERON-TB Gold	T-SPOT.TB	TST
Antigens	ESAT-6 and CFP-10	ESAT-6 and CFP-10	PPD
Positive internal control	Yes	Yes	No
Effect of repeated testing	No booster response	No booster response	Booster response
Need for return visit	No	No	Yes
Time required for results	16–24 h	16–20 h	48–72 h
Setting of test	In vitro	In vitro	In vivo
Interpretation of test	Objective (instrument-based)	Objective (instrument-based)	Subjective (operator-based)
Readout units	International units of IFN-γ	IFN-γ spot-forming cells	Millimeters of induration
Technology platform	ELISA	ELISpot	NA
Test substrate	Whole blood	Peripheral blood mononuclear cells	NA
Outcome measure	Serum concentration of IFN-γ produced by T cells	Number of IFN-γ-producing T cells	NA
Readout system	Measurement of optical density values using an automated reader	Enumeration of spots by naked eye, magnifying lens, or automated reader	Palpable induration
Cost	Expensive test	Expensive test	Cheap test

NA not applicable

has a higher sensitivity than the TST in immunocompetent subjects with active TB. Comparative studies of the two blood assays performed in large population samples have demonstrated a higher sensitivity of the T-SPOT.TB [214, 215].

The impact of treatment on the blood test results has been studied by the ELISpot in patients with TB and in those with LTBI. In general, the magnitude of ELISpot responses is significantly reduced after treatment in both patients with active TB [216, 217] and those with LTBI [218, 219]. However, due to considerable inter-individual variations in the rate of decline of the response, and the fact that only a minority of subjects becomes negative at the end of treatment, the assay cannot be used for treatment monitoring or as a "test of cure" [209]. Nevertheless, the simultaneous measurement of IL-2 and IFN-γ secretion by *M. tuberculosis*-specific T cells is correlated with the results of treatment and offers a new paradigm for monitoring [220].

2.9 Histopathology

The initial non-specific inflammatory alterations give rise, after 3–6 weeks, to the characteristic tubercle. At this stage bacilli are rarely observable, even if cultures may be positive.

A fully formed tubercle consists of a focus of epithelioid cells containing a variable but usually low number of Langhans' giant cells, and a surrounding infiltrate of mononuclear cells. The center of the tubercle undergoes caseation necrosis and sometimes calcification. As the necrosis proceeds, the perivascular and endovascular alterations around the tubercle become more marked and are accompanied by cellular reactions that lead to fibrosis.

The granulomas are highly variable in appearance, depending on the virulence of the bacilli, the size of the inoculum and the host immune response. In cases with impaired cellular immunity, as well as HIV infection and in subjects taking cytotoxic and corticosteroid therapy, the histological picture is less granulomatous, due to the small number of activated macrophages, whereas there are much larger quantities of bacilli.

Histochemical studies have demonstrated that the mononuclear cells of the tubercle are blood-derived monocytes with a high content of lysosomal enzymes. They evolve to macrophages that, following T-cell activation, give rise to epithelioid cells, some of which fuse to become multinucleated giant cells [221, 222]. The caseation necrosis is caused by the death and degeneration of the epithelioid cells and is likely mediated by cytokines such as TNF and macrophage protease.

Some specific histological pictures are dependent on the bacillary load and the immunological response. The tuberculous chancre, that is a manifestation of the primary inoculation of TB, initially features an acute neutrophil inflammation with necrosis and the presence of very many bacilli; after 3-6 weeks, the infiltrate becomes granulomatous, with caseation, and the bacilli disappear. Instead, in miliary and orificial forms, the typical tubercle does not form or is necrotic; there are large numbers of bacilli except in modest forms of neonatal miliary TB [223].

In scrofuloderma, the cutis is destroyed by non specific abscesses and ulceration; tubercles and caseation necrosis are evident at the borders, and there may also be some bacilli. In warty TB, there will be hyperkeratosis, acanthosis and papillomatosis (that is sometimes pseudoepitheliomatous); at the dermal level there is an infiltrate consisting of neutrophils, lymphocytes and a few giant cells; bacilli are rare and the typical tubercle with caseation is not often observed.

The histological findings of lupus vulgaris are variable and sometimes difficult to diagnose. A typical picture is that of a tubercle with epithelioid cells and lymphocytes; the epidermis may sometimes present the same alterations as in warty TB. The caseation may be marked or minor; bacilli are rarely demonstrable but can sometimes be shown in culture. As the lesion resolves, the fibrosis will increase. Squamous and basal cell epitheliomas may develop on the old lesions.

It is not possible to make a differential diagnosis with other mycobacterial infections on the basis of the histological findings. In sarcoidosis, all the TB alterations may be present except for caseation necrosis; as compared to the picture in lupus vulgaris, the epithelioid cells are more scattered and better defined, and are surrounded by a smaller number of lymphocytes. In tuberculoid leprosy, the only reliable differential finding is the presence of neural and perineural involvement. Tertiary syphilis shows more intense vascular changes and a plasma cell infiltrate. In leishmaniasis and blastomycosis it is important to identify the causal agent. A non-specific tuberculoid infiltrate, with irregular clusters of epithelioid cells in an inflammatory infiltrate but without the formation of the typical tubercles, is observed also in the rosacea form.

2.10 Cutaneous Tuberculosis

The wide clinical spectrum of cutaneous TB depends on the route of infection (exogenous or endogenous), the host immune response and whether the subject has had previous sensitization to TB. *M. tuberculosis* is the main organism responsible for cutaneous TB; *M. bovis* can occasionally be implicated and, more rarely, the bacille Calmette-Guérin, an attenuated form of *M. bovis*.

TB must always be considered a systemic disease, even when it is localized at the skin and even when the skin is the entry portal of the tubercle bacillus. The immuno-allergic response of the organism following on from the skin infection by mycobacteria is proof of the systemic involvement that follows the localized disease [224].

2.10.1 Epidemiology

Worldwide, there are more cases of TB nowadays than in any other period in the history of humanity [225]. The WHO estimates that every year, 1.5–2 million people die of TB. In 1999, the WHO estimated a staggering 8,417,000 new cases of TB globally, revealing a reverse of the steady decline in incidence that had occurred during the latter half of the twentieth century [225].

Cutaneous TB accounts for only a small proportion of all the cases of TB, actually less than 1–2% [226]. However, these numbers become significant in view of the high prevalence of TB in many developing countries. In India, for example, where there were 1,847,000 new cases of TB in 1999, an annual incidence of cutaneous TB of about 18,000 cases can be expected [226].

Cutaneous TB continues to be a significant medical emergency even nowadays after the advent of highly efficacious anti-tubercular drugs. Over the past 20 years, there has been a re-emergence of cutaneous TB also in European countries, due to HIV infection and deteriorating hygienic conditions of segregated people (immigrants, homeless individuals). In HIV-infected subjects, some severe or atypical cases of cutaneous TB with necrotic aspects have been reported [227–234].

The incidence of the different clinical forms of cutaneous TB varies globally. Scrofuloderma (TB colliquativa) was the commonest form in the most recent UK series [232], whereas lupus vulgaris was more common in a South African study [235]. Scrofuloderma and lupus vulgaris are the most common forms, together with an increase of tuberculids, in Japan and the Far East [236].

Scrofuloderma and primary cutaneous TB are typical of childhood and adolescence, while all the other clinical forms have a higher incidence in adulthood. Lupus vulgaris and orificial ulcerative TB have the highest incidence between the ages of 30 and 50. Tuberculids can affect all ages.

Although it is not possible to confirm a different predisposition of the different skin regions to developing tubercle infection, exposed sites (face and neck) and the limbs are those most commonly affected. Instead, the scalp seems to be quite resistant to the infection.

2.10.2 Historical Aspects

Scrofuloderma and lupus vulgaris are the oldest forms of skin TB described in the medical literature, and were known as the King's evil [225, 237]. Lupus, meaning wolf-like, was initially used to refer to an ulcerative lesion reminiscent of a wolf bite. In 1803, Robert Villand adopted the term lupus when describing the last stages of facial skin TB: this clinical description of facial lupus then gave rise to the similar terms lupus erythematosus and lupus pernio. The term tuberculosis verrucosa cutis was coined in 1869. Kaposi was the first to define mucocutaneous involvement in TB. In 1896, Darier introduced the concept of tuberculid, and later Pautrier used this term to define the papulonecrotic tuberculid [225].

2.10.3 Classification

There is still no entirely satisfactory classification, illustrating the difficulties encountered when attempting to classify a disease whose manifestations depend on various different factors. In 1896, Darier distinguished between forms of true TB and forms regarded as "tuberculids". With the advent of active anti-tubercle drugs, the failure of these so-called tuberculids to respond and their tendency to resolve spontaneously led to a critical assessment of their etiology. Thanks to new methods of detecting the *M. tuberculosis* complex, the position of tuberculids was finally better elucidated.

The most widely accepted classification of cutaneous TB is based on its propagation mechanisms via direct inoculation, through a contiguous infection, or by hematogenous dissemination (Table 2.9) [238]. According to this classification, skin involvement can occur through exogenous inoculation (in non-previously sensitized hosts, with the occurrence of regional adenopathy), by contagious spread from a focus underlying the skin (from osteomyelitis, epididymitis, and lymphadenitis), and by hematogenous spread from a distant focus (Table 2.10) [234, 239, 240].

Another useful classification then introduced the concept of "bacterial load", similar to the one described by Ridley-Jopling for Hansen's disease; cutaneous TB was thus classified as either a multibacillary or paucibacillary form [241]. The multibacillary forms include tuberculous chancre (by direct inoculation), scrofuloderma and orificial TB (by contiguity), and acute miliary TB and gumma (by hematogenous spread). These clinical pictures feature abundant bacilli, that can be seen by direct visualization or isolated in culture. Paucibacillary forms include TB verrucosa cutis and lupus vulgaris (by direct inoculation or through re-exposure), and some other forms of lupus vulgaris (by hematogenous dissemination). In these forms there are few bacilli, and they are difficult to isolate in culture. In this classification, tuberculids are included at the extreme end of the paucibacillary spectrum (Table 2.11) [225].

Table 2.9 Classification of cutaneous tuberculosis

Bacillary form	Method of inoculation	Host immune status	Clinical disease
Multibacillary forms	Direct exogenous source:		
	Primary inoculation	Naïve	Primary inoculation tuberculous chancre
	Endogenous source:		
	Contiguous spread	Low	Scrofuloderma
	Autoinoculation	Low	Orificial tuberculosis
	Hematogenous spread	Low	Acute miliary tuberculosis
			Tuberculous gumma
Paucibacillary forms	Direct post-primary inoculation	Immune	Tuberculosis verrucosa cutis
			Lupus vulgaris (occasionally)
	Hematogenous spread	High	Lupus vulgaris
			Tuberculids

Table 2.10 Clinical features of cutaneous tuberculosis

	Tuberculous chancre	Scrofuloderma	Warty TB	Orificial TB	Lupus vulgaris	Miliary TB	Tuberculous gumma
Synonyms	Cutaneous primary complex Primary inoculation tuberculosis	TB colliquativa cutis	TB verrucosa cutis Anatomist's wart Prosector's wart Butcher's wart Verruca necrogenica	Acute tuberculous ulcer Orificial ulcerative TB	TB luposa	TB cutis disseminata TB cutis acuta generalisata	Metastatic tuberculous abscess
Incidence	1–2% of cutaneous TB	Common in immigrants from developing countries Children	Most common form of cutaneous TB	Rare	10-15% of cutaneous TB Most often women	Rare Children	Immunocompromised subjects Children
Transmission	Cutaneous or mucosal inoculation in previously uninfected subject	Contiguous cutaneous involvement usually from a lymph node or bone	Cutaneous involvement in previously infected subject with moderate or high immunity	Cutaneous or mucosal autoinoculation to natural orifices from internal TB	Hematogenous or lymphatic spread Direct extension	Hematogenous dissemination from primary lung TB in subject with low immunity	Acute hematogenous dissemination from primary lung TB Low resistance
Histopathology	Initially: non specific neutrophilic inflammation with necrosis and bacilli Later: granulomatous inflammation with central caseation, epithelioid and Langhans cells; no bacilli	Granulomatous infiltrate, caseation necrosis; bacilli may be isolated	Epidermal pseudoepitheliomatous hyperplasia; microabscesses in upper dermis; occasionally bacilli	Aspecific inflammatory infiltrate; necrosis; some tubercles with caseation; bacilli	Tubercles with scanty caseation; usually no bacilli	Necrosis and aspecific infiltrate surrounded by macrophages; abundant bacilli	Necrosis and abscesses; abundant bacilli

(continued)

Table 2.10 (continued)

	Tuberculous chancre	Scrofuloderma	Warty TB	Orificial TB	Lupus vulgaris	Miliary TB	Tuberculous gumma
Clinical presentation	Papular/nodular lesions with ulcerative evolution Regional lymphadenopathy	Painless dermal-hypodermal nodule Colliquative ulceration	Warty papules evolving to verrucosa plaque with inflammatory areola	Painful shallow ulcer with undermined bluish edges	Micronodules in plaques with very slow evolution and ill-defined scarring	Papules, vesicles, pustules and nodules with necrotic ulcerative evolution	Subcutaneous nodule/fluctuating abscess
Predominant sites	Hands, face	Lateral-cervical region	Dorsum of hands	Natural orifices	Face, neck, buttocks	Trunk and limbs	Limbs
Tuberculin skin test	Initially negative, later positive	Positive	Positive	Usually positive; negative in late stages	Positive	Usually negative in late stages	Usually positive; may be negative
Differential diagnosis	Syphilitic chancre, lymphogranuloma, sporotrichosis, actinomycosis, non specific pyogenic ulcers, tularemia, *M. marinum* granuloma	Lymphomas, syphilitic gumma, abscesses, actinomycosis, suppurative hidradenitis	Common warts, hypertrophic lichen planus, nontuberculous mycobacterial infection, vegetating pyodermitis, chromomycosis	Anal chancre, condylomata acuminata, herpes simplex chronicus, lip carcinoma	Sarcoidosis, discoid lupus erythematous, leishmaniasis, dimorphic fungal infection, lymphocytoma, tertiary syphilis, tuberculoid leprosy, Bowen's disease, squamous cell carcinoma	Viral exanthema	Panniculitis, syphilitic gumma, hidradenitis suppurativa

TB tuberculosis

Table 2.11 Tuberculids

Micropapular	Lichen scrofulosorum
Papular	Papulonecrotic tuberculid
Nodular	Erythema induratum of Bazin
	Nodular tuberculid
	Erythema nodosum (occasionally)

2.10.4 Primary Inoculation Tuberculosis

This form (synonyms: *tuberculous chancre, tuberculous primary complex*) is due to direct cutaneous inoculation of *M. tuberculosis* in an individual lacking natural or artificially acquired immunity to the organism. The initial lesion contains numerous bacilli (multibacillary form).

Because acid-fast bacilli cannot penetrate the normal intact skin barrier, to foster the onset of the infection some form of injury of this defense is needed. The entry portal is usually through minor skin injuries like abrasions, hangnail wounds, impetigo, and furuncles. The inoculation may occur via various mechanisms but in the majority of cases will affect subjects working in medical-related professions (Laënnec described his own "prosector's wart" in 1826). Tuberculous chancres have followed mouth-to-mouth respiration [242], circumcision [243, 244], infections due to inadequately sterilized syringes [245], wounds [246], operations [247], ear-piercing [242], intramuscular injections given by a nurse with active TB [248], and tattooing [249]. In areas with a high TB prevalence in the community, lesions may occur anywhere on the body, from contact with sputum or following insect bites [250] or pyococcal infections of the skin. Sexual transmission has also been reported [251, 252].

The sites most frequently involved are the face and limbs, and manifestations are more often seen in children [253–262]. This form of skin TB is considered uncommon [238] but the incidence is likely underestimated, especially in areas with a high TB prevalence.

In one third of cases there is mucocutaneous involvement, and the conjunctival [239] are also affected, or the oral cavity after tooth extraction or after drinking non-pasteurized milk infected by *M. bovis* [234, 263–265].

After 1–4 weeks incubation, at the inoculation site a brownish-red papular-nodular lesion develops, that evolves into a painless, firm, non tender ulcer with undermined edges and a granular hemorrhagic base. In time, an adherent crust develops. After 1–2 months from the inoculation the onset of regional lymphadenopathy is observed, with the lymph nodes tending to adhere to the skin. These lymph nodes soften in a few weeks and can break down after the formation of a fistula, from which purulent matter with a bacillary content is discharged. The ulcers heal in a few weeks. Occasionally, lupoid nodules develop around the healed ulcer. The lymphadenopathy may persist for a long period. Lesions closely simulating paronychia may affect the fingers [254]. The combination of the tuberculous chancre and regional adenopathy is the cutaneous analogue of the primary tubercular infection of the lung, the Gohn complex. Within 2–3 years, calcification may be found in draining nodes [240].

The early histological changes are those of an acute neutrophilic reaction, with areas of necrosis and numerous bacilli. After 3–6 weeks the infiltrate becomes granulomatous, with epithelioid cells and Langhans cells (but typical tubercles are absent), and caseation necrosis, coinciding with the disappearance of the bacilli, becomes evident. At the same time as the bacilli reduce, the tuberculin test, that was initially negative, generally becomes intensely positive.

As regards diagnosis, the suspicion must be borne in mind in the case of any painless, non-healing ulcer or lesion with regional lymphadenopathy, especially in children. Acid-fast bacilli can be demonstrated in the primary skin lesion and in draining nodes in the early stages of disease. Anti-tubercular treatment must be started without awaiting the results of any further tests. At this stage, differential diagnosis is with scrofuloderma, syphilitic chancre, lymphogranuloma (Nicolas-Favre disease), tularemia, sporotrichosis, and actinomycosis [259]. Bartonellosis and especially *M. marinum* skin infections closely resemble primary TB, but the distribution, clinical course and culture characteristics show distinctive differences.

At the site of the original lesions, lupus vulgaris may develop. Occasionally, hematogenous spread of the bacilli can occur, and TB develop in other sites, including miliary TB [266]. In some cases it may follow the onset of erythema nodosum [267].

2.10.5 Tuberculosis Verrucosa

Tuberculosis verrucosa (*warty TB*) occurs due to a reinfection by exogenous tubercle bacilli in subjects who have developed a moderate-high grade of immunity to *M. tuberculosis*. There are few bacilli in such lesions (paucibacillary form).

Three possible types of manifestation can be observed. The first is by accidental superinfection from exogenous sources: physicians, pathologists, and post-mortem attendants are traditionally at risk (hence the terms "anatomist's warts", "prosector's warts", "verruca necrogenica") [268, 269]. The second occurs through inoculation from sputum of a patient with active TB. The third is observed in already infected children and young adults, who have developed some degree of immunity but can be reinfected by sputum after sitting on the ground or walking barefoot where bacilli are present [270, 271].

Tuberculosis verrucosa can also often be caused by *M. bovis*, especially in workers who come in contact with infected cattle (milkmen/maids, veterinarians, butchers).

Given the exogenous origin of the infection, the sites exposed to external contact are typically affected, such as the hands (dorsum, fingers and particular thumbs) and the extensor surfaces of the wrists. While it is the hands that are most often affected in Europe, in Asia it is the knees, ankles, feet, and buttocks [271, 272].

The "anatomical tubercle" is the prototype TB verrucosa: it is an occupational disease resulting from minor injuries occurring during autopsies or surgery on individuals with TB or while handling meat from infected animals. After a few days of incubation, the lesion starts as a small, symptomless, indurated warty papule with a slight inflammatory halo. It gradually extends to form a verrucous plaque, which

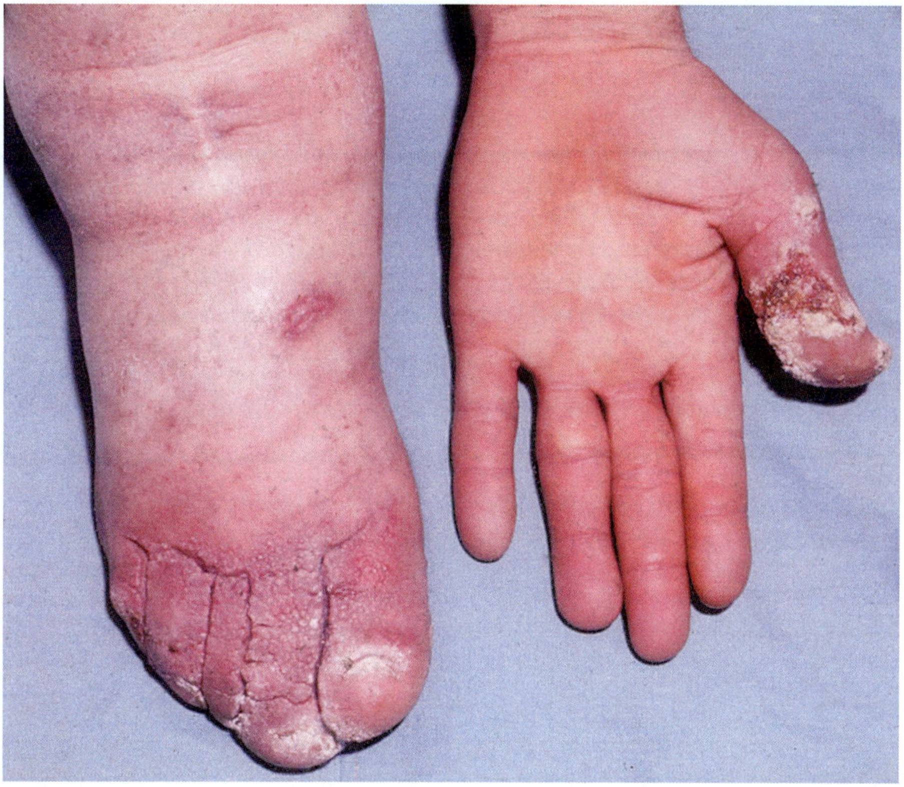

Fig. 2.1 Tuberculosis verrucosa. Warty plaques; ulcerative evolution on the thumb

may have irregular margins with finger-like projections (Fig. 2.1). Lesions undergoing the rapid development phase, that may be single or multiple, rounded or irregular, show three distinct zones: a reddish-purple flat peripheral zone; a more raised middle zone, purple or brown, papillomatous or verrucous, which may feature scattered small ulcerations covered with adherent crusts, from which a few drops of pus can leak; a central zone mostly filled with warty protrusions. The center of the lesion may undergo involution, leaving a white atrophic scar.

Tuberculosis verrucosa has a very slow evolution and cannot heal spontaneously. The lesions last for years; they may resemble lupus vulgaris, but the sites are different. They can also be psoriasiform or keloidal in appearance. Rarely, a sporotrichoid spread and tuberculous lymphadenitis have been reported [273]. Deeply destructive papillomatous and sclerotic forms can cause deformities of the limbs [274]. In Hong Kong and Singapore an exuberant granulomatous form has been described [271, 272]. Tumor-like forms can also occur [275].

At the histopathology level, the epidermis presents acanthosis, hyperkeratosis and papillomatosis. These changes can be so marked as to simulate pseudoepitheliomatous hyperplasia. In the superficial derma there is an inflammatory infiltrate with neutrophils and lymphocytes, and often abscess formations. In the middle derma there are generally tuberculoid structures with a low grade of caseous necrosis. The vessels are dilated and the connective tissues edematous [276]. Bacilli are only occasionally observed.

Digital and subungueal lesions must be differentiated from warts, and those on the hands from keratoses. Blastomycosis and actinomycosis can simulate exuberant forms. Hypertrophic lichen planus and giant lichenifications are different in terms of appearance, multiplicity of the lesions and itching. Lupus vulgaris is not usually hyperkeratotic and shows apple-jelly nodules on diascopy. Lesions induced by non-tuberculous mycobacteria can be differentiated by microbiological culture, although fishtank granuloma forms with a unique plaque due to *M. marinum* are particularly difficult to differentiate. Vegetating pyodermitis has an acute and rapid evolution (weeks): the inflammatory process is more acute, the suppuration is abundant, the margins are bright red, and the consistency is softer. It heals quickly with local antiseptic therapy.

Tuberculosis verrucosa responds to anti-tubercular treatment but unless this is administered the disease may persist for months or years [274, 277, 278], although spontaneous remission can occur, leaving atrophic scars. It is always recommended to seek for concomitant infection of the bone or lungs; miliary tuberculosis has also been reported [279].

2.10.6 Scrofuloderma

The term scrofuloderma or scrofula (from the Latin "little sow") was adopted in analogy with tumors affecting the lymph nodes of the affected sow, and that spread by contiguity to the skin, causing an ulcer.

Scrofuloderma (*tuberculosis colliquativa cutis*) results from the involvement and breakdown of the skin overlying a contiguous TB focus. This is usually a lymph gland, an infected bone or joint, or the epididymis [280]. This form is observed above all in children and adolescents [281–283], or in young adulthood [232], and is very rare in the elderly. The disease shows a slight predilection for the female gender. It is usually observed in malnourished children [284] and immunosuppressed adults [285].

This form of TB is preferentially localized in the lateral-cervical region (Figs. 2.2 and 2.3) [286]. It can also affect the axillary, supraclavicular (Fig. 2.4), epitrochlear, retroauricular, and inguinal regions (Fig. 2.5) [287, 288].

A painless dermo-hypodermal nodule with an increased consistency, indistinct margins and varying in size from a few millimeters to 1–2 cm overlies the infected gland or joint. It slowly increases in volume, involving and infiltrating the overlying skin, which becomes bluish-red. As the infiltrate softens, the mass becomes fluctuating and a cold purulent collection develops in the subcutaneous tissue. The skin can ulcerate in one or more areas and the nodule will discharge its content outside. At this stage, TB colliquativa shows an ulceration with a granulating base. The edges of the ulcer are infiltrated, bluish and irregularly

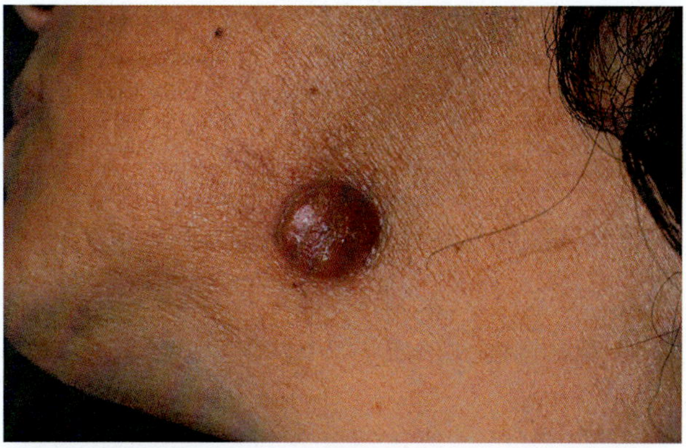

Fig. 2.2 Lateral-cervical scrofuloderma

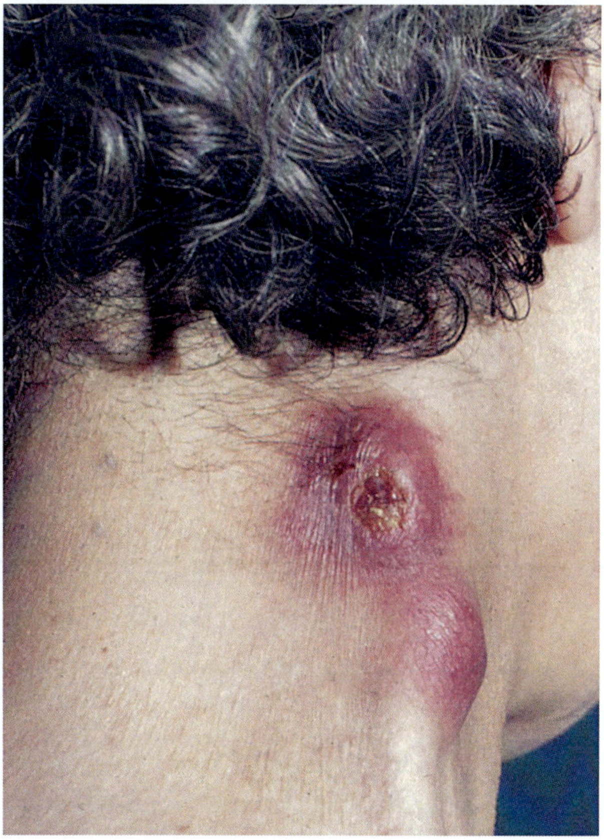

Fig. 2.3 Lateral-cervical scrofuloderma with ulcerative lesion

shaped. Adjacent multiple nodules can merge through subcutaneus fistulas and produce large, irregular ulcerations. An exuberant granulation tissue may give rise to granulomatous and fibrous pseudotumoral formations [289]. Sporotrichoid spread has been reported [290].

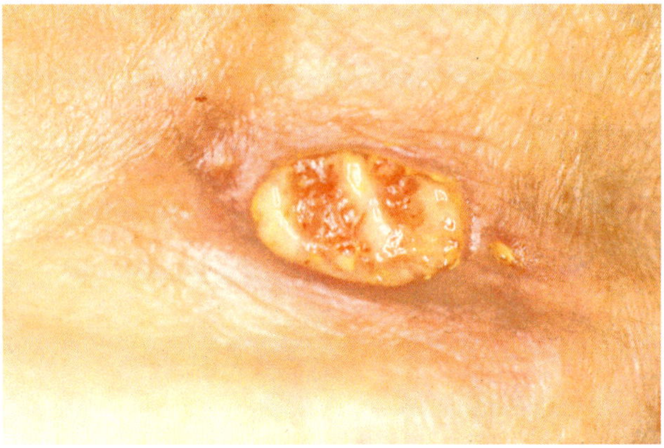

Fig. 2.4 Supraclavicular ulcerated scrofuloderma

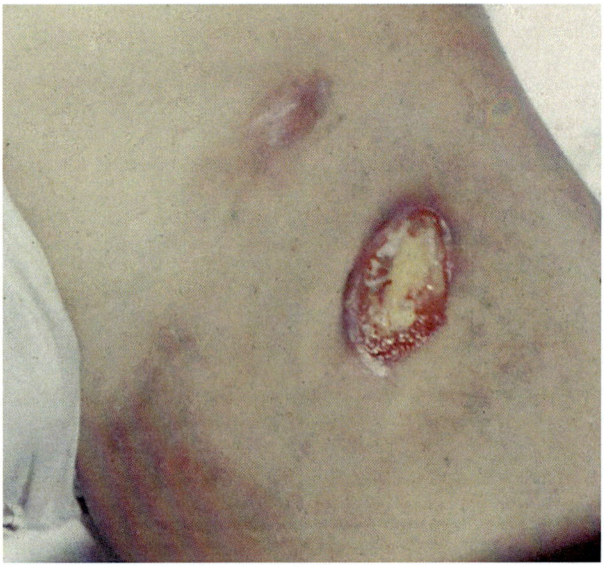

Fig. 2.5 Inguinal ulcerated scrofuloderma

Scrofuloderma which manifests as contiguous involvement of the skin overlying a site of TB of the bones and joints is not common. Any bone or joint may be affected but the most frequent site is the spine, involved in half the cases, followed in frequency by the large joints of the lower limb (hip, knee and ankle) and upper limb (shoulder, elbow and wrist), and then the small joints of the hands and feet (Figs. 2.6, 2.7, and 2.8). It is important to consider, however, that in case of spinal TB, also termed Pott's disease (after Sir Percivall Pott, 1713–1788), the "cold" abscesses may emerge well away from the site of bone disease: for example, abscesses secondary to disease in the lumbar vertebrae may emerge in the thigh below the inguinal ligament, as well as TB of the cervical spine may present as a retropharyngeal abscess.

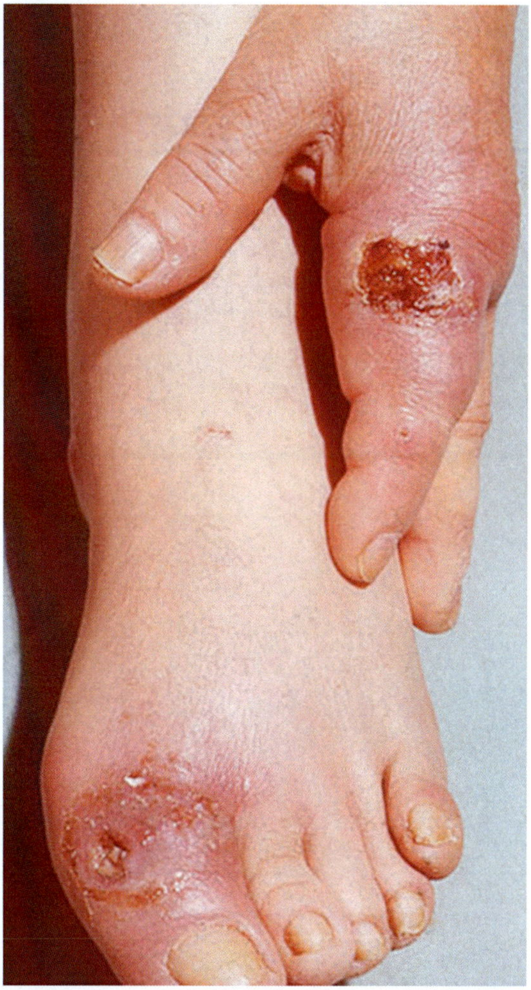

Fig. 2.6 Tubercular oteoarthropathy of the hand and feet with cutaneous involvement

In case of tuberculous epididymitis or orchitis, secondary to TB of the kidney or due to direct hematogenous spread from primary foci of disease, scrofuloderma may involve the scrotum (Fig. 2.9).

Histologically, the nodules consist of granulomatous infiltrates composed of epithelioid cells, Langhans giant cells, and lymphocytes. Marked caseation necrosis is present in deeper structures. Tubercle bacilli can usually be detected in the pus.

After a long, slow healing process, these lesions leave typical irregular and hypertrophic keloid-type scars. Sweet's syndrome has been reported in association with scrofuloderma [291]. Scrofuloderma of the neck and submandibular regions can extend to the face and upper chest. The tuberculin skin test is variable, but usually positive [292]. The response to anti-tubercular treatment is generally good;

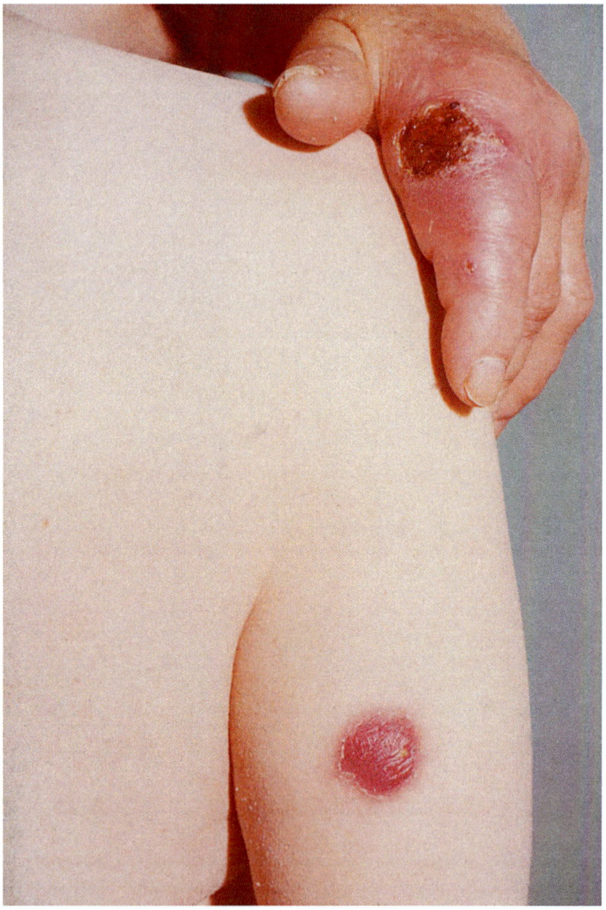

Fig. 2.7 The same patient as in Fig. 2.6. Lupus vulgaris of the arm

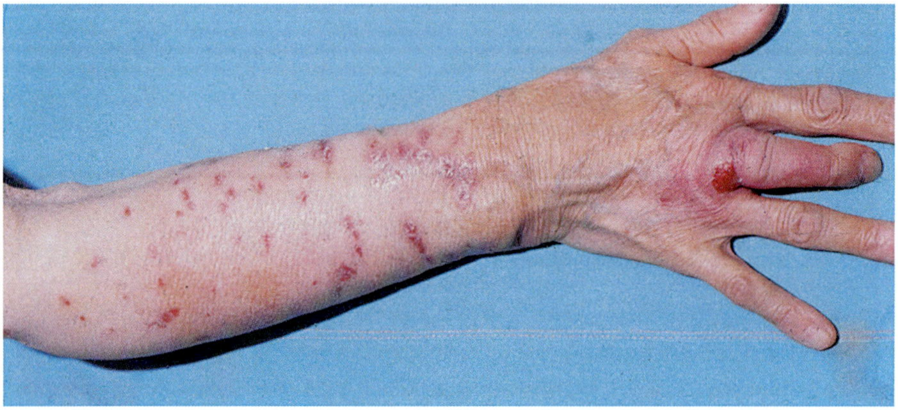

Fig. 2.8 Tubercular oteoarthropathy of the third finger of the right hand and lichen scrofulosorum

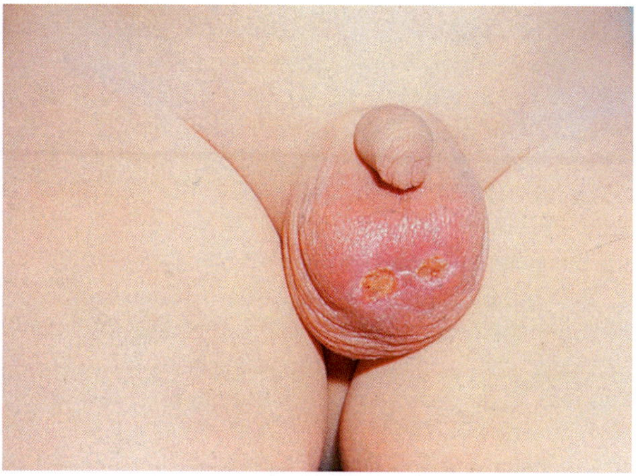

Fig. 2.9 Tuberculous epididymitis with cutaneous involvement

some authors recommend wide surgical removal of affected tissue, combined with the specific therapy.

Non-ulcerated lesions must be differentiated from lymphomas, syphilitic gummas (with a harder consistency and rarer in children), pyodermitis (abscesses, furuncles), suppurative hydroadenitis, and fungal nodules (actinomycosis, sporotricosis). Ulcerated lesions are distinguished from ulcerated syphilitic gummas: the ulcer is regular in shape, with sharp perpendicular edges, and evolves more rapidly than tuberculous lesions. Tuberculous lesions on the lower limbs should be differentiated from erythema nodosum of Bazin, B cell-lymphoma, and pyoderma gangrenosum.

2.10.7 Orificial Ulcerative Tuberculosis

This form (*orificial tuberculosis*, *acute tuberculous ulcer*) involves the mucous membranes of natural orifices and the periorificial skin of subjects affected by advanced visceral TB. It is a multibacillary form of cutaneous TB. Nowadays, it is extremely rare.

Tuberculous ulcers occur in the oral mucosa, on the lips, around the mouth, in the perianal region, and in the genital mucosa of individuals with active foci in the lungs, intestine, and genito-urinary apparatus, respectively. In these locations, ulcers result from direct self inoculation of bacilli, that are copiously eliminated from these foci. Occasionally, ulcers can have an exogenous origin due to direct inoculation of bacilli [293].

Most of these patients have a low tuberculin reactivity and the tissue reactivation is of anergic type. This form is relatively rare thanks to the strong resistance of the intact skin and mucosa to the penetration of mycobacteria. Dental caries or a trauma may favor the inoculation.

Subjects with orificial TB are generally severely ill adults with advanced internal TB and impaired cell-mediated immunity. Lesions occur most commonly in the mouth. The initial lesion is an edematous reddish nodule that rapidly breaks down to form painful, shallow ulcers with undermined bluish edges. The ulcers rarely exceed 2 cm in diameter and show no tendency to heal spontaneously. They are irregularly shaped with a hard edge; the base is irregular and yellowish, covered with a purulent and necrotic discharge; after removal of this discharge, the base of the ulcer shows a granulating, hemorrhagic surface.

Pain is the cardinal feature. There is usually evidence of infection of other organs; 79% of patients in one series had associated pulmonary TB [294]. The confirmation of the diagnosis is bacteriological and by PCR [295]. The tuberculin skin test is variable; in the later stages at least, the patient is often anergic.

In a series of 42 patients with orificial disease, 69% had oral ulcers, 21% bone involvement and 10% salivary gland and/or lymph node involvement [294]. Other sites include the genitals [296], and around the anus.

The histological changes are variable: there can be a non specific inflammatory infiltrate, or else the presence of tuberculoid nodules with caseous necrosis. In all cases, tubercle bacilli are present and easily demonstrated.

The ulcer of the lower lip can simulate a carcinoma due to the hard and infiltrated base and to concomitant submaxillary adenopathy. In perianal localizations, the differential diagnosis is with anal chancre, condylomata acuminata, and herpes simplex chronicus. The prognosis is usually serious and depends on the concomitant visceral TB and on the immunological conditions.

2.10.8 Miliary Tuberculosis

This is a rare, disseminated and multibacillary form of cutaneous TB; it occurs in association with generalized miliary TB [297] and is due to acute hematogenous dissemination of mycobacteria into the skin. It is rare and usually affects young children or immunocompromised patients, such as those with concomitant HIV infection [298–309] or following viral infection such as scarlet fever or measles [310].

The skin lesions are often acute generalized profuse crops of minute reddish-brown or purplish papules, vesicles, pustules, or hemorrhagic manifestations in an already ill patient. The vesicles may become necrotic and form small ulcers [311]. Erythematous nodules have also been reported [312]. The lesions are scattered on the trunk and limbs and, rarely, on the face. The underlying disease may not be manifest, and the diagnosis is only made at histology showing acid-fast bacilli [313]. It is always wise to seek for signs of internal infection [314].

The histology shows numerous microabscesses containing neutrophils or non-specific inflammatory infiltrates with foci of necrosis and acid-fast bacilli. The tuberculin skin test is usually positive, although it may become negative in the late stages of the disease. The development of an unusual exanthematic rash in an ill subject with known TB or tuberculous contact must suggest the diagnosis.

Anti-tubercular treatment should be started immediately in cases of a strong suspicion. The prognosis is poor, even if treatment response does sometimes occur.

2.10.9 Lupus Vulgaris

This is a chronic, progressive, post-primary, paucibacillary form of cutaneous TB in subjects with a moderate or high degree of immunity. The characteristic lesion is a plaque consisting of soft, reddish-brown papules. Such lesions will sometimes extend in some areas but heal, leaving scarring, in others. Over many years, considerable tissue destruction can occur.

Lupus vulgaris usually starts in young adulthood and is only exceptionally observed after the age of 60 years. Women are more commonly affected than men. Currently, lupus vulgaris is more frequent in northern Europe than in Mediterranean countries. In India, South Africa and Pakistan, it is the most common form of TB in adults [235, 315, 316]. In Tunisia, there has recently been an increase in the number of cases, probably reflecting a greater immunity to TB in the community [317, 318].

2.10.9.1 Pathogenesis

Lupus vulgaris originates from an underlying TB focus, typically in a bone, joint or lymph node, and arises either by contiguous extension of the disease from underlying affected tissue or by hematogenous or lymphatic spread. The underlying focus is not always evident; such cases result from a reactivation of a latent skin focus secondary to a previously silent bacteremia [319]. Lupus vulgaris can also arise due to exogenous inoculation during tattooing [320] or as a complication of the BCG vaccination [321].

Lupus vulgaris is a paucibacillary form of skin TB, and so culture of the bacilli obtained from the lesions is often extremely difficult. In a study of 4000 patients, bacilli could be cultured in only 6% of the cases [322]. A concomitant diagnosis made by PCR has been reported [323]. The bacilli will be destroyed as a result of the local tissue reaction, thanks to the good level of specific immunity in these patients.

2.10.9.2 Histopathology

The histopathological features are variable. Usually, tubercles constituted by epithelioid cells, multinucleated giant cells and lymphocytes are present in the superficial dermis. Within them, caseous necrosis is absent or at most scanty (Figs. 2.10 and 2.11). There may be an inflammatory infiltrate with giant cells at the superficial and dermal level, with rare tuberculoid structures, and it may also involve the muscular fascia, muscles, and cartilage. There will be fragmentation of the elastic fibers and destruction of the skin appendices. The epidermis may be atrophic or, more rarely, show acanthosis and hyperkeratosis; it is sometimes ulcerated. In cases of severe acanthosis there is pseudoepitheliomatous hyperplasia; this picture must be differentiated from squamous cell carcinoma [324]. Only exceptionally is it possible to demonstrate tubercle bacilli in histological sections [325].

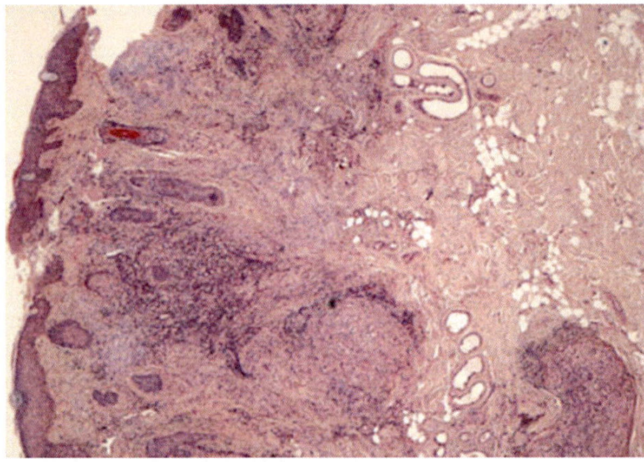

Fig. 2.10 Dermo-hypodermic tuberculoid granulomatous infiltrate (Hematoxylin-eosin – ×40)

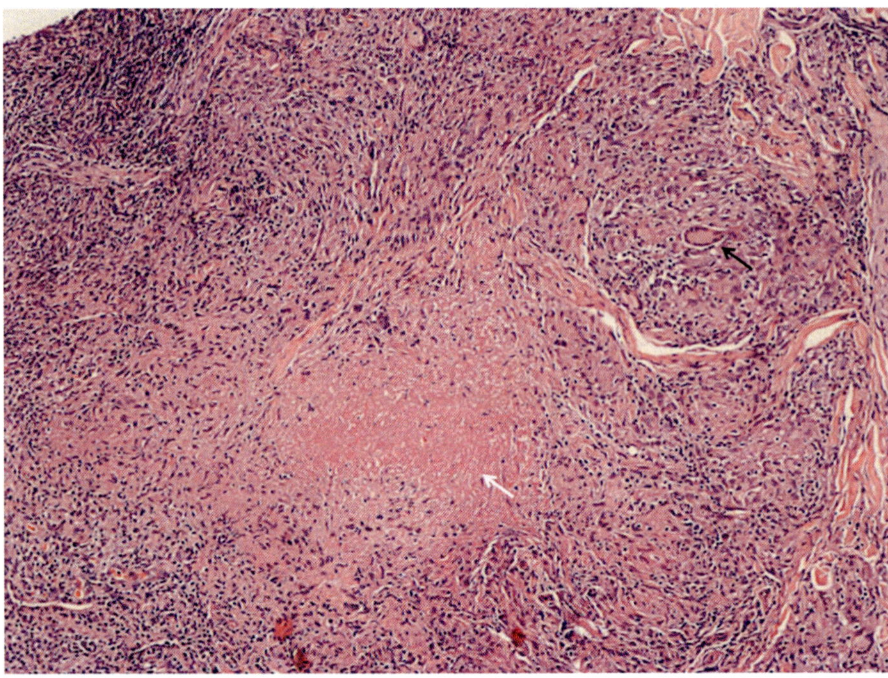

Fig. 2.11 Granulomatous infiltrate with giant Langhans cells (*black arrow*) and caseation necrosis (*white arrow*) (Hematoxylin-eosin – ×100)

2.10.9.3 Clinical Features

Lupus vulgaris can develop anywhere on the skin surface, but is prevalently localized (80-90% of cases) on the face (nose, cheeks, eyelids, lips, and ear pavilions) (Figs. 2.12, 2.13, 2.14, 2.15, 2.16, 2.17, 2.18, 2.19, 2.20, 2.21, 2.22, 2.23, 2.24, 2.25, 2.26, and 2.27). Other possible sites involved are the neck (Figs 2.28, 2.29, and 2.30), buttocks (Figs. 2.31, 2.32, and 2.33), thighs, genitalia, perianal skin, legs and back of the hands (Fig. 2.34) and forearms (Fig. 2.35). The trunk is more rarely involved.

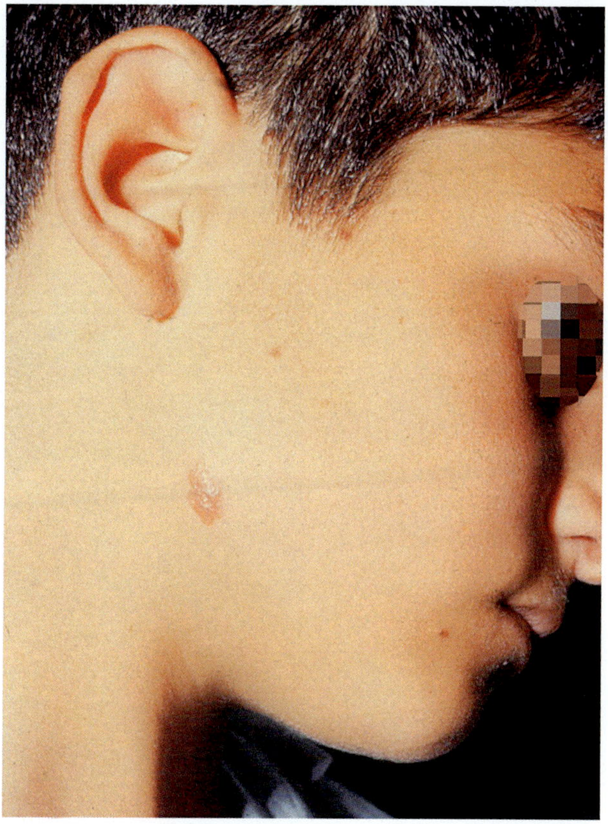

Fig. 2.12 Lupus vulgaris. Erythemato-yellowish plaque

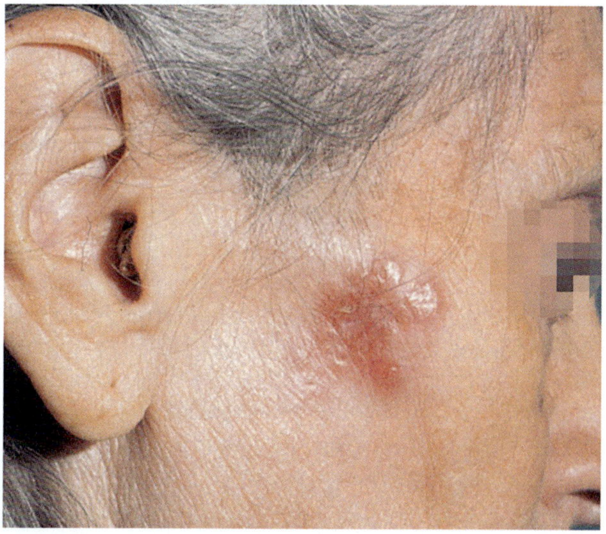

Fig. 2.13 Lupus vulgaris. Erythemato-yellowish plaque

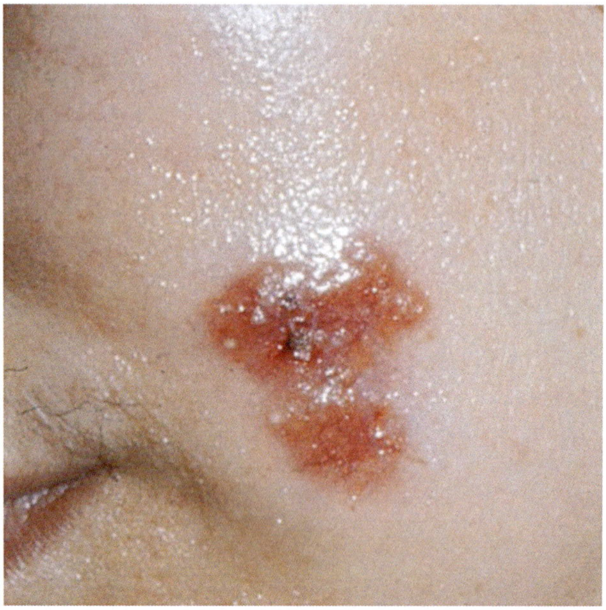

Fig. 2.14 Lupus vulgaris. Erythemato-yellowish plaque

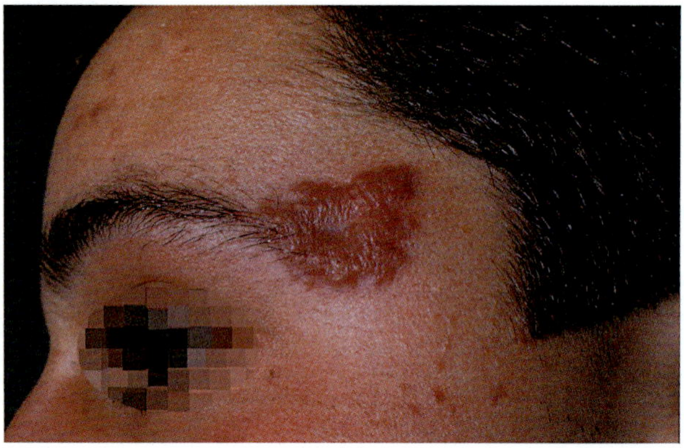

Fig. 2.15 Lupus vulgaris. Central atrophic scar

The characteristic lesion is a plaque, consisting of small dermal nodules (lupomas), that will extend gradually over the years. Apart from destroying the tissues, this lesion induces the formation of ill-defined scarred areas. The lupoma is a tiny brown nodule, ranging in size from a pin-head to a lentil, that may be slightly raised or embedded in the skin. Sometimes, it is so minimally infiltrated that on palpation it may feel like a macule. Its yellowish color gives the plaque its characteristic "apple-jelly" appearance. This shade of color is often masked by the erythematous

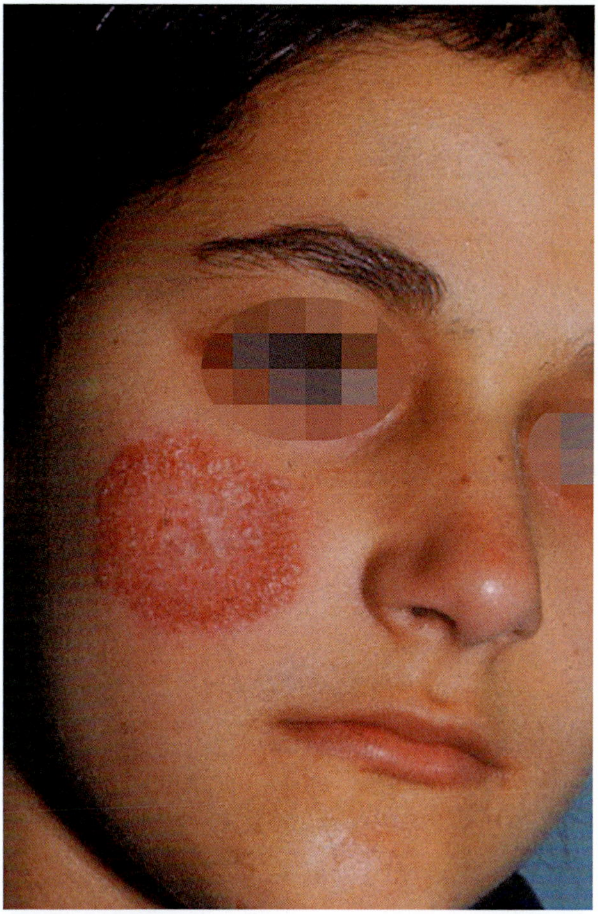

Fig. 2.16 Lupus vulgaris. Central atrophic scar

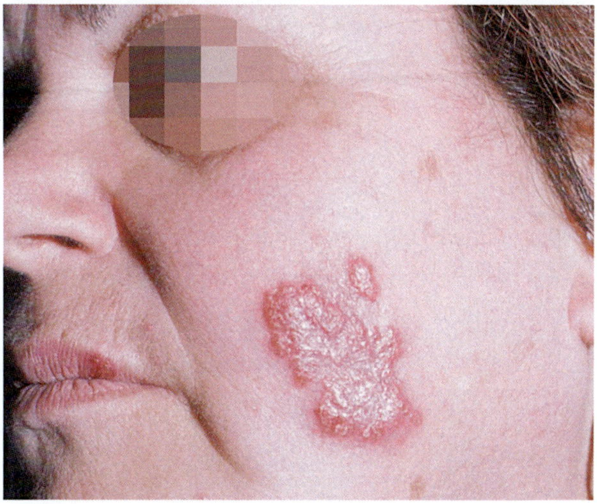

Fig. 2.17 Lupus vulgaris. Central atrophic scar

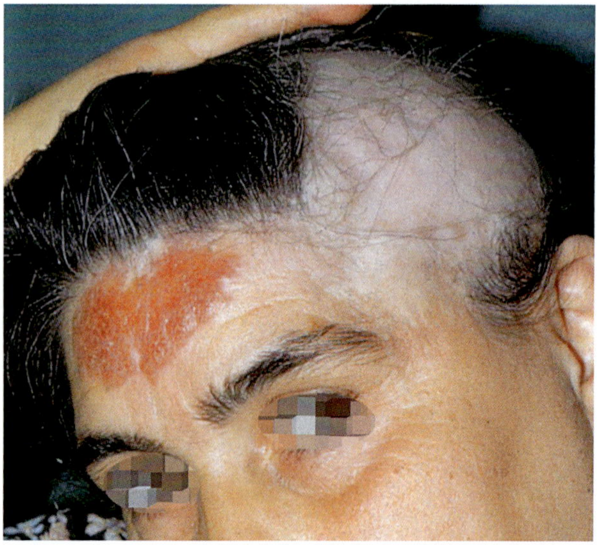

Fig. 2.18 Lupus vulgaris of the forehead. Scar of previous lupus vulgaris on the scalp

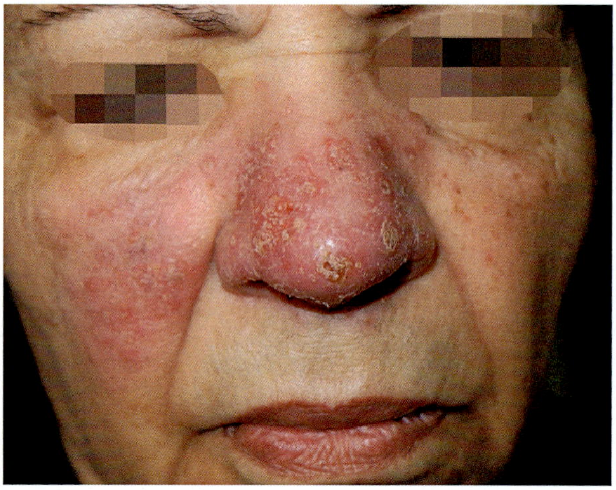

Fig. 2.19 Lupus vulgaris of the nose and cheek

and slightly scaly component of the overlying skin. Lupomas can be revealed at the edges of the plaque by inducing temporary ischemia of the lesion by diascopy (Fig. 2.36). In fact, they are evident because of their yellowish color against the off-white surrounding skin [289].

Another characteristic of lupomas is their relatively soft consistency, that can be appreciated by pressing them with a probe. The tip of a blunt probe will, in fact, easily penetrate the lesion if gentle pressure is used (Fig. 2.37). The minor consistency of lupomas is due to destruction of the connective and elastic fibers of the dermis by the tuberculous infiltration.

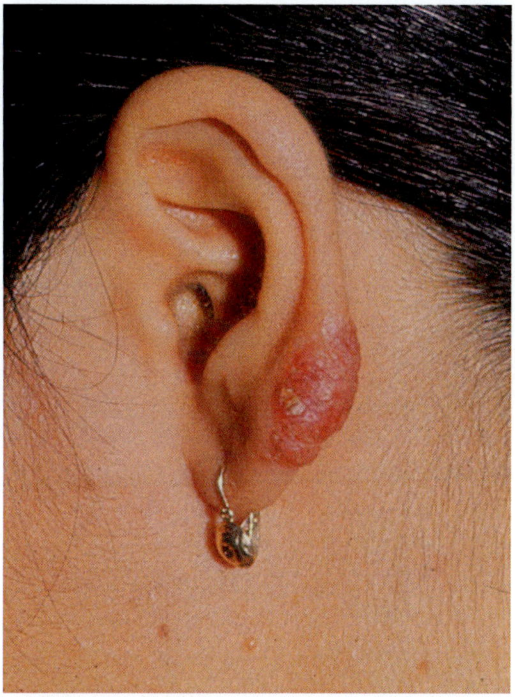

Fig. 2.20 Lupus vulgaris of the auricular lobe

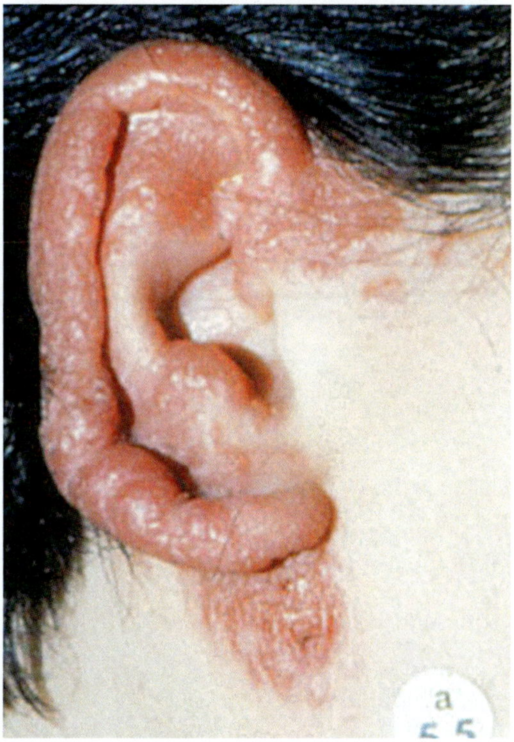

Fig. 2.21 Lupus vulgaris of the ear

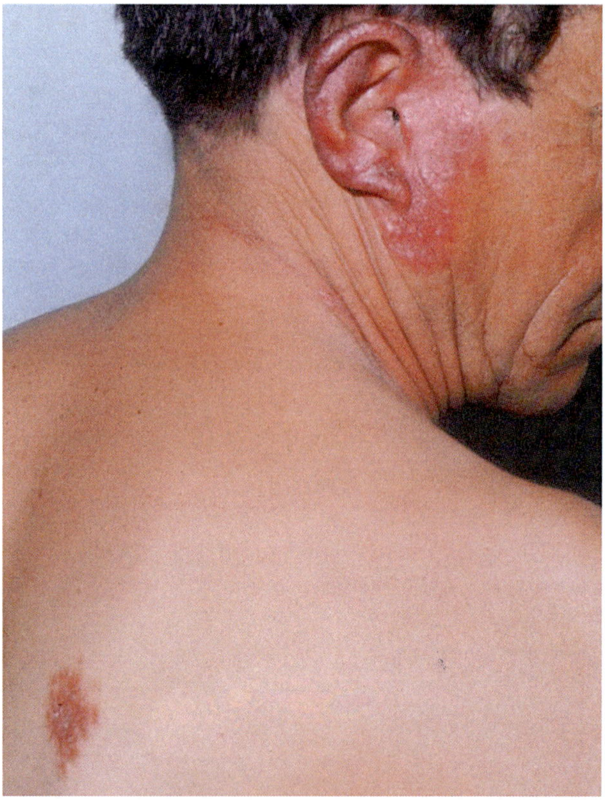

Fig. 2.22 Multiple lesions of lupus vulgaris

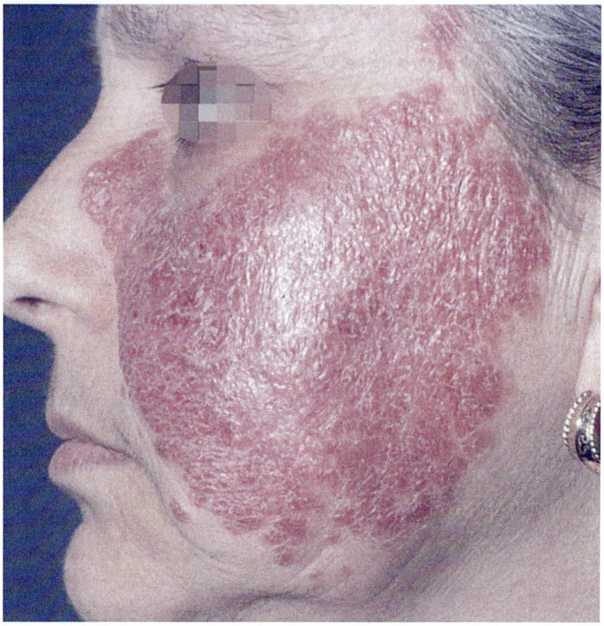

Fig. 2.23 Lupus vulgaris. Active nodular lesions at the borders of the vast plaque

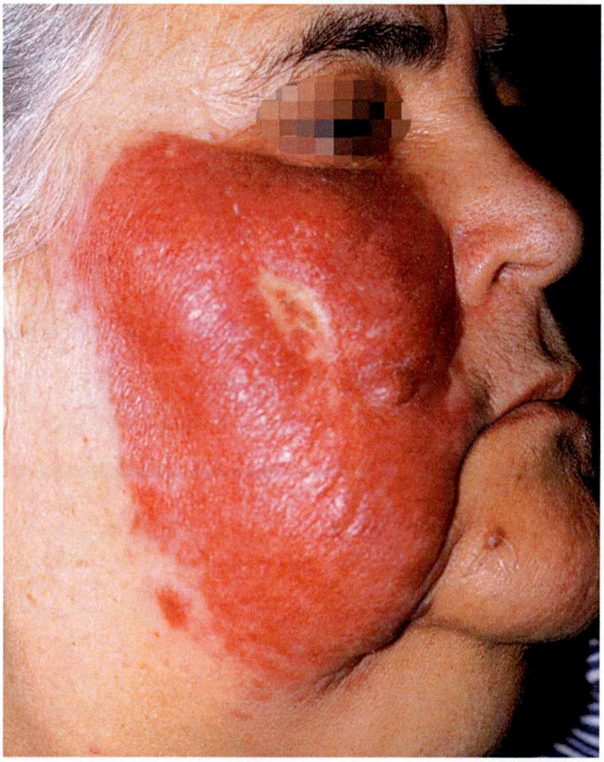

Fig. 2.24 Lupus vulgaris. Active nodular lesions at the borders of the vast plaque

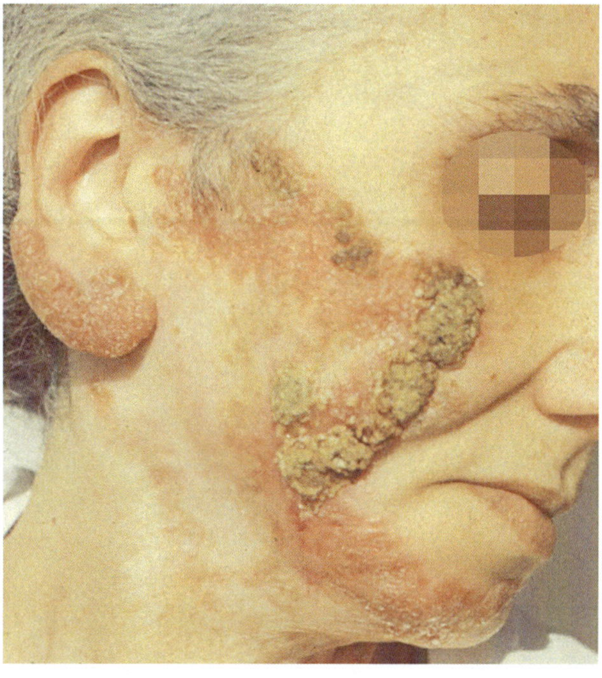

Fig. 2.25 Lupus vulgaris. Active nodular lesions with scaly component and atrophic scar

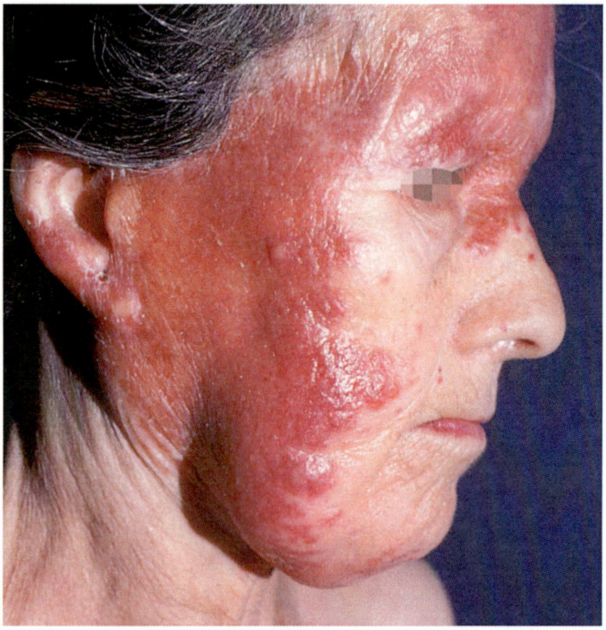

Fig. 2.26 Lupus vulgaris. Active nodular lesions at the borders of the vast plaque

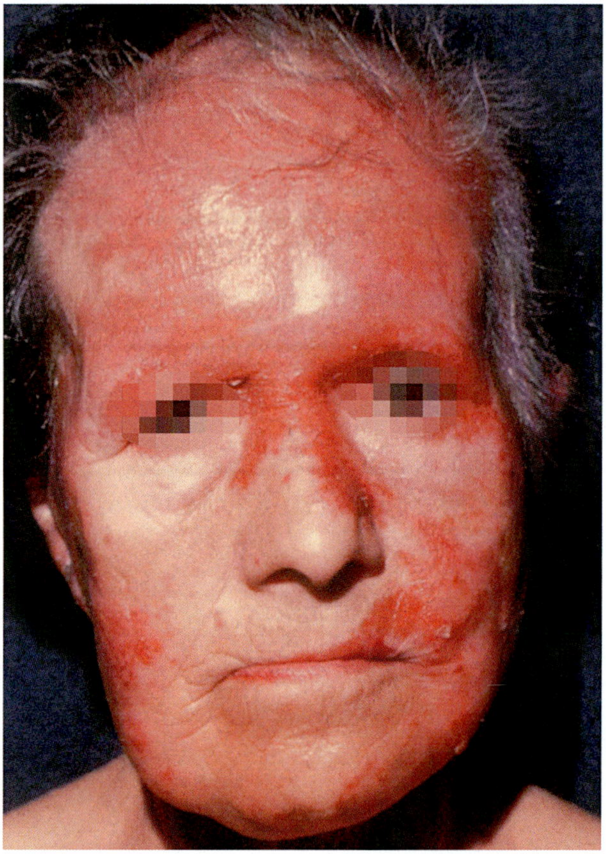

Fig. 2.27 Lupus vulgaris. Active nodular lesions at the borders of the vast plaque

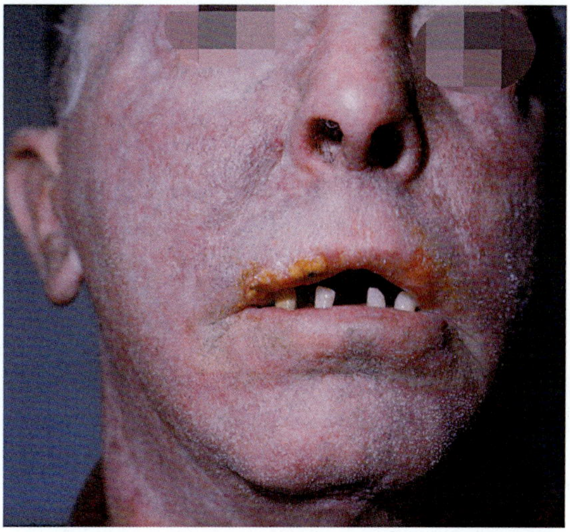

Fig. 2.28 Lupus vulgaris of the face and neck

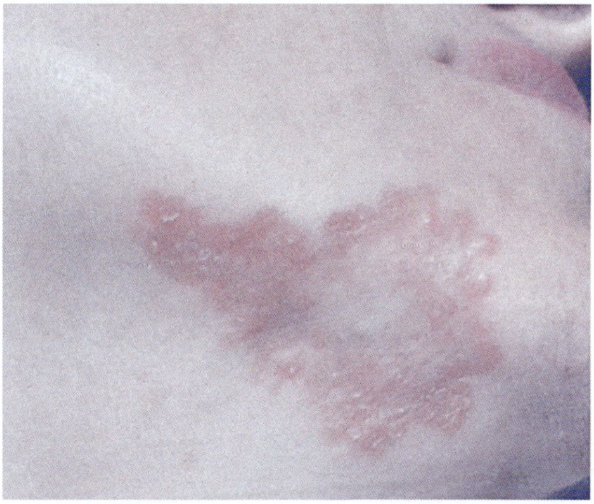

Fig. 2.29 Lupus vulgaris. Central atrophic scar

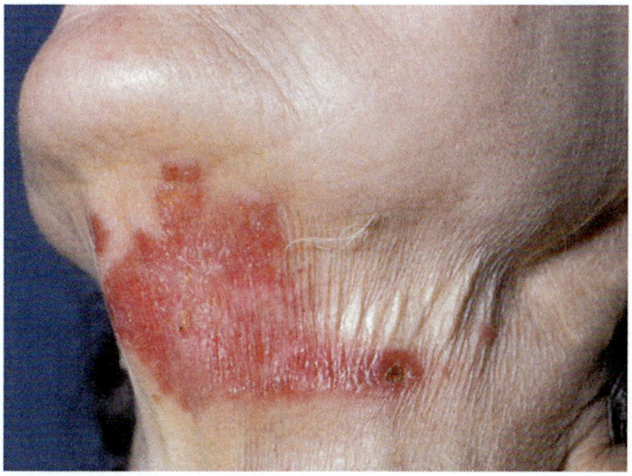

Fig. 2.30 Lupus vulgaris of the neck with atrophic scar

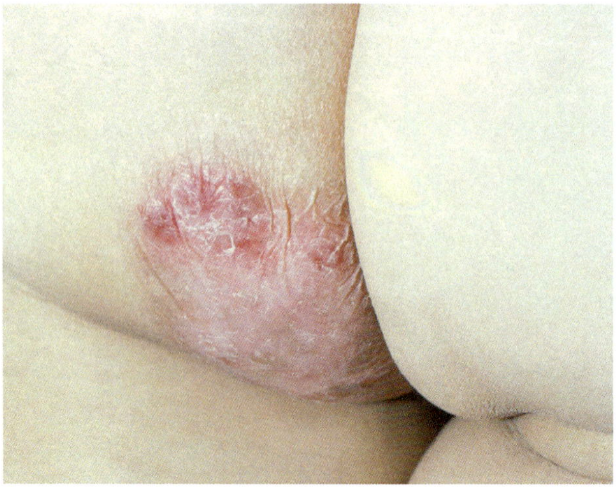

Fig. 2.31 Lupus vulgaris of the buttock with atrophic scar

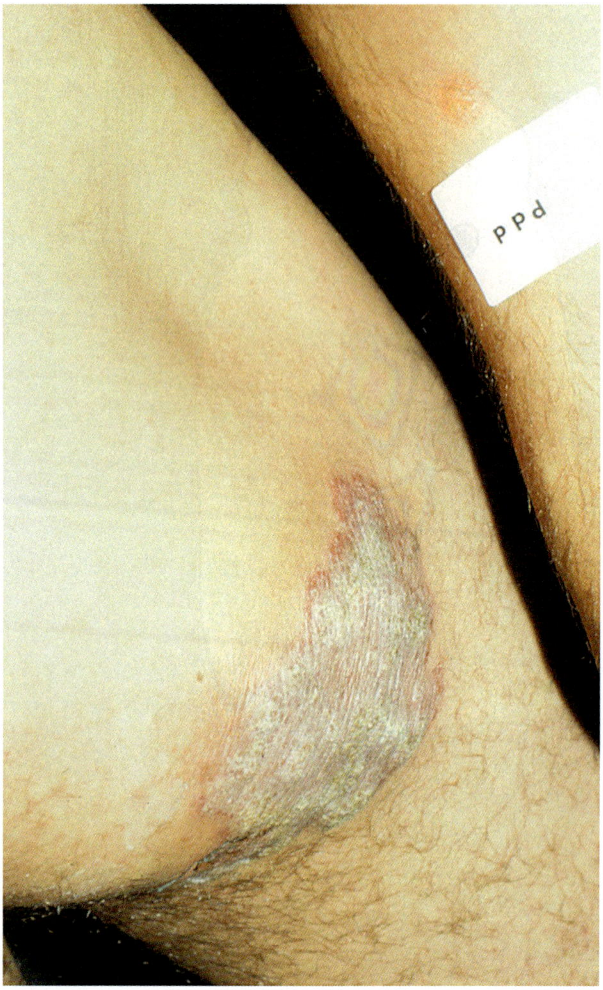

Fig. 2.32 Lupus vulgaris of the buttock with scaly component and strong positive PPD

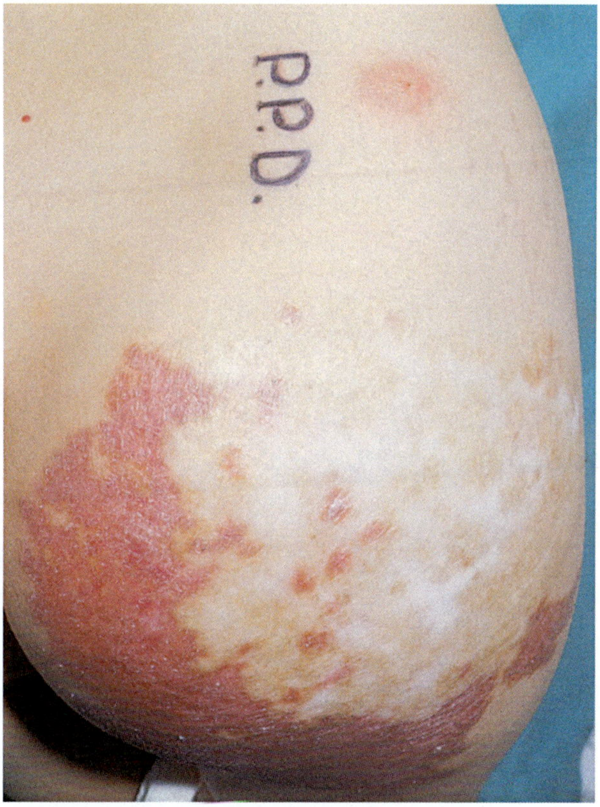

Fig. 2.33 Lupus vulgaris of the buttock with atrophic scar and strong positive PPD

The plaques vary in size and shape. Another characteristic is the tendency of the lupomas to relapse at the lesion margins and within the scarring areas (Figs. 2.38 and 2.39). Necrosis can sometimes cause superficial, slowly evolving ulcers. There is usually only one lesion except in the disseminated forms associated with active pulmonary TB [326]. Sporotrichoid-like forms have also been reported [290].

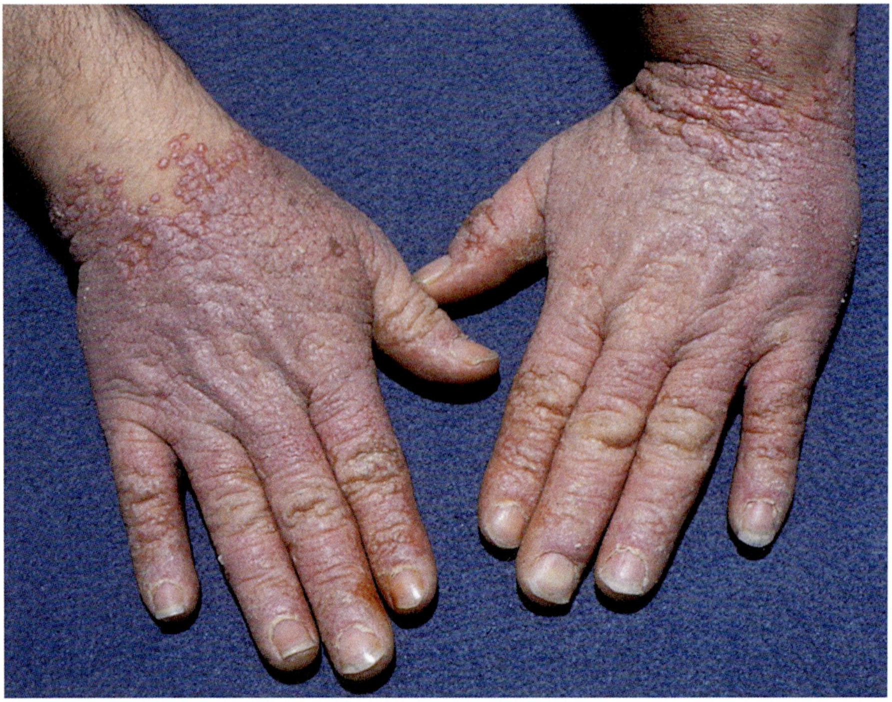

Fig. 2.34 Lupus vulgaris of the back of the hands

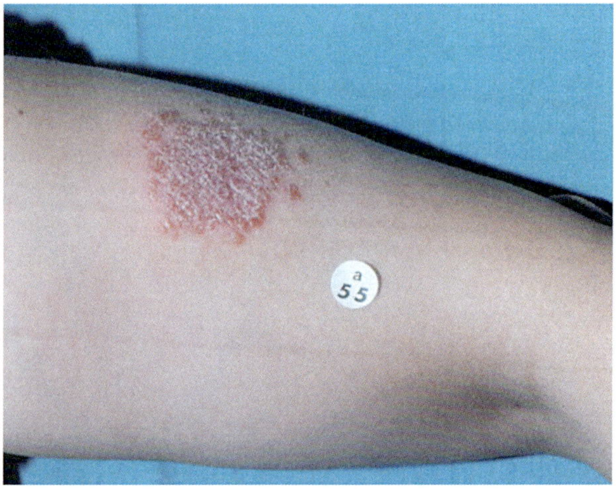

Fig. 2.35 Lupus vulgaris of the arm

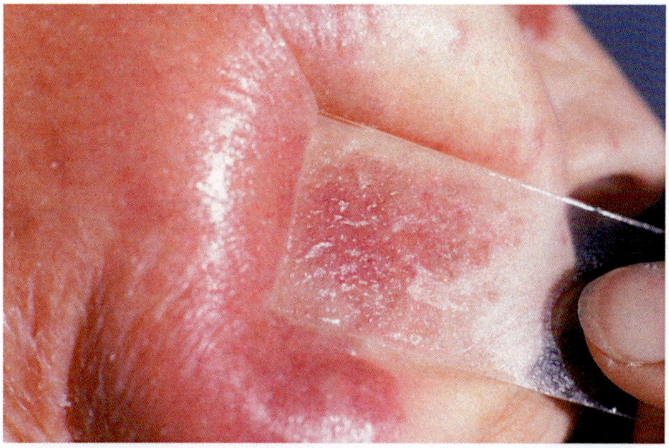

Fig. 2.36 The same case as in Fig. 2.26. Diascopy at the border of the plaque

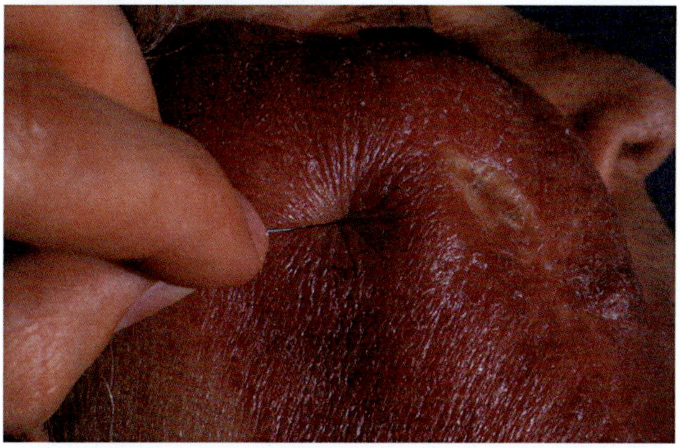

Fig. 2.37 The same patient as in Fig. 2.24. Soft consistency of the lupomas pointed out by a blunt probe

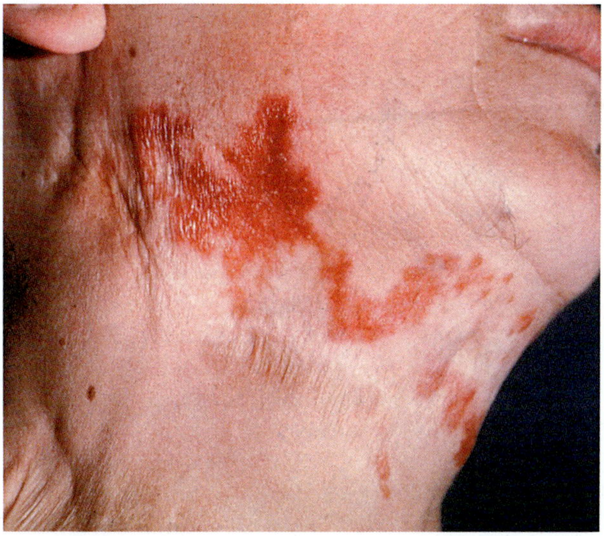

Fig. 2.38 Lupus vulgaris. Relapse on atrophic scar

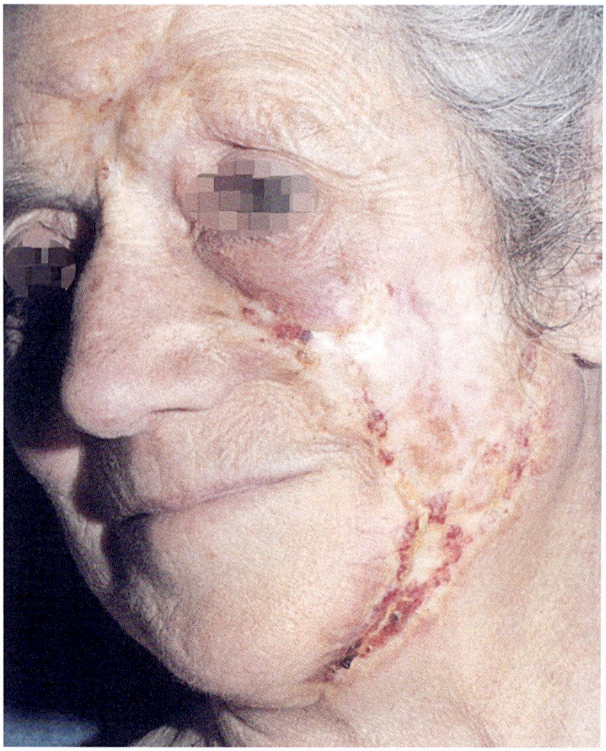

Fig. 2.39 Lupus vulgaris. Relapse on atrophic scar

2.10.9.4 Clinical Forms

Clinical forms of this cutaneous TB are very different from case to case and depend on tissue response to infection. There are five clinical patterns, some of which feature ulceration while others do not. Atypical forms and transition forms between one and another clinical form are also common.

The *plaque form* is the most common clinical variant on the face. The lesions, formed by the coalescence of lupomas, are raised; they have a smooth surface, or else are covered with a psoriasiform scale, and show irregular, tortuous margins. These lesions, whose lupomas are visible on the margins at diascopy, extend slowly, leaving irregular scars at their centers.

Ulcerative and mutilating forms (lupus exedens) are characterized by ulceration and scarring (Figs. 2.40, 2.41, 2.42, and 2.43). The ulcers are covered by crusts with a greater or lesser adherence. The skin ulceration process may extend to the deep tissues, cartilage and bones. Destruction and necrosis of the ear pavilion and nasal pyramid (Fig. 2.44) cause mutilation and permanent deformities. The ulcers do not tend to resolve but form scarring areas, often of contracting type, that typically persist and show the development of new lupomas.

Vegetating forms are hypertrophic forms characterized by a marked tendency to ulcerate (Figs. 2.45 and 2.46) and to form phagedenic necrosis areas. There is severe infiltration at the dermal level with minimal scarring. The mucous membranes are

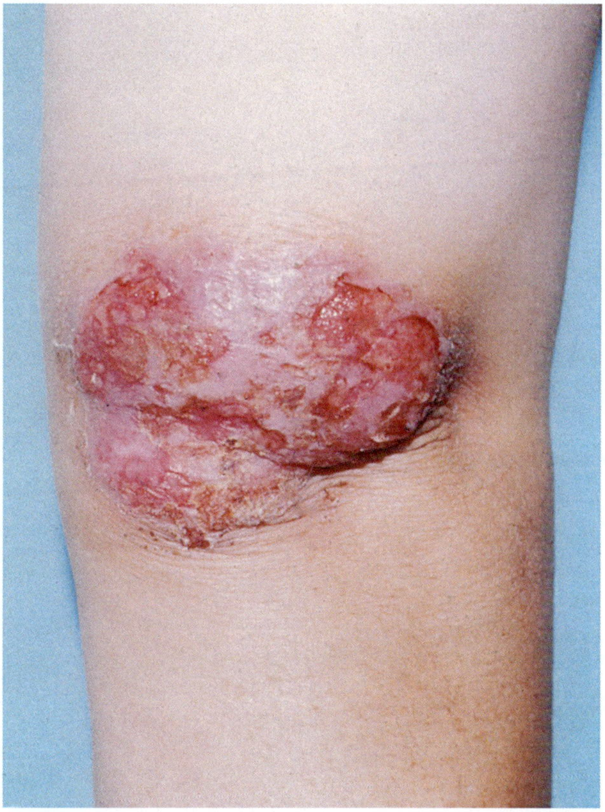

Fig. 2.40 Ulcerative lupus vulgaris of the elbow

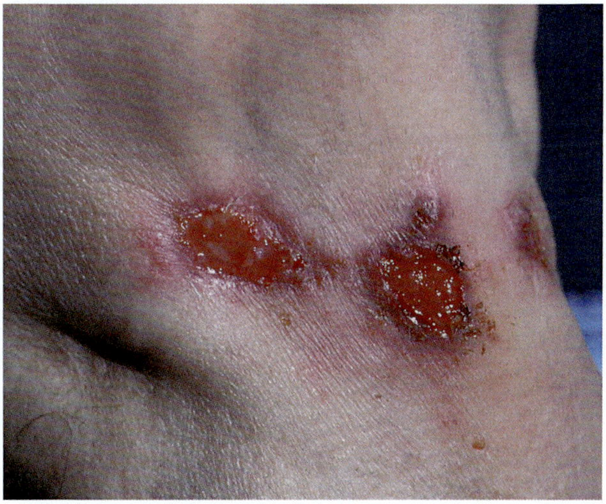

Fig. 2.41 Ulcerative lupus vulgaris of the neck

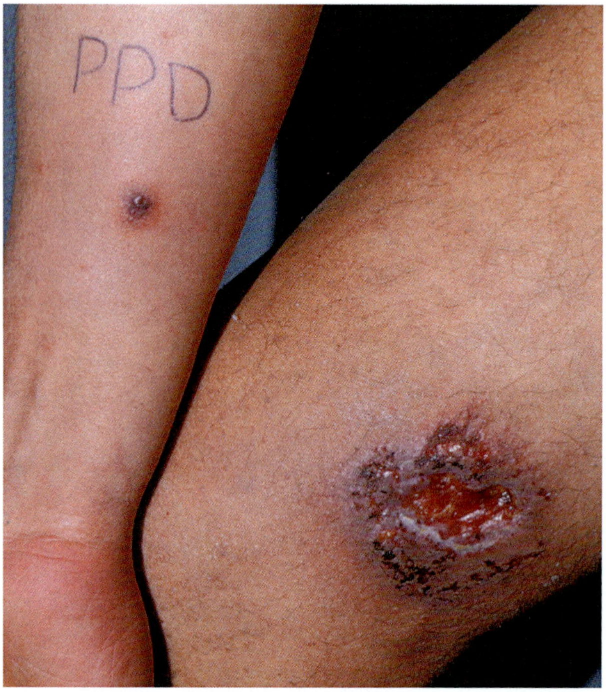

Fig. 2.42 Ulcerative lupus vulgaris of the thigh with positive PPD

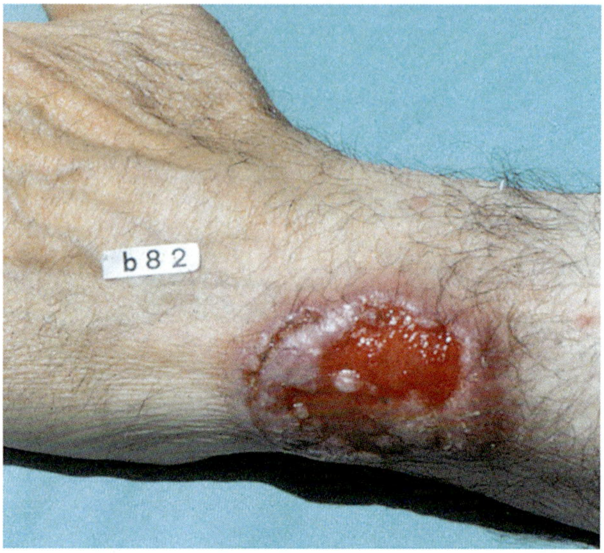

Fig. 2.43 Ulcerative lupus vulgaris of the wrist

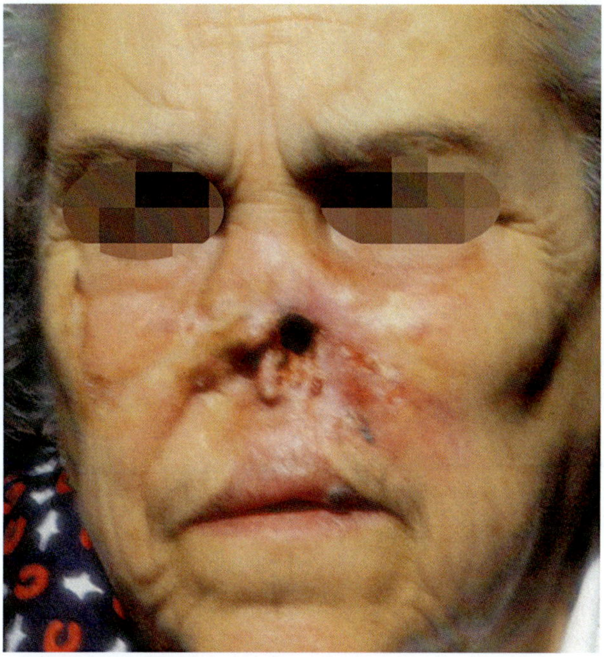

Fig. 2.44 Mutilation of the nasal pyramid due to previous lupus vulgaris

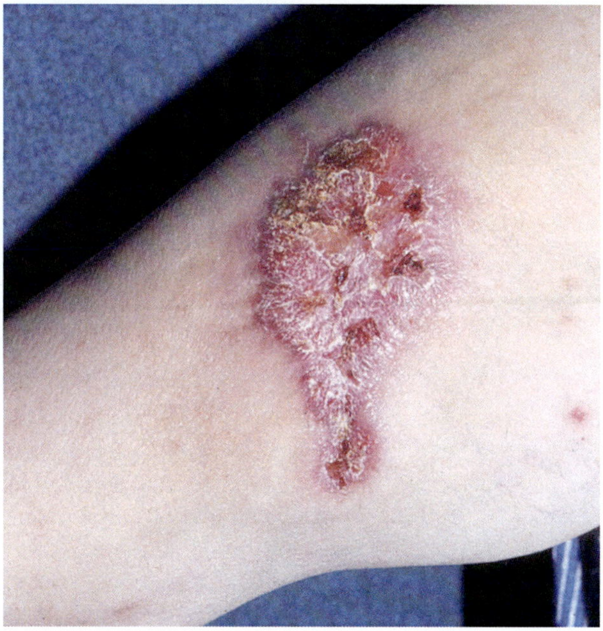

Fig. 2.45 Vegetating lupus vulgaris

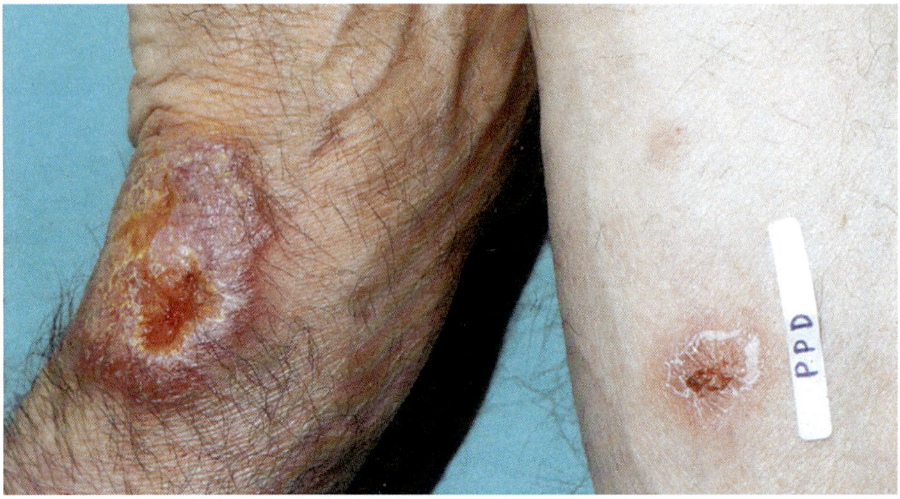

Fig. 2.46 Vegetating lupus vulgaris with positive PPD

Fig. 2.47 Lupus vulgaris mixomatous

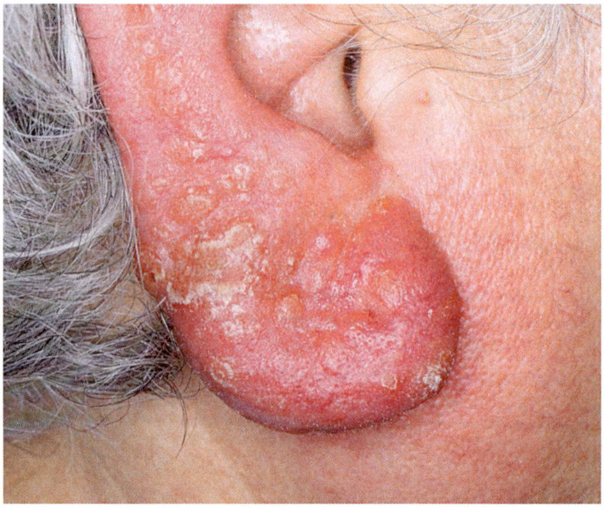

often affected and the cartilage is slowly destroyed. When the nasal or auricular cartilage is involved there will be extensive destruction and disfigurement.

Tumor-like forms are characterized by large nodules, often clustered and soft, with minor scarring. Huge soft, reddish tumors develop on the ear lobes, which become grossly enlarged ("lupus mixomatous") (Figs. 2.47, 2.48, 2.49, 2.50, and 2.51). Lymphedema and vasodilation are marked.

Papular and nodular forms present with multiple lesions arising simultaneously in disseminated lupus ("miliary lupus"). These clinical pictures arise after a temporary immunosuppression condition following childhood exanthems (measles) ("lupus miliaris post-exanthematicus").

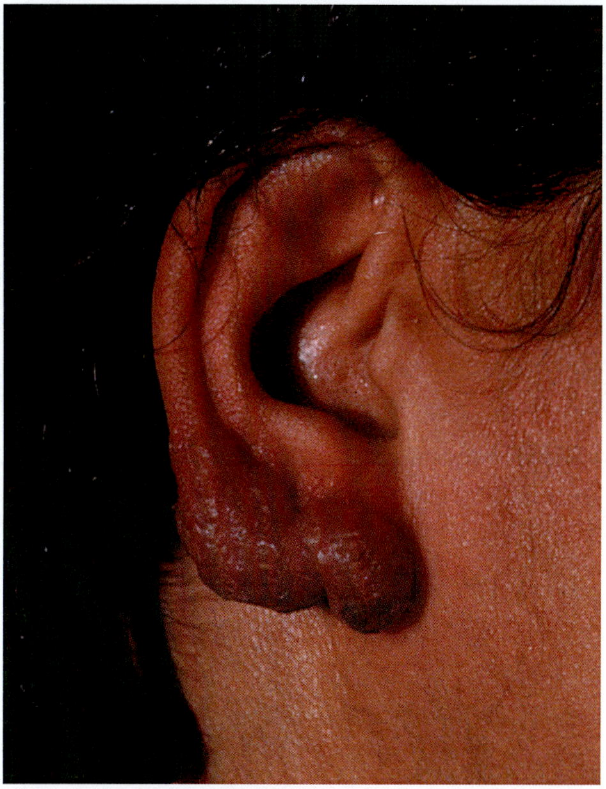

Fig. 2.48 Lupus vulgaris mixomatous

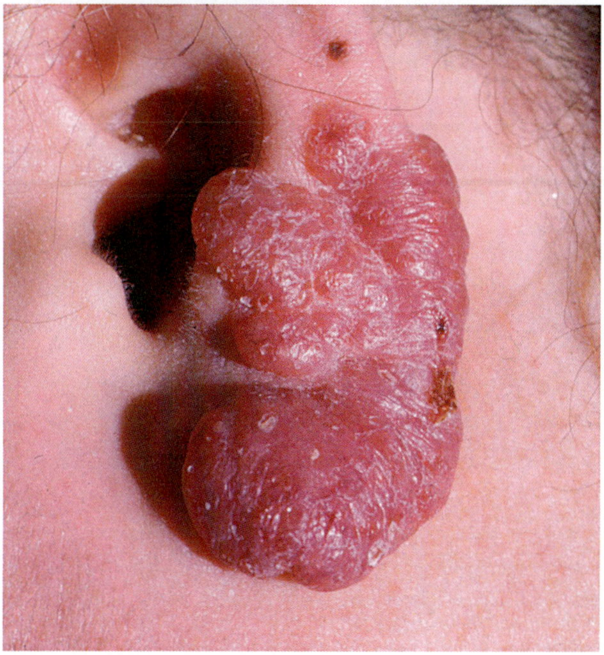

Fig. 2.49 Lupus vulgaris mixomatous

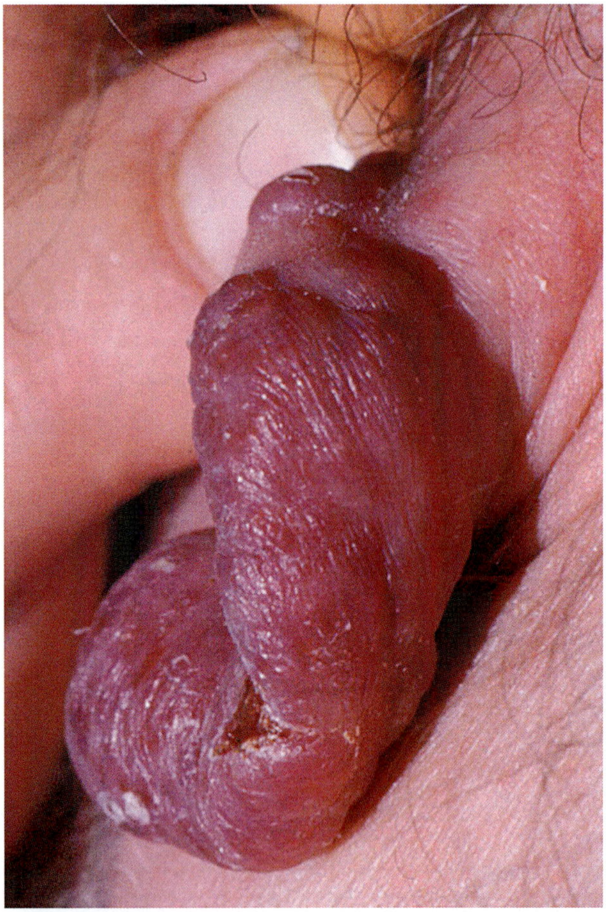

Fig. 2.50 The same patient as in Fig. 2.49

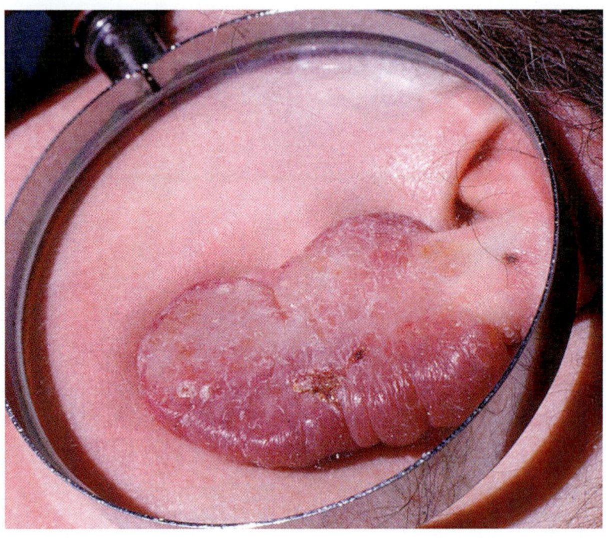

Fig. 2.51 The same patient as in Fig. 2.49. Diascopy of the lesion

2.10.9.5 Mucosal Involvement

The mucosa most often involved are the nasal, lip, oral, and conjunctival mucosa. There may be primary involvement with papules and nodules, or otherwise spread from a contiguous skin lesion. Nasal nodules bleed very easily and then ulcerate, causing destruction of the cartilage. Granulating, vegetating or ulcerating lesions of the buccal mucosa, palate, gingiva or oropharynx may occur by direct extension or by lymphatic spread from the nasal lesions. They can provoke stenosis of the larynx and scarring deformities of the soft palate.

2.10.9.6 Prognosis and Complications

The course of lupus vulgaris is chronic and progressive; if untreated, the disease will persist indefinitely and cause major tissue destruction. Long periods of apparent quiescence will alternate with periods of exacerbation. Ulcerative forms and those with a tendency to scar bring about severe facial mutilation. The destruction of the auricular cartilage causes shrinkage of the ear, and of the nasal cartilage leads to narrowing and deformation of the nostrils and alae nasi. Contraction of the peribuccal and palpebral tissues causes microstomia and ectropion, respectively.

Pyodermitis, followed by lymphangitis and lymphadenitis, is a frequent complication in ulcerative and vegetating forms. The most severe complication is the development of squamous cell carcinoma ("lupus carcinoma") (Figs. 2.52, 2.53, and 2.54). This originates at the margins of ulcerative and cicatricial lesions that have been present for many years or decades. The onset of basal cell carcinomas or sarcomas is less common. This neoplastic complication, that may mimic a relapse of lupus, is observed in 8% of patients [327, 328].

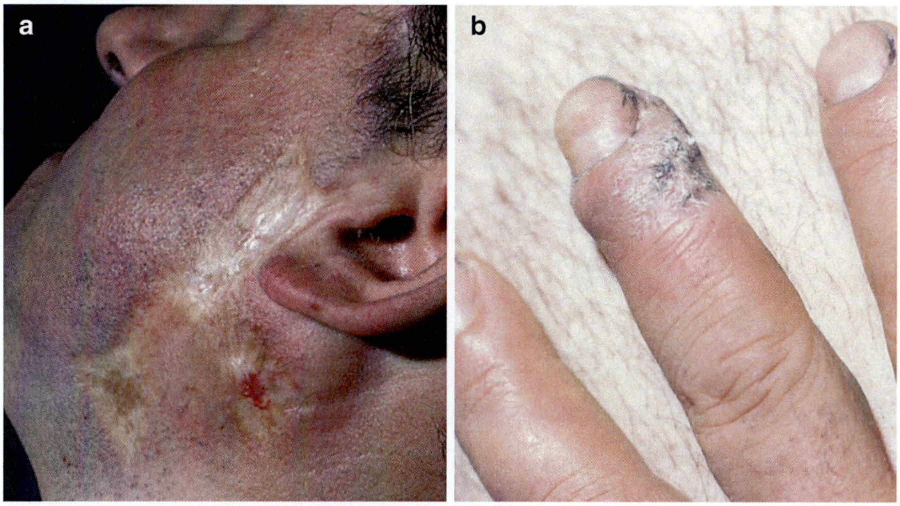

Fig. 2.52 (**a**) Lupus carcinoma with adenopathy on scar of previous lupus vulgaris. (**b**) Same patient with hyperkeratosic lupus vulgaris of the third finger

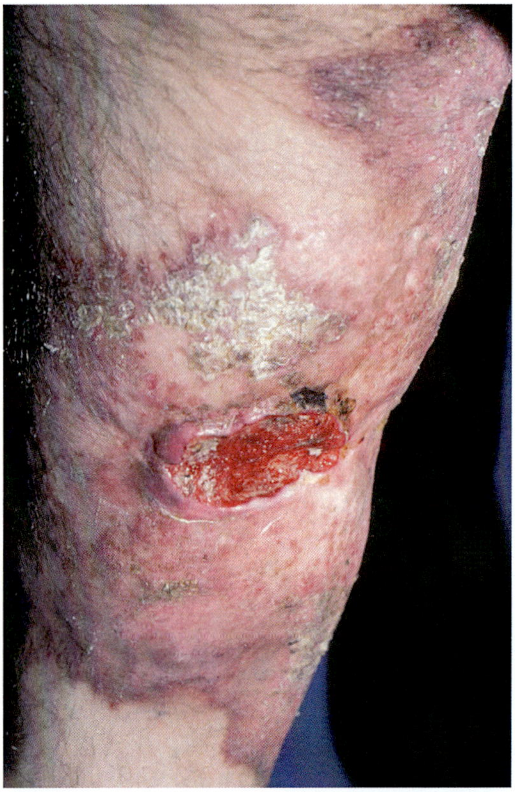

Fig. 2.53 Lupus carcinoma

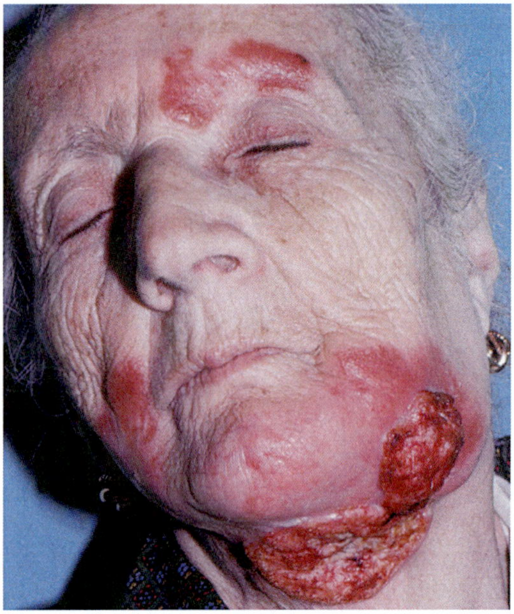

Fig. 2.54 Lupus carcinoma

2.10.9.7 Diagnosis

When the plaques are well defined with central scarring there is little diagnostic difficulty. In the initial phases the lupus may be confused with lymphocytoma or lupus erythematosus. It may be impossible to clinically distinguish the lupoid form of leishmaniasis. On the face, lupus may be mistaken for rosacea or for a port-wine stain [329], and on the limbs, for other mycobacterial infections. The serology and medical history are useful to make a differential diagnosis with some manifestations of tertiary syphilis. Tuberculoid leprosy can present similar clinical and histological findings to lupus: the patient's origin from endemic areas and the lesion anesthesia can orient the diagnosis. Histological examination will differentiate lupus vulgaris from Bowen's disease, psoriasis, and some deep mycoses. Tuberculosis verrucosa differs in terms of the marked hyperkeratosis as well as of the areas involved. The sarcoidosis nodules resemble grains of sand (the color is often grayish) rather than "apple jelly".

A trial of anti-tuberculosis therapy may be considered in cases of diagnostic difficulties, although a clinical response will be obtained only after 4–6 weeks [330, 331].

2.10.10 Tuberculous Gumma

This form of cutaneous TB (*metastatic tuberculous abscess*), that manifests with one or more lesions, is linked to hematogenous spread of a primary focus in subjects with a lowered resistance. It is most commonly observed in malnourished children after trauma [332] and in association with lymphoma [333].

Histology demonstrates suppurative granulomata with non-specific infiltrates. Direct examination of the pus will usually demonstrate tubercle bacilli.

Tuberculous gumma can present as a firm subcutaneous nodule or as a fluctuating abscess. The limbs are more often affected than the trunk. The overlying skin may ulcerate, often with sinuses [333, 334]. Multiple abscesses have been reported as a rare observation during the treatment of miliary TB [335], as well as lesions presenting as carpal tunnel syndrome [336]. The tuberculin skin test is usually positive, but may be negative if the patient is in poor general conditions. The diagnosis must be confirmed by culture.

2.10.11 Unusual Forms of Cutaneous Tuberculosis

These forms are difficult to fit into any of the above-described clinical pictures. The morphology and histology may resemble lupus vulgaris, but not as regards the site or behavior [337]. Gangrenous or vegetating forms with underlying lung or glandular disease have been described [338]. HIV-positive patients may present atypical and diffuse skin lesions [303]. Cases with cellulitis-like lesions have also been reported [339, 340], as well as patients with multifocal guttate TB verrucosa cutis and necklace lupus vulgaris [341].

A high suspicion index is necessary to make a correct diagnosis in such cases: the finding of acid-fast bacilli is not sufficient and biopsy, culture and PCR must be performed. Trial anti-tubercular treatment may be necessary to test the diagnosis, while awaiting the results of specific tests [330].

2.10.12 Tuberculids

In 1896, Darier grouped various apparently dissimilar skin manifestations under the heading of tuberculids, suggesting that they could be caused by microbial embolism from visceral tuberculous foci. Unlike true cutaneous TB, tuberculids were considered a hypersensitivity reaction to *M. tuberculosis* or its products in a subject with a significant immune status. The characteristics of tuberculids are a positive tuberculin skin test, evidence of past or manifest TB, and a positive response to anti-tuberculous treatment. In addition, there is almost always absence of bacilli in skin biopsies, and culture is negative, although PCR can detect mycobacterial DNA in some forms.

In the past, various clinical pictures were included among tuberculids that nowadays are classified as variants of rosacea. True tuberculids are listed in Table 2.11.

The pathogenesis of tuberculids is still poorly understood. They are believed to be linked to hematogenous spread of bacilli in subjects with a moderate or high grade of immunity against *M. tuberculosis*. However, it is not possible to find bacilli in these forms because they are present only in fragmented form or are destroyed at the tuberculid site by immunological mechanisms [341]. PCR is positive in some papulo-nodular forms [342–344], but not in the micropapular, lichen scrofulosorum form [341]. It has therefore been suggested that papulo-nodular forms should be considered as forms of true post-primary TB [343].

Fluctuations in the patient's immunological status can allow the development of the eruption. The onset of lichen scrofulosorum has been reported after the start of specific treatment, probably due to a shift in the patient's cell-mediated immune status [341]. Papulonecrotic tuberculid developed in one patient with HIV infection after an increase in CD4 T cells following the introduction of a second antiretroviral drug [230]. In a recent study of 131 patients with cutaneous tuberculids, the most frequent form was erythema induratum (96%), followed by papulonecrotic tuberculid (3%) [345].

2.10.12.1 Lichen Scrofulosorum

First described by Hebra in 1868, this is a lichenoid eruption of minute papules, observed above all in children and adolescents with TB. It is generally associated with a strongly positive tuberculin reaction. The eruption has been reported in association with lymph nodes TB, bone TB, and even after BCG vaccination [346]. Lichen scrofulosorum has also been reported with *M. avium* [347] and *M. szulgai* [348] infection.

In the past this tuberculid was common but today it is rarely observed in Europe except among immigrants. In 1976, four cases were reported in the UK [348]. Two series have recently been reported, of 8 [349] and 39 [350] patients in Northern India. In the second series, with 39 cases, this tuberculid accounted for 76% of all the cases of cutaneous TB over a 7-year period; 84% were aged under 15 years, while 72% presented an associated underlying TB focus at the level of the lymph nodes, lung, or bone [350–352].

The clinical picture is considered to be the result of an immune response to hematological spread from an underlying tuberculous focus. A strong positive reaction is elicited to the PPD, often measuring 18 mm or larger. Lichen scrofulosorum can coexist with other TB forms like lupus vulgaris, tuberculous gumma, and tuberculosis verrucosa cutis [353].

At the superficial derma level, around hair follicles and sweat ducts, there will be granulomas consisting of epithelioid cells, lymphocytes and occasional giant cells. There is generally no caseation. No bacilli are observed in histological sections, cultures are negative, and in general mycobacterial DNA is not demonstrable by PCR.

Clinically, the eruption manifests as asymptomatic, closely grouped lichenoid papules measuring 0.3–3 mm (Figs. 2.55 and 2.56). The papules may be skin colored or yellowish or reddish-brown, grouped in clusters or in an annular arrangement, or

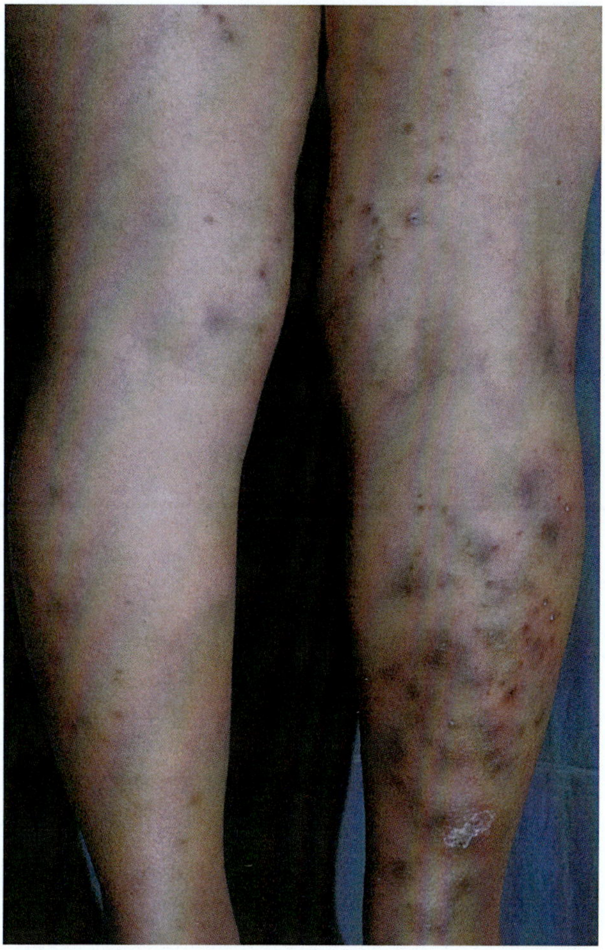

Fig. 2.55 Lichen scrofulosorum

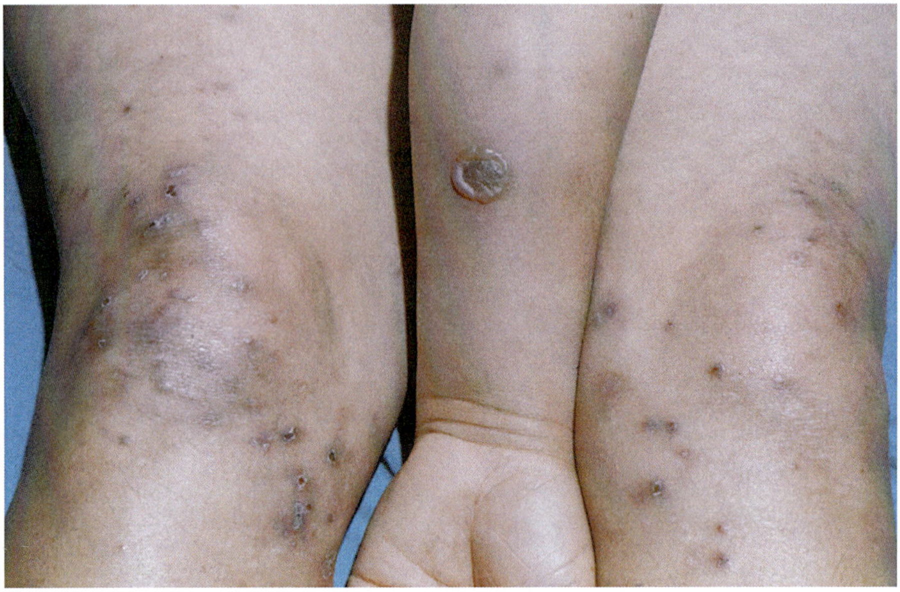

Fig. 2.56 The same patient as in Fig.2.55. Strong positive PPD

in plaques, at perifollicular sites. The surface may be smooth, slightly scaly, or with a small pustule center. They are mainly localized on the abdomen, chest and back and the origins of the limbs. One case of localization at the vulva was reported in a young girl [354].

A high suspicion index is needed for diagnosis. A TB focus elsewhere on the body should be sought. Differential diagnosis must be made with all asymptomatic eruptions of follicular papules showing a tendency to cluster. In lichen nitidus the lesions are more shiny and tend to be peripheral; keratosis spinulosa presents with spiny projections over lichenoid papules. Keratosis pilaris features non inflammatory lesions, generally on the upper thighs and arms. Differential diagnosis must also include lichenoid sarcoidosis, secondary syphilis and some drug eruptions. In one patient with AIDS, the PPD was negative [355].

Anti-tubercular treatment generally leads to resolution within 4–8 weeks without scarring.

2.10.12.2 Papulonecrotic Tuberculid

The eruption is characterized by asymmetrical crops of papulous elements located above all on the extensor surface of the limbs. The lesions tend to necrotize and resolve with varioliform scarring.

In about 40–75% of cases an associated TB focus is demonstrated [356–358]. The rapid response to anti-tubercular treatment leaves no room for doubt as to the etiology in cases in which it is not possible to demonstrate a tuberculous focus. In a study of 91 patients, papulonecrotic tuberculid evolved to lupus vulgaris in four cases [356]. This has also been observed after BCG vaccination [359–361], showing a possible hematogenous spread of the bacilli. Mycobacteria are rarely identified in the lesions; in one study, two cases of an association with lupus vulgaris were reported [356]. *M. tuberculosis* DNA has been revealed in skin lesions by PCR [342]. Papaulonecrotic tuberculid has been observed with *M. avium* complex in a subject with HIV infection [362]. The PPD is positive and often elicits a severe necrotic reaction after 8–12 h.

The eruption is more frequent in children and young adults with active or past systemic manifestations of TB. The sites most commonly affected are the extensor surface of the limbs, the hands (fingers), shoulders, buttocks, penis (sometimes the only site) [363–365] and also the face. In general, the lesions are symmetrically distributed and characterized by crops of scattered papules with a diameter of about 1 cm, being deep red and with an increased consistency, embedded in the dermis (Figs. 2.57 and 2.58). The eruption may continue for months or even years: the papules ulcerate and are covered by a blackish crust; then they leave pigmented, sometimes atrophic varioliform scars lasting a few weeks. The ulcers may last for some months [357]. The eruption is subjectively asymptomatic. Transition forms [356] and coexistence with lupus vulgaris [326] and with erythema induratum [366, 367] have been described.

The primary alteration of this papulous lesion is an endovasculitis that can lead to obliteration of dermal vessels. Around these vessels there is a nonspecific cellular infiltrate, above all of lymphocytes and occasionally of epithelioid cells and giant cells. The superficial dermis and the epidermis above the infiltrate undergo necrosis, which is responsible for the vesicopustule that precedes the crust. Histologically, a palisade is seen around larger lesions [358].

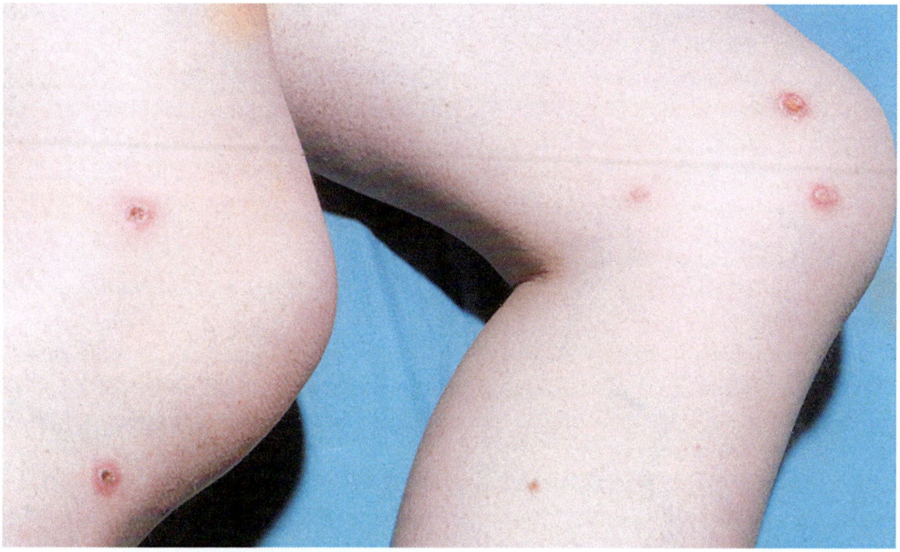

Fig. 2.57 Papulonecrotic tuberculid

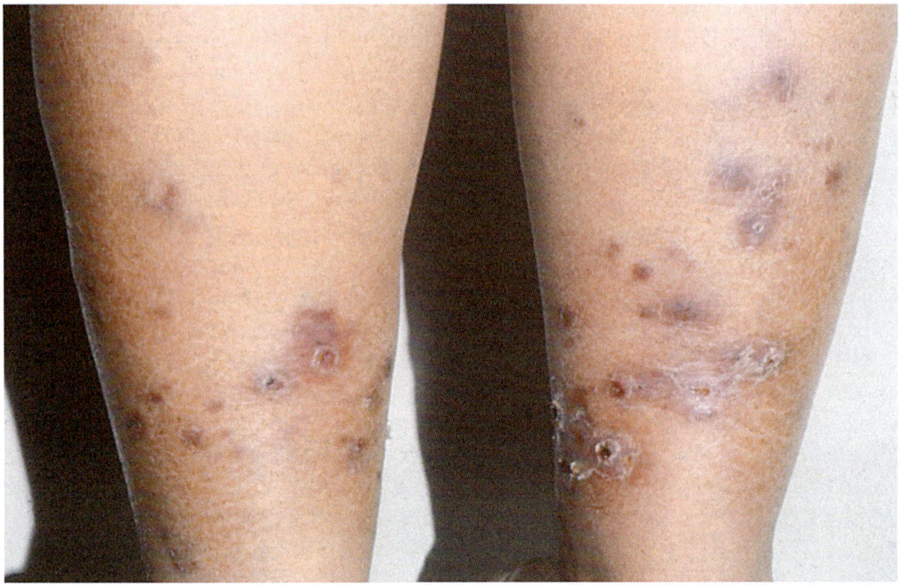

Fig. 2.58 Papulonecrotic tuberculid

Differential diagnosis includes acute pityriasis lichenoides varioliformis, usually more extensive, involving the trunk and palmoplantar surfaces and a histological picture of lymphocytic vasculitis. Biopsy and tuberculin test must be performed in all cases; PCR may be useful. An interferon-γ-base assay can aid diagnosis when PCR is negative [368]. Specific anti-tubercular treatment is decisive in doubtful cases.

2.10.12.3 Nodular Tuberculids

Erythema induratum of Bazin [369], considered a true nodular tuberculid, affects the subcutaneous fat. It has recently been termed "nodular tuberculid", a non-ulcerated nodular form with histological involvement of the dermis and subcutaneous fat junction [370]. Finally, other pictures such as erythema nodosum and nodular vasculitis can occasionally be linked to TB.

Erythema Induratum of Bazin

This picture was described by Antoine Bazin in 1861. It describes a condition that generally affects the legs, and is characterized by chronic relapsing nodular lesions. It is almost exclusively observed in young or middle-aged women (90%) and resolves after anti-tubercular treatment. A high percentage of patients has a history of TB. The incidence of the disease has reduced remarkably in most developed countries, in line with the decreased incidence of TB.

The tuberculin test is positive. *M. tuberculosis* is rarely evidenced in the lesions but mycobacterial DNA can be found in up to 77% of biopsies [344]. It has been suggested that purified protein derivative-specific T cells that produce IFN-γ may be involved, as a type of delayed hypersensitivity response to mycobacterial antigens at the site of skin lesions [371].

The dermatosis typically affects the mid and lower third of the legs, especially the posterior external surfaces and, more rarely, the thighs, abdomen and buttocks. The eruption is generally painless, characterized by palpable, purplish-red, ill-defined rounded nodules in the dermis-hypodermis (Figs. 2.59, 2.60, 2.61, 2.62, and 2.63). The lesions may sometimes be associated with pain of the affected limb. The lesions are isolated or few, rarely being numerous. The skin overlying the nodules is generally purplish and sometimes desquamating (scaly collarette). They have a variable evolution, sometimes regressing spontaneously whereas in other cases they soften in the center and turn into torpid, irregularly shaped ulcers, that are mostly superficial although sometimes there is deep loss of substance, with perpendicular walls ("*erythema induratum of the Hutchinson*" type) (Figs. 2.64, 2.65, 2.66, and 2.67). The affliction has a chronic course, persists for months or years, and generally relapses in winter. In fact, the cold is a predisposing factor and in many cases the disease onset is observed on skin affected by erythrocyanosis, or on cutis marmorata. Resolution is slow even with adequate treatment [372].

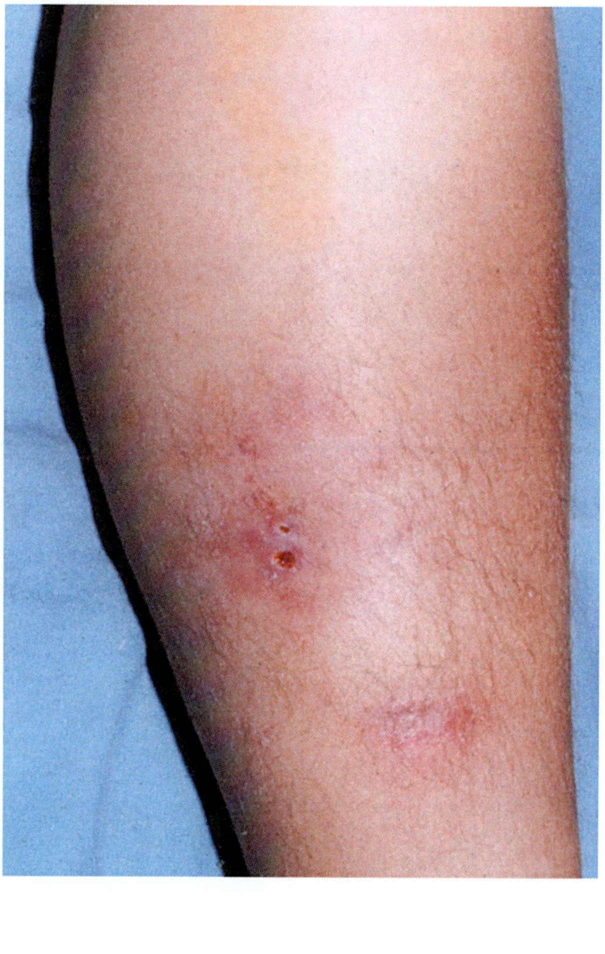

Fig. 2.59 Erythema induratum of Bazin

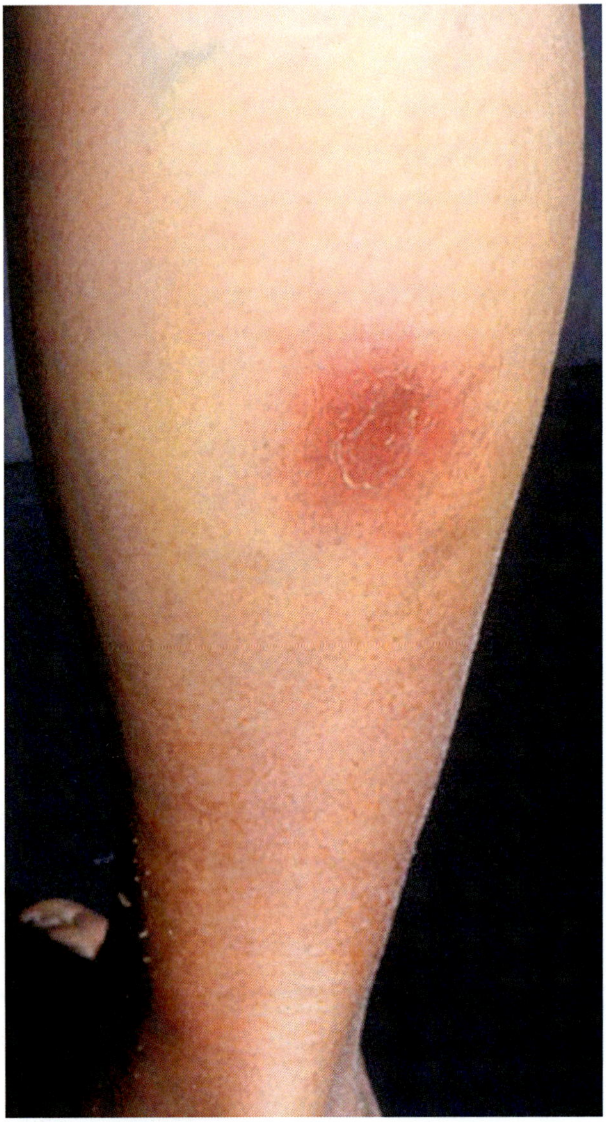

Fig. 2.60 Erythema induratum of Bazin

The early lesions are confined to subcutaneous tissue, but then ulcerative lesions will develop also in the dermis and the epidermis. The histological pattern is variable but there are two or three aspects in common in all cases, apart from the tubercular infiltrate: septal panniculitis, vasculitis of subcutaneous arteries and veins, necrosis of adipocytes, and an epithelioid infiltrate. To demonstrate these lesions the biopsy must be deep. Vascular alterations include swelling of the endothelium and

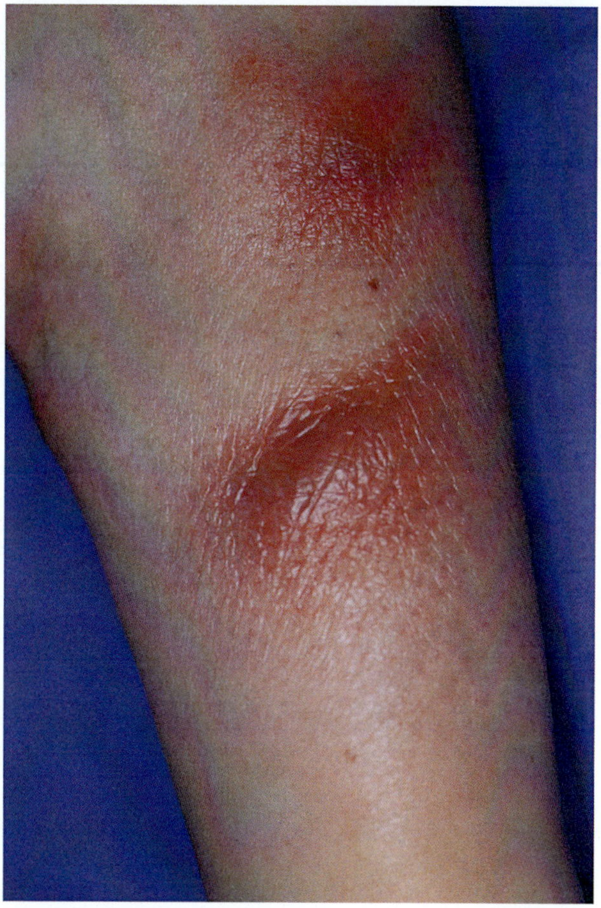

Fig. 2.61 Erythema induratum of Bazin

hypertrophy of the vessels, and even occlusion (thrombosis) of the lumen, with fibrinoid necrosis. The granulomatous reaction can be non-specific or tuberculoid: it consists of epithelioid cells, lymphocytes and foreign body or Langhans-type giant cells. This infiltrate can invade the adipose tissue and in part replace it. Venous occlusion causes necrosis of the infiltrate cells with the formation of areas of eosinophilic necrosis that resemble caseous necrosis. Epithelioid cells sometimes surround necrosis foci, causing these structures to look like tubercles; in other cases it looks like a panniculitis with lymphocytes, plasma cells, and polymorphonuclear cells. In the infiltrate zone, collagen tissue, elastic fibers, and adipocytes are destroyed. The final stage is fibrosis, which follows on after atrophy of the subcutaneous fat [289, 373, 374].

A positive tuberculin test cannot be regarded as definitive proof for the diagnosis. The only certain criterion is the demonstration of mycobacteria via PCR or culture.

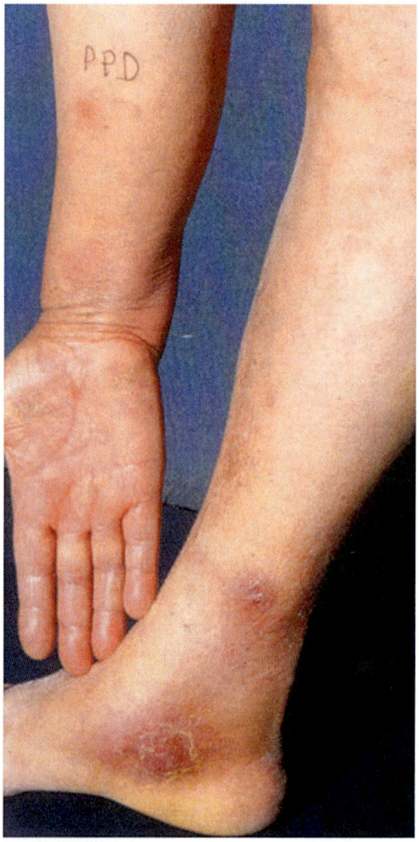

Fig. 2.62 Erythema induratum of Bazin. Strong positive PPD

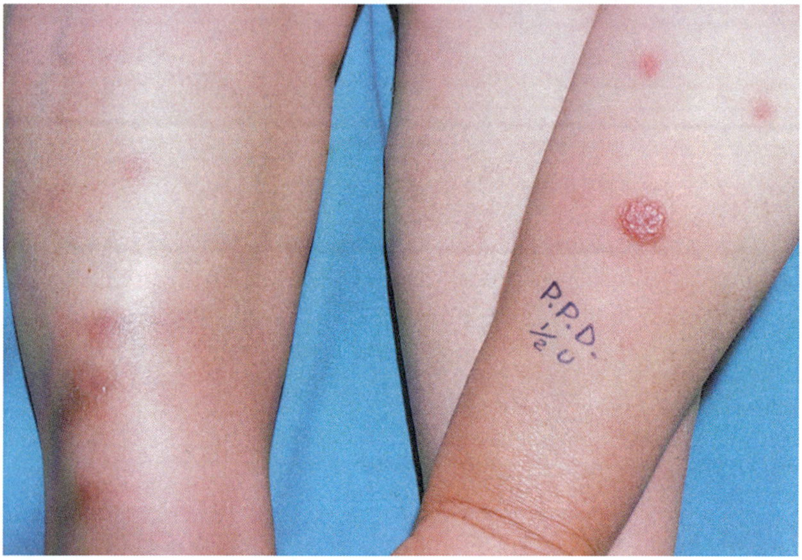

Fig. 2.63 Erythema induratum of Bazin. Strong positive PPD

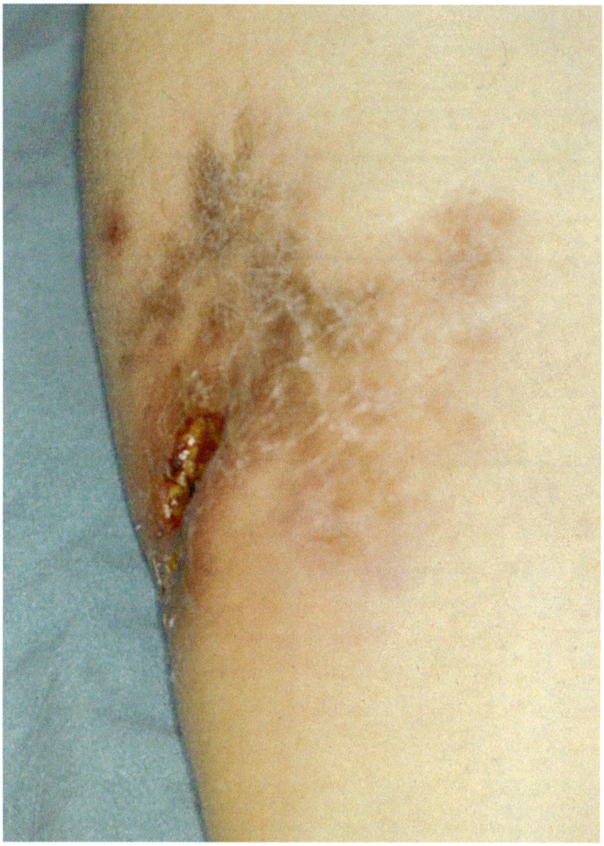

Fig. 2.64 Erythema induratum of the Hutchinson type

Dermal-hypodermal nodules in the lower third of the leg in women with erythrocyanosis are pathognomonic for the clinical diagnosis. For some authors, all cases in which the Koch bacillus is not demonstrated should be considered as nodular vasculitis not tuberculous erythema induratum. In a recent study, about 10% of cases were positive for *M. tuberculosis* by PCR [375]. The therapeutic *ex juvantibus* criterion can also be valid. In all cases an accurate search for active TB foci is essential [376, 377].

The histological criterion is useful for diagnostic purposes when typical tuberculoid structures are evident. However, in all recent lesions there is only a non-specific granulomatous infiltrate with mononuclear cells and degeneration of subcutaneous fat, even if the PPD is positive.

Differential diagnosis is made with erythema nodosum and nodular panniculitis. The onset of erythema nodosum is more acute and the disease involves the anterior surface of the legs; the lesions are painful at palpation and the patient suffers from general malaise. The cellular infiltrate of erythema nodosum is less dense, generally consisting of few scattered cell clusters. Caseous necrosis is absent. The presence of giant cells and vascular changes can also be found in erythema nodosum, although

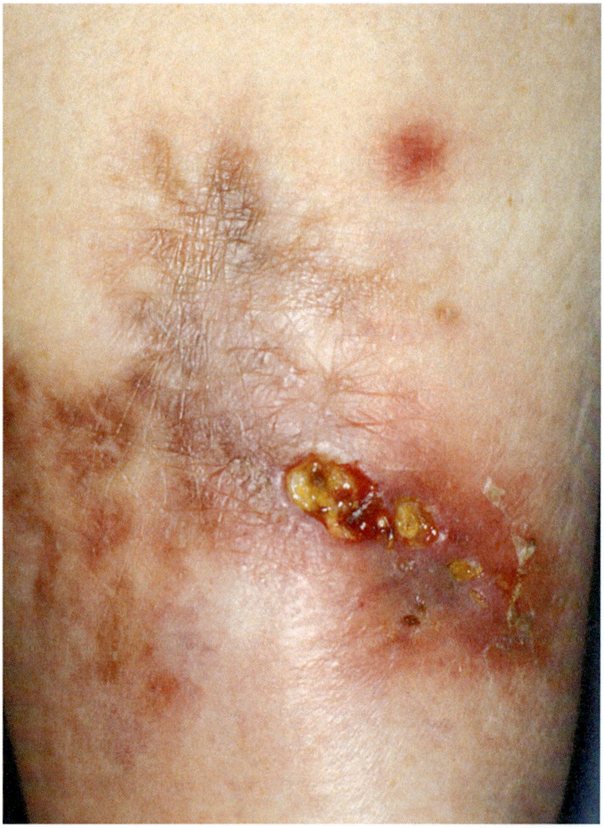

Fig. 2.65 Erythema induratum of the Hutchinson type

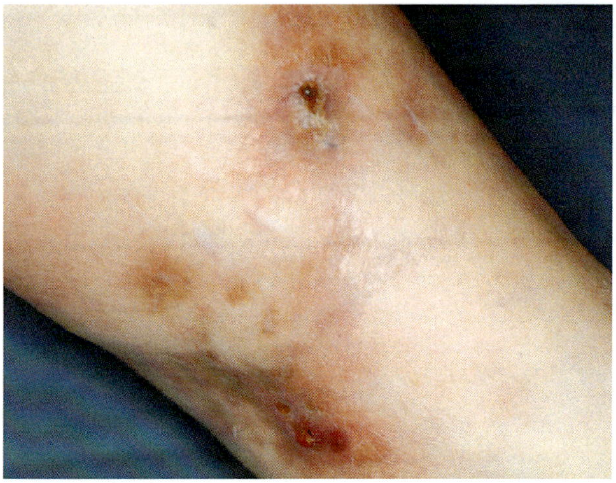

Fig. 2.66 The same patient as in Fig. 2.65

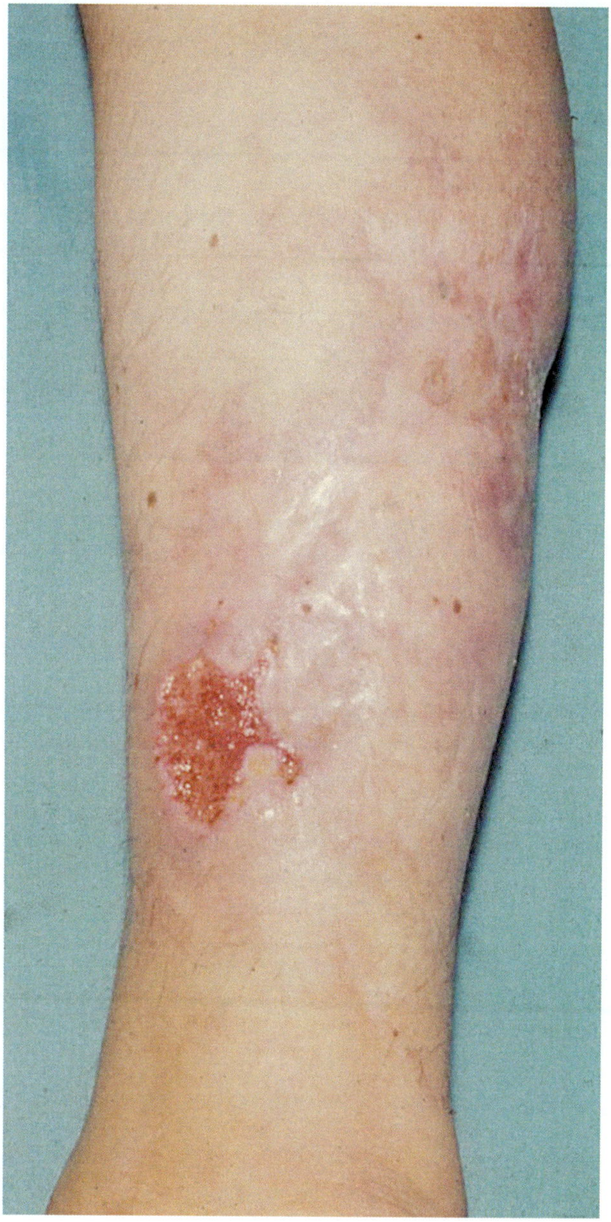

Fig. 2.67 Erythema induratum of the Hutchinson type

the vasculitis will be limited to smaller veins and will not affect the arteries. Clinical and histological findings and specific laboratory tests allow the differentiation of panniculitis (pancreatic lobular panniculitis, drug-induced mixed panniculitis, panniculitis in granulomatous vasculitis, and venous thrombosis) from erythema induratum and erythema nodosum.

Nodular Tuberculid

In four female patients, dull red or bluish-red non-tender, non ulcerating nodules were observed, about 1 cm in diameter, located on the lower legs. The histological alterations of the granulomatous vasculitis were localized in the junction between the deep dermis and the adjacent subcutaneous fat. The Mantoux test was strongly positive; in two patients there was associated pulmonary TB. In all cases the disease resolved with full anti-tubercular treatment [370]. Other similar cases have since been reported [378, 379].

Erythema Nodosum

TB is now a very rare cause of erythema nodosum in Western Europe and the USA, but is still observed in countries where TB is common. In children it is always important to exclude TB: this was the cause in 9 of 113 children with extrapulmonary forms reported in the UK in 1978–79 [380].

2.10.12.4 Other Possible Tuberculids

Granulomatous mastitis is a very rare inflammatory disease of the breast with a multiple etiology. Clinically and radiologically it may mimic breast cancer. It is often unilateral, and consists of ulcerative plaques, nodules or abscess in the female breast [381]. It has a chronic course and does not respond to antibiotic treatment. In endemic TB areas, some cases of granulomatous mastitis have a tubercular nature. PCR may be positive and the PPD strongly positive [382, 383]. There is an excellent response to anti-tubercular treatment in these patients [225, 384].

Lupus miliaris disseminatus faciei is generally considered as a variant of rosacea. However, in endemic areas with a high TB prevalence, patients with papulonecrotic lesions of the face and ear pavilions leading to varicelliform scarring can be observed. In these lesions, that show a granulomatous histology, it is sometimes possible to isolate mycobacteria. The tuberculin skin test is positive and anti-tubercular treatment is efficacious. These cases should be classified as true lupus miliaris of the face [225]. A high suspicion index is needed to make a correct diagnosis.

2.11 Tuberculosis of the Oral Cavity

Oral manifestations of TB are uncommon, being seen in only 0.5–1.5% of patients with TB [265, 287–292]. They may be primary but are more frequently secondary, linked to auto-infection from the sputum, or to hematogenous or lymphatic spread of the bacilli [385].

It is believed that an intact oral mucosa, the constant flow of saliva and its antibacterial properties, protect the oral tissues from the invasion of tubercle bacilli, but any local trauma can favor the onset of the infection. Other local predisposing factors are poor oral hygiene, hyperkeratosis disorders (leukoplakia), oral mucosa inflammation or dental extraction [386–392].

Table 2.12 Characteristics of primary and secondary oral tuberculosis (modified, by [265])

	Primary oral tuberculosis	Secondary oral tuberculosis
Occurrence	Very rare, predominantly in children	More frequent, especially in middle-aged and elderly patients
Risk factors	Oral traumas, tobacco smoking, hyperkeratotic disorders, poor oral hygiene, immunodeficiency (diabetes, neoplasms, alcoholism, HIV infection, prolonged corticosteroid therapy)	
Clinical features	Ulcer superficial or deeper and covered with granular tissue	Ulcer with undermined irregular edges covered with Trelat granules
Local lymph node	Enlarged, painful	Enlarged or not, usually not painful
Pain	No	Yes

The site most commonly affected is the tongue, followed by the labial mucosa, hard palate, gingival and buccal mucosa [393, 394]. In primary oral TB forms, the gingival and buccal mucosa are usually affected.

Ulcers are the most common manifestations. In primary TB, a non-painful ulcer is accompanied by submandibular, submental or cervical lymph nodes. Primary forms are more common in children and secondary forms in the middle-aged and elderly [395]. In the secondary forms the ulcers are extremely painful. They are normally single but can be multiple, superficial or deep, oval or long, and the base is covered by necrotic tissue. The ulcer margins are irregular, indistinct and indurated. These tubercular ulcerations show no tendency to heal and gradually grow, over a long period. The base of these secondary ulcers may be covered by yellowish or bluish Trelat granules [388, 396] (Table 2.12).

Oral TB can exceptionally manifest in lupoid form: pinkish or yellowish granules appear on an inflamed base. These form aggregates that then undergo ulceration, and will heal leaving scarring. Apart from these types of lesions, nodules, papules, and periapical granulomas have been described [388, 392, 396, 397]. The tubercular process may also extend to the craniofacial bones; in these rare circumstances, extraoral fistulas can develop on the cheeks.

It must be borne in mind that oral TB manifestations are highly infectious. Differential diagnosis must be made with syphilis, actinomycosis, histoplasmosis, epithelial cancer, recurrent aphthous stomatitis, erosive forms of lichen planus, Crohn's disease and sarcoidosis. Tubercular ulcers are persistent, do not respond to topical treatment and are generally single and painful. Instead, syphilitic lesions are indolent and have smooth, indurated margins. Oral cancer develops slowly and may take on a cauliflower appearance; the margins are firm and raised, and the base is infiltrated. Initially, neoplastic ulcers are not painful but are prone to bleeding. It should be noted that in 3% of cases of oral TB there is coexistent oral malignancy [393, 396]. Multiple, painful and recurrent ulcers may indicate aphthae or mucocutaneous diseases (ulcerative lichen planus, pemphigoid).

The final diagnosis is confirmed by histology, that may reveal the presence of granulomatous infiltration with Langhans giant cells and lymphocytes; foci of caseous necrosis can be observed. Mycobacteria may be demonstrated. The tuberculin skin test is positive.

2.12 Cutaneous Tuberculosis in Pediatric Age

There are a number of differences between TB in adults and in infants, children and adolescents. In most cases, in the adult TB is linked to a reactivation of dormant bacilli lodged in the lung apexes, whereas in childhood it is generally a complication of the initial infection. In the adult, the interval between the infection and the onset of the clinical disease is very long, years or even decades, whereas in small children it is often only weeks or months. Children more frequently develop extrapulmonary forms. Due to these differences in the pathophysiology, the approach to diagnosis, treatment and infection and disease prevention in children is different [398].

The contacts investigations, i.e. making a close examination of subjects who have had contacts with a suspected case of TB including the tuberculin skin test, chest radiography, and physical examination, is the most important community measure in order to prevent TB in children [399]. The most frequent settings for exposure in a child are, of course, above all the household, the school, daycare centers or other closed environments. Hypersensitivity to tuberculin takes up to 3 months to develop, and for this reason the WHO recommends that at the exposure stage, children under the age of 5 years should be treated to prevent the rapid development of severe forms of TB [398]. It must be borne in mind, in fact, that an immunocompetent adult with an untreated TB infection has an approximately 5–10% risk of developing the disease in a lifetime, while in an immunocompetent infant the risk is 40% within 1–2 years from the infection and the resulting disease forms are often very severe and life-threatening [398]. Moreover, while in the adult the infection and the disease are distinct events because of the long interval between them, in the child the two stages are a continuum, and often immediately consecutive [400].

It is estimated that worldwide, each year there are 1.5 million cases of TB in children and 500,000 deaths [401]. About 60% of TB cases are in infants and children less than 5 years of age. By contrast, in the range between 5 and 16 years, often called the "favored age", children generally have the lowest rates of disease in any population. The clinical expression of TB in children also differs according to age: while miliary, meningeal and lymphatic forms are observed between the ages of 1 and 5, all the extrapulmonary forms are more common in older children and adolescents [398].

The distribution by gender varies in different studies but is in general 1:1, unlike in adults, where there is a predominance in the male sex [281, 398, 402–407]. In children, like in adults, the risk of TB is increased in cases of diabetes mellitus [408] and immunocompromising conditions. The TB rates are highest between January and June in the Northern Hemisphere, likely because of closer contact with infected adults in the colder seasons.

In the United States, where 70% of TB cases affect children under 5 [409], the highest incidence is among ethnic and racial minority groups and the foreign-born, as opposed to Caucasians [410]. In fact, about 88% of cases are observed among African American, Hispanic, Asian and Native American children, reflecting the risk of transmission in the living environment of these children [409, 411]. At all ages, about 50% of the cases of TB seen in foreign-born individuals are observed within 5 years of immigration.

Most children are infected at home, but outbreaks occur in elementary and high schools, nursery schools, churches, school buses, and stores: a high risk adult working in the area is frequently a source in these outbreaks [398].

Various studies have shown that the increased incidence of TB in children is also associated with a simultaneous increase of HIV infection among adults in the community [399].

In terms of transmission, children are generally infected by an adult or adolescent in the immediate household, usually a relative, grandparent, or older sibling. Chance contacts outside the family are much more rare; nevertheless, babysitters, schoolteachers, nurse teachers, school bus drivers, nurses and parishioners can be implicated in single cases and in mini-epidemics within limited population groups [412].

Children with TB rarely infect another child [413] and the few that do show adult type TB characteristics [414]. This is because in tuberculous children there are relatively few bacilli in endobronchial secretions, and a productive cough is not a feature of endobronchial TB or the miliary form [415]. Also children lack the expectorant force of adults when coughing. Guidelines drawn up by Centers of Disease Control and Prevention have established that children with TB do not require isolation in hospital unless they have an uncontrolled productive cough, a cavitary lesion, or acid-fast organisms-positive sputum smears [416]. Instead, adolescents with a typical reactivated pulmonary TB transmit the infection in the same way as adults do.

In children the entry portal is the lung in more than 95% of cases. Then the infection follows the same pathway as in adults. Extrapulmonary TB forms are observed in 25-35% of children; the most common form is localized in the lymph nodes of the neck [417–419]. The most severe forms are disseminated miliary disease and meningitis.

Interpretation of the Mantoux skin test should be similar in children and adults (Table 2.13) [195, 420]. The American Academy of Pediatrics (AAP) has suggested that 10 mm should be the cut-off point for all children aged less than 4 years [421], not because of the reduced ability to mount an induration reaction in children but in order to minimize false-negative reactions in small children at increased risk of developing life-threatening forms of TB when infected. For more information about the influence of the different factors on the accuracy of tuberculin skin testing, and the recommendations regarding gamma interferon release assays in children, interested readers should consult the reference list [398, 421–425].

Table 2.13 Interpretation of the Mantoux skin test (modified, by [398])

Reaction size (mm)	Factors
≥5	Contact with an infected case
	Abnormal X ray or clinical findings
	HIV infection or immunosuppression
≥10	Previous residence in a high-prevalence area
	Contact with a high-risk adult
	Residence in a long-term care facility
	Age <4 years
≥15	Absence of risk factors

The incidence of pediatric cutaneous TB is variable, ranging from 0.36 to 31.6%. In a study based on a hospital survey, cutaneous TB accounted for 1.67% of 7005 cases of pulmonary and extrapulmonary TB: the most common forms were lupus vulgaris and tuberculosis verrucosa cutis, and the incidence in children under 10 was 18.3% of the total cases in these same clinical forms [426]. In an Indian study, the cutaneous TB population in patients less than 16 years was 18.7% [281]. A higher prevalence, 31.6%, was recorded in another hospital-based survey from India [406], while in another study it was 0.36% of all pediatric outpatients [407]. In Ethiopia, pediatric cutaneous TB accounted for 24.2% of cutaneous TB cases [427]. In a Tunisian study, among 26 patients with cutaneous TB observed over a period of 20 years, 6 (23%) were under 12 years of age [428].

Overall, the clinical presentation in childhood is similar to that in adults, but the tendency to disseminate is higher in children. In a prospective study of 103 patients (aged <19 years), the most common clinical patterns of cutaneous TB were scrofuloderma (36.9%), lichen scrofulosorum (33%), and lupus vulgaris (21.3%). There was a lower incidence of TB verrucosa cutis (3.9%), papulonecrotic tuberculid (3.9%), and erythema nodosum (2.9%). Systemic associations were observed in 53.4% of cases [402]. In another Indian study, of 75 children (≤16 years) with cutaneous TB, the most common clinical form was scrofuloderma (53.3%) [281]. According to the authors, this is probably due to the consumption of unboiled/unpasteurized milk, a common habit in India that can cause infection of cervical lymph nodes by *M. bovis* via the tonsils [281].

2.12.1 Bacillus Calmette-Guérin-Induced Skin Lesions

BCG is injected at birth and after 3 months, and at the inoculation site the child develops an erythematous papule. The papule then crusts over and subsides at 9–12 months of age leaving an atrophic scar. Apart from the papule, some complications can develop. If the vaccine is injected subcutaneously by mistake (not intradermally), an abscess or BCGoma can develop [402], and give rise to a possible regional suppurative lymphadenitis.

Localized forms of cutaneous TB, such as lupus vulgaris, are rarely observed in immunocompetent infants [429], whereas a disseminated BCG infection or BCGiosis [430] is possible in immunodeficient children. BCGiosis is seen in children under the age of 2 years and is more common in males. It responds poorly to anti-tubercular treatment [431].

2.13 Diagnosis and Prognosis

Classically, the absolute criteria for the diagnosis of TB are a positive culture of *M. tuberculosis* from the lesion, successful guinea-pig inoculation, and mycobacterial DNA identification by PCR. Inoculation in the guinea-pig is no longer done today because identical results can be obtained with multiple cultures. With the BACTEC system a rapid culture diagnosis is possible in 2-6 days [432].

The in vitro amplification of specific DNA sequences by PCR has become a valid means for making a rapid identification of slow-growing organisms such as *M. tuberculosis*. Recently, several systems using PCR for the molecular detection of mycobacterial DNA have been reported, using different parts of the genome to generate highly sensitive and specific probes [433–439]. Some systems have amplified the insertion sequence IS6110 because of the repetitive nature of this element in the *M. tuberculosis* genome [438]. The use of two different primer pairs targeting the gene encoding for 16S ribosomal RNA (common to all mycobacteria), as well as the insertion sequence IS6110, specific for the *M. tuberculosis* complex, may further increase the sensitivity of detection [439].

As few as two colony-forming units of *M. tuberculosis* cells, or as little as 15 fg of DNA can be detected [344]. PCR positivity has been demonstrated in all the clinical forms of cutaneous TB and in two forms of tuberculids, namely papulonecrotic tuberculid and erythema induratum [293, 323, 342, 344, 440], The technique helps to make a rapid diagnosis and may be particularly useful in paucibacillary forms like lupus vulgaris. Moreover, the test can be done on various pathological specimens, including archival formalin-fixed tissue sections. The limitation of PCR is its minor sensitivity [439].

Other lesser diagnostic criteria are: active, proven TB in other body sites; the presence of acid-fast bacilli in the lesions (but the same bacilli are also present in infections by other mycobacteria); the histopathology; the clinical history and physical signs; a positive tuberculin skin test; and the effect of the specific therapy.

Differential diagnosis must be made with some forms of leprosy, syphilis, leishmaniasis, deep mycoses, infections with non-tuberculous mycobacteria, and sarcoidosis.

The prognosis depends on an early, accurate diagnosis. Generalized and meningeal TB have a doubtful prognosis. In patients with HIV infection and TB the mortality is higher than in HIV-negative patients [441, 442]. In infants and young children TB is always a very serious disease. Cutaneous TB generally shows a good response to treatment, with an evident clinical response within 4–6 weeks; lupus vulgaris responds more rapidly than scrofuloderma.

2.14 Management

2.14.1 General Measures and Principles of Chemotherapy

In each case of cutaneous TB it is essential to manage the disease from the perspective of the patient's condition overall, as well as making an accurate search for underlying disease foci and coexistent infections [399]. Owing to the increased incidence of drug-resistant TB, it is vitally important to obtain bacteriological confirmation of the diagnosis if possible, and to carry out susceptibility tests. If the patients comes from a risk area or from a background with an increased risk of HIV infection, HIV testing and counseling should be considered, after obtaining informed consent.

To treat active TB effectively, the selected drugs must be able to reach the bacilli in the various compartments [441, 442], in other words the bacilli within the extracellular environment that actively multiply in the liquid caseous debris of pulmonary cavities (this large population of organisms is the prime location for the natural selection of drug resistant bacilli), the slow growing bacilli within macrophages (these organisms are few but the acid environment and the lack of reproductive activity limit the utility of many anti-TB medicaments), and the slow growing organisms within the solid caseous material (here the penetration of drugs is hindered by a limited blood flow).

Treatment must be continued for long enough to ensure the eradication of all the vital bacilli. The simultaneous administration of several active drugs can create a statistically effective barrier against the onset of resistance, since the resistance mutations of each specific drug occur independently.

The current first-line regimens consist of three or four drugs that, by acting together, can eradicate the bacilli in the various compartments and prevent the development of drug resistance. For instance, rifampicin (rifampin in the USA) is bactericidal against all three populations; isoniazid is bactericidal against extracellular organisms; streptomycin and the aminoglycosides are bactericidal against extracellular organisms, while ethambutol lacks a bactericidal activity [443].

The standard treatment regimens are divided into two phases. The first consists of 8 weeks of treatment, the second of another 4–7 months, depending on the response to the treatment. The first phase relies on rifampicin, isoniazid and pyrazinamide, the second on isoniazid and rifampicin.

Adherence to treatment is obviously highly important in view of the length of the treatment and the possible development of resistance. For this reason, the American Thoracic Society, CDC Infectious Diseases Society of America [444] and NICE 2011 guidelines [445] recommend direct observation therapy (DOT, that is supervision by the physician of the adherence to treatment of all patients). Effective intermittent dosing regimens (twice or thrice weekly) can facilitate these efforts. DOT, where the ingestion of every drug dose is witnessed, has been shown to improve cure rates in various countries [446]. DOT is recommended for all patients, especially those unlikely to show good compliance (the homeless, alcoholics, drug abusers, drifters, the seriously mentally ill, as well as patients with multiple drug resistance) [447].

2.14.2 Drugs

Rifampicin, isoniazid, pyrazinamide, ethambutol, and streptomycin are the standard first-line medicaments. Fluoroquinolones, with a bactericidal activity against *M. tuberculosis*, are used in cases of drug resistance and when first line drugs are not tolerated [441].

2.14.2.1 Isoniazid

Its bactericidal activity interferes with the production of the tubercle bacilli cell wall component, mycolic acid [446]. Available in oral and parenteral formulations, it is metabolized by the liver and has a half-life of 1–3 h. Dosage may be daily, or twice or three times weekly.

The most common adverse events are elevated transaminases (up to five times the upper limit of normal, and normalizing after the treatment is suspended) in 10–20% of cases, hepatitis (rare, but serious) in less than 1% of cases and peripheral neuropathy in 0.2% of patients. Isoniazid-related hepatitis is associated with older age, alcohol consumption, and is more common when it is administered together with rifampicin. Other rare events are a rash, hematological abnormalities, and a lupus-like syndrome [441].

2.14.2.2 Rifampicin

This is a potent bactericidal agent and inhibits the DNA-dependent RNA polymerase of *M. tuberculosis*. It has a half-life of 1.5–5 h, penetrates most tissues, and is available in oral and intravenous formulations but drug–drug interactions with various antiretroviral agents limit their contemporary use, so it is often replaced with rifabutin.

Hepatotoxicity linked to rifampicin is uncommon and manifests with a cholestatic presentation, increased bilirubin and alkaline phosphatase. A rash with pruritus is observed in 6% of cases but is transitory [448]. Rifampicin causes a temporary benign orange tinge of urine and tears.

2.14.2.3 Pyrazinamide

This is bactericidal and exerts its activity by disrupting membrane activity and transport functions [449]. It is used in the first 2 months of treatment, is available in an oral formulation, has a half-life of 9–10 h, and is cleared through the kidneys. Pyrazinamide failure to act in this regimen means that the treatment needs to be prolonged for at least 9 months [441].

The most serious adverse event is hepatotoxicity, observed in 1% of patients. High uric acid is a common occurrence but does not require treatment suspension except in patients suffering from gout. Other side effects are nausea, vomiting, cutaneous photosensitivity, and a mild rash.

2.14.2.4 Ethambutol

This bacteriostatic agent is employed with rifampicin and pyrazinamide when isoniazid is not tolerated or is resistant. It has a half-life of about 4 h, is available in an oral formulation, and is excreted through the kidneys.

An dose-related event is optic neuritis when the dosage is more than 15 mg/kg of body weight [450]: the loss of red-green color discrimination can be an early manifestation. The sight must be checked before starting treatment and monthly during the treatment. If the sight does become affected, suspension of the drug is generally enough to solve the problem.

2.14.2.5 Streptomycin

This bactericidal aminoglycoside acts on the protein synthesis of the tubercle bacillus. It is excreted through the kidneys and care must be taken when using it in patients with renal failure. It is available in parenteral formulations. Primary resistance to streptomycin is observed in high-incidence countries.

In 10% of cases ototoxicity (vestibular disorders and hearing loss) has been reported, especially at cumulative doses of more than 100 g [451]. In 2% of cases there is renal toxicity.

2.14.3 Alternative Drugs in First-Line Regimens

Rifabutin has a similar mechanism of action to that of rifampicin but being more lipid-soluble, it has a half-life of about 45 h. It can be safely used with various antiretroviral regimens. Adverse effects include hepatitis, leukopenia in 2% of cases, uveitis, and arthralgias. Like rifampicin, rifabutin stains the body fluids.

Rifapentine also has a similar activity to that of rifampicin; it is contraindicated in HIV-infected patients due to the development of rifampicin-resistance. It has the same adverse side effects as rifampicin.

The aminoglycosides kanamycin, amikacin, and capreomycin can be used instead of streptomycin. *M. tuberculosis* strains that are resistant to streptomycin may be susceptible to other aminoglycosides, but the susceptibility to each drug must be confirmed by resistance testing. Resistance to kanamycin indicates resistance also to amikacin. These agents are available only in parenteral formulations, and the side effects are the same as with streptomycin [441].

Fluoroquinolones are potent bactericides against *M. tuberculosis* [452] and when the disease is susceptible, are an important reserve in cases of MDR. They can also be used as first-line drugs in cases of intolerance or resistance. In cases of rifampicin monoresistance or intolerance, a fluoroquinolone can be used as a component of the 12–18 months regimen that includes isoniazid and ethambutol, and at least 2 months of pyrazinamide. Those most commonly employed are moxifloxacin, levofloxacin, and ofloxacin. Fluoroquinolones are available in both oral and parenteral formulations. Side effects include nausea, QT prolongation, neuropsychiatric disorders, and tendon rupture. Their use is not recommended in children and in pregnancy due to their action on developing bone and cartilage.

2.14.4 Second-Line Drugs

Apart from those mentioned above as alternative drugs in first line regimens, other second-line drugs are cycloserine, ethionamide, and *p*-aminosalicylic acid, and various others. These drugs are less active than the first-line drugs and have more adverse effects [453].

Cycloserine is bacteriostatic and acts on the mycobacteria cell wall synthesis. It is taken by mouth and rapidly absorbed. The most common adverse effects are on the central nervous system (psychosis, mania, depression, seizures, and other emotional disturbances). They are dose-dependent (rare under a dosage of 30 μg/ml), and are mostly observed in subjects with previous neurological or psychiatric problems. The adult dosage is 750 mg/day in 2–3 doses; the starting dose is 500 mg daily. Serum levels must be checked before increasing the drug dosage [453].

Ethionamide is similar to isoniazid in terms of mechanism of action and structure, and is bactericidal. The most common side effects are gastrointestinal: nausea, epigastric pain, and a metallic taste; in 4.3% of cases significant hepatitis develops. Hypothyroidism is another common adverse effect. The drug can be used in association with other drugs at an initial dosage of 250 mg daily, to reach 500–1000 mg/day during the first 7–10 days of treatment [453].

para-Aminosalicylic acid (PAS) has a bacteriostatic action, is rapidly absorbed and spreads in caseous TB lesions; it does not penetrate non-inflamed meninges. The dosage is 8–12 g/day split into several doses. Side effects include nausea, vomiting, anorexia, and diarrhea (the latter at the beginning of treatment, often improving after the first weeks). A starting dose of 4 g daily is recommended, gradually increasing over 10 days. Especially in association with ethionamide, PAS causes hypothyroidism [453].

Clofazimine, a compound also used in leprosy, is active in TB although its mechanism of action is unknown. It is generally well tolerated except for some gastrointestinal symptoms and the problem of skin staining.

Linezolid is an oxazolidinone with a modest or minimal bactericidal activity; instead, it acts by blocking ribosomal protein synthesis. It is used in cases of XDR-TB, at a dosage of 600 mg twice daily. However, to limit toxicity, some authors have used 600 or 300 mg just once a day. Side effects include myelosuppression, peripheral and optic neuropathy (that may persist even after suspension of the therapy), and lactic acidosis. It is associated with the serotonin syndrome in 25% of cases (in fact, it is important to avoid food and beverages with a high tyramine content) [453].

Imipenem is listed by the WHO as a third-line agent for the treatment of TB. It does have a bactericidal activity, albeit not strong, and its clinical efficacy has still to be determined.

2.14.5 Treatment Regimens

A short-course regimen of 26 weeks (6 months) is the treatment of choice in newly diagnosed subjects never previously treated for TB. The entire treatment should be with DOT. This regimen involves an initial phase of 8 weeks (2 months) using four drugs: isoniazid, rifampicin, pyrazinamide, plus ethambutol or streptomycin. The latter drugs (ethambutol is generally preferred) must be administered in the initial phase until results on the susceptibility to isoniazid, rifampicin and pyrazinamide are obtained. Then ethambutol can be discontinued. After the first phase, isoniazid and rifampicin will be continued for a further 4 months (18 weeks).

During the initial phase, daily administration is recommended for the first 2 weeks, and to follow, a twice-weekly or thrice-weekly schedule is a valid option. In HIV-coinfected patients intermittent treatment is not advised.

Dosages in adults and in children are reported in Tables 2.14 and 2.15, respectively [399, 441, 444]. All drugs must be taken on an empty stomach.

Table 2.14 Drugs commonly used for the treatment of tuberculosis in adults

Drug	Dose/day	Time of treatment (months)
Isoniazid	300 mg	6
Rifampicin	450 mg (weight <50 kg) 600 mg (weight >50 kg)	6
Pyrazinamide	1.0 g (weight <50 kg) 2.0 g (weight >50 kg)	2
Ethambutol	800 mg (weight <50 kg) 1.6 g (weight >50 kg)	2

Table 2.15 Drugs commonly used for the treatment of tuberculosis in children

Drug	Daily dose (mg/kg)	Maximum daily dose
Isoniazid	10–15	300 mg
Rifampicin	10–20	600 mg
Pyrazinamide	15–30	2 g
Ethambutol	15–20	1 g
Streptomycin[a]	20–40	1 g

[a]Intramuscular administration

This standard 6-months regimen has also been shown effective to treat cutaneous TB: in one patients series, in which 50% had a coexisting disease elsewhere, a good clinical response was obtained with no post-treatment relapses [232]. In the past, some forms of cutaneous TB were treated with isoniazid alone but nowadays this monotherapy is no longer acceptable owing to the risk of developing drug resistance.

If diagnosed in the early phase, the excision of small lupus vulgaris or warty TB lesions may be effective. Surgery is helpful in scrofuloderma, also in order to reduce the duration of chemotherapy.

2.14.6 Treatment Failure and Relapse

In 95% of patients receiving appropriate first-line treatment cultures become negative within 3 months. Should negativity fail to develop, the possible causes of a delayed response must be considered, namely non compliance, drug resistance, malabsorption, and laboratory error (contamination). The susceptibility tests must be repeated on the last culture specimens, and any resistance to rifampicin and isoniazid established using sensitive molecular assays [454].

Treatment failure is defined as a positive culture after 4 months of appropriate treatment [441]. To prevent further resistance a single drug should never be added to a failing regimen. Empirical addition of a fluoroquinolone and an additional oral agent (PAS, ethionaminde, or cycloserine) may be a valid measure [444].

Relapse is classified as the reappearance of TB in a successfully treated subject; it must be differentiated from exogenous reinfection. The relapse may be due to a lack of sterilization of residual TB organisms; it is generally observed in subjects with a heavy disease burden and delayed culture negativity, and occurs within 6–12 months of the end of the therapy. Susceptibility tests need to be repeated to verify the activity of the first-line drugs. In cases of drug resistance, three new active agents must be included in the retreatment regimen [444].

2.14.7 Treatment in Special Circumstances

The standard 6-months regimen, if properly supervised, is effective also in HIV-positive subjects [455]. The response rate is the same as in non-HIV-infected patients but the drug reactions are stronger and the reinfection rates higher.

Treatment is similar in children and adults, except for a lower use of ethambutol in the former; it will last 6 months [398].

Treating congenital TB poses a greater risk than treating pregnant women with active TB. Streptomycin is the only documented teratogenic drug. Even if the data on the teratogenicity of pyrazinamide are incomplete, the drug is not recommended by the WHO in the treatment of pregnant women in the United States. The starting treatment can be with isoniazid, rifampicin and ethambutol and mothers can suckle their infants when receiving this regimen. The doses in the breast milk are not sufficient to treat the child, that must receive supplemental pyridoxine, because this vitamin is inhibited by the isoniazid dosage in breast milk [441].

2.14.8 Therapy of Multidrug Resistant Tuberculosis

Multidrug-resistant TB (MDR-TB), due to strains that are resistant to at least isoniazid and rifampicin [456], is difficult to treat and requires the use of expensive, more toxic and less effective drugs. In 2006, the definition of extensive XDR-TB was revised to: TB resistant to isoniazid, rifampicin, a second-line injectable drug (kanamycin, amikacin, or capreomycin), and any fluoroquinolones [457]. This new definition identifies a group with a poorer outcome and high mortality rates [458].

In 2009, the WHO reported an estimated 440,000 cases of MDR-TB, 50,000 cases of XDR-TB, and 150,000 deaths due to MDR-TB [453]. This is probably an underestimate bearing in mind the lack of laboratory facilities for performing susceptibility tests, especially for second-line drugs, in many developing countries. The nations with the highest numbers of cases are India, China, the Russian Federation, South Africa, and Bangladesh. The increase in MDR-TB and XDR-TB is also linked to HIV infection, for various reasons [459].

Molecular studies have shown that MDR-TB strains form as a result of sequential resistance mutations to single drugs [460].

The resistance that develops during or after a treatment cycle was initially labeled "acquired drug resistance" but now the WHO has labeled it "resistance among previously treated cases". The resistance that arises without any previous TB-treatment was called "primary drug resistance", now changed to "resistance among new cases". Thus, "new cases" are those individuals who have never received anti-tubercular drugs or have taken them for less than 1 month, while "previously treated cases" are those who have undergone at least one month of treatment [461].

Causes of resistance include: inadequate primary treatment regimens, addition of a single drug to a failing treatment regimen, failure to recognize resistance, failure to recognize or ensure adherence, and inappropriate isoniazid monotherapy of TB infection. These treatment errors are more common in patients cared for by private providers [453]. Therefore, it is best for treatment to be started during an initial period of hospital stay, also in order to supervise more closely any side effects that may develop.

The treatment for MDR-TB must include several drugs and be administered for long periods (18–24 months or more). Obviously, whenever possible the treatment must be based on susceptibility tests. It should preferably be started with 6, or not less than four drugs with a proven susceptibility, two of which must be bactericidal [462]. The standard approach is to use any first-line drug to which the bacilli isolated are shown to remain susceptible (even if they were a part of a previously ineffective regimen), add an injectable drug, add a fluoroquinolone (levofloxacin or moxifloxacin), and select the remaining drugs in order to complete the regimen of five or preferably six drugs. These additional drugs should be chosen among second-line and third-line drugs (linezolid, amoxicillin-clavulanic acid, imipenem, clarithromycin, and clofazimine).

The treatment duration will depend on the disease entity, the number of bactericidal drugs included in the regimen, the patient's immunological and nutritional status and the clinical and bacteriological response to therapy.

Even if there are insufficient data on safety in pregnancy for various second-line drugs, some studies have reported favorable outcomes for the mother and fetus. Women of fertile age should be helped to avoid pregnancy during treatment for MDR-TB [463].

The treatment for XDR-TB is still more difficult. Both first and second-line drugs need to be used after having made susceptibility tests also for all the injectable drugs, ethionamide and newer-generation fluoroquinolones. The principles are the same as for MDR-TB treatment. The regimen must include at least six drugs selected among first-, second- and third-line, both injectable and oral, and will be quite long, even if definitive guidelines are not yet available [464]. Linezolid can be considered in such cases, but has significant toxicity.

In HIV-infected subjects with MDR-TB and XDR-TB a regimen based as far as possible on susceptibility tests is recommended, generally consisting of seven or eight drugs. Naturally, during such aggressive treatment regimens the patient must be closely monitored from the clinical and toxicological standpoints.

2.15 Chemoprophylaxis

This issue is highly debated in the control of TB. Strictly speaking, the term should be applied to the prevention of TB in uninfected subjects at high risk of infection and development of the disease, such as children exposed to a source case in the home. More usually, the term is used to refer to the treatment of latent infection to prevent the onset of active TB. That being so, in some nations like the USA, where

TB is very uncommon and BCG vaccination is no longer used, chemoprophylaxis is given to tuberculin reactors. In such circumstances, starting from the assumption that very few viable bacilli are present and the risk of mutation to isoniazid resistance is likely low, isoniazid is given as monotherapy, generally for one year. This treatment has proven effective and protective in the long term. The problems arising with isoniazid monotherapy include poor compliance, hepatic complications and the onset of resistance. Because of the risk of liver damage, some authors believe that only subjects aged less than 35 years should receive chemoprophylaxis [465].

In general, the role of chemoprophylaxis in high TB incidence areas has not played an important role in the control of the disease. However, since the advent of the HIV/AIDS pandemic its role has been revised: various studies of isoniazid monotherapy have found it effective in co-infected patients [466, 467]. Unfortunately, the effect is short term and ends when the treatment is suspended. The best results are obtained in tuberculin-positive subjects with a relatively high lymphocyte count. For these reasons the WHO has recommended that prophylaxis be confined to tuberculin-positive HIV-positive subjects.

In HIV-positive subjects, 9 months' treatment with isoniazid is sufficient and prolonging it for 12 months adds very little. Assessments have also been made of 4 months of rifampicin and 2 months of rifampicin and pyrazinamide but the only advantage is the shorter treatment duration. It is important that HIV-positive subjects receiving chemoprophylaxis do not have active TB. In any case, policies for the use of chemoprophylaxis vary from one nation to another.

2.16 Vaccination

Vaccination is unable to prevent the establishment of TB [468] and can only prevent disease progression after the formation of a microscopic tubercle [128]. After one or two years from the BCG vaccination, all but a small residue of the BCG has been eliminated. The difference between vaccinated and non vaccinated subjects is that the former show an accelerated formation of the tubercle. In other words, there is a rapid local recruitment of lymphocytes and macrophages, that are quickly activated. This accelerated immune response often arrests the early focus of infection, thus preventing the progression to clinical disease [150]. Instead, in non vaccinated subjects the lymphocytes and macrophages activation is much slower and so the risk of active clinical infection is higher.

The challenge for researchers studying vaccines is to find antigens that are "more potent" than BCG in producing T-cell populations that activate macrophages to destroy the bacilli (CMI) and antigens that are "less potent" than BCG in producing T-cell populations that cause caseous necrosis and liquefaction [469], considered "pathological" as a tissue-damaging DTH. In short, a vaccine must produce a higher "CMI/tissue-damaging DTH ratio" than the currently available BCG vaccines do. A vaccine that is better than the current BCG strains must induce a strong CMI with little or no sensitivity to tuberculin [470]. The antigen fractions favoring the tubercle bacillus (probably protein complexes and carbohydrates and lipids) may stimulate CMI with minimal tissue-damaging DTH, while those that do not favor them (probably the tuberculoproteins that cause the tuberculin reaction) may produce more tissue-damaging DTH (caseation and liquefaction) with less CMI [128]. The tuberculoproteins that induce the tuberculin reaction have never been shown to have a protective action [471]. Indeed, they can induce severe necrosis in the tuberculin-positive host if concentrations rise beyond certain limits. Other fractions may have beneficial immunogenic effects without inducing tuberculin sensitivity, although these principles have still to be confirmed [472].

It is possible that recombinant vaccines may be better than the existing BCG vaccines [473–477]. To produce them, the DNAs for additional antigens are added to the BCG genome. These recombinant BCG strains seem to produce high CMI with little or no sensitivity to tuberculin, and so should be more efficacious than those currently available. The vaccines should expand the T-cell population that produces CMI together with little expansion of the T-cell population that produces DTH (caseous necrosis).

References

1. Daniel TM (2006) The history of tuberculosis. Respir Med 100:1862
2. Daniel TM (2011) Tuberculosis in history: did it change the way we live? In: Schlossberg D (ed) Tuberculosis and nontuberculous mycobacterial infections, 6th edn. ASM Press, Washington, DC, p 3
3. van Zy L, du Plessis J, Viljoen J (2015) Cutaneous tuberculosis overview and current treatment regimens. Tuberculosis (Edinb) 95:629
4. Gutierrez MC, Brisse S, Brosch R et al (2005) Ancient origin and gene mosaicism of the progenitor of *Mycobacterium tuberculosis*. PLoS Pathog 1:e5
5. Kapur V, Whittam TS, Musser JM (1994) Is *Mycobacterium tuberculosis* 15,000 years old? J Infect Dis 170:i348
6. Brosch R, Gordon SV, Marmiesse M et al (2002) A new evolutionary scenario for the *Mycobacterium tuberculosis* complex. Proc Natl Acad Sci U S A 99:3684
7. Sreevatsan S, Pan X, Stockbauer KE et al (1997) Restricted structural gene polymorphism in the *Mycobacterium tuberculosis* complex indicates evolutionarily recent global dissemination. Proc Natl Acad Sci U S A 94:9869
8. Gagneux S, DeRiemer K, Van T et al (2006) Variable host-pathogen compatibility in *Mycobacterium tuberculosis*. Proc Natl Acad Sci U S A 103:2869
9. Hirsh AE, Tsolaki AG, DeRiemer K et al (2004) Stable association between strains *of Mycobacterium tuberculosis* and their human host populations. Proc Natl Acad Sci U S A 101:4871
10. Morse D, Brothwell DR, Ucko PJ (1964) Tuberculosis in ancient Egypt. Am Rev Respir Dis 90:524
11. Zimmerman MR (1979) Pulmonary and osseous tuberculosis in an Egyptian mummy. Bull N Y Acad Med 55:604
12. Nerlich AG, Haas CJ, Zink A et al (1997) Molecular evidence for tuberculosis in an ancient Egyptian mummy. Lancet 350:1404
13. Crubézy E, Ludes B, Poveda JD et al (1998) Identification of *Mycobacterium* DNA in an Egyptian Pott's disease of 5,400 years old. C R Acad Sci III (Paris) 321:941
14. Morse D (1967) Tuberculosis. In: Brothwell D, Sandison AT (eds) Disease in antiquity. A survey of the diseases, injuries and surgery of early populations. Charles C Thomas, Springfield

15. Daniel VS, Daniel TM (1999) Old testament biblical references to tuberculosis. Clin Infect Dis 29:1557
16. Daniel TM (1997) Captain of death: the story of tuberculosis. University of Rochester Press, Rochester
17. Allison MJ, Mendoza D, Pezzia A (1973) Documentation of a case of tuberculosis in pre-Columbian America. Am Rev Respir Dis 107:985
18. Salo WL, Aufderheide AC, Buikstra J et al (1994) Identification of *Mycobacterium tuberculosis* DNA in a pre-Columbian Peruvian mummy. Proc Natl Acad Sci U S A 91:2091
19. Arriaza BT, Salo W, Aufderheide AC et al (1995) Pre-Columbian tuberculosis in northern Chile: molecular and skeletal evidence. Am J Phys Anthropol 98:37
20. Daniel TM (2000) The origins and precolonial epidemiology of tuberculosis in the Americas: can we figure them out? Int J Tuberc Lung Dis 4:395
21. Robert CA, Buikstra JE (2003) The bioarcheology of tuberculosis. A global view on a reemerging disease. University of Florida Press, Gainesville
22. Daniel TM (2004) René Theophile Hyacinthe Laënnec and the founding of pulmonary medicine. Int J Tuberc Lung Dis 8:517
23. Laënnec RTH (1962) A treatise on the disease of the chest. (Translated by Forbes J). Hafner Publishing Company, New York
24. Daniel TM (2005) Robert Koch and the pathogenesis of tuberculosis. Int J Tuberc Lung Dis 9:1181
25. von Pirquet C (1907) Der Diagnostiche wert der Kutanen Tuberculin-Reaktion bei der Tuberkulose des Kindesalters auf grund von 100 Sektionen. Wien Medizin Wchnschr 20:1123
26. von Pirquet C (1907) Die Allergieprobe zur Diagnose der Tuberkulose in Kindessalter. Wien Medizin Wchnschr 28:1369
27. Sakula A (1983) BCG: who were Calmette and Guérin? Thorax 38:806
28. Daniel TM (2005) Leon Charles Albert Calmette and BCG vaccine. Int J Tuberc Lung Dis 9:944
29. Calmette A (1928) On preventive vaccinaton of the new-born against tuberculosis by B.C.G. Br J Tuberc 22:161
30. Schatz A, Bugie E, Waksman SA (1944) Streptomycin, a substance exhibiting antibiotic activity against Gram-positive and Gram-negative bacteria. Proc Exp Biol Med 55:66
31. Espinal MA, Raviglione MC (2011) Tuberculosis – a World Health Organization perspective. In: Schlossberg D (ed) Tuberculosis and nontuberculous mycobacterial infections, 6th edn. ASM Press, Washington, DC, p 182
32. World Health Organization (1994) 47th World Health Assembly: Provisional Agenda Item 19. Tuberculosis Programme. Progress Report by the Director-General. WHA47/1994/A47/12.World Health Organization. World Health Organization, Geneva
33. Dye C, Maher D, Weil D et al (2006) Targets for global tuberculosis control. Int J Tuberc Lung Dis 10:460
34. World Health Organization (2009) Global Tuberculosis Control. A short update to the 2009 report. WHO/HTM/TB/2009.426. World Health Organization, Geneva
35. Kato-Maeda M, Luetkemeyer A, Small PM (2011) Tuberculosis associated with HIV infection. In: Schlossberg D (ed) Tuberculous and nontuberculous mycobacterial infections, 6th edn. ASM Press, Washington, DC, p 481
36. UNAIDS (2010) UNAIDS Report on the global AIDS epidemic. UNAIDS, Geneva
37. Vynnycky E, Fine PE (1997) The natural history of tuberculosis: the implications of age-dependent risks of disease and the role of reinfection. Epidemiol Infect 119:183
38. World Health Organization (2009) Global Tuberculosis Control 2009: epidemiology, strategy, financing. World Health Organization, Geneva
39. Selwyn PA, Hartel D, Lewis VA et al (1989) A prospective study of the risk of tuberculosis among intravenous drug users with human immunodeficiency virus infection. N Engl J Med 320:545

40. Bocchino M, Galati D, Sanduzzi A et al (2005) Role of mycobacteria-induced monocyte/macrophage apoptosis in the pathogenesis of human tuberculosis. Int J Tuberc Lung Dis 9:375
41. Patel NR, Swan K, Li X et al (2009) Impaired *M. tuberculosis*-mediated apoptosis in alveolar macrophages from HIV+ persons: potential role of IL-10 and BCL-3. J Leukoc Biol 86:53
42. Burman WJ, Jones BE (2003) Clinical and radiographic features of HIV-related tuberculosis. Semin Respir Infect 18:263
43. Schluger NW, Rom WN (1998) The host immune response to tuberculosis. Am J Respir Crit Care Med 157:679
44. Moore D, Liechty C, Ekwaru P et al (2007) Prevalence, incidence and mortality associated with tuberculosis in HIV-infected patients initiating antiretroviral therapy in rural Uganda. AIDS 21:713
45. Schluger NW, Perez D, Liu YM (2002) Reconstitution of immune responses to tuberculosis in patients with HIV infection who receive antiretroviral therapy. Chest 122:597
46. Sutherland R, Yang H, Scriba TJ et al (2006) Impaired IFN-gamma-secreting capacity in mycobacterial antigen-specific CD4 T cells during chronic HIV-1 infection despite long-term HAART. AIDS 20:821
47. Toossi Z (2003) Virological and immunological impact of tuberculosis on human immunodeficiency virus type 1 disease. J Infect Dis 188:1146
48. Goletti D, Weissman D, Jackson RW et al (1996) Effect of *Mycobacterium tuberculosis* on HIV replication. Role of immune activation. J Immunol 157:1271
49. Toossi Z, Mayanja-Kizza H, Hirsch CS et al (2001) Impact of tuberculosis on HIV-1 activity in dually infected patients. Clin Exp Immunol 123:233
50. Mayanja-Kizza H, Wu M, Aung H et al (2009) The interaction of monocyte chemoattractant protein-1 and tumor necrosis factor-alpha in *Mycobacterium tuberculosis*-induced HIV-1 replication at sites of active tuberculosis. Scand J Immunol 69:516
51. Sunderam G, McDonald RJ, Maniatis T et al (1986) Tuberculosis as a manifestation of the acquired immunodeficiency syndrome (AIDS). JAMA 256:362
52. Small PM, Schecter GF, Goodman PC et al (1991) Treatment of tuberculosis in patients with advanced human immunodeficiency virus infection. N Engl J Med 324:289
53. Kaplan JE, Benson C, Holmes KK et al (2009) Guidelines for prevention and treatment of opportunistic infections in HIV-infected adults and adolescents: recommendations from CDC, the National Institutes of Health, and the HIV Medicine Association of the Infectious Diseases Society of America. MMWR Recomm Rep 58:1
54. Hesseling AC, Cotton MF, Fordham von Reyn C et al (2008) Consensus statement on the revised World Health Organization recommendations for BCG vaccination in HIV-infected infants. Int J Tuberc Lung Dis 12:1376
55. Bannister C, Bennett L, Carville A et al (2009) Evidence behind the WHO guidelines: hospital care for children: what is the evidence that BCG vaccination should not be used in HIV-infected children? J Trop Pediatr 55:78
56. Hesseling AC, Johnson LF, Jaspan H et al (2009) Disseminated Bacille Calmette-Guérin disease in HIV-infected South African infants. Bull World Health Organ 87:505
57. Lotte A, Wasz-Hockert O, Poisson N et al (1988) Second IUATLD study on complications induced by intradermal BCG-vaccination. Bull Int Union Tuberc Lung Dis 63:47
58. Mansoor N, Scriba TJ, de Kock M et al (2009) HIV-1 infection in infants severely impairs the immune response induced by Bacille Calmette-Guérin vaccine. J Infect Dis 199:982
59. Grouge JM, Zumla A (2003) Tuberculosis. In: Cook GC, Zumla A (eds) Manson's tropical diseases, 21st edn. WB Saunders, London, p 995
60. World Health Organization (2009) Guidelines for surveillance of drug resistance in tuberculosis, 4th ed. WHO/HTM/STB,2009,422. World Health Organization, Geneva
61. World Health Organization (2010) Multidrug and extensively drug resistant TB (M/XDR-TB) 2010 global report on surveillance and response. WHO/HTM/TB/2010.3. World Health Organization, Geneva

62. Singh N, Paterson DL (1998) *Mycobacterium tuberculosis* infection in solid-organ transplant recipients: impact and implications for management. Clin Infect Dis 27:1266
63. Muñoz P, Rodríguez C, Bouza E (2005) *Mycobacterium tuberculosis* infection in recipients of solid organ transplants. Clin Infect Dis 40:581
64. Aguado JM, Singh N (2011) Tuberculosis and organ transplantation. In: Schlossberg D (ed) Tuberculosis and nontuberculous mycobacterial infections, 6th edn. ASM Press, Washington, DC, p 498
65. Bravo C, Roldán J, Roman A et al (2005) Tuberculosis in lung transplant recipients. Transplantation 79:59
66. Morales P, Briones A, Torres JJ et al (2005) Pulmonary tuberculosis in lung and heart-lung transplantation: fifteen years of experience in a single center in Spain. Transplant Proc 37:4050
67. Torre-Cisneros J, Doblas A, Aguado JM et al (2009) Tuberculosis after solid-organ transplant: incidence, risk factors, and clinical characteristics in the RESITRA (Spanish Network of Infection in Transplantation) cohort. Clin Infect Dis 48:1657
68. Basiri A, Hosseini-Moghaddam SM, Simforoosh N et al (2008) The risk factors and laboratory diagnostics for post renal transplant tuberculosis: a case-control, country-wide study on definitive cases. Transpl Infect Dis 10:231
69. Qunibi WY, Al-Sibai MB, Taher S et al (1990) Mycobacterial infection after renal transplantation-report of 14 cases and review of the literature. Q J Med 77:1039
70. Aguado JM, Herrero JA, Gavaldá J et al (1997) Clinical presentation and outcome of tuberculosis in kidney, liver, and heart transplant recipients in Spain. Spanish Transplantation Infection Study Group, GESITRA. Transplantation 63:1278
71. Woeltje KF, Mathew A, Rothstein M et al (1998) Tuberculosis infection and anergy in hemodialysis patients. Am J Kidney Dis 31:848
72. Dutt AK (2011) Epidemiology and host factors. In: Schlossberg D (ed) Tuberculosis and nontuberculous mycobacterial infections, 6th edn. ASM Press, Washington, DC, p 11
73. Gomez Reino JJ, Carmona L, Valverde VR et al (2003) Treatment of rheumatoid arthritis with tumor necrosis factor inhibitors may predispone to significant increase in tuberculosis risk: a multicenter active surveillance report. Artritis Rheum 48:2122
74. Bass JB Jr, Farer LS, Hopewell PC et al (1994) Treatment of tuberculosis and tuberculosis infection in adults and children. American Thoracic Society and the Centers for Disease Control and Prevention. Am J Respir Crit Care Med 149:1359
75. American Thoracic Society, Centers for Disease Control Society (1994). Treatment of tuberculosis and tuberculosis infection in adults and children. Am J Respir Crit Care Med 149:1359
76. Joint Statement of the American Thoracic Society (ATS) and the Centers for Disease Control and Prevention (CDC) (2000) Targeted tuberculin testing and treatment of latent tuberculosis infection. Am J Respir Crit Care Med 161:S221
77. Bovornkitti S, Kangsadal P, Sathirapat P et al (1960) Reversion and reconversion rate of tuberculin skin reactions in correction with the use of prednisone. Dis Chest 38:51
78. Schatz M, Patterson R, Kloner R et al (1976) The prevalence of tuberculosis and positive tuberculin skin tests in a steroid-treated asthmatic population. Ann Intern Med 84:261
79. Kim HA, Yoo CD, Baek HJ et al (1998) *Mycobacterium tuberculosis* infection in a corticosteroid-treated rheumatic disease patient population. Clin Exp Rheumatol 16:9
80. Jick SS, Lieberman ES, Rahman MU et al (2006) Glucocorticoid use, other associated factors, and the risk of tuberculosis. Arthritis Rheum 55:19
81. Grange JM, Ustianowski A, Zumla A (1998) Tuberculosis and pregnancy. In: Diwan V, Thorson A, Winkvist A (eds) Gender and tuberculosis. Nordic School of. Public Health, Götenberg, p 77
82. Menzies D, Fanning A, Yuan L et al (1995) Tuberculosis among health care workers. N Engl J Med 332:92
83. Menzies D, Joshi R, Pai M (2007) Risk of tuberculosis infection and disease associated with work in health care settings. Int J Tuberc Lung Dis 11:593

84. Sepkowitz KA (1994) Tuberculosis and the health care worker: a historical perspective. Ann Intern Med 120:71
85. McFarland JW, Hickman C, Osterholm M et al (1993) Exposure to *Mycobacterium tuberculosis* during air travel. Lancet 342:112
86. Driver CR, Valway SE, Morgan WM et al (1994) Transmission of *Mycobacterium tuberculosis* associated with air travel. JAMA 272:1031
87. Centers for Disease Control and Prevention (CDC) (1995) Exposure of passengers and flight crew to *Mycobacterium tuberculosis* on commercial aircraft, 1992–1995. MMWR Morb Mortal Wkly Rep 44:137
88. Comstock GW (1978) Tuberculosis in twins: a re-analysis of the Prophit survey. Am Rev Respir Dis 117:621
89. Crowle AJ, Elkins N (1990) Relative permissiveness of macrophages from black and white people for virulent tubercle bacilli. Infect Immun 58:632
90. Sead WW, Senner JW, Reddick WT et al (1990) Racial differences in susceptibility to infection by *Mycobacterium tuberculosis*. N Engl J Med 322:422
91. Delgado JC, Baena A, Thim S et al (2002) Ethnic-specific genetic associations with pulmonary tuberculosis. J Infect Dis 186:1463
92. Al-Arif LI, Goldstein RA, Attronti LF et al (1979) HLA-Bw15 and tuberculosis in a North American black population. Am Rev Respir Dis 120:1275
93. Bellamy R, Ruwende C, Corrah T et al (1998) Variations in the NRAMP1 gene and susceptibility to tuberculosis in West Africans. N Engl J Med 338:640
94. Goldfeld AE, Delgado JC, Thim S et al (1998) Association of an HLA-DQ allele with clinical tuberculosis. JAMA 279:226
95. Oeltmann JE, Kammerez JS, Pevzner ES et al (2009) Tuberculosis and substance abuse in the United States, 1997–2006. Arch Intern Med 169:189
96. Deiss RG, Rodwell TC, Garfein RS (2009) Tuberculosis and illicit drug use: review and update. Clin Infect Dis 48:72
97. Lönnroth K, Williams BG, Stadlin S et al (2008) Alcohol use as a risk factor for tuberculosis – a systematic review. BMC Public Health 8:289
98. Bates MN, Khalakdina A, Pai M et al (2007) Risk of tuberculosis from exposure to tobacco smoke: a systematic review and meta-analysis. Arch Intern Med 167:335
99. Brudney K, Dobkin J (1991) Resurgent tuberculosis in New York City. Human immunodeficiency virus, homeless, and the decline of tuberculosis control programs. Am Rev Respir Dis 144:745
100. Concato J, Rom WN (1994) Endemic tuberculosis among homeless men in New York City. Arch Intern Med 154:2069
101. Esteban J, Alonso-Rodríguez N (2011) *Mycobacterium bovis* and other uncommon members of the *Mycobacterium tuberculosis* complex. In: Schlossberg D (ed) Tuberculosis and nontuberculous mycobacterial infections, 6th edn. ASM Press, Washington, DC, p 607
102. Grange JM, Yates MD (1994) Zoonotic aspects of *Mycobacterium bovis* infection. Vet Microbiol 40:137
103. Calmate A (1936) L'infection bacillaire et la tuberculose, 4h edn. Masson et Cie, Paris
104. Aranaz A, Cousins D, Mateos A et al (2003) Elevation of *Mycobacterium tuberculosis* subsp. *caprae* Aranaz et al. 1999 to species rank as *Mycobacterium caprae* comb. nov., sp. nov. Int J Syst Evol Microbiol 53:1785
105. Cousins DV, Bastida R, Cataldi A et al (2003) Tuberculosis in seals caused by a novel member of the *Mycobacterium tuberculosis* complex: *Mycobacterium pinnipedii* sp. nov. Int J Syst Evol Microbiol 53:1305
106. Niemann S, Kubica T, Bange FC et al (2004) The species *Mycobacterium africanum* in the light of new molecular markers. J Clin Microbiol 42:3958
107. Meyer CG, Scarisbrick G, Niemann S et al (2008) Pulmonary tuberculosis: virulence of *Mycobacterium africanum* and relevance in HIV co-infection. Tuberculosis (Edinburgh). 88:482

108. de Jong BC, Adetifa I, Walther B et al (2010) Differences between tuberculosis cases infected with *Mycobacterium africanum*, West African type 2, relative to Euro-American *Mycobacterium tuberculosis*: an update. FEMS Immunol Med Microbiol 58:102
109. Aranaz A, Liébana E, Gómez-Mampaso E et al (1999) *Mycobacterium tuberculosis* subsp. *caprae* subsp. nov.: a taxonomic study of a new member of the *Mycobacterium tuberculosis* complex isolated from goats in Spain. Int J Syst Bacteriol 49:1263
110. Prodinger WM, Brandstätter A, Naumann L et al (2005) Characterization of *Mycobacterium caprae* isolates from Europe by mycobacterial interspersed repetitive unit genotyping. J Clin Microbiol 43:4984
111. Kubica T, Rüsch-Gerdes S, Niemann S (2003) *Mycobacterium bovis* subsp. *caprae* caused one-third of human *M. bovis*-associated tuberculosis cases reported in Germany between 1999 and 2001. J Clin Microbiol 41:3070
112. Rodríguez E, Sánchez LP, Pérez S et al (2009) Human tuberculosis due to *Mycobacterium bovis* and *M. caprae* in Spain, 2004–2007. Int J Tuberc Lung Dis 13:1536
113. Kremer K, van Soolingen D, van Embden J et al (1998) *Mycobacterium microti*: more widespread than previously thought. J Clin Microbiol 36:2793
114. van Soolingen D, van der Zanden AG, de Haas PE et al (1998) Diagnosis of *Mycobacterium microti* infections among humans by using novel genetic markers. J Clin Microbiol 36:1840
115. Foudraine NA, van Soolingen D, Noordhoek GT et al (1998) Pulmonary tuberculosis due to *Mycobacterium microti* in a human immunodeficiency virus-infected patient. Clin Infect Dis 27:1543
116. Kiers A, Klarenbeek A, Mendelts B et al (2008) Transmission of *Mycobacterium pinnipedii* to humans in a zoo with marine mammals. Int J Tuberc Lung Dis 12:1469
117. van Soolingen D, Hoogenboezem T, de Haas PE et al (1997) A novel pathogenic taxon of the *Mycobacterium tuberculosis* complex, Canetti: characterization of an exceptional isolate from Africa. Int J Syst Bacteriol 47:1236
118. Miltgen J, Morillon M, Koeck JL et al (2002) Two cases of pulmonary tuberculosis caused by *Mycobacterium tuberculosis* subsp *canettii*. Emerg Infect Dis 8:1350
119. Wells WF (1934) On airborne infection: study 11, droplets and droplet nuclei. Am J Hyg 20:611
120. Louden RG, Roberts RM (1966) Droplet expulsion from the respiratory tract. Am Rev Respire Dis 95:435
121. Ayele WY, Neill SD, Zingstag J et al (2004) Bovine tuberculosis: an old disease but a new threat to Africa. Int J Tuberc Lung Dis 8:924
122. LoBue PA, Betancourt W (2003) peter C. Epidemiology of *Mycobacterium bovis* disease in San Diego Country, 1994-2000. Int J Tuberc Lung Dis 7:180
123. Hlvasa MC, Moonan PK, Cowan LS et al (2008) Human tuberculose due to *Mycobacterium bovis* in the United States, 1995-2005. Clin Infect Dis 47:1608
124. Frampton MW (1992) An outbreak of tuberculosis among hospital personnel caring for a patient with a skin ulcer. Ann Intern Med 117:312
125. Templeton GL, Illing LA, Young L et al (1995) The risk for transmission of *Mycobacterium tuberculosis* at the bedside and during autopsy. Ann Intern Med 122:922
126. Sutherland I (1976) Recent studies in the epidemiology of tuberculosis, based on the risk of being infected with tubercle bacilli. Adv Tuberc Res 19:1
127. Styblo K (1984) Epidemiology of tuberculosis. VEB Gustav Fisher Verlag Jena, Hague, p 82
128. Dannenberg AM Jr, Converse PJ (2011) Pathophysiology and immunology. In: Schlossberg D (ed) Tuberculosis and nontuberculous mycobacterial infections, 6th edn. ASM Press, Washington, DC, p 29
129. Dannenberg AM Jr (1978) Pathogenesis of pulmonary tuberculosis in man and animals: protection of personnel against tuberculosis. In: Montali R (ed) Mycobacterial infections of zoo animals. Smithsonian Institution Press, Washington, DC, p 65
130. Jensen PA, Lambert LA, Iademarco MF et al (2005) Guidelines for preventing the transmission of *Mycobacterium tuberculosis* in health-care settings, 2005. MMWR Recomm Rep 54:1

131. Fleischmann RD, Alland D, Eisen JA et al (2002) Whole-genome comparison of *Mycobacterium tuberculosis* clinical and laboratory strains. J Bacteriol 184:5479
132. Brodin P, Eiglmeier K, Marmiesse M et al (2002) Bacterial artificial chromosome-based comparative genomic analysis identifies *Mycobacterium microti* as a natural ESAT-6 deletion mutant. Infect Immun 70:5568
133. Manabe YC, Scott CP, Bishai WR (2002) Naturally attenuated, orally administered *Mycobacterium microti* as a tuberculosis vaccine is better than subcutaneous *Mycobacterium bovis* BCG. Infect Immun 70:1566
134. Behr MA, Small PM (1999) A historical and molecular phylogeny of BCG strains. Vaccine 17:915
135. Behr MA, Wilson MA, Gill WP et al (1999) Comparative genomics of BCG vaccines by whole-genome DNA microarray. Science 284:1520
136. Domenech P, Reed MB (2009) Rapid and spontaneous loss of phthiocerol dimycocerosate (PDIM) from *Mycobacterium tuberculosis* grown in vitro: implications for virulence studies. Microbiology 155:3532
137. Converse PJ, Eisenach KD, Theus SA et al (2010) The impact of mouse passaging of *Mycobacterium tuberculosis* strains prior to virulence testing in the mouse and guinea pig aerosol models. PLoS One 5:e10289
138. Lurie MB, Dannenberg AM (1965) Macrophage function in infectious disease with inbred rabbits. Bacteriol Rev 29:466
139. Stead WW (2001) Variation in vulnerability to tuberculosis in America today: random, or legacies of different ancestral epidemics? Int J Tuberc Lung Dis 5:807
140. Dannenberg AM Jr (1993) Immunopathogenesis of pulmonary tuberculosis. Hosp Pract (Off Ed) 28:51
141. Bellamy R, Ruwende C, Corrah T et al (1999) Tuberculosis and chronic hepatitis B virus infection in Africans and variation in the vitamin D receptor gene. J Infect Dis 179:721
142. Casanova JL, Abel L (2002) Genetic dissection of immunity to mycobacteria: the human model. Annu Rev Immunol 20:581
143. Malik S, Schurr E (2002) Genetic susceptibility to tuberculosis. Clin Chem Lab Med 40:863
144. Goldberg MF, Saini NK, Porcelli SA (2014) Evasion of innate and adaptive immunity by *Mycobacterium tuberculosis*. Microbiol Spectr 2:MGM2-0005-2013
145. Sia JK, Georgieva M, Rengarajan J (2015) Innate immune defenses in human tuberculosis: an overview of the interactions between *Mycobacterium tuberculosis* and innate immune cells. J Immunol Res 2015:747543
146. Lerner TR, Borel S, Gutierrez MG (2015) The innate immune response in human tuberculosis. Cell Microbiol 17:1277
147. Chaves AS, Rodriguez MF, Mattos AM et al (2015) Challenging *Mycobacterium tuberculosis* dormancy mechanisms and their immunodiagnostic potential. Braz J Infect Dis 19:636
148. Amaral EP, Lasunaskaia EB, D'Império-Lima MR (2016) Innate immunity in tuberculosis: how the sensing of mycobacteria and tissue damage modulates macrophage death. Microbes Infect. 18(1):11–20
149. Dannenberg AM Jr (2006) Pathogenesis of human tuberculosis: insights from the rabbit model. ASM Press, Washington, DC
150. Dannenberg AM Jr (2010) Perspectives on clinical and preclinical testing of new tuberculosis vaccines. Clin Microbiol Rev 23:781
151. Wahl SM, McCartney-Francis N, Hunt DA et al (1987) Monocyte interleukin 2 receptor gene expression and interleukin 2 augmentation of microbicidal activity. J Immunol 139:1342
152. Toossi Z, Sedor JR, Lapurga JP et al (1990) Expression of functional interleukin 2 receptors by peripheral blood monocytes from patients with active pulmonary tuberculosis. J Clin Invest 85:1777
153. Moncada S, Palmer RM, Higgs EA (1991) Nitric oxide: physiology, pathophysiology, and pharmacology. Pharmacol Rev 43:109

154. Green SJ, Nacy CA, Meltzer MS (1991) Cytokine-induced synthesis of nitrogen oxides in macrophages: a protective host response to *Leishmania* and other intracellular pathogens. J Leukoc Biol 50:93
155. Fenton MJ, Riley LW, Schlesinger LS (2005) Receptor-mediated recognition of *Mycobacterium tuberculosis* by hosts cells. In: Cole ST, Eisenach KD, McMurray DN et al (eds) Tuberculosis and the tubercle bacillus. ASM Press, Washington, DC, p 405
156. Means TK, Wang S, Lien E et al (1999) Human Toll-like receptors mediate cellular activation by *Mycobacterium tuberculosis*. J Immunol 163:3920
157. North RJ, Jung YJ (2004) Immunity to tuberculosis. Annu Rev Immunol 22:599
158. Russel DG (2005) *Mycobacterium tuberculosis*: the indigestible microbe. In: Cole ST, Eisenach KD, McMurray DN et al (eds) Tuberculosis and the tubercle bacillus. ASM Press, Washington, DC, p 427
159. Armstrong JA, Hart PD (1971) Response of cultured macrophages to *Mycobacterium tuberculosis*, with observations on fusion of lysosomes with phagosomes. J Exp Med 134:713
160. Peters J (2001) Entry and survival of pathogenic mycobacteria in macrophages. Microbes Infect 3:249
161. Russell DG (2001) *Mycobacterium tuberculosis*: here today, and here tomorrow. Nat Rev Mol Cell Biol 2:569
162. Tsolaki AG (2009) Innate immune recognition in tuberculosis infection. Adv Exp Med Biol 653:185
163. Nouailles G, Dorhoi A, Koch M et al (2014) CXCL5-secreting pulmonary epithelial cells drive destructive neutrophilic inflammation in tuberculosis. J Clin Invest 124:1268
164. Harriff MJ, Cansler ME, Toren KG et al (2014) Human lung epithelial cells contain *Mycobacterium tuberculosis* in a late endosomal vacuole and are efficiently recognized by $CD8^+$ T cells. PLoS One 9:e97515
165. Altare F, Durandy A, Lammas D et al (1998) Impairment of mycobacterial immunity in human interleukin-12 receptor deficiency. Science 280:1432
166. Altare F, Lammas D, Revy P et al (1998) Inherited interleukin 12 deficiency in a child with Bacille Calmette-Guérin and *Salmonella enteritidis* disseminated infection. J Clin Invest 102:2035
167. Picard C, Fieschi C, Altare F et al (2002) Inherited interleukin-12 deficiency: IL12B genotype and clinical phenotype of 13 patients from six kindreds. Am J Human Genetics 70:336
168. Fieschi C, Dupuis S, Catherinot E et al (2003) Low penetrance, broad resistance, and favorable outcome of interleukin 12 receptor beta1 deficiency: medical and immunological implications. J Exp Med 197:527
169. Velez DR, Wejse C, Stryjewski ME et al (2010) Variants in toll-like receptors 2 and 9 influence susceptibility to pulmonary tuberculosis in Caucasians, African-Americans, and West Africans. Hum Genet 127:65
170. Ma X, Liu Y, Gowen BB et al (2007) Full-exon resequencing reveals toll-like receptor variants contribute to human susceptibility to tuberculosis disease. PLoS One 2:e1318
171. Davila S, Hibberd ML, Hari Dass R et al (2008) Genetic association and expression studies indicate a role of toll-like receptor 8 in pulmonary tuberculosis. PLoS Genet 4:e1000218
172. Bellamy R, Ruwende C, Corrah T et al (1998) Assessment of the interleukin 1 gene cluster and other candidate gene polymorphisms in host susceptibility to tuberculosis. Tuber Lung Dis 79:83
173. Wilkinson RJ, Patel P, Llewelyn M et al (1999) Influence of polymorphism in the genes for the interleukin (IL)-1 receptor antagonist and IL-1beta on tuberculosis. J Exp Med 189:1863
174. Wilkinson RJ, Llewelyn M, Toossi Z et al (2000) Influence of vitamin D deficiency and vitamin D receptor polymorphisms on tuberculosis among Gujarati Asians in West London: a case-control study. Lancet 355:618
175. Fabri M, Stenger S, Shin DM et al (2011) Vitamin D is required for IFN-gamma-mediated antimicrobial activity of human macrophages. Sci Transl Med 3:104ra102

176. Rook GA, Steele J, Fraher L et al (1986) Vitamin D3, gamma interferon, and control of proliferation of *Mycobacterium tuberculosis* by human monocytes. Immunology 57:159
177. Martineau AR, Wilkinson KA, Newton SM et al (2007) IFN-gamma and TNF-independent vitamin D-inducible human suppression of mycobacteria: the role of cathelicidin LL-37. J Immunol 178:7190
178. Procop GW, Roberts GD (2011) Laboratory diagnosis and susceptibility testing. In: Schlossberg D (ed) Tuberculosis and nontuberculous mycobacterial infections, 6th edn. ASM Press, Washington, DC, p 66
179. Goto M, Oka S, Okuzumi K et al (1991) Evaluation of acridinium-ester-labeled DNA probes for identification of *Mycobacterium tuberculosis* and *Mycobacterium avium-Mycobacterium intracellulare* complex in culture. J Clin Microbiol 29:2473
180. Alcaide F, Benítez MA, Escribà JM et al (2000) Evaluation of the BACTEC MGIT 960 and the MB/BacT systems for recovery of mycobacteria from clinical specimens and for species identification by DNA AccuProbe. J Clin Microbiol 38:398
181. Sandin RL (1996) Polymerase chain reaction and other amplification techniques in mycobacteriology. Clin Lab Med 16:617
182. Shrestha NK, Tuohy MJ, Hall GS et al (2003) Detection and differentiation of *Mycobacterium tuberculosis* and nontuberculous mycobacterial isolates by real-time PCR. J Clin Microbiol 41:5121
183. Moore DF, Curry JI, Knott CA et al (1996) Amplification of rRNA for assessment of treatment response of pulmonary tuberculosis patients during antimicrobial therapy. J Clin Microbiol 34:1745
184. Piersimoni C, Scarparo C (2003) Relevance of commercial amplification methods for direct detection of *Mycobacterium tuberculosis* complex in clinical samples. J Clin Microbiol 41:5355
185. Bergmann JS, Woods GL (1996) Clinical evaluation of the Roche AMPLICOR PCR *Mycobacterium tuberculosis* test for detection of *M. tuberculosis* in respiratory specimens. J Clin Microbiol 34:1083
186. Catanzaro A, Davidson B, Fujiwara PL et al (1997) Rapid diagnostic tests for tuberculosis: what is the appropriate use? American Thoracic Society Workshop. Am J Respir Crit Care Med 155:1804
187. Centers for Disease Control and Prevention (CDC) (2009) Updated guidelines for the use of nucleic acid amplification tests in the diagnosis of tuberculosis. MMWR Morb Mortal Wkly Rep 58:7
188. Procop GW (2007) Molecular diagnostics for the detection and characterization of microbial pathogens. Clin Infect Dis 45:S99
189. Roberts GD, Goodman NL, Heifets L et al (1983) Evaluation of the BACTEC radiometric method for recovery of mycobacteria and drug susceptibility testing of *Mycobacterium tuberculosis* from acid-fast smear-positive specimens. J Clin Microbiol 18:689
190. Blanchard JS (1996) Molecular mechanisms of drug resistance in *Mycobacterium tuberculosis*. Annu Rev Biochem 65:215
191. García de Viedma D (2003) Rapid detection of resistance in *Mycobacterium tuberculosis*: a review discussing molecular approaches. Clin Microbiol Infect 9:349
192. Torres MJ, Criado A, Ruiz M et al (2003) Improved real-time PCR for rapid detection of rifampin and isoniazid resistance in *Mycobacterium tuberculosis* clinical isolates. Diagn Microbiol Infect Dis 45:207
193. Richeldi L (2006) An update on the diagnosis of tuberculosis infection. Am J Respir Crit Care Med 174:736
194. Siebert FB, Glenn JT (1944) Tuberculin purified protein derivate: preparation and analyses of a large quantity for standard. Am Rev Tuberc 44:9
195. Huebner RE, Schein MF, Bass JB Jr (1993) The tuberculin skin test. Clin Infect Dis 17:968
196. Andersen P, Doherty TM (2005) The success and failure of BCG – implications for a novel tuberculosis vaccine. Nat Rev Microbiol 3:656

197. Wang L, Turner MO, Elwood RK et al (2002) A meta-analysis of the effect of Bacille Calmette-Guérin vaccination on tuberculin skin test measurements. Thorax 57:804
198. Yates VM (2010) Mycobacterial infections. In: Burnst T, Breathnach S, Cox N et al (eds) Rook's textbook of dermatology, 8th edn. Wiley-Blackwell, Oxford, p 6
199. Comstock GW, Woolpert SF (1978) Tuberculin conversions: true or false? Am Rev Respir Dis 118:215
200. Thompson NJ, Glassroth JL, Snider DE Jr et al (1979) The booster phenomenon in serial tuberculin testing. Am Rev Respir Dis 119:587
201. Menzies D (1999) Interpretation of repeated tuberculin tests. Boosting, conversion, and reversion. Am J Respir Crit Care Med 159:15
202. Barnes PF, Mistry SD, Cooper CL et al (1989) Compartmentalization of a CD4+ T lymphocyte subpopulation in tuberculous pleuritis. J Immunol 142:1114
203. Barnes PF, Fong SJ, Brennan PJ et al (1990) Local production of tumor necrosis factor and IFN-gamma in tuberculous pleuritis. J Immunol 145:149
204. Toossi Z, Gogate P, Shiratsuchi H et al (1995) Enhanced production of TGF-beta by blood monocytes from patients with active tuberculosis and presence of TGF-beta in tuberculous granulomatous lung lesions. J Immunol 154:465
205. The Global Plan to Stop Tuberculosis (2003). http://www.who.int/gtb/publications/stb/cds_stb_2003_23/globalplan.en.pdf.203
206. Barnes PF (2001) Diagnosing latent tuberculosis infection: the 100-year upgrade. Am J Respir Crit Care Med 163:807
207. Barnes PF (2004) Diagnosing latent tuberculosis infection: turning glitter to gold. Am J Respir Crit Care Med 170:5
208. Kunst H (2006) Diagnosis of latent tuberculosis infection: the potential role of new technologies. Respir Med 100:2098
209. Lalvani A (2007) Diagnosing tuberculosis infection in the 21st century. New tools to tackle an old enemy. Chest 131:1898
210. Mahairas GG, Sabo PJ, Hickey MJ et al (1996) Molecular analysis of genetic differences between *Mycobacterium bovis* BCG and virulent *M. bovis*. J Bacteriol 178:1274
211. Lalvani A, Pathan AA, McShane H et al (2001) Rapid detection of *Mycobacterium tuberculosis* infection by enumeration of antigen-specific T cells. Am J Respir Crit Care Med 163:824
212. Chapman AL, Munkanta M, Wilkinson KA et al (2002) Rapid detection of active and latent tuberculosis infection in HIV-positive individuals by enumeration of *Mycobacterium tuberculosis*-specific T cells. AIDS 16:2285
213. Mazurek GH, Jereb J, Lobue P et al (2005) Guidelines for using the QuantiFERON-TB Gold test for detecting *Mycobacterium tuberculosis* infection, United States. MMWR Recomm Rep. 54(RR-15):49
214. Ferrara G, Losi M, D'Amico R et al (2006) Use in routine clinical practice of two commercial blood tests for diagnosis of infection with *Mycobacterium tuberculosis*: a prospective study. Lancet 367:1328
215. Lee JY, Choi HJ, Park IN et al (2006) Comparison of two commercial interferon-gamma assays for diagnosing *Mycobacterium tuberculosis* infection. Eur Respir J 28:24
216. Pathan AA, Wilkinson KA, Klenerman P et al (2001) Direct ex vivo analysis of antigen-specific IFN-gamma-secreting CD4 T cells in *Mycobacterium tuberculosis*-infected individuals: associations with clinical disease state and effect of treatment. J Immunol 167:5217
217. Lalvani A, Nagvenkar P, Udwadia Z et al (2001) Enumeration of T cells specific for RD1-encoded antigens suggests a high prevalence of latent *Mycobacterium tuberculosis* infection in healthy urban Indians. J Infect Dis 183:469
218. Ewer K, Millington KA, Deeks JJ et al (2006) Dynamic antigen-specific T-cell responses after point-source exposure to *Mycobacterium tuberculosis*. Am J Respir Crit Care Med 174:831
219. Chee CB, Khinmar KW, Gan SH et al (2007) Latent tuberculosis infection treatment and T-cell responses to *Mycobacterium tuberculosis*-specific antigens. Am J Respir Crit Care Med 175:282

220. Millington KA, Innes JA, Hackforth S et al (2007) Dynamic relationship between IFN-gamma and IL-2 profile of *Mycobacterium tuberculosis*-specific T cells and antigen load. J Immunol 178:5217
221. Elder DE, Elenitsas R, Johnson BL Jr et al (2005) Lever's histopathology of the skin, 9th edn. Lippncott Williams and Wilkins, Philadelphia, p 561
222. Adams DO (1975) The structure of mononuclear phagocytes differentiating in vivo. II. The effect of *Mycobacterium tuberculosis*. Am J Pathol 80:101
223. McCray MK, Esterly NB (1981) Cutaneous eruptions in congenital tuberculosis. Arch Dermatol 117:460
224. Fadda G (2012) Tuberculosis: novel approaches to an old disease. J Infect Dev Ctries 6:4
225. Bravo FG, Gotuzzo E (2007) Cutaneous tuberculosis. Clin Dermatol 25:173
226. Camminero J (2003) Guia de la tuberculosis para medicos specialists. International Union Against Tuberculosis and Respiratory Diseases, Paris, p 35
227. Morrone A, Muscardin LM, Bartoli F et al (1988) Imported dermatoses in Italy. J Eur Acad Dermatol Venereol 11:306
228. Laurenti P, Bruno S, Quaranta G et al (2012) Tuberculosis in sheltered homeless population of Rome: an integrated model of recruitment for risk management. Scientific World J 2012:396302
229. High WA, Evans CC, Hoang MP (2004) Cutaneous miliary tuberculosis in two patients with HIV infection. J Am Acad Dermatol 50:S110
230. Alsina M, Campo P, Toll A et al (2000) Papulonecrotic tuberculid in a human immunodeficiency virus type 1-seropositive patient. Br J Dermatol 143:232
231. Fernandes C, Maltez F, Lourenço S et al (2004) Papulonecrotic tuberculid in a human immunodeficiency virus type-1 patient with multidrug-resistant tuberculosis. J Eur Acad Dermatol Venereol 18:369
232. Yates VM, Ormerod LP (1977) Cutaneous tuberculosis in Blackburn district (UK): a 15 years prospective series. Br J Dermatol 136:483
233. Sehgal VN, Jani MK, Srivastaria G (1989) Changing patterns of cutaneous tuberculosis. Int J Dermatol 28:231
234. Sehgal VN, Wagh SA (1990) Cutaneous tuberculosis: current concept. Int J Dermatol 29:237
235. Visser AJ, Heyl T (1993) Skin tuberculosis as seen at Ga-Rankuwa Hospital. Clin Exp Dermatol 18:507
236. Hamada M, Urobe K, Moroi Y et al (2004) Epidemiology of cutaneous tuberculosis in Japan: a retrospective study from 1906 to 2002. Int J Dermatol 43:727
237. Sierra X (1995) Historia de la tuberculosis cutánea. Piel 10:118
238. Beyt BE Jr, Ortbals DW, Santa Cruz DJ et al (1981) Cutaneous mycobacteriosis: analysis of 34 cases with a new classification of the disease. Medicine (Baltimore) 60:95
239. Dinning WJ, Marston S (1985) Cutaneous and ocular tuberculosis: a review. J R Soc Med 78:576
240. Hill MK, Sanders CV (2011) Cutaneous tuberculosis. In: Schlossberg D (ed) Tuberculosis and nontuberculous mycobacterial infections, 6th edn. ASM Press, Washington, DC, p 409
241. Tigoulet F, Fournier V, Caumes E (2003) Clinical form of the cutaneous tuberculosis. Bull Soc Pathol Exot 96:362
242. Heilman KM, Muschenheim C (1965) Primary cutaneous tuberculosis resulting from mouth-to-mouth respiration. N Engl J Med 273:1035
243. Hole LE (1913) Tuberculosis acquired through ritual circumcision. JAMA 61:99
244. Bolgert M (1967) La tubercolose cutanée. Historique, clinique et evolution thérapeutique. Semin Hosp Paris 43:868
245. Valledor T, Exposito L, Costales F et al (1954) Tuberculosis primaria de la piel en la infancia. Rev Cubana Pediatr 26:147
246. Ara M, Seral C, Baselga C et al (2000) Primary tuberculous chancre caused by *Mycobacterium tuberculosis* after goring with a bull's horn. J Am Acad Dermatol 43:535
247. Scuderi G, Cardia L (1964) Nodular tuberculosis of the skin of the lids and the regional lymph glands. Rev Bras Oftal 23:183

248. Heycock JB, Noble TC (1961) Four cases of syringe-transmitted tuberculosis. Tubercle 42:25
249. Horney DA, Gaither JM, Cauer R et al (1985) Cutaneous inoculation tuberculosis secondary to jailhouse tattoing. Arch Dermatol 121:648
250. Nenoff P, Rytter S, Schubert H et al (2000) Multilocular inoculation tuberculosis of the skin after stay in Africa: detection by mycobacterial DNA using polymerase chain reaction. Br J Dermatol 143:226
251. Bjornstad R (1947) Tuberculous primary infection of the genitalia. Acta Dermatol Venereol (Stockh) 27:106
252. Angus BJ, Yates M, Conlon C et al (2001) Cutaneous tuberculosis of the penis and sexual transmission confirmed by molecular typing. Clin Infect Dis 33:E132
253. Fisher I, Orkin M (1966) Primary tuberculosis of the skin. JAMA 195:314
254. Goette DK, Jacobson KW, Doty DR (1978) Primary cutaneous inoculation tuberculosis of the skin. Arch Dermatol 114:567
255. Hoyt EM (1981) Primary inoculation tuberculosis. JAMA 245:1556
256. Kramer F, Sasse S, Simms J et al (1993) Primary cutaneous tuberculosis after a needlestick injury from a patient with AIDS and undiagnosed tuberculosis. Ann Intern Med 119:549
257. Minkowitz S, Brandt IJ, Rapp Y et al (1969) "Prosector's Wart" (cutaneous tuberculosis) in a medical student. Am J Clin Pathol 51:260
258. O'Donnell TF, Jurgenson FF, Weyerich NH (1971) An occupational hazard-tuberculosis paronychia. Arch Surg 103:757
259. Pereira CA, Webber B, Orson JM (1976) Primary tuberculosis complex of the skin. JAMA 235:942
260. Rytel MW, Davis ES, Prebil KJ (1970) Primary cutaneous inoculation tuberculosis. Am Rev Respir Dis 102:264
261. Sahn SA, Pierson DJ (1974) Primary cutaneous inoculation drug-resistant tuberculosis. Am J Med 57:676
262. Strand S (1946) Tubercular primary lesion on penis-cancer, penis venereal tuberculosis. Acta Dermatol Venereol 26:461
263. Shengold MA, Sheingold H (1951) Oral tuberculosis. Oral Surg 4:239
264. Weaver RA (1987) Tuberculosis of the tongue. JAMA 235:2418
265. Krawiecka E, Szponar E (2015) Tuberculosis of the oral cavity: an uncommon but still a live issue. Postępy Dermatol Alergol 32:302
266. Aquilar I, Graudos E, Palacios R et al (2007) Fatal case of tuberculosis chancre in a patient with AIDS. J Infect 54:137
267. Miller FJW, Cashman JM (1955) Peripheral tuberculosis lymphadenitis associated with a visible primary focus. Lancet i:1286
268. Grange JM, Noble WC, Yates MD et al (1988) Inoculation mycobacterioses. Clin Exp Dermatol 13:211
269. Lundgren R, Norman E, Asbert I (1987) Tuberculosis infection transmitted at autopsy. Tubercle 68:147
270. Mitchell PG (1954) Tuberculosis verrucosa cutis among Chineses in Hong Kong. Br J Dermatol 66:444
271. Wong KO, Lee KP, Chin SF (1968) Tuberculosis of the skin in Hong Kong. Br J Dermatol 80:424
272. Goh YS, Ong BH, Rajan VS (1974) Tuberculosis cutis in Singapore: a two year experience. Sing. Med J 15:223
273. Pereira MB, Gnomes MK, Pereira F (2000) Tuberculosis verrucosa cutis associated with tuberculous lymphadenitis. Int J Dermatol 39:856
274. Foo CCI, Tan HH (2005) A case of tuberculosis verrucosa cutis undiagnosed for 44 years and resulting in fixed-flexion deformity of the arm. Clin Exp Dermatol 30:149
275. Iizwa O, Aiba S, Tagami H (1991) Tuberculosis verrucosa cutis in a tumor like form. Br J Dermatol 125:79
276. Montgomery H (1937) Histopathology of various types of cutaneous tuberculosis. Arch Dermatol Syph 35:698

277. Massellis P, Gasparini G, Caputo R et al (1955) Tuberculosis verrucosa cutis which remained undiagnosed for forty-three years. Dermatology 191:145
278. Gruber PC, Whittam LR, du Vivier A (2002) Tuberculosis verrucosa cutis on the sole of the foot. Clin Exp Dermatol 27:188
279. Padmavathy L, Lakshmana RL, Ethirajan N et al (2007) Tuberculosis verrucosa cutis (TBVC)-foot with miliary tuberculosis. Ind J Tuberc 54:145
280. Tur E, Brenner S, Meiron Y (1996) Scrofuloderma (tuberculosis colliquativa cutis). Br J Dermatol 134:350
281. Kumar B, Rai R, Kaur I et al (2001) Childhood cutaneous tuberculosis: a study over 15 years from northen India. Int J Dermatol 40:26
282. Phandi D, Reddy BSN, Chowdhary S et al (2004) Cutaneous tuberculosis in Indian children: the importance of screening for involvement of internal organs. J Eur Acad Dermatol Venereol 18:546
283. Vashist P, Sahoo B, Kurana K et al (2007) Cutaneous tuberculosis in children and adolescents: a clinicohistological study. J Eur Acad Dermatol Venereol 21:40
284. Singal A, Sonthalia S (2010) Cutaneous tuberculosis in children: the Indian perspective. Indian J Dermatol Venereol Leprol 76:494
285. Barbagallo J, Tager P, Ingleton R et al (2002) Cutaneous tuberculosis: diagnosis and treatment. Am J Clin Dermatol 3:319
286. Kim GW, Park HJ, Kim HS et al (2012) Delayed diagnosis of scrofuloderma misdiagnosed as a bacterial abscess. Ann Dermatol 24:70
287. Sehgal VN, Srivastava G, Khurana VK et al (1987) An appraisal of epidemiologic, clinical, bacteriologic, histopathologic and immunologic parameters in cutaneous tuberculosis. Int J Dermatol 26:521
288. Ramesh V, Misra RS, Jain RK (1987) Secondary tuberculosis of the skin: clinical features and problems in laboratory diagnosis. Int J Dermatol 26:578
289. Cerimele D, Ena P (2013) Tuberculosis of the skin. In: Giannetti A, Del Forno C (eds) Textbook of dermatology and sexually transmitted diseases. Padova, Piccin Nuova Libreria, p 483
290. Ramesh V (2007) Sporotrichoid cutaneous tuberculosis. Clin Exp Dermatol 32:680
291. Mahaisaviriya P, Chaiprasert A, Manonukul J et al (2002) Scrofuloderma and Sweet's syndrome. Int J Dermatol 41:28
292. Deklotz C, Deklotz T (2012) Scrofuloderma. New Engl J Med 366:2215
293. Ratcliff DP (1973) Tuberculosis of the mandible. Br Deut J 135:122
294. Mignogna MD, Muzio LL, Favia G et al (2000) Oral tuberculosis: a clinical evaluation of 42 cases. Oral Dis 6:25
295. Nachbar F, Classen V, Nachbar T et al (1996) Oral tuberculosis: detection by polymerase chain reaction. Br J Dermatol 135:106
296. Fejer A (1989) Sur la question de la tuberculose des organes genitaux: à propos de deux cas très rares. Ann Dermatol Vénéréol 29:488
297. Sharma SK, Mohan A (2011) Miliary tuberculosis. In: Schlossberg D (ed) Tuberculosis and nontuberculous mycobacterial infections, 6th edn. ASM Press, Washington, DC, p 415
298. Libraty DH, Byrd TF (1996) Cutaneous miliary tuberculosis in AIDS era: case report and review. Clin Infect Dis 23:706
299. High WA, Evans CL, Hoang MP (2004) Cutaneous miliary tuberculosis in two patients with HIV infection. J Am Acad Dermatol 50(Suppl 5):S100
300. Stack RJ, Bickley LK, Coppel IG (1990) Miliary tuberculosis presenting as skin lesions in a patient with acquired immunodeficiency syndrome. J Am Acad Dermatol 23:1031
301. Rohatgi PK, Palazzolo JV, Saini NB (1992) Acute miliary tuberculosis of the skin in acquired immunodeficiency syndrome. J Am Acad Dermatol 26:356
302. Bassiri A, Chan NB, McLeod A et al (1993) Disseminated cutaneous infection due to *Mycobacterium tuberculosis* in a person with AIDS. Can Med Assoc J 148:577
303. Inwald D, Nelson M, Cramp M et al (1994) Cutaneous manifestations of mycobacterial infection in patients with AIDS. Br J Dermatol 130:111

304. Corbett EL, Crossley I, De Cook KM et al (1995) Disseminated cutaneous *Mycobacterium tuberculosis* in a patient with AIDS. Genitourin Med 71:308
305. Antinori S, Galimberti L, Tadini GL et al (1995) Tuberculosis cutis miliaris disseminata due to multidrug-resistant *Mycobacterium tuberculosis* in AIDS patients. Eur J Clin Microbiol Infect Dis 14:911
306. Hudson CP, Wood R, O'Keefe EA (1997) Cutaneous miliary tuberculosis in the AIDS era: case report and review. Clin Infect Dis. 25:1484
307. Antinori S, Bini T, Galimberti L et al (1997) Cutaneous miliary tuberculosis in a patient infected with human immunodeficiency virus. Clin Infect Dis 25:1484
308. Esquivel SP, Vigua L, Velazquez J et al (1998) Tuberculosis diseminada con manifestaciones cutànes en pacientes con sida. A proposito de 4 observaciones. Enferm Infecc Microbiol Clin 16:31
309. Daikos GL, Uttamchandani RB, Tuda C et al (1998) Disseminated miliary tuberculosis of the skin in patients with AIDS: report of four cases. Clin Infect Dis 27:205
310. Schermer DR, Simpson CG, Haserick JR et al (1969) Tuberculosis cutis miliaris acuta generalisata. Arch Dermatol 99:64
311. del Giudice P, Bernard E, Perrin C et al (2000) Unusual cutaneous manifestations of miliary tuberculosis. Clin Infect Dis 30:201–204
312. Kounis NG, Constantinidis K (1979) Unusual tuberculous skin manifestations. Practitioner 222:390
313. Kennedy C, Knowles GK (1975) Miliary tuberculosis presenting with skin lesions. Br Med J 3:356
314. Rietbroek RC, Dahlmans RP, Smedts F et al (1991) Tuberculosis cutis miliaris disseminata as a manifestation of miliary tuberculosis: literature review and report of a case of recurrent skin lesions. Rev Infect Dis 13:265
315. Kumar B, Muralidhar S (1999) Cutaneous tuberculosis: a twenty-year prospective study. Int J Tuberc Lung Dis 3:494
316. Bhutto AM, Solangi A, Khaskhely NM et al (2002) Clinical and epidemiological observations of cutaneous tuberculosis in Larkana, Pakistan. Int J Dermatol 41:159
317. Fenniche S, Ben Jennet S, Marrak H et al (2003) Cutaneous tuberculosis: anatomoclinical features and clinical course. Ann Dermatol Vénéréol 130:1021
318. Hay RT (2005) Cutaneous infection with *Mycobaterium tuberculosis*: how has this altered with the changing epidemiology of tuberculosis? Curr Op Infect Dis 18:93
319. Marcoval J, Servitje O, Moreno A et al (1992) Lupus vulgaris. Clinical, histopathologic, and bacteriologic study of 10 cases. J Am Acad Dermatol 26:404
320. Ghorpade A (2006) Tattoo inoculation lupus vulgaris in two Indian ladies. J Eur Acad Dermatol Venereol 20:476
321. Tan HH, Seow CS (2002) A review of cutaneous granulomas and lupus vulgaris following BCG vaccination in a skin hospital in Singapore. Ann Acad Med Singapore 31:663
322. Horwitz O (1960) The localization of lupus vulgaris of the skin. Acta Tuberc Scand 39(Suppl. 49):1
323. Steidl M, Neubert U, Volkenandt M et al (1993) Lupus vulgaris confirmed by polymerase-chain reaction. Br J Dermatol 129:314
324. McKee PH (1966) Pathology of the skin, 2nd edn. Mosby-Wolfe, St. Louis, p 36
325. Duhra P, Grattan CE, Ryatt KS (1988) Lupus vulgaris with numerous tubercle bacilli. Clin Exp Dermatol 13:31
326. Seuol M, Ozcan A, Aydin A et al (2000) Disseminated lupus vulgaris and papulonecrotic tuberculid: case report. Pediatr Dermatol 17:133
327. Motswaledi MH, Doman C (2007) Lupus vulgaris with squamous cell carcinoma. J Cutan Pathol 34:939
328. Forstrum L (1969) Carcinomatous changes in lupus vulgaris. Ann Clin Res 1:213
329. Cotterill JA (1988) Lupus vulgaris simulating a port-wine stain. Br J Dermatol 119:127
330. Ramam M, Mittal R, Ramesh V (2005) How soon does cutaneous tuberculosis respond to treatment? Implications for a therapeutic test of diagnosis. Int J Dermatol 44:121

331. Maejima H, Arai S, Ebata T et al (2007) Tuberculous gumma associated with idiopathic thrombocytopaenic purpura: report of a Japanese female patient. J Dermatol 34:86
332. Vidal D, Barnadas M, Pérez M et al (2001) Tuberculous gumma following venepuncture. Br J Dermatol 144:601
333. Kalaria VG, Kapila R, Schwartz RA (2000) Tuberculous gumma (cutaneous metastatic tuberculous abscess) with underlying lymphoma. Cutis 66:277
334. Difonzo EM, Lotti L, Salvini C et al (2006) Tuberculous gumma in a patient with cervical lymphadenitis. Int J Dermatol 45:1467
335. Mert A, Bilir M, Osturk R et al (2000) Tuberculous subcutaneous abscesses developing during miliary tuberculosis therapy. Scand J Infect Dis 32:37
336. Lee KE (1985) Tuberculosis presenting as carpal tunnel syndrome. J Hand Surg Am 10:242
337. Brown FS, Anderson RH, Burnett JW (1982) Cutaneous tuberculosis. J Am Acad Dermatol 6:101
338. Dogliotti M, Leibowitz M, Smith E (1979) Lupus vulgaris. An unusual fungating and ulcerated form in a black South African. Int J Dermatol 18:749
339. Lee NH, Choi EH, Lee WS et al (2000) Tuberculous cellulitis. Clin Exp Dermatol 25:222
340. Sehgal UN, Srivastava G, Ahuja P et al (1988) Unusual clinical manifestations of cutaneous tuberculosis. J Dermatol 15:334
341. Thami GP, Kaur S, Kanwar AJ et al (2002) Lichen scrofulosorum: a rare manifestation of a common disease. Pediatr Dermatol 19:122
342. Victor T, Jordaan HF, Van Niekerk DJ et al (1992) Papulonecrotic tuberculid. Identification of *Mycobacterium tuberculosis* DNA by polymerase chain reaction. Am J Dermatopathol 14:491
343. Degitz K, Steidl M, Thomas P et al (1993) Aetiology of tuberculids. Lancet 341:239
344. Baselga E, Margall N, Barnadas MA et al (1997) Detection of *Mycobacterium tuberculosis* DNA in lobular granulomatous panniculitis (erythema induratum, nodular vasculitis). Arch Dermatol 133:457
345. Ho CK, Ho MH, Chong LY (2006) Cutaneous tuberculosis in Hong Kong: an update. Hong Kong Med J 12:272
346. Evans RG, Warner J (1967) Lichen scrofulosorum following BCG. Arch Dis Child 42:448
347. Komatsu H, Terunuma A, Tabata N et al (1999) *Mycobacterium avium* infection of the skin associated with lichen scrofulosorum: report of three cases. Br J Dermatol 141:554
348. Ross GL, Chong H, Collyns T et al (2007) Lichen scrofulosorum caused by *Mycobacterium szulgai*: a new cause of a tuberculide reaction. Br J Dermatol 156:586
349. Beena KR, Ramesh V, Mukherjee A (2000) Lichen scrofulosorum – a series of eight cases. Dermatology 201:272
350. Singal A, Bhattacharya SN (2005) Lichen scrofulosorum: a prospective study of 39 patients. Int J Dermatol 44:489
351. Hudson PM (1976) Tuberculide (lichen scrofulosorum) secondary to osseous tuberculosis. Clin Exp Dermatol 1:391
352. Graham-Brown RAC, Sarkany I (1980) Lichen scrofulosorum with tuberculous dactylitis. Br J Dermatol 103:561
353. Torrelo A, Valverde E, Mediero IG et al (2000) Lichen scrofulosorum. Pediatr Dermatol 17:373
354. Pandhi D, Mehta S, Singal A (2007) Genital tuberculid in a female child: a new entity (childhood vulval tuberculid). Pediatr Dermatol 24:573
355. Aranayagam AV, Ash S, Russel Jones R (1994) Lichen scrofulosorum in a patient with AIDS. Clin Exp Dermatol 19:74
356. Morrison JGL, Fourile ED (1974) The papulonecrotic tuberculid: from Arthus reaction to lupus vulgaris. Br J Dermatol 91:263
357. Wilson-Jones E, Winkelmann RK (1986) Papulonecrotic tuberculid: a neglected disease in Western countries. J Am Acad Dermatol 14:815
358. Jordan HF, Van Niekerk DJ, Louw M (1994) Papulonecrotic tuberculid: a clinical, histopathological and immunohistochemical study of 15 patients. Am J Dermatopathol 16:474

359. De Bruyne JI, Van Creveld S, Prakken JR (1953) Papular tuberculid after BCG vaccination. Acta Derm Venereol (Stockh) 33:385
360. Figuereido A, Poiares-Baptista A, Branco M et al (1987) Papular tuberculid post-BCG vaccination. Int J Dermatol 26:291
361. Muto J, Kuroda K, Tajima S (2006) Papular tuberculides post-BCG vaccination: case report and review of the literature in Japan. Clin Exp Dermatol 31:611
362. Williams JT, Pulitzer DR, De Villez RL (1995) Papulonecrotic tuberculid secondary to disseminated *Mycobacterium avium* complex. Int J Dermatol 34:217
363. Nishigori C, Taniguchi S, Hayakawa M et al (1986) Penis tuberculides: papulonecrotic tuberculides on the glans penis. Dermatologica 172:93
364. Kumar B, Sharma VK (1987) Papulonecrotic tuberculides on glans penis. Dermatologica 174:151
365. Srivastava N, Solanski LS, Singh SP et al (2007) Papulonecrotic tuberculid on the glans: worm-eaten appearance. Int J Dermatol 46:1324
366. Milligan A, Chen K, Groham-Brown RAC (1990) Two tuberculides in one patient: a case report of papulonecrotic tuberculide and erythema induratum occurring together. Clin Exp Dermatol 15:21
367. Chuang YH, Kuo TT, Wang CM et al (1997) Simultaneous occurence of papulonecrotic tuberculid and erythema induratum and identification of *Mycobacterium tuberculosis* DNA by polymerase chain reaction. Br J Dermatol 137:276
368. Tanaka R, Matsuura H, Kobashia Y (2007) Clinical utility of an interferon-γ-based assay for mycobacteral detection in papulonecrotic tuberculid. Br J Dermatol 156:169
369. Bazin APE (1861) Leçons théoretiques et cliniques sur la scrofula, 2nd edn. Delahaye, Paris, p 146
370. Jordan HF, Schneider JW, Abdulla EAK (2000) Nodular tuberculid: a report of four patients. Pediatr Dermatol 17:183
371. Koga T, Kubota Y, Kiryu H et al (2001) Erythema induratum in a patient with active tuberculosis of the axillary lymph node: IFN-gamma release of specific T cells. Eur J Dermatol 11:48
372. Förström L, Hannuksela M (1970) Antituberculous treatment of erythema induratum of Bazin. Acta Derm Venereol (Stockh) 50:143
373. Schneider JW, Jordaan HF (1997) The histopathologic spectrum of erythema induratum of Bazin. Am J Dermatopathol 19:323
374. Chen YH, Yan JJ, Chao SC et al (2001) Erythema induratum: a clinicopathologic and polymerase chain reaction study. J Formos Med Assoc 100:244
375. Vieites B, Suárez-Peñaranda JM, Pérez Del Molino ML et al (2005) Recovery of *Mycobacterium tuberculosis* DNA in biopsies of erythema induratum–results in a series of patients using an improved polymerase chain reaction technique. Br J Dermatol 152:1394
376. Yagi M, Kawabata I, Izaki S et al (1994) Primary tuberculosis of the nasopharynx with erythema induratum of Bazin. J Otorhinolaryngol Relat Spec 56:291
377. Del Moral RF, Ereno C, Arrinda JM et al (1994) Erythema induratum of Bazin and active renal tuberculosis. J Am Acad Dermatol 31:288
378. Friedman PC, Husain S, Grossman ME (2005) Nodular tuberculid in a patient with HIV. J Am Acad Dermatol 53:S154
379. Motswaledi HM, Schultz EJ (2006) Superficial thrombophlebitic tuberculide. Int J Dermatol 45:1337
380. Medical Research Council Tuberculosis and Chest Disease Unit (1982) Tuberculosis in children in a national survey of notifications in England and Wales 1978–9. Arch Dis Chil 57:734
381. Tse GM, Poon CS, Ramachandram K et al (2004) Granulomatous mastitis: a clinicopathological review of 26 cases. Pathology 36:254
382. Elsiddig KE, Khalil EA, Elhag IA et al (2003) Granulomatous mammary disease: ten years' experience with fine needle aspiration cytology. Int J Tuberc Lung Dis 7:365
383. Mirsaeidi SM, Masjedi MR, Mansouri SD et al (2007) Tuberculosis of the breast: report of 4 clinical cases and literature review. East Mediterr Health J 13:670

384. Bani-Hani KE, Yaghan RJ, Matalka II et al (2004) Idiopathic granulomatous mastitis: time to avoid unnecessary mastectomies. Breast J 10:318
385. Ebenezer J, Samuel R, Mathew GC et al (2006) Primary oral tuberculosis: report of two cases. Indian J Dent Res 17:41
386. Nanda KDS, Mehta A, Marwaha M et al (2011) A disguised tuberculosis in oral buccal mucosa. Dent Res J. 8:154
387. Khammissa RA, Wood NH, Meyerov R et al (2011) Primary oral tuberculosis as an indicator of HIV infection. Patholog Res Int 2011:893295
388. Kakisi OK, Kechagia AS, Kakisis IK et al (2010) Tuberculosis of the oral cavity: a systematic review. Eur J Oral Sci 118:103
389. Awasthi S, Singh V, Nizamuddin M (2010) Tuberculosis of oral mucosa. Internet J Infect Dis 8, Number 2
390. Mohanapriya T, Singh KB, Arulappan T et al (2012) Lingual tuberculosis. Indian J Tuberc 59:39
391. Von Arx DP, Husain A (2001) Oral tuberculosis. Br Dent J 190:420
392. Dixit R, Sharma S, Nuwal P (2008) Tuberculosis of oral cavity. Indian J Tuberc 55:51
393. Kannan S, Thakkar P, Dcruz AK (2011) Tuberculosis masquerading as oral malignancy. Indian J Med Paediatr Oncol 32:180
394. Sorris ST, Fazio RC, Fang L (2002) Oral medicine secrets. Hannley & Belrus, Philadelphia, p 85
395. Kamala R, Sinha A, Srivastava A et al (2011) Primary tuberculosis of the oral cavity. Indian J Dermatol Res 22:835
396. Ram H, Kumar S, Mehrotra S et al (2012) Tubercular ulcer mimicking squamous cell carcinoma of buccal mucosa. J Maxillofac Oral Surg 11:105
397. Sureshchandra B, Naveen Kumar N (2001) Detection of presence or absence of *Mycobacterium tuberculosis* in infected and uninfected pulp using a microbiological culture method-case series. Endodontology 23:6
398. Starke JR (2011) Tuberculosis in infants and children. In: Schlossberg D (ed) Tuberculosis and nontuberculous mycobacterial infections, 6th edn. ASM Press, Washington, DC, p 456
399. Kimerling M, Barker J, Bruce F et al (2000) Preventable childhood tuberculosis in Alabama: implications and opportunity. Pediatrics 105:e53
400. Khan EA, Starke JR (1995) Diagnosis of tuberculosis in children. Increased need for better methods. Emerg Infect Dis 1:115
401. Nelson LJ, Wells CD (2004) Global epidemiology of childhood tuberculosis. Int J Tuberc Lung Dis 8:636
402. Vashisht P, Sahoo B, Khurona N et al (2007) Cutaneous tuberculosis in children and adolescents: a clinicohistological study. J Eur Acad Dermatol Venereol 21:40
403. Kathuria S, Ramesh U (2010) Clinical profile of cutaneous tuberculosis in pediatric age. G Ital Dermatol Venereol 145:289
404. Newton SM, Brent AJ, Anderson S et al (2008) Paediatric tuberculosis. Lancet Infect Dis 8:498
405. Brent AJ, Anderson ST, Kampmann B et al (2008) Childhood tuberculosis: out of sight, out of mind? Trans R Soc Trop Med Hyg 102:217
406. Ramesh V, Misra RS, Beena KR et al (1999) A study of cutaneous tuberculosis in children. Pediatr Dermatol 16:264
407. Arya L, Koranne RV, Deb M (1999) Cutaneous tuberculosis in children a clinico-microbiological study. Indian J Dermatol Venereol Leprol 65:137
408. Webb EA, Hesseling AC, Schaaf HS et al (2009) High prevalence of *Mycobacterium tuberculosis* infection and disease in children and adolescents with type 1 diabetes mellitus. Int J Tuberc Lung Dis 13:868
409. Nelson LJ, Schneider E, Wells CD et al (2004) Epidemiology of childhood tuberculosis in the United States, 1993–2001: the need for continued vigilance. Pediatrics 114:333

410. Stout JE, Saharia KK, Nageswaran S et al (2006) Racial and ethnic disparities in pediatric tuberculosis in North Carolina. Arch Pediatr Adolesc Med 160:631
411. Ussery XT, Valway SE, McKenna M et al (1996) Epidemiology of tuberculosis among children in the United States: 1985 to 1994. Pediatr Infect Dis J 15:697
412. Lincoln EM (1965) Epidemics of tuberculosis. Bibl Tuberc 21:157
413. Wallgren A (1937) On contagiousness of children tuberculosis. Acta Pediatr 22:229
414. Curtis A, Ridzon R, Vogel R et al (1999) Extensive transmission of *Mycobacterium tuberculosis* from a child. N Eng J Med 341:1491
415. Starke RJ (2001) Transmission of *Mycobacterium tuberculosis* to and from children and adolescents. Seminar Pediatr Infect Dis 12:115
416. Centers for Disease Control and Prevention (2005) Guidelines for preventing the trasmission of *Mycobacterium tuberculosis* in health-care facilities. MMWR Recommend Rep 54(RR-17):1
417. Marais BJ, Wright CA, Schaaf HS et al (2006) Tuberculous lymphadenitis as a cause of persistent cervical lymphadenopathy in children from a tuberculosis-endemic area. Pediatr Infect Dis J 25:142
418. Wright CA, Hesseling AC, Banford C et al (2009) Fine-needle aspiration biopsy: a first-line diagnostic procedure in paediatric tuberculosis suspects with peripheral lymphadenopathy? Int J Tuberc Lung Dis 13:1373
419. Wright CA, Warren RM, Marais BJ (2009) Fine-needle aspiration biopsy: an undervalued diagnostic modality in paediatric mycobacterial disease. Int J Tuberc Lung Dis 13:1467
420. Shingadia D, Novelli V (2003) Diagnosis and treatment of tuberculosis in children. Lancet Infect Dis 3:624
421. American Academy of Pediatrics (2009) Red book: report of the Committe on Infections Diseases, 28th edn. American Academy of Pediatrics, Elk Grove Village
422. Connell TG, Ritz N, Paxton GA et al (2008) A three-way comparison of tuberculin skin testing, QuantiFERON-TB gold, and T-SPOT.TB in children. PLoS One 3:e2624
423. Bianchi L, Galli L, Moriondo M et al (2009) Interferon-gamma release assay improves the diagnosis of tuberculosis in children. Pediatr Infect Dis J 28:510
424. Nicol MP, Dauies MA, Wood K et al (2009) Comparison of T-SPOT.TB assay and tuberculin skin test for the evaluation of young children at high risk for tuberculosis in a community setting. Pediatrics 123:38
425. Lewinsohn DA, Lobato MN, Jereb JA (2010) Interferon-gamma release assays: new diagnostic tests for *Mycobacterium tuberculosis* infection and their use in children. Curr Opin Pediatr 22:71
426. Padmavathy L, Lakshmana Rao L, Pari T et al (2008) Lupus vulgaris and tuberculosis verrucosa cutis (TBVC)–a clinical, pathological and epidemiological study of 71 cases. Indian J Tuberc 55:203
427. Terranova M, Padovese V, Fornari U et al (2008) Clinical and epidemiological study of cutaneous tuberculosis in Northern Ethiopia. Dermatology 217:89
428. Mlika RB, Tounsi J, Fenniche S et al (2006) Childhood cutaneous tuberculosis: a 20-year retrospective study in Tunis. Dermatol Online J 12:11
429. Farsinejad K, Daneshpazhooh M, Sairafi H et al (2009) Lupus vulgaris at the site of BCG vaccination: report of three cases. Clin Exp Dermatol 34:e167
430. Sadeghi-Shabestari M, Rezaci N (2009) Disseminated Bacille Calmette-Guérin in Iranian children with severe combined immunodeficiency. Int J Infect Dis 13:e420
431. Talbot EA, Perkins MD, Silva SF et al (1997) Disseminated bacille Calmette-Guérin disease after vaccination: case report and review. Clin Infect Dis 24:1139
432. Neff TA (1986) Bronchoscopy and Bactec for the diagnosis of tuberculosis. State of the art, or a brief dissertation on the efficient search for the tubercle bacillus? Am Rev Respir Dis 133:962
433. Brisson-Noël A, Gicquel B, Lecossier D et al (1989) Rapid diagnosis of tuberculosis by amplification of mycobacterial DNA in clinical samples. Lancet ii:1069

434. Hance AJ, Grandchamp B, Lévy-Frébault V et al (1989) Detection and identification of mycobacteria by amplification of mycobacterial DNA. Mol Microbiol 3:843
435. Thierry D, Brisson-Noël A, Lévy-Frébault V et al (1990) Characterization of a *Mycobacterium tuberculosis* insertion sequence, IS6110, and its application in diagnosis. J Clin Microbiol 28:2668
436. Altamirano M, Kelly MT, Wong A et al (1992) Characterization of a DNA probe for detection of *Mycobacterium tuberculosis* complex in clinical samples by polymerase chain reaction. J Clin Microbiol 30:2173
437. Lee BW, Tan JA, Wong SC et al (1994) DNA amplification by the polymerase chain reaction for the rapid diagnosis of tuberculous meningitis. Comparison of protocols involving three mycobacterial DNA sequences, IS6110, 65 kDa antigen, and MPB64. J Neurol Sci 123:173
438. Eisenach KD, Cave MD, Bates JH et al (1990) Polymerase chain reaction amplification of a repetitive DNA sequence specific for *Mycobacterium tuberculosis*. J Infect Dis 161:977
439. Hsiao PF, Tzen CY, Chen HC et al (2003) Polymerase chain reaction based detection of *Mycobacterium tuberculosis* in tissues showing granulomatous inflammation without demonstrable acid-fast bacilli. Int J Dermatol 42:281
440. Penneys NS, Craig L, Leonardi MD et al (1993) Identification of *Mycobacterium tuberculosis* DNA in a case of lupus vulgaris. Arch Dermatol 129:1594
441. Dobbs TE, Webb RM. Chemotherapy of tuberculosis. In: Schlossberg D (ed) Tuberculosis and nontuberculous mycobacterial infections. 6th ed, Washington, DC, ASM Press, 2011:211:107
442. Grosset J (1980) Bacteriologic basis of short-course chemotherapy of tuberculosis. Clin Chest Med 1:231
443. Mitchinson D (1979) Basic mechanism of chemotherapy. Chest 76:s771
444. American Thoracic Society, Centers for Disease Control and Prevention, and Infections Diseases Society of America (2003) Treatment of tubercuolosis. MMWR Morb Mortal WKly Rep 52(RR11):1
445. National Collaborating Centre for Chronic Conditions (UK); Centre for Clinical Practice at NICE (UK). Royal College of Phisycians. Tuberculosis (2011) Clinical diagnosis and management of tuberculosis and measures for its prevention and control. Royal College of Physicians, London
446. Morse DI (1996) Directly observed therapy for tuberculosis. BMJ 312:719
447. Wang L, Takayama K (1972) Relationship between the uptake of isoniazid and its action on in vivo mycolic acid synthesis in *Mycobacterium tuberculosis*. Antimicrob Agents Chemother 2:438
448. Villarino ME, Ridzon R, Weismuller PC et al (1997) Rifampin preventive therapy for tuberculosis infection: experience with 157 adolescents. Am J Respir Crit Care Med 155:1735
449. Zhang Y, Wade MM, Scorpio A et al (2003) Mode of action of pyrazinamide: disruption of *Mycobacterium tuberculosis* membrane transport and energetics by pyrazinoic acid. J Antimicrob Chemother 52:790
450. Leibold JE (1966) The ocular toxicity of ethambutol and its relation to dose. Am NY Acad Sei 135:904
451. Feldman WH (1954) Streptomycin: some historical aspects of its development as a chemotherapeutic agent in tuberculosis. Am Rev Tuber 89:859
452. Moadebi S, Harder CK, Fitzgerald MJ et al (2007) Fluoroquinolones for the treatment of pulmonary tuberculosis. Drugs 67:2077
453. Seaworth BJ, Longfield RN (2011) Therapy of multidrug-resistant and extensively drug-resistant tuberculosis. In: Schlossberg D (ed) Tuberculosis and nontuberculous mycobacterial infections, 6th edn. ASM Press, Washington, DC, p 120
454. Lacoma A, Garcia-Sierra N, Prat C et al (2008) GenoType MTBDRplus assay for molecular detection of rifampin and isoniazid resistance in *Mycobacterium tuberculosis* strains and clinical samples. J Clin Microbiol 46:3660
455. Perriëns JH, St Louis ME, Mukadi YB et al (1995) Pulmonary tuberculosis in HIV-infected patients in Zaire. A controlled trial of treatment for either 6 or 12 months. N Engl J Med 332:779
456. Iseman MD (1993) Treatment of multidrug-resistant tuberculosis. N Engl J Med 329:784

457. Centers for Disease Control and Prevention (2006) Notice to readers: revised definition of extensively drug-resistant tuberculosis. MMWR Morb Mortal Wkly Rep 55:1176
458. Raviglione MC, Smith IM (2007) XDR tuberculosis–implications for global public health. N Engl J Med 356:656
459. Runsen ID, Harries AD, Heldad E et al (2010) Drug supply shortage in 2010: the inexcusable failure of global tuberculosis control. Int J. Tuber Lung Dis 16:253
460. Ramaswamy S, Musser JM (1998) Molecular genetic basis of antimicrobial agent resistance in *Mycobacterium tuberculosis*: 1998 update. Tuber Lung Dis 79:3
461. Dye C, Scheele S, Dolin P et al (1999) Consensus statement. Global burden of tuberculosis: estimated incidence, prevalence, and mortality by country. WHO Global Surveillance and Monitoring Project. JAMA 282:677
462. World Health Organization (2008) Guidelines for the programmatic management of drug-resistant tuberculosis. Emergency update 2008. World Health Organization, Geneva
463. Shin S, Guerra D, Rich M et al (2003) Treatment of multidrug-resistant tuberculosis during pregnancy: a report of 7 cases. Clin Infect Dis 36:996
464. Tam CM, Yew WW, Yuen KY (2009) Treatment of multidrug-resistant and extensively drug-resistant tuberculosis: current status and future prospects. Expert Rev Clin Pharmacol 2:405
465. Israel HL (1993) Chemoprophylaxis for tuberculosis. Respir Med 87:81
466. World Health Organization Global Tuberculosis Programme and UNAIDS (1988) Policy statement on preventive therapy against tuberculosis in people living with HIV. WHO, Geneva
467. Hawken HP, Muhindi DW (1999) Tuberculosis preventive therapy in HIV-infected persons: feasibility issues in developing countries. Int J Tuberc Lung Dis 3:646
468. Sutherland I, Lindgren I (1979) The protective effect of BCG vaccination as indicated by autopsy studies. Tubercle 60:225
469. Dannenberg AM Jr (2009) Liquefaction and cavity formation in pulmonary TB: a single method in rabbit skin to test inhibitors. Tuberculosis (Edinburgh) 89:243
470. Comstock GW (1988) Identification of an effective vaccine against tuberculosis. Am Rev Respir Dis 138:479
471. Crowle AJ (1988) Immunization against tuberculosis: what kind of vaccine? Infect Immun 56:2769
472. Seibert FB (1960) A theory of immunity in tuberculosis. Perspect Biol Med 3:264
473. Andersen P (2001) TB vaccines: progress and problems. Trends Immunol 22:160
474. Collins HL, Kaufmann SH (2001) Prospects for better tuberculosis vaccines. Lancet Infect Dis 1:21
475. Chara N, Yamada T (2001) Recombinant BCG vaccines. Vaccine 19:4089
476. Britton WJ, Palendira V (2003) Improving vaccines against tuberculosis. Immunol Cell Biol 81:34
477. Horwitz MA, Harth G, Dillon BJ et al (2005) Enhancing the protective efficacy of *Mycobacterium bovis* BCG vaccination against tuberculosis by boosting with *Mycobacterium tuberculosis* major secretory protein. Infect Immunol 73:4676

Mycobacterium bovis Skin Infection

3

Domenico Bonamonte, Angela Filoni, and Gianni Angelini

The bovine tubercle bacillus must firstly be placed in context among the other agents of tuberculosis [1–5]. In the early decades of the twentieth century, bacteriologists recognized four varieties of tubercle bacilli (human, bovine, avian and cold-blooded), depending on the life forms from which they were isolated. By the middle of the century, only two varieties were still recognized as agents of human and bovine tuberculosis (TB), namely *Mycobacterium tuberculosis* and *M. bovis* [6], respectively.

In the 1960s, another TB agent was isolated in Africa, and named *M. africanum* [7], but this was later seen to include two varieties [8]. Finally, in the 1980s it was found that two varieties of *M. tuberculosis* itself could also be distinguished: classical and Asian [9]. This group of organisms, to which *M. microti*, *M. pinnipedii*, *M. canettii*, and *M. caprae* were later added, is denominated the *M. tuberculosis* complex (Table 3.1). The bacillus Calmette-Guérin (BCG) was classed with *M. bovis* [10]. The avian and cold-blooded tubercle bacilli were then classified separately: the first, that includes *M. avium* and *M. intracellulare*, is included in the *M. avium* complex (together with *M. lepraemurium* and *M. paratuberculosis*), while the second includes *M. chelonae* and *M. fortuitum* [11].

D. Bonamonte, MD, PhD (✉)
Department of Biomedical Science and Human Oncology, University of Bary "Aldo Moro", Bari, Italy
e-mail: domenico.bonamonte@uniba.it

A. Filoni, MD
University of Bary "Aldo Moro", Bari, Italy

G. Angelini, MD
Professor of Dermatology, Former Professor and Chairman, University of Bary "Aldo Moro", Bari, Italy

D. Bonamonte, G. Angelini (eds.), *Mycobacterial Skin Infections*,
DOI 10.1007/978-3-319-48538-6_3

Table 3.1 *Mycobacterium tuberculosis* complex: some species and variants

Species	Variants	Common name
M. tuberculosis	Classical	Human tubercle bacillus
	Asian	
M. bovis	Classical	Bovine tubercle bacillus
	BCG	
M. africanum	Type I	African tubercle bacillus
	Type II	
M. microti		Vole bacillus

3.1 The Organism

A few years after Koch's discovery of the tubercle bacillus (1882), the American Theobald Smith demonstrated that there were constant phenotypical differences between the tubercule bacilli of human origin and those isolated from cattle, and so introduced a subdivision of the two species [12–13]. Much later, in 1970, the bovine tubercle bacillus was named *M. bovis* [6].

M. bovis (from Latin bos: bue) grows at the ideal temperature of 37°C in 21 or more (between 24 and 40) days. It is an ancient pathogen that causes disease in humans, as well as the majority of cases of TB in cattle and a large number of domesticated and wild mammal species [1, 14, 15]. For many years it was believed that in origin, the first pathogen was the bovine bacillus, while the human *M. tuberculosis* was a descendant that adapted to life in the human host around 10,000–15,000 years ago, associated with cattle domestication [3, 16]. Recent studies, however, have demonstrated that *M. bovis*, together with the other members of the *M. tuberculosis* complex, belong to a separate lineage of bacteria that shares a common ancestor with *M. tuberculosis* [16, 17].

M. bovis has a greater number of potential hosts than *M. tuberculosis*. Domestic cattle are considered its natural hosts and the principal reservoir of infections for humans and other animals [13, 18]. However, wild animals also have a potential role in the maintenance and spread of the disease [19]. At the beginning of the twentieth century, 20–40% of cattle in European herds were tuberculous [20]. Some of the most recent examples of infection from wild animals are from the badger in the United Kingdom and the Republic of Ireland [21, 22], the possum and the ferret in New Zealand [23], the red deer and wild boar in Spain [24], the Cape buffalo in parts of South Africa [25], and the white-tailed deer in Michigan (USA) [19]. Other demonstrated animal hosts of *M. bovis* infection include antelopes, camels, cats, dogs, pig, sheep, bison, hare, alpaca, llama, equines, foxes, goat, marsupials, mink, moles, and rats [1, 3, 20, 26].

Owing to being closely related, there are relatively few differences between *M. bovis* and *M. tuberculosis*, and so identifying the former is not easy [27, 28], even if culture differences between *M. tuberculosis* and *M. bovis* have been recognized since the discovery of both organisms. *M. bovis* requires pyruvate supplemental media because it is not able to use glycerol as a carbon source. For this reason it shows poor growth in pyruvate-free media like Löwenstein-Jensen, the medium

Table 3.2 Identification of species within the *Mycobacterium tuberculosis* complex (modified, by [28])

Species	Variant	TCH	NO_3	O_2	PZA	Niacin acc
M. bovis	Classical	Sens	Neg	Mic	Res	Neg
	BCG	Sens	Neg	Aer	Res	Neg
M. tuberculosis	Classical	Res	Pos	Aer	Sens	Pos
	Asian	Sens	Pos	Aer	Sens	Pos

TCH susceptibility to thiophene-2-carboxylic acid hydrazide, NO_3 nitratase reductase, *Niacin acc* niacin accumulation, O_2 oxygen preference for growth, *PZA* susceptibility to pyrazinamide, *Sens* sensitive, *Res* resistant, *Pos* positive, *Neg* negative, *Mic* microaerophylic, *Aer* aerobic

most commonly used for mycobacterial culture. In this medium, *M. bovis* shows disgonic colonies, which has led microbiologists to believe that it may be an *M. bovis* isolate. *M. bovis* can also be cultured in different Middlebrook media (both liquid and solid), with good results [29].

Various biochemical tests are available to differentiate *M. tuberculosis* and *M. bovis* [11, 13], such as nitrate reductase (positive for *M. tuberculosis* and negative for *M. bovis*), susceptibility to thiophene-2-carboxylic acid hydrazide (*M. bovis* is susceptible, *M. tuberculosis* is resistant), susceptibility to pyrazinamide (*M. bovis* is resistant, *M. tuberculosis* is usually susceptible), and niacin accumulation (positive for *M. tuberculosis*, negative for *M. bovis*) (Table 3.2). Moreover, *M. bovis* is microaerophilic, and grows well in sites with low oxygen levels (e.g., in tissue), whereas *M. tuberculosis* is aerobic, preferring sites where there is an abundance of oxygen (e.g., the lungs) [3]. However, these tests need to be performed and interpreted by experienced operators, and are not easy to carry out in medium-size and small clinical mycobacteriology laboratories. Another disadvantage of these phenotypical tests is that some *M. bovis* isolates show similar characteristics to those of *M. tuberculosis* [30].

Since the complete genome sequence of *M. bovis* became known, the search for specific genetic markers has been ongoing [17]: *M. bovis* strains lack the *mtp40* sequence found in *M. tuberculosis*, lack the chromosomal regions RD7, RD8, RD9 and RD10 [16], and carry a particular mutation at position 169 in the *pncA* gene conferring pyrazinamide resistance [31]. A specific mutation at position 285 in the *oxyR* gene [32] and the absence of spacers 3, 9, 16 and 39 to 43 in the DR locus [33] are also characteristic of *M. bovis*. However, the use of these markers is confined to reference or research laboratories. A system based on PCR and hybridization has been introduced into routine laboratory practice in recent years, and permits easy identification of the species of the *M. tuberculosis* complex [34].

3.2 Molecular Typing Methods

To be able to institute efficacious control measures of TB, a knowledge of the dynamics of transmission of the pathogen and of the factors involved is required; molecular epidemiology data are helpful in this context. Unlike in *M. tuberculosis*, restriction fragment length polymorphism (RFLP) typing based on the insertion sequence IS*6110* (IS*6110* RFLP), the gold standard for *M. tuberculosis* genotyping, provides only limited discrimination among *M. bovis* isolates because this species usually has only one or few IS*6110* copies, especially in isolates from cattle [35]. In fact, the resolution of the IS*6110* RFLP method is known to be inversely proportional to the number of IS*6110* copies, due to the existence of IS*6110* insertion hot spots, and so patterns with six or fewer bands are not appropriate to establish recent transmission [36].

Various other epidemiological genotyping methods have recently been considered for *M. bovis* strains [5] but no standardized tests are yet available.

3.3 Epidemiology and Transmission

It is estimated that 0.3–7.2% of cases of TB in humans in developed countries are due to *M. bovis* [15, 27, 28, 37–44]. Instead, the percentage of cases in most developing countries is not known, in part because of the use of inappropriate isolation and identification methods of this pathogen, but is surely much higher (10–15%) than in industrialized areas, and poses a major threat to public health [18, 37, 45–48].

At the Congress on Tuberculosis held in London in 1901, Koch stated that the bovine tubercle bacillus posed a very limited danger to humans, and that steps to eradicate the disease from cattle were unnecessary [49]. But on the basis of present knowledge Koch was incontrovertibly in error [50]: the bovine tubercle bacillus does pose a threat to human health [3]. Now that human TB is a re-emergent disease, there is evidence that *M. bovis* poses a greater threat to human health than was popularly believed. This threat, like that of the disease caused by *M. tuberculosis*, may be exacerbated by the human immunodeficiency virus pandemic [3]. In 1992, the European Union included TB caused by *M. bovis* as one of the four main zoonoses requiring specific surveillance and investigation [51]. In these circumstances, an effective linkage between veterinary and human public health services has been recommended, and should be still further strengthened [3].

In agricultural folklore, various names are used to refer to cattle diseases, such as wens, grape disease, pearl disease wasters, piners, and snoters, but all of these can be identified as TB [3].

In the past it was thought that *M. bovis* was a highly resistant organism, surviving in cow feces for at least 5 months in winter and 2 months in summer, and in soil for up to 2 years [52]. Subsequent evidence suggested, instead, that *M. bovis* disappears from the environment much more quickly [53], and that the activity of sunlight and of other bacteria, protozoa and fungi which normally contribute to the breakdown of feces, appears to destroy tubercle bacilli [3].

Transmission of *M. bovis* can occur between domestic and wild animals, from animals to humans, and, more rarely, from humans to animals or between humans [1, 3, 13, 54–56]. The infection is acquired by aerosol inhalation (through the inhalation of small droplets, just like human TB), ingestion, or direct contact with infected animals [13, 15]. Bovine TB in cattle is a respiratory disease above all, and aerosol spread of bacilli is the main source of infection from other animals to humans [54–57].

Human infection has often been associated with the ingestion of unpasteurized milk and milk products from animals with infected udders. A link between tuberculous cervical adenitis and the consumption of milk from diseased cattle had already been established in 1946 by Klenke [3]: the bacilli can enter the body through the tonsils and then affect the cervical lymph nodes. Both milk-borne and meat-borne bacilli can cause intestinal TB, and hematogenous spread to other organs is possible. Although only 1% of tuberculous cows had infected udders, it was clear that their milk posed a serious public health threat, and so programs were instituted to control the disease eradication in cattle, and to inspect meat and the pasteurization of milk. However, these controls are still often lacking in many developing countries. In Argentina, where the prevalence of TB in the cattle population is relatively high, despite the pasteurization of milk combined with a high standard of meat inspection, most of the patients infected with *M. bovis* are workers at slaughterhouses or in rural areas [1, 58].

More rarely, man can be infected through the ingestion of insufficiently cooked bovine meat. However, as pointed out above, nowadays these sources of infection are present only in developing countries where bovine TB is prevalent, control measures are not applied, and pasteurization of milk is rarely practiced [37, 47]. Inevitably, in these same developing countries, the rates of bovine TB are higher in rural populations [3]. In developed countries, instead, the incidence of infection has declined remarkably and most cases observed nowadays are in older people, being a reactivation of infection acquired in the past when the animal infection was still common [13, 55].

The transmission of *M. bovis* to man from various animals other than cattle is sporadic and largely associated with specific jobs, such as in farmers, veterinarians, abattoir workers, animal handlers, and hunters [41, 59–63]. There is also evidence of sporadic transmission from humans to animals [1, 13, 64], and among humans associated with nosocomial outbreaks [65–70]. In these cases an important role in the host susceptibility is played by immune suppression due to HIV-coinfection, cancer therapy, alcohol misuse, and insulin-dependent diabetes mellitus.

3.4 Clinical Features

Human disease caused by *M. bovis* is clinically and histologically indistinguishable from that of *M. tuberculosis* [37, 39, 64–75]. According to various authors, *M. bovis* induces above all extrapulmonary TB forms [37, 43, 71, 73, 75], whereas others have observed above all pulmonary forms [1, 72, 74]. In any case, the clinical manifestations depend on the transmission pathway: ingesting milk contaminated with *M. bovis* induces lymph nodes and intestinal forms, whereas contagion through the respiratory tract leads to TB of the lungs.

Other relatively frequent extrapulmonary forms are genitourinary and osteoarticular. In adults, pulmonary forms are generally due to a reactivation of old infections. Pulmonary TB is the most common form in immunocompromised subjects. In children, lymph nodes and intestinal infections are more common, likely reflecting contagion through foodstuffs.

Infection through skin wounds causes cutaneous [76], tendon and localized lymph nodes lesions in personnel who handle infected carcasses, and in veterinarians exposed during surgical or other occupational procedures [28, 44].

We observed seven cases of occupational warty TB in farmhands milking cattle affected by tubercular mastitis. In six cases the clinical manifestations involved the dorsum of the hands and in one, the flexor surface of the right wrist. The complaint presented with confluent papules forming plaques with a hyperkeratosic surface (Figs. 3.1, 3.2, 3.3, 3.4, 3.5, 3.6, 3.7, and 3.8). In all cases the

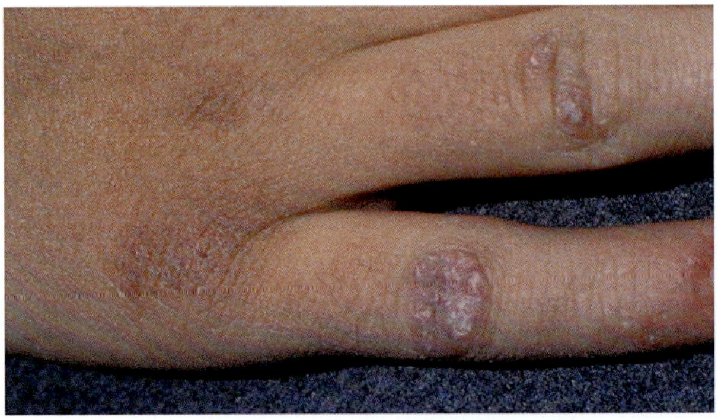

Fig. 3.1 Occupational warty tuberculosis in milker

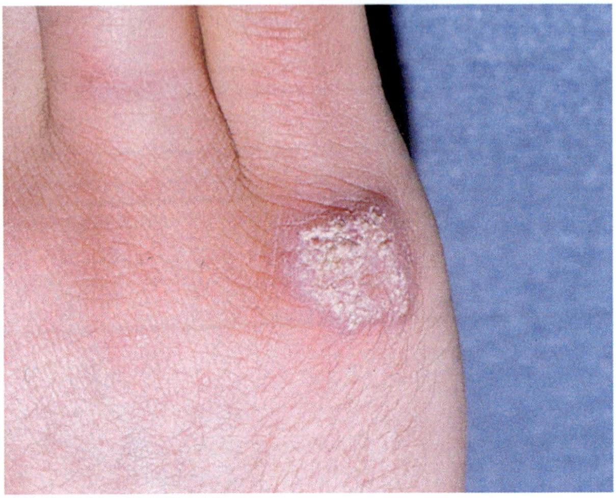

Fig. 3.2 Occupational warty tuberculosis in milker

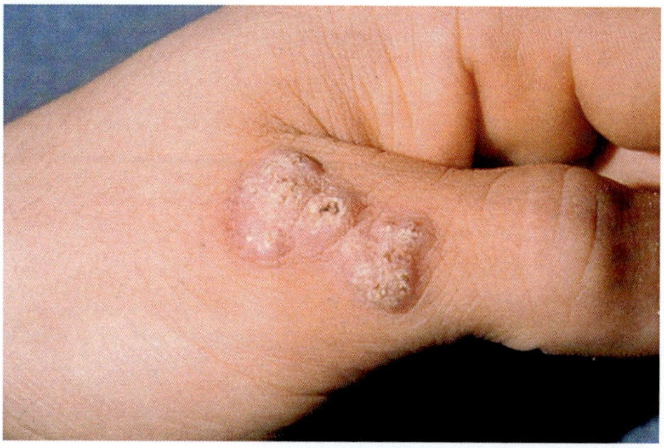

Fig. 3.3 Occupational warty tuberculosis in milker

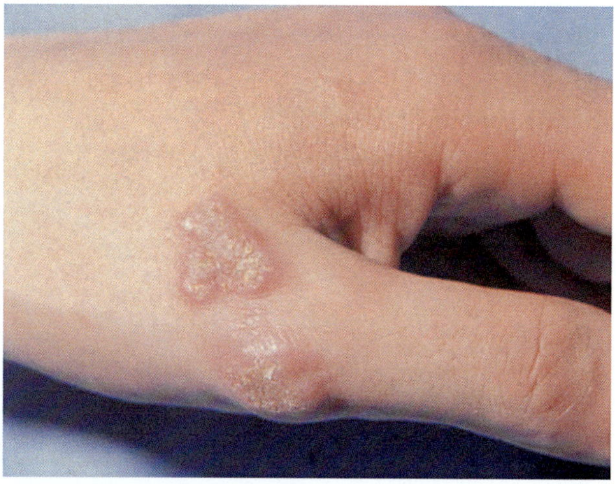

Fig. 3.4 Occupational warty tuberculosis in milker

histopathological finding was a granulomatous tubercular infiltrate with giant Langhans-type cells and no sign of central caseation (Figs. 3.9 and 3.10). No acid-fast bacilli were seen at histology. All the patients were immunocompetent and there were no associated systemic symptoms. The personal and family history for TB due to *M. tuberculosis* was negative. The PPD reaction was strongly positive in all cases. The complaint resolved in all the patients after 4–6 months of treatment with a 3-drug regimen, isoniazid (300 mg/day), rifampicin (600 mg/day), and ethambutol (15 mg/kg/day).

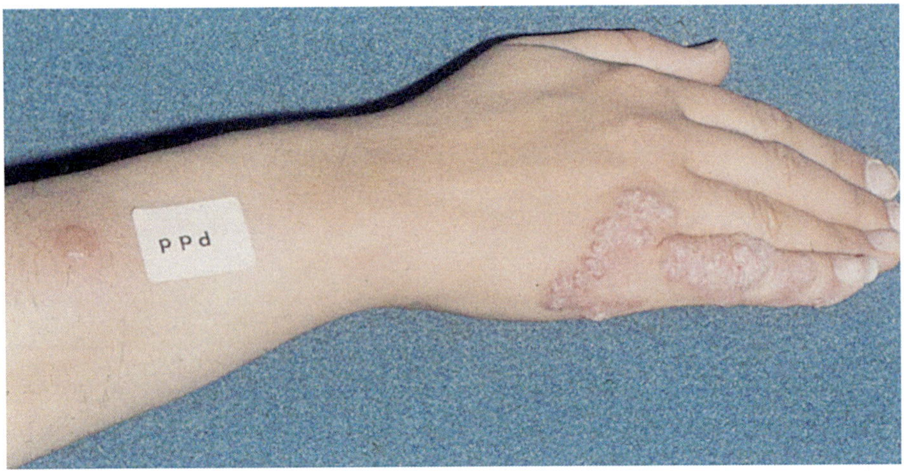

Fig. 3.5 Occupational warty tuberculosis in milker. Strong positive PPD

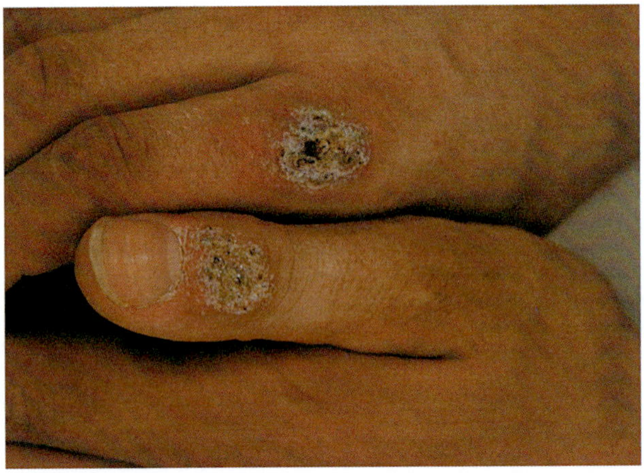

Fig. 3.6 Occupational warty tuberculosis in milker

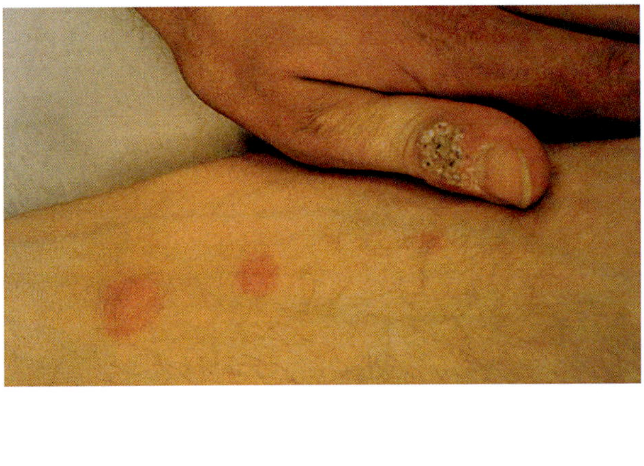

Fig. 3.7 The same patient as in Fig. 3.6. Positive reactions to PPD of various mycobacteria

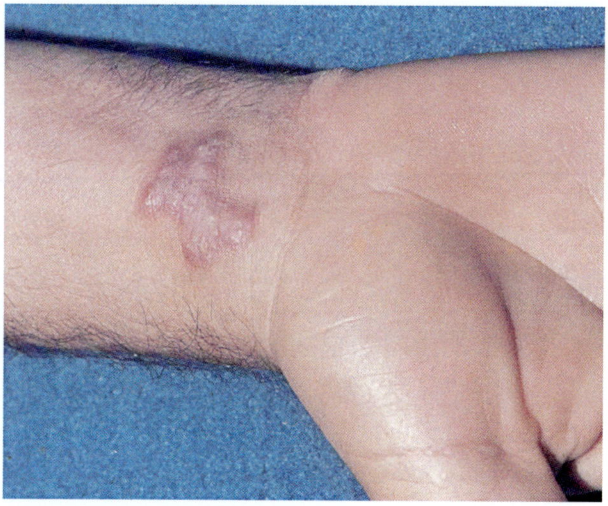

Fig. 3.8 Occupational warty tuberculosis in milker

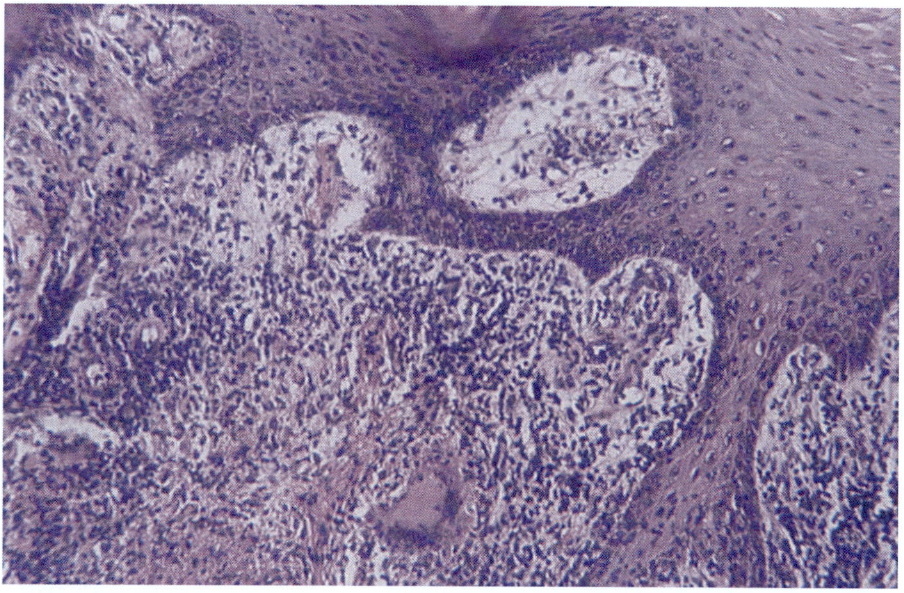

Fig. 3.9 Hyperkeratosis, acanthosis, and papillomatosis of the epidermis. Granulomatous inflammation of the dermis with giant Langhans cells (Hematoxylin-eosin – ×100)

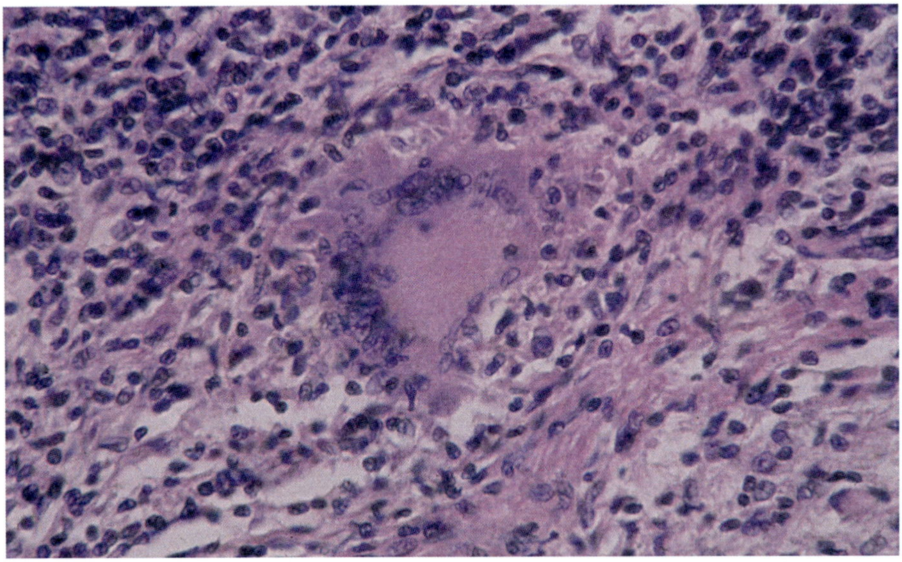

Fig. 3.10 Tubercular granulomatous infiltrate with epithelioid cells, lymphocytes and Langhans cell (Hematoxylin-eosin – ×200)

3.5 Susceptibility and Treatment

M. bovis infection is treated with the same antibiotic regimens, for the same duration, as in the treatment of TB infection by *M. tuberculosis*. However, *M. bovis* resistance to pyrazinamide, a key characteristic for the microbiological identification of the strains, should be borne in mind.

Resistance in vitro of *M. bovis* to other drugs seems to be rare; the most common type is to isoniazid (in the past this was used alone to treat bovine TB). Nevertheless, due to the risk of resistant strains it is always wise to perform susceptibility tests using the same methods as for *M. tuberculosis*.

Treatment should be started with isoniazid, rifampicin and ethambutol: if the isolate is sensitive to rifampicin and isoniazid, these two drugs should be continued for a total of 9 months. In cases of isoniazid-resistance, rifampicin and ethambutol should be administered for 12 months [5].

Multidrug (MDR) *M. bovis* resistant strains and extensive-multidrug (XDR) *M. bovis* resistant strains are rare, even if an outbreak of XDR *M. bovis* strains was described among HIV-infected patients in Spain in the mid-1990s [77]. This outbreak started in a hospital in Madrid and spread to other hospitals in Spain and in other countries [72, 77]. The strain was resistant to all first- and second-line drugs, and posed a great challenge in these patients, who were mostly HIV-infected subjects. The use of alternative drugs like linezolid or amoxicillin-clavulanic acid, yielded good results in some patients, especially HIV-negative subjects [72, 78].

3.6 Control and Recommendations

In agreement with Moda and Coll [28] and Collins [79], various control measures need to be adopted. Reliable and economic systems of veterinary surveillance must be implemented: abattoir controls have a key role in controlling the prevalence of bovine TB. It is important to acquire accurate information about *M. bovis* infection in humans and animals from farmers and those involved in slaughtering and marketing meat. Infected animals must be eliminated to limit the spread of the infection, and heat treatment of milk (pasteurization) promoted in all nations.

References

1. O'Reilly LM, Daborn CJ (1995) The epidemiology of *Mycobacterium bovis* infections in animals and man: a review. Tuber Lung Dis 76(Suppl 1):1
2. Cassidy JP, Bryson DG, Pollock JM et al (1999) Lesions in cattle exposed to *Mycobacterium bovis*-inoculated calves. J Comp Pathol 121:321
3. Collins CH (2000) The bovine tubercle bacillus. Br J Biomed Sci 57:234
4. Pollock JM, Buddle BM, Andersen P (2001) Towards more accurate diagnosis of bovine tuberculosis using defined antigens. Tuberculosis (Edinburgh) 81:65
5. Esteban J, Alonso-Rodriguez N (2011) *Mycobacterium bovis* and other uncommon members of the M*ycobacterium tuberculosis* complex. In: Schlossberg D (ed) Tuberculosis and nontuberculous mycobacterial infections, 6th edn. ASM Press, Washington, DC, p 607
6. Karlson AG, Lessel EF (1970) *Mycobacterium bovis* nom. nov. Int J Syst Bact 20:273
7. Castets M, Rist N, Boisvert H (1969) La varieté africaine du bacille tuberculeux humaine. Med Afrique Noir 16:321
8. David HL, Johan MT, Lessel EF (1978) Numerical taxonomy analysis of *Mycobacteruym africanum*. Int J Syst Bact 48:46
9. Yates MD, Collins CH, Grange JM (1982) "Classical" and "Asian" variants of *Mycobacterium tuberculosis* isolated in South East England, 1977–1980. Tubercle 63:55
10. Grange JM, Gibson J, Osborn TW et al (1983) What is BCG? Tubercle 64:129
11. Collins CH, Grange JM, Yates MD (1997) Tuberculosis bacteriology: organization and practice, 2nd edn. Butterworth-Heinemann, Oxford
12. Smith T (1898) A comparative study of bovine tubercle bacilli and of human bacilli from sputum. J Exp Med 3:451
13. Grange JM, Yates MD (1994) Zoonotic aspects of *Mycobacterium bovis* infection. Vet Microbiol 40:137
14. Cousins DV (2001) *Mycobacterium bovis* infection and control in domestic livestock. Rev Sci Tech 20:71
15. de la Rua-Domenech R (2006) Human *Mycobacterium bovis* infection in the United Kingdom: incidence, risks, control measures and review of the zoonotic aspects of bovine tuberculosis. Tuberculosis (Edinburgh) 86:77
16. Brosch R, Gordon SV, Marmiesse M et al (2002) A new evolutionary scenario for the *Mycobacterium tuberculosis* complex. Proc Natl Acad Sci U S A 99:3684
17. Garnier T, Eiglmeier K, Camus JC et al (2003) The complete genome sequence *of Mycobacterium bovis*. Proc Natl Acad Sci U S A 100:7877
18. Cleaveland S, Shaw DJ, Mfinanga SG et al (2007) *Mycobacterium bovis* in rural Tanzania: risk factors for infection in human and cattle populations. Tuberculosis (Edinburgh) 87:30
19. de Lisle GW, Mackintosh CG, Bengis RG (2001) *Mycobacterium bovis* in free-living and captive wildlife, including farmed deer. Rev Sci Tech 20:86
20. Francis J (1947) Bovine tuberculosis. Staples, London

21. Nolan A, Wilesmith JW (1994) Tuberculosis in badgers (*Meles meles*). Vet Microbiol 40:179
22. Gallagher J, Muirhead RH, Daykin JM et al (2005) Bovine tuberculosis and badgers. Vet Rec 156:555
23. Coleman JD, Cooke MM (2001) *Mycobacterium bovis* infection in wildlife in New Zealand. Tuberculosis (Edinburgh) 81:191
24. Aranaz A, De Juan L, Montero N et al (2004) Bovine tuberculosis (*Mycobacterium bovis*) in wildlife in Spain. J Clin Microbiol 42:2602
25. Michel AL, Bengis RG, Keet DF et al (2006) Wildlife tuberculosis in South African conservation areas: implications and challenges. Vet Microbiol 112:91
26. Lepper AWD, Corner LA (1983) Naturally-occurring mycobacterioses of animals. In: Ratledge C, Stanford JL (eds) The biology of the mycobacteria. Academic, London, p 417
27. Grange JM, Yates MD (1995) Guidelines for specification within the *Mycobacterium tuberculosis* complex. World Health Organization, Geneva. (Unpublished document WHO/Zoon.94.174)
28. Moda G, Daborn CJ, Grange JM et al (1996) The zoonotic importance of *Mycobacterium bovis*. Tuber Lung Dis 77:103
29. Hines N, Payeur JB, Hoffman LJ (2006) Comparison of the recovery of *Mycobacterium bovis* isolates using the BACTEC MGIT 960 system, BACTEC 460 system, and Middlebrook 7H10 and 7H11 solid media. J Vet Diagn Invest 18:243
30. Kubica T, Agzamova R, Wright A et al (2006) *Mycobacterium bovis* isolates with *M. tuberculosis* specific characteristics. Emerg Infect Dis 12:763
31. Scorpio A, Zhang Y (1996) Mutations in *pncA*, a gene encoding pyrazinamidase/nicotinamidase, cause resistance to the antituberculous drug pyrazinamide in tubercle bacillus. Nat Med 2:662
32. Sreevatsan S, Escalante P, Pan X et al (1996) Identification of a polymorphic nucleotide in *oxyR* specific for *Mycobacterium bovis*. J Clin Microbiol 34:2007
33. Haddad N, Masselot M, Durand B (2004) Molecular differentiation of *Mycobacterium bovis* isolates. Review of main techniques and applications. Res Vet Sci 76:1
34. Richter E, Weizenegger M, Fahr AM et al (2004) Usefulness of the GenoType MTBC assay for differentiating species of the *Mycobacterium tuberculosis* complex in cultures obtained from clinical specimens. J Clin Microbiol 42:4303
35. Skuce RA, Brittain D, Hughes MS et al (1996) Differentiation of *Mycobacterium bovis* isolates from animals by DNA typing. J Clin Microbiol 34:2469
36. Kremer K, van Soolingen D, Frothingham R et al (1999) Comparison of methods based on different molecular epidemiological markers for typing of *Mycobacterium tuberculosis* complex strains: interlaboratory study of discriminatory power and reproducibility. J Clin Microbiol 37:2607
37. Cosivi O, Grange JM, Daborn CJ et al (1998) Zoonotic tuberculosis due to *Mycobacterium bovis* in developing countries. Emerg Infect Dis 4:59
38. Cousins DV, Dawson DJ (1999) Tuberculosis due to *Mycobacterium bovis* in Australian populations: cases recording during 1970–1994. Int J Tuberc Lung Dis 3:715
39. Ojo O, Sheehan S, Corcoran GD et al (2008) *Mycobacterium bovis* strains causing smear-positive human tuberculosis. Southwest Ireland. Emerg Infect Dis 14:1931
40. Robert J, Boulahbal F, Trystram D et al (1999) A national survey of human *Mycobacterium bovis* infection in France. Network of Microbiology Laboratories in France. Int J Tuberc Lung Dis 3:711
41. Rodríguez E, Sánchez LP, Pérez S et al (2009) Human tuberculosis due to *Mycobacterium bovis* and *M. caprae* in Spain, 2004–2007. Int J Tuberc Lung Dis 13:1536
42. Cotter TP, O'Shaughnessy E, Sheehan S et al (1996) Human *Mycobacterium bovis* infection in the south-west of Ireland 1983–1992: a comparison with *M. tuberculosis*. Ir Med J 89:62
43. Hlavsa MC, Moonan PK, Cowan LS et al (2008) Human tuberculosis due to *Mycobacterium bovis* in the United States, 1995-2005. Clin Infect Dis 47:168
44. Mertoğlu A, Biçmen C, Karaarslan S et al (2016) Pulmonary tuberculosis due to *Mycobacterium bovis* revealed by skin lesion in slaughterhouse worker. Clin Respir J, Apr 7.

45. Cosivi O, Meslin FX, Daborn C et al (1995) Epidemiology of *Mycobacterium bovis* infection in animals and humans, with particular reference to Africa. Rev Sci Tech 14:733
46. Ashford DA, Whitney E, Raghunathan P et al (2001) Epidemiology of selected mycobacteria that infect humans and other animals. Rev Sci Tech 20:325
47. Ayele WY, Neill SD, Zinsstag J et al (2004) Bovine tuberculosis: an old disease but a new threat to Africa. Int J Tuberc Lung Dis 8:924
48. de Kantor IN, Ambroggi M, Poggi S et al (2008) Human *Mycobacterium bovis* infection in ten Latin American countries. Tuberculosis (Edinburgh) 88:358
49. British Congress on Tuberculosis (1901) Transactions of the British Congress on tuberculosis, vol 1–3. Cowers, London, p 1902
50. The Stationary Office (1911) Royal Commission on tuberculosis. Final report. The Stationary Office, London
51. European Union (1993) Council Directive 29/117/EEC of 17 December 1992. Off J Eur Comm L62:38
52. Wray C (1975) Survival and spread of pathogenic bacteria of veterinary importance within the environment. Vet Bull 45:543
53. Duffield BJ, Young DA (1985) Survival of *Mycobacterium bovis* in defined environmental conditions. Vet Microbiol 10:193
54. Morris RS, Pfeiffer DU, Jackson R (1994) The epidemiology of *Mycobacterium bovis* infections. Vet Microbiol 40:153
55. Palmer MV (2007) Tuberculosis: a reemerging disease at the interface of domestic animals and wildlife. Curr Top Microbiol Immunol 315:195
56. Thoen C, Lobue P, de Kantor I (2006) The importance of *Mycobacterium bovis* as a zoonosis. Vet Microbiol 112:339
57. Menzies FD, Neill SD (2000) Cattle-to-cattle transmission of bovine tuberculosis. Vet J 160:92
58. Ritacco V, de Kantor I (1992) Zoonotic tuberculosis in Latin America. J Clin Microbiol 30:3299
59. Fanning A, Edwards S (1991) *Mycobacterium bovis* infection in human beings in contact with elk (*Cervus elaphus*) in Alberta, Canada. Lancet 338:1253
60. Dalovisio JR, Stetter M, Mikota-Wells S (1992) Rhinoceros' rhinorrhea: cause of an outbreak of infection due to airborne *Mycobacterium bovis* in zookeepers. Clin Infect Dis 15:598
61. Liss GM, Wong L, Kittle DC et al (1994) Occupational exposure to *Mycobacterium bovis* infection in deer and elk in Ontario. Can J Public Health 85:326
62. Thompson PJ, Cousins DV, Gow BL et al (1993) Seals, seal trainers, and mycobacterial infection. Am Rev Respir Dis 147:164
63. Wilkins MJ, Bartlett PC, Frawley B et al (2003) *Mycobacterium bovis* (bovine TB) exposure as a recreational risk for hunters: results of a Michigan Hunter Survey, 2001. Int J Tuberc Lung Dis 7:1001
64. Sjögren I, Hillerdal O (1978) Bovine tuberculosis in man-reinfection or endogenous exacerbation. Scand J Respir Dis 59:167
65. Blázquez J, Espinosa de Los Monteros LE, Samper S et al (1997) Genetic characterization of multidrug-resistant *Mycobacterium bovis* strains from a hospital outbreak involving human immunodeficiency virus-positive patients. J Clin Microbiol 35:1390
66. Gori A, Marchetti G, Catozzi L et al (1998) Molecular epidemiology characterization of a multidrug-resistant *Mycobacterium bovis* outbreak amongs HIV-positive patients. AIDS 12:445
67. Guerrero A, Cobo J, Fortún J et al (1997) Nosocomial transmission of *Mycobacterium bovis* resistant to 11 drugs in people with advanced HIV-1 infection. Lancet 350:1738
68. Palenque E, Villena V, Rebollo MJ et al (1998) Transmission of multidrug-resistant *Mycobacterium bovis* to an immunocompetent patient. Clin Infect Dis 26:995
69. Waecker NJ Jr, Stefanova R, Cave MD et al (2000) Nosocomial transmission of *Mycobacterium bovis* bacille Calmette-Guérin to children receiving cancer therapy and to their health care providers. Clin Infect Dis 30:356

70. Rivero A, Márquez M, Santos J et al (2001) High rate of tuberculosis reinfection during a nosocomial outbreak of multidrug-resistant tuberculosis caused by *Mycobacterium bovis* strain B. Clin Infect Dis 32:159
71. Dankner WM, Waecker NJ, Essey MA et al (1993) *Mycobacterium bovis* infections in San Diego: a clinicoepidemiologic study of 73 patients and a historical review of a forgotten pathogen. Medicine (Baltimore) 72:11
72. Esteban J, Robles P, Soledad Jiménez M et al (2005) Pleuropulmonary infections caused by *Mycobacterium bovis*: a re-emerging disease. Clin Microbiol Infect 11:840
73. Byarugaba F, Charles-Etter EM, Godreuil S et al (2009) Pulmonary tuberculosis and *Mycobacterium bovis*. Uganda. Emerg Infect Dis 15:124
74. Evans JT, Smith EG, Banerjee A et al (2007) Cluster of human tuberculosis caused by *Mycobacterium bovis*: evidence for person-to-person transmission in the UK. Lancet 369:1270
75. Mignard S, Pichat C, Carret G (2006) *Mycobacterium bovis* infection, Lyon. France. Emerg Infect Dis 12:1431
76. Lhote R, Raskine L, Gottlieb J et al (2016) Tuberculose cutanée de l'oreille à *Mycobacterium bovis*. Ann Dermatol Venereol 143:611
77. Samper S, Martín C, Pinedo A et al (1997) Transmission between HIV-infected patients of multidrug-resistant tuberculosis caused by *Mycobacterium bovis*. AIDS 11:1237
78. Fortún J, Martín-Dávila P, Navas E et al (2005) Linezolid for the treatment of multidrug-resistant tuberculosis. J Antimicrob Chemother 56:180
79. Collins JD (2006) Tuberculosis in cattle: strategic planning for the future. Vet Microbiol 112:369

Bacillus Calmette-Guérin

4

Domenico Bonamonte, Angela Filoni, and Gianni Angelini

Approximately one third of the world population is infected by *Mycobacterium tuberculosis*, and a greater and continuing factor that is bolstering the ongoing tuberculosis (TB) epidemic is the human immune deficiency virus (HIV). Further complicating the issue, multidrug resistance (MDR) has arisen worldwide, and by early 2010, 58 countries had reported at least one case of extensively drug resistant TB [1]. For all these reasons, TB prevention through vaccination is a key global health priority [2].

Various vaccines have been shown to reduce the risk of disease and mortality due to TB in man, but only one has been used in global immunization programs: the *M. bovis* bacillus Calmette-Guérin (BCG). BCG is an attenuated live vaccine administered at birth to children in most countries where TB is endemic. It is the vaccine most widely used all over the world, and an estimated three billion doses have been administered to date [3]. Despite having reduced the burden of TB in many zones, the BCG has various limitations and so the development of more efficacious vaccines against TB is an extremely urgent issue [4, 5]. The ideal vaccine should prevent both the initial tubercle infection and the development of active disease, or reactivation in previously infected healthy hosts as well as in particularly vulnerable populations (HIV-infected and other immunocompromised individuals) [2].

D. Bonamonte, MD, PhD (✉)
Department of Biomedical Science and Human Oncology, University of Bary "Aldo Moro", Bari, Italy
e-mail: domenico.bonamonte@uniba.it

A. Filoni, MD
University of Bary "Aldo Moro", Bari, Italy

G. Angelini, MD
Professor of Dermatology, Former Professor and Chairman, University of Bary "Aldo Moro", Bari, Italy

D. Bonamonte, G. Angelini (eds.), *Mycobacterial Skin Infections*,
DOI 10.1007/978-3-319-48538-6_4

Table 4.1 Protection against tuberculosis (modified, by [2])

1- Naturally acquired mycobacterial infection:
Mycobacterium tuberculosis
Nontuberculous mycobacteria
2- Vaccine-induced mycobacterial infection:
BCG (live)
Mycobacterium microti (live)
Whole-cell mycobacterial vaccines (inactivated), including *Mycobacterium vaccae*

4.1 Immunoprotection Against Tuberculosis

A prior mycobacterial infection, either naturally acquired or vaccine-induced, offers some immune protection, albeit partial (Table 4.1). Epidemiological and experimental studies in animals suggest that a previous infection by *M. tuberculosis* confers a relative protection against the development of later disease due to re-exposure [6]. However, this protection is lower in cases of cellular immunodeficiency, as demonstrated in HIV-infected subjects [7].

Skin test studies in humans suggest that also a previous infection by nontuberculous mycobacteria (NTM), acquired naturally through exposure to colonized water or soil, confers protection against TB [8, 9]. The same protection, gained from NTM, has been experimentally demonstrated [9, 10]. NTM infections, that are common in various parts of the world, are generally acquired in childhood [11]. In the United States, about 40% of adults show positive reactions to skin tests with the *M. avium* complex (MAC), while most of them have negative skin tests to tuberculin [12]. Naturally acquired NTM infections can induce equal protection levels against TB to the BCG levels, and this may explain the lack of efficacy of BCG in some zones where there are many NTM infections [9]. Previous mycobacterial infections can also reduce the efficacy of BCG by limiting its replication, as demonstrated in mice [13].

In 1950, a study with a live mycobacterial vaccine, *M. microti* (the vole bacillus) was conducted: a single dose demonstrated a 5-year efficacy of 84% in 54,239 tuberculin-negative British adolescents [14]. This shows that antigens other than those to *M. tuberculosis* and *M. bovis* can protect against TB.

Inactivated whole-cell mycobacterial vaccines had been tested before the spread of BCG, and proved efficacious in preventing TB [15].

4.2 BCG Vaccine

M. bovis BCG was developed by Leon Calmette, a physician, and Camille Guérin, a veterinarian: in 1902, they began by passing a strain of *M. bovis* isolated from a cow with tuberculous mastitis in culture every 3 weeks for a total of 230 passages. Inoculation of this attenuated *M. bovis* strain in calves and guinea pigs did not elicit evidence of infection. Then protection was demonstrated also in other animals (pigs, rabbit, and horses), and after immunized cows had been challenged with a wild-type, virulent strain of *M. bovis* and showed no sign of infection, in 1921 the vaccine was administered orally to humans [2].

The first recipient was a 3-day-old infant whose mother had died of TB a few hours after delivery. The grandmother, who took over the care of the child, was also affected by TB. The baby suffered no ill effects from the vaccine and did not develop TB. Between 1921 and 1924, 600 more children were vaccinated without any serious complications. Among them were Calmette's own grandchildren [16]. In 1928, the vaccine was certified as safe by the League of Nations.

The original BCG strains were distributed and maintained in different laboratories, and so gave rise to several genetically distinct strains. The first randomized, controlled trial of vaccine efficacy was conducted by Aronson between 1935 and 1938 [17]. In 1947, the World Health Organization (WHO) launched a TB control program that included spreading the use of the BCG. From the 1950s to 1997 the vaccine lots were under the direction of the WHO and administered by the Danish State Serum Institute in Copenaghen, Denmark. Since then, the manufacturers have been responsible for the vaccine manufacture and quality. Four strains (Glaxo, Danish, Pasteur, and Tokio), account for over 90% of vaccines currently administered [2, 18].

4.3 Immune Response to BCG Vaccination

The BCG vaccine induces a mild systemic infection in healthy hosts. Autopsy studies of recently immunized children who died of other causes showed a widespread granuloma formation [19]. This attenuated infection elicits both a cell-mediated and a humoral immune response to mycobacterial antigens. In vaccinated subjects there is a lymphocyte proliferation response to proteins secreted by BCG and *M. tuberculosis* [20, 21], as well as a variety of cytokines responses outside the Th1 cells [22–24]. As to the humoral response, BCG induces both IgG and IgM responses [25, 26].

Most tuberculin-negative subjects immunized with BCG develop a positive tuberculin skin test after some weeks. This effect declines over time and so the current recommendation is to consider reactions of >10 mm present several years after the vaccination as a latent infection by *M. tuberculosis* rather than a persistent effect of the BCG. It should also be borne in mind that BCG-induced tuberculin reactions can be boosted by repeated skin tests and that although the issue has not been rigorously studied, it is generally believed that the development of a BCG-induced tuberculin sensitivity is not a surrogate for protective immunity against TB [2].

4.4 Efficacy of BCG

Although in the United States the problem of the efficacy of the BCG is somewhat controversial, it is widely accepted that childhood immunization is effective [2].

As stated above, a prior infection with *M. tuberculosis* or NTM confers a comparable anti-TB protection to the BCG. Indeed, some studies have shown that skin test-negative subjects demonstrate cellular and humoral immune responses to mycobacteria, and so are not mycobacteria naïve [23, 26, 27]. For this reason, the efficacy of the vaccine should be assessed in mycobacterium-naïve hosts, that is newborns. Prospective studies of this type have revealed an efficacy of 73% against disease and 97% against death [17, 28–30]. Many BCG trials have been conducted also in older children and adults (including subjects already infected by *M. tuberculosis* or NTM), and these studies, too, confirmed the protective efficacy of BCG immunization [17, 31].

Instead, trials in HIV infection have yielded contrasting results [32, 33]. Nevertheless, because BCG immunization in HIV-infected infants carries a risk of disseminated BCG disease, the vaccine should not be administered to infants with known HIV infection [32–35].

It has also been suggested that the BCG could reduce the risk of active TB infection [36, 37]. BCG re-vaccination in tuberculin-negative children (nowadays, booster doses of vaccine are still administered only in few countries) does not confer an additional protection against TB disease [38–40], despite the enhancement of IFN-γ responses to mycobacterial antigens [41].

The BCG vaccine has been found effective also against other diseases. Various studies have shown an efficacy ranging from 50% to 80% against *M. leprae*. The BCG is effective in preventing infection by *M. ulcerans* in about 50% of cases, and is protective also against osteomyelitis [42]. The BCG also offers cross protection against childhood lymphadenitis due to MAC [43], whereas failure to vaccinate is associated with a marked increase of this infection [44]. For immunotherapy purposes, the BCG is used in the management of superficial and *in situ* transitional cell carcinoma of the bladder, usually, instilled into the bladder on a monthly basis [45]. Primary infection of the glans penis by *M. bovis*-BCG has been described after intravesical BCG treatment [46]. Distant cutaneous granulomas have been described after BCG immunotherapy for malignant melanoma [47, 48].

4.5 Administration and Side Effects of BCG

The Tice vaccine (Organon), the only one used in the United States, is a mixture of killed and live bacilli ranging from 37,500 to 3,000,000 CFU per dose: 0.2–0.3 ml of vaccine reconstituted in 1.0 ml of sterile water is administered in the lower deltoid area by the multiple-puncture technique (0.2–0.3 ml reconstituted in 2 ml of sterile water for infants less than 1 year of age) [49]. Tuberculin skin test conversion usually occurs 6–12 weeks after vaccination.

The side effects of the vaccination depend on the BCG strain, dose, method of administration, and recipient [50]. Newborns suffer more complications than older children and adults. Among the strains in current use, the Pasteur and Danish cause the highest rates of side effects: lymphadenitis, for example, is more common with the Pasteur strain than the Tokyo or Brazil strains [51]. The average amount (CFU) of viable bacilli varies from strain to strain, and many vaccines also contain nonviable bacilli. Intradermal inoculation is associated with a higher risk of local

Table 4.2 Side effects of parenteral BCG vaccination (modified, by [2])

Reaction	Incidence	Comment
Mild		
Induration, erythema, pain at the injection site	95%	All vaccines
Ulceration at inoculation site	70%	Varies according to strain
Lymphadenopathy	1–2%	
Serious		
Osteomyelitis	0.01–300/million	Varies according to strain
Disseminated infection	0.19–1.56/million	Associated with immunocompromised state

reactions but while the multiple-puncture technique has a lower rate of local reactions, it is more costly, less precise and more technically demanding [51].

The most common side effect of the BCG is a local reaction at the inoculation site, with pain, swelling, and erythema. This reaction is observed in 95% of vaccinated subjects, persists for several weeks and generally resolves after three months without complications other than scar formation [52]. In 75% of cases there is also myalgia; 70% have ulceration with drainage at the vaccination site, 2% an abscess and 1–2% lymphadenitis [53]. In cases of adenitis, ulceration and drainage may be observed, above all when the lesion develops rapidly, within 2 months of the vaccination. Indolent forms and those with a delayed onset must be kept under observation. The role of adjunctive antimycobacterial therapy is controversial [54] (Table 4.2).

Osteomyelitis is reported to occur in 0.01 per million vaccines in Japan (multiple-puncture technique) and 300 per million in Finland (intradermal technique) [55]. The treatment relies on isoniazid and rifampicin (like *M. bovis*, the BCG is resistant to pyrazinamide).

Disseminated disease, including a fatal outcome, is reported after 0.19–1.56 per million vaccines. Dissemination, that generally starts with the above described local signs, then evolves after weeks or months to fever, weight loss, and multiorgan disease with elevated nonspecific inflammatory markers [56–58]. The disease has an ominous outcome and mortality exceeds 40–50% despite proper therapy. Although these complications are more commonly observed in children, some cases among HIV patients have recently been reported, that occurred some years after the vaccination [59]. Because of these severe complications, the BCG vaccine is contraindicated in HIV-positive and other immunosuppressed patients, as are other live vaccines [60].

The treatment of the mild complications of vaccination, like abscesses, includes drainage, needle aspiration, and erythromycin (250 mg/6 h) or isoniazid (5 mg/kg daily) for 3 months [60].

Disseminated disease therapy includes the use of isoniazid and rifampicin for a minimum of 6 months, with the addition of ethambutol, ethionamide, cycloserine, streptomycin, or a quinolone during the first 2 months of therapy. It is wise to prolong the therapy for at least 9 months [57, 60]. The addition of corticosteroids (prednisone, 40 mg daily) has proven useful in severe disease [60].

Specific complications of BCG include tuberculous processes. Lupus vulgaris may develop at the vaccination site, generally between a few months to 3 years after immunization [61, 62]; it is more common after multiple vaccinations [63]. Scrofuloderma [64] and tuberculids [65], and erythema induratum of Bazin have also been reported [66]. Since these are hypersensitivity reactions to *M. bovis*, anti-tubercular treatment is unnecessary except in immunocompromised patients. The onset of basal cell carcinoma on the BCG scar has also been described [67]. The keloid formation seens common after the BCG vaccination [50, 68–71].

4.6 Current Use of BCG

BCG is routinely administered to newborns in TB-endemic countries [72]. In countries with endemic HIV infection, the WHO recommends testing infants for HIV infection before administering the BCG [35].

The BCG is still administered universally at birth in some developed countries, and is administered selectively to high-risk infants in the United Kingdom [73–75], Finland [76], and Sweden [77]. By contrast, in the United States it has never been routinely administered; in the past it was used in health care workers. Because the U.S. policy for TB prevention attributes a great importance to tuberculin skin testing and the treatment of latent infection, and because the BCG can interfere with the tuberculin skin test, there has always been great reluctance to administer the BCG to all potential high-risk groups. Current guidelines recommend the BCG in children with continual exposure to an untreated or ineffectively treated TB victim that cannot undergo anti-tubercular treatment. In addition, the BCG is recommended in children exposed to a subject with multidrug resistant TB, if they cannot be removed from such contact [2]. Additional recommended BCG recipients are health care workers exposed to contagious multidrug resistant TB, tuberculin-negative homeless subjects, and infants or tuberculin-negative adults moving to TB-endemic countries [78–80].

In Italy, the most recent guidelines limit the indications for vaccination only to health workers at high risk of exposure to multidrug resistant tubercular strains, or that operate in high risk environments, and who cannot undergo preventive therapy in cases of cuticonversion owing to clinical contraindications to the use of specific drugs [81].

4.7 New Vaccines Against Tuberculosis

The BCG is highly efficacious against TB when administered to newborns but the protection declines with age, and little or no protection against TB reactivation remains in adults. BCG boosters are ineffective (Table 4.3) [40]. For this reason there is an ample consensus that a booster vaccine to follow BCG immunization needs to be developed, or else a completely novel two-vaccine booster regimen. Obviously, it is also important to reduce the risk of side effects and improve the

Table 4.3 Favorable and unfavorable characteristics of BCG (modified, by [2])

Favorable characteristics	In newborns, reduction of disease and death due to tuberculosis
	In newborns, reduction of the risk of meningeal and miliary tuberculosis
	In newborns, reduction of the risk of nontuberculous lymphadenitis, leprosy, and *Mycobacterium ulcerans* infection
	Low cost
Unfavorable characteristics	Limited efficacy against reactivation of tuberculosis
	Limited efficacy in mycobacteria-experienced children and adults
	Uncertain efficacy in HIV infection
	Limited duration of efficacy
	Local side effects
	Risk of adenitis and osteomyelitis
	Risk of disseminated BCG in HIV-infected recipients
	Absence of booster effect
	Effect on tuberculin skin test reaction
	Requirement for parenteral immunization
	Unknown immune correlate of protection

duration of protection [2]. Since HIV-associated TB now accounts for more than 50% of global cases of TB, another important goal is a safe and durable vaccine for the prevention of HIV-associated TB [82, 83]. Many new vaccines currently undergoing testing in humans have been reported by Lahey and von Reyn [2]. They are based on selected antigens (leading subunit antigens include *M. tuberculosis* Ag85, ESAT, CFP 10, and Mtb72t) [84], whole-cell inactivated vaccines [85, 86], and recombinant versions of the BCG [87].

References

1. World Health Organization (2010) Multidrug and extensively drug-resistant TB (M/XDR-TB): 2010 Global report on surveillance and response. World Health Organization, Geneva
2. Lahey T, von Reyn CF (2011) *Mycobacterium bovis* BCG and new vaccines against tuberculosis. In: Schlossberg D (ed) Tuberculosis and nontuberculous mycobacterial infections, 6th edn. ASM Press, Washington, DC, p 162
3. Fine PE, Carneiro IA, Milstien JB et al (1999) Issue relating to the use of BCG in immunization programs: a discussion document. Department of Vaccines and Biologicals, World Health Organization, Geneva
4. Andersen P (2001) TB vaccines: progress and problems. Trends Immunol 22:160
5. Brennan MJ, Fruth U (2002) Global forum on TB vaccine research and development. Word Health Organization, June 7–8, 2001, Geneva. Tuberculosis (Edinburgh) 81:365
6. Ziegler JE, Edwards ML, Smith DW (1985) Exogenous reinfection in experimental airborne tuberculosis. Tubercle 66:121
7. Sonnenberg P, Murray J, Glynn JR et al (2001) HIV-1 and recurrence, relapse, and reinfection of tuberculosis after cure: a cohort study in South African mineworkers. Lancet 358:1687
8. Edwards LB, Palmer CE (1968) Biology of the mycobacterioses. Identification of the tuberculous-infected by skin tests. Am N Y Acad Sci 154:140
9. Fine PE (1995) Variation in protection by BCG: implications of and for heterologous immunity. Lancet 346:1339

10. Edwards ML, Goodrich JM, Muller D et al (1982) Infection with *Mycobacterium avium-intracellulare* and the protective effects of Bacille Calmette-Guérin. J Infect Dis 145:733
11. Fairchok MP, Rouse JH, Morris SL (1995) Age-dependent humoral responses of children to mycobacterial antigens. Clin Diagn Lab Immunol 2:443
12. von Reyn CF, Horsburgh CR, Olivier KN et al (2001) Skin test reactions to *Mycobacterium tuberculosis* purified protein derivative and *Mycobacterium avium* sensitin among health care workers and medical students in the United States. Int J Tuberc Lung Dis 5:1122
13. Brandt L, Feino Cunha J, Weinreich Olsen A et al (2002) Failure of the *Mycobacterium bovis* BCG vaccine: some species of environmental mycobacteria block multiplication of BCG and induction of protective immunity to tuberculosis. Infect Immun 70:672
14. Hart PD, Sutherland I (1977) BCG and vole bacillus vaccines in the prevention of tuberculosis in adolescence and early adult life. Br Med J 2:293
15. Weiss DW (1959) Vaccination against tuberculosis with nonliving vaccines. I. The problem and its historical background. Am Rev Respir Dis 80:676
16. Sakula A (1983) BCG: who were Calmette and Guérin? Thorax 38:806
17. Aronson JD (1948) Protective vaccination against tuberculosis with special reference to BCG vaccination. Am Rev Tuberc 58:255
18. Behr MA (2001) Correlation between BCG genomics and protective efficacy. Scand J Infect Dis 33:249
19. Trevenen CL, Pagtakhan RD (1982) Disseminated tuberculoid lesions in infants following BCG vaccination. Can Med Assoc J 127:502
20. Lowry PW, Ludwig TS, Adams JA et al (1998) Cellular immune responses to four doses of percutaneous bacille Calmette-Guérin in healthy adults. J Infect Dis 178:138
21. Surekha Rani H, Vijaya Lakshmi V, Sumanlatha G et al (2005) Cell-mediated immune responses in children towards secreted proteins of *Mycobacterium bovis* BCG. Tuberculosis (Edinburgh) 85:89
22. Kemp EB, Belshe RB, Hoft DF (1996) Immune responses stimulated by percutaneous and intradermal bacille Calmette-Guérin. J Infect Dis 174:113
23. Ravn P, Boesen H, Pedersen BK et al (1997) Human T cell responses induced by vaccination with *Mycobacterium bovis* bacillus Calmette-Guérin. J Immunol 158:1949
24. Lalor MK, Smith SG, Floyd S et al (2010) Complex cytokine profiles induced by BCG vaccination in UK infants. Vaccine 28:1635
25. Rota S, Beyazova U, Karsligil T et al (1994) Humoral immune response against antigen 60 in BCG-vaccinated infants. Eur J Epidemiol 10:713
26. Hoft DF, Kemp EB, Marinaro M et al (1999) A double-blind, placebo-controlled study of *Mycobacterium*-specific human immune responses induced by intradermal bacille Calmette-Guérin vaccination. J Lab Clin Med 134:244
27. von Reyn CF, Williams PL, Lederman HM et al (2001) Skin test reactivity and cellular immune responses to *Mycobacterium avium* sensitin in AIDS patients at risk for disseminated *M. avium* infection. Clin Diagn Lab Immunol 8:1277
28. Levine MI, Sackett MF (1948) Results of BCG immunization in New York City. Am Rev Tuberc 53:517
29. Rosenthal SR, Loewinsohn E, Graham ML et al (1961) BCG vaccination in tuberculous households. Am Rev Respir Dis 84:690
30. Rosenthal SR, Loewinsohn E, Graham ML et al (1961) BCG vaccination against tuberculosis in Chicago. A twenty-year study statistically analyzed. Pediatrics 28:622
31. Aronson NE, Santosham M, Comstock GW et al (2004) Long-term efficacy of BCG vaccine in American Indians and Alaska Natives: a 60-year follow-up study. JAMA 291:2086
32. Marsh BJ, von Reyn CF, Edwards J et al (1997) The risks and benefits of childhood bacille Calmette-Guérin immunization among adults with AIDS. International MAC Study Groups. AIDS 11:669
33. Waddell RD, Lishimpi K, von Reyn CF et al (2001) Bacteremia due to *Mycobacterium tuberculosis* or *M. bovis* Bacille Calmette-Guérin (BCG) among HIV-positive children and adults in Zambia. AIDS 15:55

34. Hesseling AC, Schaaf HS, Hanekom WA et al (2003) Danish bacille Calmette-Guérin vaccine-induced disease in human immunodeficiency virus-infected children. Clin Infect Dis 37:1226
35. Hesseling AC, Marais BJ, Gie RP et al (2007) The risk of disseminated Bacille Calmette-Guérin (BCG) disease in HIV-infected children. Vaccine 25:14
36. Soysal A, Millington KA, Bakir M et al (2005) Effect of BCG vaccination on risk of *Mycobacterium tuberculosis* infection in children with household tuberculosis contact: a prospective community-based study. Lancet 366:1443
37. Eisenhut M, Paranjothy S, Abubakar I et al (2009) BCG vaccination reduces risk of infection with *Mycobacterium tuberculosis* as detected by gamma interferon release assay. Vaccine 27:6116
38. Leung CC, Tam CM, Chan SL et al (2001) Efficacy of the BCG revaccination programme in a cohort given BCG vaccination at birth in Hong Kong. Int J Tuberc Lung Dis 5:717
39. Cunha SS, Alexander N, Barreto ML et al (2008) BCG revaccination does not protect against leprosy in the Brazilian Amazon: a cluster randomised trial. PLoS Negl Trop Dis 2:e167
40. Rodrigues LC, Pereira SM, Cunha SS et al (2005) Effect of BCG revaccination on incidence of tuberculosis in school-aged children in Brazil: the BCG-REVAC cluster-randomised trial. Lancet 366:1290
41. Barbosa T, Arruda S, Fernandes BD et al (2003) BCG (Bacille of Calmette-Guérin) revaccination leads to improved in vitro IFN-gamma response to mycobacterial antigen independent of tuberculin sensitization in Brazilian school-age children. Vaccine 21:2152
42. Portaels F, Aguiar J, Debacker M et al (2004) *Mycobacterium bovis* BCG vaccination as prophylaxis against *Mycobacterium ulcerans* osteomyelitis in Buruli ulcer disease. Infect Immunol 72:62
43. Katila ML, Brander E, Backman A (1987) Neonatal BCG vaccination and mycobacterial cervical adenitis in childhood. Tubercle 68:291
44. Romanus V, Hallander HO, Wåhlén P et al (1995) Atypical mycobacteria in extrapulmonary disease among children. Incidence in Sweden from 1969 to 1990, related to changing BCG-vaccination coverage. Tuber Lung Dis 76:300
45. Brincks EL, Risk MC, Griffith TS (2013) PMN and anti-tumor immunity. The case of bladder cancer immunotherapy. Semin Cancer Biol 23:183
46. Ribera M, Bielsa J, Manterola JM et al (1995) *Mycobacterium bovis*-BCG infection of the glans penis: a complication of intravesical administration of bacillus Calmette-Guérin. Br J Dermatol 132:309
47. Caplan SE, Kauffman CL (1996) Primary inoculation tuberculosis after immunotherapy for malignant melanoma with BCG vaccine. J Am Acad Dermatol 35:783
48. Moff SL, Corey GR, Gottfredsson M (1999) Distant cutaneous granulomas after bacille Calmette-Guérin immunotherapy for malignant melanoma: case for direct infection. Clin Infect Dis 29:1569
49. Smith KC, Starke JR (1999) Bacille Calmette-Guérin vaccine. In: Plotkin SA, Orenstein WA (eds) Vaccines. W.B. Saunders, Philadelphia, p 121
50. Lotte A, Wasz-Höckert O, Poisson N et al (1984) BCG complications. Estimates of the risks among vaccinated subjects and statistical analysis of their main characteristics. Adv Tuberc Res 21:107
51. Praveen KN, Smikle MF, Prabhakar P et al (1990) Outbreak of Bacillus Calmette-Guérin-associated lymphadenitis and abscesses in Jamaican children. Pediatr Infect Dis J 9:890
52. Brewer MA, Edwards KM, Palmer PS et al (1994) Bacille Calmette-Guérin immunization in normal healthy adults. J Infect Dis 170:476
53. Turnbull FM, McIntyre PB, Achat HM et al (2002) National study of adverse reactions after vaccination with bacille Calmette-Guérin. Clin Infect Dis 34:447
54. Goraya JS, Virdi VS (2001) Treatment of Calmette-Guérin bacillus adenitis: a metaanalysis. Pediatr Infect Dis J 20:632
55. Kröger L, Korppi M, Brander E et al (1995) Osteitis caused by bacille Calmette-Guérin vaccination: a retrospective analysis of 222 cases. J Infect Dis 172:574
56. Abramowsky C, Gonzales B, Sorensen RU (1993) Disseminated bacillus Calmette-Guérin infections in patients with primary immunodeficiencies. Am J Clin Pathol 100:52

57. Casanova JL, Blanche S, Emile JF et al (1996) Idiopathic disseminated bacillus Calmette-Guérin infection: a French national retrospective study. Pediatrics 98:774
58. Talbot EA, Perkins MD, Silva SF et al (1997) Disseminated bacille Calmette-Guérin disease after vaccination: case report and review. Clin Infect Dis 24:1139
59. van Deutekom H, Smulders YM, Roozendaal KJ et al (1996) Bacille Calmette-Guérin (BCG) meningitis in an AIDS patient 12 years after vaccination with BCG. Clin Infect Dis 22:870
60. Grange JM (1998) Complications of bacille Calmette-Guérin (BCG) vaccination and immunotherapy and their management. Commun Dis Public Health 1:84
61. Izumi AK, Matsunaga J (1982) BCG vaccine-induced lupus vulgaris. Arch Dermatol 118:171
62. Handjani F, Delir S, Sodaifi M et al (2001) Lupus vulgaris following bacille Calmette-Guérin vaccination. Br J Dermatol 144:444
63. Horwitz O, Meyer J (1957) The safety record of BCG vaccination and untoward reactions observed after vaccination. Bibl Tuberc 13:245
64. Atasoy M, Aliağaoğlu C, Erdem T et al (2005) Scrofuloderma following BCG vaccination. Pediatr Dermatol 22:179
65. Muto J, Kuroda K, Tajima S (2006) Papular tuberculides post-BCG vaccination: case report and review of the literature in Japan. Clin Exp Dermatol 31:611
66. Inoue T, Fukumoto T, Ansai S et al (2006) Erythema induratum of Bazin in an infant after Bacille Calmette-Guerin vaccination. J Dermatol 33:268
67. Nielsen T (1979) Basal cell epithelioma in a BCG vaccination scar. Arch Dermatol 115:678
68. Sanders R, Dickon MG (1982) BCG vaccination scars: an avoidable problem? Br Med J 285:1679
69. Fang JW, Ko BM, Wilson JA (1993) BCG vaccination scars: incidence and acceptance amongst British high-school children. Child Care Health Dev 19:37
70. Kwamanga D, Githui W, Agwanda R et al (1993) BCG scar survey among primary school children in Kenya (1986–1990). East Afr Med J 70:568
71. Boran C, Coban YK, Sasmaz S et al (2003) Huge keloid formation after BCG vaccination. Pediatr Dermatol 20:460
72. Tala E, Romans V, Tala-Heikkilä M (1997) Bacille Calmette-Guérin vaccination in the 21st century. Eur Respir Mon 4:327
73. United Kingdom Health Deparments (1996) Immunization against infections diseases. HMSO, London
74. Department of Health (1996) Tuberculosis: two reports from the Interdepartmental Working Group on Tuberculosis. Executive Lett 93:51
75. Rodrigues LC, Noel Gill O, Smith PG (1991) BCG vaccination in the first year of life protects children of Indian subcontinent ethnic origin against tuberculosis in England. J Epidemiol Community Health 45:78
76. Salo EP (2006) BCG in Finland: changing from a universal to a selected programme. Euro Surveill 11:18
77. Romanus V, Svensson A, Hallander HO (1992) The impact of changing BCG coverage on tuberculosis incidence in Swedish-born children between 1969 and 1989. Tuber Lung Dis 73:150
78. Brewer TF, Heymann SJ, Krumplitsch SM et al (2001) Strategies to decrease tuberculosis in US homeless populations: a computer simulation model. JAMA 286:834
79. Centers for Disease Control and Prevention (1996) The role of BCG vaccine in the prevention and control of tuberculosis in the United States. A joint statement by the Advisory Council for the Elimination of Tuberculosis and the Advisory Committee on Immunization Practices. MMWR Recomm Rep 45:1
80. Cobelens FG, van Deutekom H, Draayer-Jansen IW et al (2000) Risk of infection with *Mycobacterium tuberculosis* in travellers to areas of high tuberculosis endemicity. Lancet 356:461
81. Ministero della Salute (2013) Prevenzione della tubercolosi negli operatori sanitari e soggetti ad essi equiparati. Ministero della Salute. Direzione Generale della Prevenzione, Ufficio V, Malattie Infettive e Profilassi Internazionale. 7 febbraio

82. von Reyn CF, Vuola JM (2002) New vaccines for the prevention of tuberculosis. Clin Infect Dis 35:465
83. Doherty TM, Andersen P (2000) Tuberculosis vaccines: developmental work and the future. Curr Opin Pulm Med 6:203
84. Alderson MR, Bement T, Day CH et al (2000) Expression cloning of an immunodominant family of *Mycobacterium tuberculosis* antigens using human CD4+ T cells. J Exp Med 191:551
85. Waddell RD, Chintu C, Lein AD et al (2000) Safety and immunogenicity of a five-dose series of inactivated *Mycobacterium vaccae* vaccination for the prevention of HIV-associated tuberculosis. Clin Infect Dis 30(Suppl 3):S309
86. Manabe YC, Scott CP, Bishai WR (2002) Naturally attenuated, orally administered *Mycobacterium microti* as a tuberculosis vaccine is better than subcutaneous *Mycobacterium bovis* BCG. Infect Immun 70:1566
87. Grode L, Seiler P, Baumann S et al (2005) Increased vaccine efficacy against tuberculosis of recombinant *Mycobacterium bovis* bacille Calmette-Guérin mutants that secrete listeriolysin. J Clin Invest. 115:2472

Leprosy

5

Domenico Bonamonte, Angela Filoni, Pietro Verni,
Paolo Romita, and Gianni Angelini

Leprosy (synonyms: Hansen's disease, Hanseniasis, Hansenosis, Lepra) (from the Latin word *lepra*, which means "scaly" and the Greek *lepo* meaning "to scale") is a chronic infective granulomatous disease caused by the bacillus *Mycobacterium leprae*, an intracytoplasmic parasite of Schwann cells and macrophages. It mainly affects the peripheral nervous system, skin, and other tissues such as the reticuloendothelial system, mucous membranes, the eyes, testes, bones and joints, muscles, and adrenal glands [1–10]. Among communicable diseases, leprosy is one of the leading causes of permanent physical disability worldwide. The disease and resulting visible deformities contribute to the intense social stigma associated with this affliction, that provokes discrimination and avoidance of any contact with patients and their families. Pathogenic transmission occurs via person-to-person contact, especially through the nasorespiratory route, although there is some possibility of transplacental infection [11]. Recently, zoonotic infections have also been reported [12, 13].

Once distributed worldwide, leprosy is now seen primarily in the tropical and subtropical regions of Asia, Africa, and Central and South America. This geographic distribution is likely due more to the poor living standards and hygiene than to the warmer climate [2, 3]. Although it can exceptionally be fatal, leprosy is still one of the most serious long term health problems in developing countries [14, 15].

D. Bonamonte, MD, PhD (✉)
Department of Biomedical Science and Human Oncology,
University of Bari "Aldo Moro", Bari, Italy
e-mail: domenico.bonamonte@uniba.it

A. Filoni, MD • P. Verni, MD • P. Romita, MD
University of Bari "Aldo Moro", Bari, Italy

G. Angelini, MD
Professor of Dermatology, Former Professor and Chairman,
University of Bari "Aldo Moro", Bari, Italy

D. Bonamonte, G. Angelini (eds.), *Mycobacterial Skin Infections*,
DOI 10.1007/978-3-319-48538-6_5

The host immune response is responsible for the variable clinical features of the disease, ranging from forms with only mild signs and a good immune response, to diffuse, very severe forms with little or no immune response.

5.1 History

Leprosy is an ancient disease. The first written records are in the Indian Veda books dating back to 600 B.C., although recent archeological findings in India have revealed a skeleton dated 2000 B.C. with evident signs of leprosy [16, 17]. In China, the most ancient description of the disease is to be found in a classic tome of Chinese medicine dating back to 400 B.C., the "Nei Jing" [18].

Instead, the cases mentioned in the Bible actually refer to psoriasis, vitiligo and other skin disorders not leprosy. In fact, for many years the biblical term *tzaraat* was taken to refer to leprosy; however, the disease or diseases described under this name has no relation to leprosy as it was known in the Middle Ages, nor even in its current form. Leprosy was associated with the biblical leprosy as a result of two inaccurate translations: the Hebrew *tzaraat* was first translated in Greek as leprosy in the sixth century (because there was no equivalent for *tzaraat* in Greek), and then the word leprosy was translated into Arabic as lepra in the ninth century [19]. There is a growing consensus that the term leprosy used in the Bible to define a group of skin diseases has no connection to Hansen's disease as it is known today [20–25]: in fact, the skin manifestations reported in the Bible are very different from those characterizing Hansen's disease today [22, 24].

In the eastern Mediterranean the disease was carried by the Jews in their flight from Egypt, where it had been introduced by the slaves carried off from modern-day Ethiopia [18]. It was then brought in from India by soldiers marching with Alexander the Great between 327–326 B.C., and spread throughout the Greek and Roman Empires [6]. The first scientific evidence of leprosy was found in an Egyptian skeleton and two Coptic mummies from the second century B.C. and the fifth century A.D., respectively [6].

The Phoenician traders were the first to spread leprosy along the western Mediterranean coasts. In ancient Greece, in fact, leprosy was known as "the Phoenician canker" or "canker of Tyre". In the seventh and eighth centuries A.D. leprosy already posed a social problem, and indeed, in Italy and then in France laws were passed to isolate sufferers [18]. The disease became endemic in Europe in the Middle Ages, between the twelfth and thirteenth centuries, owing to both military forays and trade routes between Asia and Europe. The environmental conditions in the various European cities at the time, where both individual and collective hygiene were extremely poor, contributed to foster the spread.

In the Middle Ages it was the Church that took charge of identifying and isolating lepers, this being the only way to protect the community from contagion, since no effective treatment was discovered until 1942. In a ceremony held in church, the patient, robed in a dark tunic, was officially declared a leper; provided with a sack, a stick, a water container, gloves, a cup and a bell to ring as a warning to people to keep away, the sufferer was then banished from society [26]. Some behavioral rules were dictated: patients should use the stick to indicate what object they wished to buy, only use their own cup for drinking, should never speak to anyone unless standing downwind (in order to prevent transmission because it was already known to be contracted by contact and through the airways). Patients should live at least 1/3 of a mile away from the city walls. At that time lepers rapidly became invalids, went blind and declined slowly toward death [25].

In the 12th century, the first leper asylums appeared in the west, to keep them away from the community. By 1200 there were 19,000–20,000 asylums in Europe. The disease had by then spread even to very cold countries like Iceland and Greenland, and affected all social classes. With the passing of centuries and the spread of tuberculosis, leprosy became less common in Europe, and reduced to rare epidemics in poor areas with high promiscuity and poor hygiene [26]. Outbreaks became more and more rare in Europe as from 1700, whereas in southern Europe (Italy, Spain, Greece, Malta) they did not disappear until the 1970s.

In the United States of America, where leprosy did not exist in the pre-Columbian era, the disease was introduced as from the 18th and 19th centuries by the French and Norwegian immigrants and remained active until the 1950s, while in the islands of Oceania and New Guinea, it appeared in the 20th century. A true regression of the disease occurred only after 1950 with the introduction of sulfone [26].

During the 19th century, Daniel Cornelius Danielssen (1815–1894) and Carl W. Boeck (1808–1875) reported the first modern description of leprosy [6], and in the 1870s, a third Norwegian, Gerhard Henrik Armauer Hansen (1841–1912), conducted microbiological and epidemiological studies of *M. leprae*, publishing his results on the discovery of the bacillus in 1874 [27–31]. Mitsuda then devised the skin test for leprosy in 1919 [9, 32]. The importance of sulfones to treat leprosy was reported by Faget and Coll in 1942 [33].

In 1960, Shepard published results on the sensitivity of mice to leprosy, demonstrating a limited proliferation of mycobacteria taken from human tissue specimens and inoculated in mouse footpads to test their sensitivity to drugs [34]. In 1966, Ridley and Jopling suggested a classification of leprosy based on the immunologic status of the patient [35]. Since the 1970s, studies of the proliferation of *M. leprae* have been made on nine-banded armadillos, which contract leprosy [36]. Finally, in 2001, the sequencing of the entire genome of *M. leprae* was reported [37].

Over the course of time, leprosy has not only posed a challenge to medicine but also to social and charitable activities [38]. Among the great philanthropists who dedicated their professional and family lives to dealing with leprosy patients, Dr. Albert Schweitzer (1875–1965), an Alsatian theologian, Lutheran minister, musicologist, and philosopher, deserves particular mention. In 1913 he founded a leprosy hospital in Lambaréné in the French Congo (now Gabon), and in 1952 he was awarded the Nobel Peace Prize [38]. Another great figure was Agnes Gonxha Bojaxhiu (1910–1997), better known by her monastic name, Maria Theresa of Child Jesus of Calcutta. At the age of 18, she left her country, Albania, and started her missionary work in Calcutta in August 1948. In 1956, Mother Theresa and the Missionaries of Charity (the name of the order she founded) established a center for leprosy patients ("Skantinagar": "City of Peace") near Asansol (Calcutta). In 1979, Mother Theresa received a Nobel Prize for her humanitarian work [38].

Among other great philanthropists was the Polish doctor Wanda Maria Bleńska (1911–2013, nicknamed the "Mother of the Lepers"), who worked in a leprosy center in Bulubie, Lake Victoria in Uganda (she often repeated that leprosy patients need vitamins, the most important of which is vitamin "L", meaning *love*), as well as the Polish missionary Marian Zelazek (1918–2006), whose missionary work was carried out in India, in particular [38].

5.2 Epidemiology

The most important source of data on the epidemiology of leprosy is the World Health Organization (WHO) and its *Weekly Epidemiologic Record*, the last of which refers to 2014 [39]. Worldwide, data have been collected since 1985, when the prevalence of leprosy was about 5 million; by 2014 it had dropped to 175,554 (number of cases recorded; prevalence/10,000 population: 0.31) [39, 40]. The goal of the "elimination of leprosy as a public health problem" policy by the WHO, declared in 1991, namely to reduce the prevalence below 1 patient per 10,000 population, has since been achieved thanks to the advent of multidrug therapy (MDT), intensive control programs, and changing case definitions [40].

The data in the latest WHO report derive from 121 countries from 5 WHO Regions: 29 countries in Africa, 31 countries from the Americas, 19 from the Eastern Mediterranean, 11 from South-East Asia, and 31 from the Western Pacific. There were no data from European countries (Table 5.1). The annual reports contain data on the number of cases administered MDT at the year's end, the new cases reported during the year, the multibacillary cases, paucibacillary cases, the number of women and children among the new cases and the new cases with a reduction of grade 2 disabilities (R2D cases) [39].

The main indicator of the outcome of the fight against leprosy, and also the nearest approximation of the disease incidence, is the number of new cases detected (NCD) in a given year. Analysis of the WHO data shows that this indicator was relatively stable between the years 1985 and 1997, ranging from 550,000 to 700,000

Table 5.1 Registered prevalence of leprosy and number of new cases in 102 countries (modified, by [39])

Region	No cases registered, first quarter of 2015 (prevalence/10.000 population)	No new cases detected in 2014 (new-case detection rate/100.000 population)
Africa	19,968 (0.26)	18,597 (2.44)
Americas	29,967 (0.33)	33,789 (3.75)
Eastern Mediterranean	2212 (0.04)	2342 (0.38)
South East Asia	119,478 (0.63)	154,834 (8.12)
Western Pacific	3929 (0.02)	4337 (0.24)
Total	175,554 (0.31)	213,899 (3.78)

cases. In the following years the number of NCD dropped, and then remained stable from 2005 (NCD: 299,036) to 2014 (NCD: 213,899). WHO information about these data are lacking [41]. Some authors believe that in the last decade, due to WHO recommendations (simplification of the anti-leprosy campaign by abolishing the microbiological assessment and establishing the diagnosis and disease classification, used to select the therapeutic regimen, only on clinical aspects, namely the number of lesions) the diagnostic sensitivity and quality of treatments have declined [10].

However, it is also true that leprosy is marked by some peculiar features: its chronic nature, particularly long incubation times, minor early symptoms and signs, and the difficulty in establishing the time of onset of the disease due to the lack of suitable diagnostic tests to verify the presence of infection in a subject. At the time when the specific treatment is begun, the patient may already have infected other subjects, who will develop the disease much later. It is therefore likely that the impact of the treatment on the reduction of the NCD will be very gradual [40].

In any case, on the basis of the number of new cases worldwide it is clear that leprosy is still a major public health problem, especially in three regions, Southeast Asia, the Americas and Africa. In 2014, Southeast Asia reported the highest number of new cases, 154,834, accounting for 72% of the global burden. The highest number of sufferers was reported in India, 125,785 cases, or 81% of the new regional cases and 59% of the new cases in the world. South America reported 33,789 cases (16% of the total), Brazil having the highest number of cases, 31,064 (92% of the regional and 15% of the global NCD). Africa reported 18,597 cases: 8.7% of the global total [39]. In 2014, 13 countries continued to report more than 1000 new cases (94% of all the NCD), with minor variations as compared to the previous years, calculated up to 2005 (Table 5.2).

Globally, 37.7% of NCD are women. Child cases indicate early, continual transmission of the infection: the proportion of children among the new cases is 8.8% globally. New G2D (reduction of grade 2 disabilities) cases, on the other hand, indicate a delayed detection of the disease: the proportion is 6.6% globally [39]. During 2014, moreover, 1312 cases of relapse were reported, in 106 countries; relapse is the result of inadequate and/or incomplete treatment [39].

Table 5.2 New cases reported in 2014 in 13 countries (modified, by [39])

Country	Number of new cases
India	125,785
Brazil	31,064
Indonesia	17,025
Ethiopia	3758
Bangladesh	3622
Democratic Republic of Congo	3272
Nepal	3046
Nigeria	2983
Myanmar	2877
Sri Lanka	2157
United Republic of Tanzania	1947
Philippines	1655
Madagascar	1617
Total	213,899

In view of the above data, it is extremely difficult to make accurate predictions of future trends for leprosy. The predicted annual decline of incidence ranges from 2 to 12%: this means that the eradication strategies are reducing transmission but the decline is still very slow [39]. It is important to have a clear understanding of the modes of transmission of the disease, also taking into account possible animal or environmental reservoirs of *M. leprae*. The global NCD trends will likely remain more or less stable over the short term. Since MDT alone is not sufficient to prevent new cases, in order to reduce the incidence of leprosy in the 21st century new preventive measures are needed, like chemoprophylaxis and immunoprophylaxis, as well as the earliest possible detection of cases [40, 42].

A predictive study of the future incidence of leprosy in three highly endemic countries, namely India, Brazil and Indonesia, which account for more than 80% of all cases worldwide, revealed that although the infection should be eliminated in the very near future at nation-level, in the highly endemic regions of these three nations (Chhattisgarh, Pará State and Madura) this same elimination will not achieved by 2020 with the current leprosy control strategy. Regional NCD rates are 2–7 times higher than at the nation level [43]. These data demonstrate an absolute need for further control measures.

5.3 Modes of Transmission

Leprosy is one of the oldest diseases in the world, and among the most dramatic. Even today sufferers are often ostracized. It is essential, therefore, that the general public be made aware that leprosy is not a genetic disorder and that it is 100% curable, and that patients, on the contrary, are in need of constant, complete social support [44].

Over time, the knowledge of the etiopathogenesis of leprosy has evolved from the original miasmic non microbial theory of the origin of disease, or anti-contagion, to the modern recognition of contagion and genetics [45]. According to the ancient miasmic theory, dating back to Hippocrates (c 460 B.C. to c 370 B.C.), a disease is caused by the miasma emanating from rotting matter coming from inside the hearth, that enters the human body and induces various diseases, including leprosy. The treatment of miasma diseases consisted of righting the imbalance among the four Hippocratic humors underlying human health, namely blood, phlegm, bile, and black bile, by means of bloodletting, and the administration of diaphoretics and emetics [44–47]. The miasma theory endured over the centuries, until it was discarded by some modern dermatologists between the end of the 18th and beginning of the 19th century [45]. As well as Jean-Louis Alibert (1768–1838), Ferdinand Hebra (1816–1880), and Louis Adolphus Duhring (1845–1913), even Jonathan Hutchinson (1828–1913) believed in the miasma theory, attributing the cause of leprosy to poor hygiene, an unbalanced diet, humid climate, and plentiful consumption of badly cured fish [48, 49].

Then, the development of histological and cytological studies began to clarify the etiology of leprosy. Daniel Cornelius Danielssen (1815–1894) was the first to describe the presence of "vacuolated" or "foamy" cells with a light yellow diaphanous mass and ill-defined borders, and containing chestnut-colored small granules [45]. These same cells were later described by Rudolf LK Virchow (1821–1902). Finally, Gerhard Armauer Hansen (1841–1912) revealed that the acid-alcohol resistant rods in lepra cells were the leprosy bacillus [27–30, 45], and attempted to culture them and inoculate them under laboratory conditions. The failure to inoculate them in laboratory animals led to rejection by medical society of the entire infectious hypothesis advanced by Hansen. Nevertheless, Hansen published his results in 1874 [27, 30]. Then he made the morally inacceptable decision to inoculate a patient with a maculoanesthetic form of the disease with material taken from a leprosy nodule of a patient with a tuberous form [29]. The same experiment had been made by Danielssen years before, when he inoculated three volunteers with material from lepromatous nodules. Fortunately both attempts yielded negative results [30].

Virchow believed that the rods observed by Hansen were nothing other than crystals of fatty acids [29] and Albert LS Neisser (1855–1916), who had been given biological material from lepromatous patients by Hansen, published his results in October 1879, claiming to be the first to observe the leprosy bacillus. Neisser also described the aggregation of the bacilli in "globes", which had not been previously reported by Hansen. After an exchange of correspondence with Hansen in 1880, however, Neisser admitted Hansen's prior discovery of the leprosy bacillus [45, 50, 51]. At the First International Congress of Leprology in 1897 in Berlin, Hansen's infective hypothesis was accepted, and the possibility of person-to-person transmission of the disease [45].

The problem of experimental inoculation in animals was finally solved in 1960 by Shepard, who demonstrated the sensitivity of mice to leprosy [34]. In 2001, Cole and Coll of the Pasteur Institute in Paris sequenced the *M. leprae* genome, and this made it possible to determine the region where the infection arose and its source, man or armadillo [52, 53].

In 2005, again at the Pasteur Institute, following a study of 175 samples from 21 countries, four polymorphisms were identified, differentiating strains of *M. leprae*: the first and rarest in Ethiopia, New Caledonia and Nepal; the second in Asia and the Pacific coasts of East Africa (Madagascar and Mozambique); the third in Europe and the Americas; the fourth in the Caribbean and West Africa [54]. Leprosy has affected every part of the world in different periods of history, but its irregular geographic distribution has always been considered an enigma. There can be no doubt that it also affects colder countries, but it is also true that in some countries (Japan, Norway, and the United States) its incidence had declined even before the advent of the specific treatment. Nowadays the five countries with the highest rates of incidence are located in (sub)tropical regions: India, Brazil, Indonesia, Bangladesh, and Ethiopia [39]. Leprosy is nonrandom in its distribution [55]. Even in endemic zones patients are not equally distributed but rather extensively clustered, and there is an unequal distribution even in focal areas [56].

Man is considered to be the main source of infection. Contact with a subject known to have leprosy is the principal risk factor, even if the mode of transmission of the microorganism from one individual to another is still uncertain [57]. It is very likely that transmission occurs through droplets via aerosols. The entry portal of bacteria in man seems to be the nasal mucosa, although the skin may also play a part.

Leprosy patients do not all transmit the disease to the same extent, and the greatest source is untreated multibacillary lepromatous patients [58, 59], who shed large quantities of bacilli from their nose. Contact with these patients poses the highest risk of contagion, 5–8-fold higher than the general population [59]. It is still not entirely clear whether paucibacillary patients are infectious in all stages of the disease, and whether those with a subclinical infection (with no clinical signs) are already infective [40]. Another source of infection may be silent carriers with bacilli in the nasal mucosa who live in endemic leprosy areas, as demonstrated in a seroepidemiology and polymerase chain reaction study that showed positivity rates among contacts and non contacts [60]. Another study revealed that in highly endemic areas not only household contact with seropositive patients but also with those in neighboring houses is more likely to induce antibodies against *M. leprae* [61]. These same Authors found that seroprevalence was higher among people who live in close proximity to seropositive patients ($\leq$75 m), and that there is an even greater increase, albeit not always, in the presence of two seropositive patients [61]. This is the "stone-in-the-pond" concept, originally developed for tuberculosis and then used for leprosy, to describe the transmission in concentric circles around a patient.

Leprosy can present with different clinical pictures according to the host immunity to Hansen's bacillus. Other factors that have an effect are genetic differences, age, nutritional and health status [62]. Various studies have reported a protective effect of BCG vaccination, at percentages ranging from 20 to 90% [63]. Even environmental mycobacteria can confer some degree of protection against leprosy [64].

The highest age incidence is between 15 and 20, while there are regional differences in sex ratios; a prevalence is often reported in the male sex, also for multibacillary forms, and males also develop serious disabilities more frequently than females [40].

Surprisingly, in endemic areas not more than 5% of exposed subjects will develop the disease in their lifetimes, even if there have been outright epidemics in some cases [65, 66]. There do not seem to be causal relations between leprosy and poverty, but malnutrition could play a role in bringing about the disease [67]. HIV infection does not seem to have altered the course of the disease in co-infected patients to any great extent [68], even if recent data indicate a higher incidence of leprosy in HIV patients in treatment with highly active antiretroviral therapy than was previously supposed [69].

5.3.1 Modes of Direct and Environmental Skin Transmission

A number of studies have been focused upon a possible transmission of leprosy through direct inoculation into the skin [70]. Relevant injuries include tattoos [71–73], falls [74, 75], injuries involving objects [76, 77], contaminated needles in a medical setting [78], thorns pricking armadillos in the nose and ears [79], vaccination scars [80, 81], general injuries [82, 83], and animal bites [84]. However, these modes of transmission must be considered exceptional and have a low frequency, even if the possible transmission through tattooing tools has important implications from the hygiene and public health standpoints.

Indirect transmission of *M. leprae* could occur through environmental reservoirs, as emerged in a case-control study conducted in Brazil [85]. *M. leprae* can survive for months outside the human body in favorable circumstances, and so could be a source of infection [86, 87]. It has been seen that *M. leprae* can be harbored in soil [88–91], in water [87], on plants [92–94], in various animal species such as amoeba [95], insects [96, 97], and fish [49, 98, 99], in primates [100], and armadillos [101, 102]. A knowledge of these sources will obviously have implications on the possibility or controlling or eradicating the disease. There are two reasons for the search for non human sources of *M. leprae*, firstly the repeated observation of infection in subjects with no apparent history of exposure to other known cases [55, 103–105], and secondly the presence of disease clusters in particular areas, like near to water sources [85, 106]. However, to date there is still no clear evidence of infection caused by environmental non-human sources. Above all, it is important to differentiate non-human reservoirs (all the studies investigating the presence of *M. leprae* in soil, water or other environmental non-human samples used molecular techniques to detect bacterial DNA or RNA) of *M. leprae* from a transient environmental presence. Lepromatous patients can spread large numbers of bacilli in the environment through bodily secretions, or while sneezing, coughing or talking [55, 107–109]. The fact that some bacilli can stay viable in certain cell-free environments for hours, days or weeks does not mean that they can persist as infectious reservoirs [110, 111]. The problem is whether the bacilli can replicate: on the basis of what we know about the *M. leprae* genoma, it is highly unlikely that leprosy bacilli can replicate in any extra-cellular environment [37]. The notion of free-living *M. leprae* persisting in the environment is therefore biologically implausible, even if it might be possible that in water the bacilli could be associated with protozoa or with aquatic invertebrates hosts, as has been suggested for *M. ulcerans* [112]. There is also debate as to whether *M. leprae* can persist in other vertebrates. In fact, the host range is very limited [88]: some species of primates appear to be only marginally susceptible to the experimental infection, and few animals develop the disease in captivity [113, 114], while in free-ranging primates the infection has never yet been reported. The predilection of *M. leprae* for cool body temperatures was recognized immediately after discovery of the bacillus, and in 1911 Couret suggested that fish could be suitable hosts for propagating the bacilli [98]. However, up to now laboratory attempts in fish have failed, and the only non-human source in which it is notoriously possible to replicate *M. leprae* is the mouse footpad (*Mus musculus*) and the nine-banded armadillo (*Dasypus novemcinctus*). In this regard it should also be noted that mouse is not a source of the bacillus outside the artificial laboratory environment: conventional mouse, in fact, is relatively resistant to *M. leprae*, can kill the bacilli after infection and does not develop the disease [115].

5.4 *Mycobacterium leprae* and Armadillos

In 1971, Kirchheimer and Storrs discovered that the nine-banded armadillo (*D. novemcinctus*) (Fig. 5.1) was susceptible to experimental infection with *M. leprae* [36], and thereby revolutionized the research field, making the armadillo the host of choice for the propagation in vivo of the leprosy bacilli [70, 88, 116]. In 1975, the existence of a natural systemic leprous infection was discovered among wild armadillos in the Southern United States [117]. It was then ascertained that the armadillo bacillus is indistinguishable from the human bacillus, that the infection is widespread among armadillos in the Southern United States [101, 118] and that in the armadillo, the infection originates by natural means [13, 102]. It has recently been confirmed that leprosy is a zoonosis in this region and that the armadillo is likely involved in up to 64% of the new human leprosy cases recorded in the United States each year [119], thus highlighting the role of these animals as a reservoir of the human infection.

Belonging to the Xenarthra order, there are 21 different species of armadillos in nine different genera [119]; the most important armadillo in leprosy research is *D. novemcinctus* (also known as the long-nosed or nine-banded armadillo). Armadillos are about the size of domestic cats, have short limbs and a hard flexible banded carapace protecting the body. Their body temperature is low, 33–35°C, a most important characteristic that has attracted the attention of leprosy researchers since as stated above, the bacillus is known to have a predilection for the cooler regions of the human body. Another important feature in the armadillo is that the bacilli multiply and give rise to a systemic infection. Experimental infection routes in the armadillo are intravenous (that can increase the number of bacilli 10,000-fold), intradermic, percutaneous and respiratory [120]. To cause infection, 1×10^3 bacilli are enough, even if the incubation times reduce with higher doses of bacilli ($1\text{–}4 \times 10^9$) injected intravenously. In the armadillo the bacilli are localized in the peripheral nerves and the cells of the reticuloendothelial system, so the infection can become generalized without causing any significant impairment of the vital organs. After 18–24 months from experimental inoculation, most of these animals develop a severe infection, with up to 10^{12} bacilli recoverable from each animal [116, 120, 121].

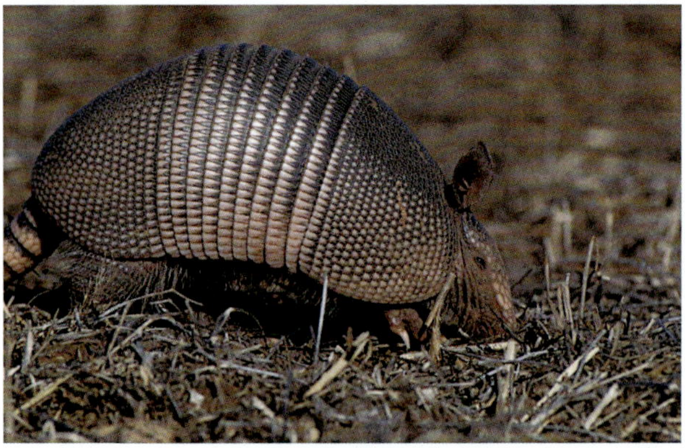

Fig. 5.1 Armadillo *Dasypus novemcinctus* (Picture under public domain. Reproduced from U.S. Fish and Wildlife Service, John and Karen Hollingsworth)

Unlike man, only 15–20% of armadillos are resistant to the infection [120]. But like in man, where is a genetic association for susceptibility to *M. leprae* [122, 123], in armadillo there will also be a comparable response to the infection in the mother and offspring, and the genetic traits in *M. leprae*-resistant animals are similar to those in resistant humans [124].

In the armadillo, skin lesions are not easy to see, while the most common symptoms are the typical plantar ulceration, and abrasions of the nose, eyes and feet and in other parts of the animal's body subject to friction [125]. Plantar ulcers show an increased severity and frequency in the advanced stages of the infection and are likely similar to those in humans, linked to a reduced sensitivity of the lower limbs [120]. Serological, histopathological tests and polymerase chain reaction of *M. leprae*-specific DNA are necessary to make the diagnosis also in the armadillo [126]. Only man and the amadillo develop a comparable intense neurological involvement by *M. leprae*, while in all other laboratory animals no involvement of the nerves has been found. The granulomatous response of the armadillo to *M. leprae* is structurally identical to that in man, with the same Ridley-Jopling histological spectrum. In about 70% of armadillos there is a response to the lepromin skin test for the lepromatous type, while the remaining responses are of borderline or tuberculoid type [127].

5.4.1 Zoonotic Leprosy

The armadillo does not easily reproduce in captivity, and needs to be taken from the wild to study the infection. In 1975, Walsh discovered that free-ranging armadillos in Louisiana were naturally affected by infection from *M. leprae*, and it was later found that the disease was widespread among North American armadillos [117]. Although the infection was perhaps originally localized in the areas of the Western Gulf of Mexico, it is certain that nowadays it occurs among armadillos all over the northern range. The highest prevalence in the USA is among animals that inhabit low-lying poorly drained areas, especially those of the southern Mississippi river valley and other bottom-lands [117].

Recent observations have demonstrated that leprosy is a zoonosis in the Southern United States, and that the armadillo can transmit *M. leprae* to man. Multiple *M. leprae* genotypic-strains have been identified in patients in the United States, confirming that the infection was introduced from different regions. However, the single unique *M. leprae* genotypic-strain (3I-2-v1) present among 88% of the wild armadillos was also found in 64% of the patients studied: it is therefore the primary strain for endemic human infection in the southern United States, where several patients actually use armadillos for food or have direct contact with these animals [13]. Leprosy was not present in the New World in pre-Colombian times but it had become widespread by 1750 in the vicinity of New Orleans. Armadillos must therefore have acquired the infection from man in the last 300 years [128].

Biomarkers of *M. leprae* have been reported in armadillos in Argentina [129], Brazil [130–132], Colombia [133], and Mexico [134]. Epidemiological studies in

Brazil have also demonstrated environmental sources for some cases of human infection, and that contact with armadillos is a significant risk factor for leprosy [85, 104]. In some parts of Texas the density of armadillos is up to 50/km^2, whereas it is very much lower in South America [135, 136]. Moreover, the armadillos in South America present less genetic diversity (that seems to make the animals more resistant to the disease) than those in the United States.

5.5 Etiology

The etiological agent of leprosy is *M. leprae* (Hansen's bacillus), a non cultivable, Gram-positive obligate intracellular, acid-fast bacillus (Fig. 5.2). In size and shape it closely resembles the bacillus of tuberculosis. Under the electron microscope the bacillus seems to show a great variety of forms; the most common is a slightly curved rod-shaped organism with parallel sides and rounded ends, 1–8 μm long and 0.3 μm in diameter. Apart from these typical aspects, degenerating elements can be seen (fragmented, granular with bipolar staining) or undergoing involution (curved, and larger than normal) in histological preparations. They stain red with the Ziehl-Neelsen method, whereas they do not react to Sudan black.

M. leprae grows at 30–33°C, with a doubling time of 12 days. The genome sequence, published in 2001 [37], is of a 3.27 Mb genome that displays an extremely reductive evolution. Less than half the genome contains functional genes: many pseudogenes are present. One hundred and sixty five genes are unique to *M. leprae*, and functions may be attributed to 29 of them. Comparing the genome sequence of *M. leprae* with that of *M. tuberculosis* reveals an extreme case of reductive evolution. Gene deletion and decay have eliminated many important activities, such as siderophore production, part of the oxidative and most of the microaerophylic and

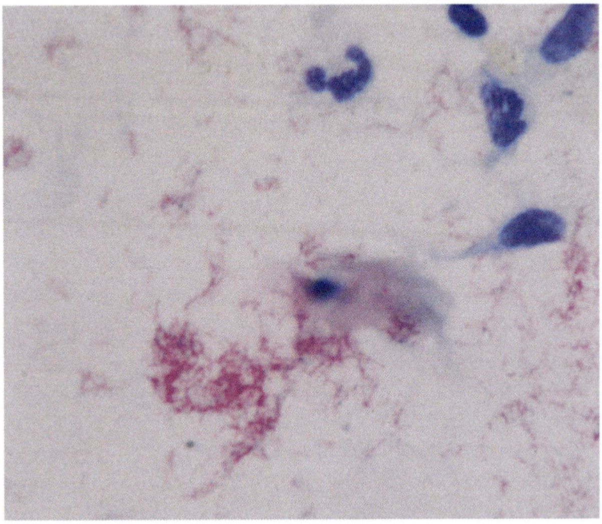

Fig. 5.2 Intact bacilli, single and in bunches, in nasal secretion of lepromatous leprosy patient

anaerobic respiratory chains, and numerous catabolic systems and their regulatory circuits [7, 8]. In total, 1500 genes are common to both *M. leprae* and *M. tuberculosis*. Comparative analysis reveals that both mycobacteria derived from a common ancestor and, at one stage, they had gene pools of similar size. Down-sizing from a genome of 4.42 Mb, such as that of *M. tuberculosis*, to one of 3.27 Mb would account for the loss of some 1200 protein coding sequences [7].

Leprosy bacilli are localized both intracellularly (macrophages, giant cells, endothelial cells, neutrophils, Schwann cells) and extracellularly: they can be isolated or grouped in parallel, as a "palisade" or as "bundles of cigars". Most striking are the intracellular and extracellular masses known as "globi", which consist of clumps of bacilli in morphocapsular material. The bacterial surface appears to be surrounded by a thick lipid membrane that permits reciprocal cohesion and determines drug resistance.

Up to now, attempts to culture the bacillus in inert media have failed. Tissue cultures (human fibroblasts) have limited use because the replication rate of the mycobacteria is much slower than that of the host cells (mitosis occurs every 20–30 days). Animal models of the infection are therefore very important, even if they are not easy to set up, for the purposes of drug screening, sensitivity studies of microorganisms isolated from patients, and experimental drug design. In vivo, the bacilli multiply if injected into the mouse footpad, the site of choice due to the microorganism's predilection for colder temperature regions of the human body (the nose, ear pavilions, fingers, testicles). Mice subjected to thymectomy or fatal irradiation present lepromatous lesions even after intravenous injection. Among animal species, those that develop a generalized infection are the armadillo and the porcupine (*Hystrix*, used in Europe), animals that have a lower body temperature (30°C–36°C).

Some distinguishing characteristics are typical of *M. leprae* (apart from failure to grow in vitro in standard culture media, the limited growth on the mouse footpad and the antigen determinants): the loss of acid-fast resistance after treatment with pyridine and the oxidation of dihydroxyphenylalanine. Treatment with pyridine of slides containing *M. leprae* deprives the bacilli of the ability to retain the stain after destaining with the Ziehl-Neelsen technique. However, fresh highly pure pyridine needs to be used. Since other mycobacteria (*M. vaccae, M. phlei*) can behave in the same way, the loss of acid-fastness must be considered an additional criterion, not a specific one. Another typical feature is the *M. leprae* ability to oxidize diphenols, and this capacity is specific to the bacillus; the substance used is D-3-4-dihydroxyphenylalanine (DOPA) [137].

As Hansen had already observed, the Ziehl-Neelsen technique does not uniformly stain all the bacteria on a skin slide. Hansen believed this was an index of bacterial degeneration. In fact, using the *M. leprae* inoculation technique on the mouse footpad, it has been shown that the irregularly stained bacteria are not vital. These findings prompted the notion of the morphological index (MI) and bacterial index (BI). The former is based on the percentage of "solidly" stained *M. leprae* in biopsies or skin strips treated with the Ziehl-Neelsen method. During the treatment, the number of non uniformly stained bacilli increases, so the MI is useful to control the effects of therapy, although this determination is fairly delicate and requires considerable experience [137]. The BI is expressed in terms of a variation in the total number of bacilli in a skin strip, regardless of their morphology. It provides a valid indication of the bacterial load and can be used for clinical classification purposes or to assess the efficacy of therapy.

Electron microscopy has revealed some characteristics aspects of *M. leprae* derived from both human and mouse and armadillo tissues. Some bands are evident on the surface of the microorganism, that are probably signs of cell wall division [138]. The cell wall is about 20 nm thick and, like other mycobacteria, is two-layered, with an inner electron-dense layer and an outer electron-transparent layer. The cytoplasm is electron-dense and contains structures that are common to Gram-positive microorganisms: DNA, mesosomes and storage granules, and a continuous plasma membrane below the cell wall. This is in clear contrast with what is seen in irregularly staining organisms where the contents are partially decomposed and badly destroyed, and the plasma membrane is incomplete [139]. The latter ultra-structural appearances support the evidence of morphological irregularities observed upon the death of the bacilli. Cell division by formation of a cross wall is the conventional process for bacteria. The wall surface has the fibrous structure common to all mycobacteria and the previously mentioned wall bands, that look like ridges surrounding the bacteria [140].

5.5.1 Biological Properties of *Mycobacterium leprae*

All the available information derives from studies conducted in the mouse footpad. *M. leprae* has a generation (doubling) time of 11–13 days during the logarithmic generation phase [141, 142]. This is the slowest known multiplication rate, even as compared to all other slow-growing mycobacteria (*M. tuberculosis* has a generation time of 20 h), that is consistent, in fact, with the chronic nature of the disease. It is important to note that there is no variation in this rate among the many strains of *M. leprae* obtained in different regions of the world, demonstrating that the leprosy type is determined by the host rather than the bacterium. Moreover, identical generation times for *M. leprae* have been reported in both healthy mice and thymectomized-irradiated T-cell deficient mice [143].

The fact that leprosy predominantly affects the skin, nasal mucosa, peripheral nerves (particularly more superficial nerves) and testicles bears witness to the fact that *M. leprae* prefers a growth temperature of less than 37°C. As is well known, this has also been demonstrated in mice, where the infection spreads predominantly to cooler sites [143], and justifies the susceptibility to the infection of the armadillo (where *M. leprae* multiplies in the liver, spleen and lymph nodes), that has a core temperature of 30–36°C [144]. In addition, Shepard has shown that the maximum growth of *M. leprae* in the footpad occurs when the mice are kept at a temperature range of 27–30°C, while distinctly lesser growth occurs at a temperature of 25°C or 36°C [145].

As regards the viability and pathogenicity of *M. leprae* isolated from patients, measured as infectivity (above all in normal or T-cell deficient mice or in the armadillo) and stability following serial passages in animals, it has been ascertained that:

1. viability is retained for 7–10 days in tissues or in tissue homogenates stored at 4°C; 2. there are no differences in the growth pattern or pathogenicity in mouse or armadillo of *M. leprae* strains isolated from patients, regardless of the clinical type of leprosy, or the race or geographic origin of the patients; 3. continuous serial passages of *M. leprae* for several years in normal mice do not increase or change the pathogenicity [139].

It has been demonstrated that acid-fast bacilli from lepromatous patients were viable following mouse footpad inoculation and that the resulting growth pattern resembled *M. leprae* [34]. This shows the importance of nasal secretion as a possible source of man-to-man infection. Moreover, quantitative assessments of the total output of *M. leprae* in nasal discharges, in the form of nose blows, from untreated lepromatous patients have demonstrated that large numbers of viable bacilli are continually discharged [107, 108].

5.5.2 Chemical Composition of *Mycobacterium leprae*

The chemical structure of the *M. leprae* wall, like that of other mycobacteria, consists of a cross-linked peptidoglycan with attached polysaccharide chains (arabinogalactan) bearing mycolic acids. The latter, having a high molecular weight, account for more than half the weight of the walls and are probably responsible for the hydrophobic nature of the mycobacteria. However, while other mycobacteria have three types of mycosides, *M. leprae* has only two, the a- and keto-mycosides. In *M. leprae*, moreover, unlike the other mycobacteria, L-alanine is completely replaced by glycine in the peptide moiety of the peptidoglycan [4, 146].

Mycobacteria are characterized by the production of a variety of unusual lipids, often wall-associated, that form the outermost layer of the bacteria or are secreted into the surrounding environment. Two of these lipids, predominantly extracellular, are specific to *M. leprae*. The first is a serologically active glycolipid of the phenol-glycol type [147], containing a unique trisaccharide (2,3-di-*O*-methylrhamnose, 3-*O*-methylrhamnose and 3,6-di-*O*-methylglucose) [148]. This glycolipid has been found in armadillo liver and in the skin of lepromatous patients, indicating that live *M. leprae* secrete the glycolipid locally, where it accumulates and may constitute the characteristic foamy material seen in the macrophages in lepromatous patients. An even more important feature of this glycolipid is its antigenicity, resulting in the production of anti-glycolipid antibodies of the IgG and IgM classes, identified by immunodiffusion [149] and ELISA techniques [150] in the serum of leprosy patients. ELISA is the more sensitive of the two methods. Antibodies, in particular of the IgM class, have been demonstrated in tuberculoid (60%) and lepromatous (90%) leprosy patients, but not in patients with tuberculosis nor those infected by *M. kansasii, M. avium,* or *M. intracellulare* [151]. These findings underline the species-specificity of the glycolipid (probably determined by the trisaccharide moiety) and its potential as a serological test for leprosy.

The second lipid of special interest from *M. leprae* is phthiocerol dimycocerosate (PDIM), that is structurally related to the glycolipid but lacks carbohydrate.

Although it has also been isolated from *M. tuberculosis* and other mycobacteria species, the PDIM isolated from *M. leprae* is chemically different [151], and is thus another lipid that could be used to identify *M. leprae*.

5.5.3 Bacteriological Aspects

Because *M. leprae* cannot be cultured, the only tests available for the diagnosis and classification of leprosy, and for monitoring response to treatment and applying control measures, are bacteriological tests of tissue from the skin and nasal mucosa.

The skin can be employed for slit-skin smears and for biopsies. Scraping smears from skin lesions, stained by the Ziehl-Neelsen method, is the standard test to estimate the number of *M. leprae* in the lesions (bacterial index, BI) and the proportion of viable bacteria (morphological index, MI, solid ratio). The skin site chosen for the smear is cleaned with spirit on a small cotton swab. After the spirit has dried, the skin is pinched up into a fold between the index finger and thumb, exerting sufficient pressure to prevent or minimize bleeding. Then, with a small sterile scalpel blade, a cut is made about 5 mm long, and deep enough (about 3 mm) to penetrate well into the infiltrated layer of the dermis. Any blood exuding is dried with a cotton swab. The scalpel blade is then rotated by 90 degrees, and with the blunt edge the side of the cut is scraped several times to obtain a tissue pulp from below the epidermis. The material on the scalpel point is then transferred onto a glass microscope slide, where it is spread with a circular movement, to produce a uniform, moderately thick smear over an area of 5–7 mm in diameter [4].

In the case of untreated lepromatous patients or those with suspected drug-resistant relapse, smears must be taken from six sites, namely both ear lobes and four active skin sites. In the case of treated lepromatous patients and those who seem to be responders, as well as patients with non-lepromatous leprosy, smears must be taken from sites previously found to be positive, from both ear lobes and from representative skin areas.

5.5.3.1 Bacterial Index

Various indexes are available to measure the BI; the most reliable and recommended method is based on a logarithmic scale [152], and extends from the presence of very many to very few alcohol-acid-fast bacilli, and the steps (1+, 2+, etc.) are regularly spaced, each additional unit indicating a ten-fold increase in the number of bacilli (Table 5.3). The measurement is carried out under oil immersion (objective lens ×100, eye-piece ×6 or ×8) determining the number of bacilli/field after examining 25–100 fields, on a logarithmic scale ranging from 0 to 6 [4]. Smears containing many red cells are discarded. All bacilli are counted, whether uniformly or irregularly stained, and the number is scored according to the scale in Table 5.3. The scores of the smears from a number of different skin sites added together and divided by the number of sites yields the patient's final BI. An untreated patient with lepromatous leprosy will have a BI in the range 6+ to 5+; the BI will be 0 to 2+ in the case of borderline tuberculoid leprosy and 0 in tuberculoid leprosy.

Table 5.3 Bacterial index score (BI) (modified, by [4])

Average number of AFB	BI[a]
>1000/field	6 +
1000-100/field	5 +
100-10/field	4 +
10-1/field	3 +
10-1/10 fields	2 +
10-1/100 fields	1 +
0/100 fields	0 +

[a]The BI for the patient is the average of the BIs at the individual sites

AFB acid-fast bacilli

5.5.3.2 Morphological Index

After staining with carbol-fuchsin, the bacilli even of untreated patients show a variable morphology: most stain irregularly and only a few show solid-staining acid-fast filaments. Under the electron microscope, the irregularly stained bacilli are organisms showing gross degenerative alterations while the solid-stained rods are the only vital ones, that are infectious for mice. On this assumption, bearing in mind that the number of irregularly stained bacilli increases with treatment, the morphological index was introduced as an indirect measure of their viability, and to measure the response to treatment [152]. On the same slit-skin smears used to measure the BI, in fields picked at random, the irregularly and regularly stained bacilli are counted among at least 100 organisms, if available. Only individual bacteria whose entire outline can be seen, and that are not touching or superimposed, are counted. The bacteria with uniform, bright staining along their entire length are counted whereas those with pale or any irregular staining are not. The MI is expressed as the proportion or % of regularly stained bacteria over the total score. In 1971, Ridley introduced a modified score, subdividing the irregularly stained bacilli into fragmented (F) and granular (G) forms and formulating the S(solid)FG index [153].

Fragmented bacilli include those with small unstained zones (bacilli with enlarged clubbed extremities or pointed extremities are not taken into account) and very short rods (less than 2 μm). Granular bacilli show two or more full thickness unstained areas in the bacillary body. The bacilli present in the globi cannot be precisely counted and so their numbers are estimated (0 = none, 1 = few, 2 = numerous, 3 = very numerous). A large globus can contain about 100 bacilli, a medium-sized globus 60 and a small one 30. In general, non clumped bacilli that can be counted are also visible in the globi. When staining smears it is very important to stain a positive control too: a negative result could be due not only to a true absence of bacilli, but also to a staining error.

The MI is theoretically of great practical use, because it can guide the determination of the infectiousness of a patient, her/his response to treatment and in a treated patient with a positive MI, it can provide early evidence of relapse. The limit to the MI is that it may provide an overestimate of viable bacteria because the interval between the degenerative alterations causing irregular staining and biological death is not known. Moreover, it must be borne in mind that the measurement of the MI is particularly demanding and requires skilled staff and optimal laboratory conditions.

5.5.3.3 Skin Biopsy Specimens

These are particularly important to determine any emergence of *M. leprae* strains that are resistant to treatment. They need to be sent to specialized centers and this requires accurate planning to ensure that the *M. leprae* are still viable when they are received for the purposes of animal inoculation. The time between the biopsy and the animal inoculation should not be longer than 7 days (preferably 5), and the biopsy tissue (placed in a sterile container without any additives) must be kept cool in a refrigerator at 4°C until it is shipped, and have sufficient wet ice in a thermos flask for the shipment duration.

5.5.3.4 Smears of Nasal Secretions

While skin smears are "closed" lesions from which few if any bacilli are discharged, because in most cases the epidermis remains intact, nasal secretions are "open" and in lepromatous leprosy large numbers of *M. leprae* are discharged (in fact, the nasal mucosa is ulcerated). In other leprosy forms, too, the nasal mucosa is infected and so nasal secretions are a valuable assessment to determine the response to treatment and the patient's potential infectiousness. Nasal lesions resolve rapidly with effective chemotherapy. The nasal secretion specimen should be obtained from an early morning "nose blow" into a sheet of cellophane: the secretion is classified as clear, watery or mucoid and in this last case it is immediately collected on a small cotton swab and mounted on a stick. At the same time, the cotton swab can be scraped over the nasal mucosa after the patient has blown her/his nose. The specimen is then spread onto a slide and stained with the Ziehl-Neelsen method.

5.5.4 Biochemistry of *Mycobacterium leprae*

The survival of *M. leprae* seems to depend largely on the host. There must therefore be mechanisms whereby it escapes the host defense system and can procure the substances needed to survive [154]. The host cells preferably parasitized by the bacillus are macrophages and Schwann cells, both of which have a phagocytic activity. In these, *M. leprae* lives and multiplies, localizing at the level of the phagosomes, phagolysosomes and the cytoplasm.

Intracellular parasites must contend with two main defense mechanisms: fusion of the lysosomes with the phagosome where the microorganisms and oxidized molecules produced by the cell in response are located. The lysosomes, cytoplasmic vesicles that are particularly abundant in the phagocytes, contain proteolytic and hydrolytic enzymes with a degrading function. Fusion of their membrane with that of the phagosomes leads to the formation of the phagolysosome where the enzymatic degradation of the phagosome content occurs. Some mycobacteria, including *M. tuberculosis*, can inhibit the fusion of this membrane when they are vital, but *M. leprae* and *M. lepraemurium* do not possess this capacity [154].

Phagocytes have another cytotoxic mechanism that is common also to polymorphonuclear leukocytes, namely the production inside the phagosome of oxygen radicals that oxidize the ingested particles. *M. leprae* cannot trigger this "respiratory burst", that shortens the life of the parasitized cell. However, there is sufficient evidence that *M. leprae* can collect nutrient matter from the host cell, like glucose, glycogen, amino acids, thymidine, purines, and inorganic phosphate. The uptake of thymidine and purines is very important in the synthesis of nucleic acid, and that of the amino acids for protein synthesis [155].

An important protective function for *M. leprae* is exerted by the cell wall, especially the surface lipids. This complex wall seems to have a protective action both in inhospitable intracellular environments and in the external environment, and is able to resist enzymatic and oxidative attacks. Phenol glycolipid I, in fact, seems to be able to neutralize the oxygen reactive molecules [154].

5.5.5 Lepromins

Lepromins prepared from *M. leprae* are used as skin-test agents. In 1919, Mitsuda described the first integral lepromin, and since 1940 this test has been applied in both leprosy patients and healthy subjects. Over the years, Mitsuda's lepromin has been modified several times, especially as regards standardization. It consists of an autoclaved emulsion of *M. leprae* obtained from skin lesions with a rich bacillary content from patients with lepromatous leprosy. However, this skin test does not have a diagnostic value because the reaction is not positive in all patients with leprosy, and in addition may be positive in some healthy subjects. A positive reaction is obtained in patients with tuberculoid leprosy and a negative reaction in those with lepromatous leprosy. The reaction differs from the one produced by tuberculin in tuberculosis because it is biphasic, with an early tuberculin-like response (the Fernandez reaction, induced by soluble *M. leprae* antigens, expressed by a palpable infiltrate some mm thick; in many individuals it is not present, and when it is, it persists only for 1–2 days) followed by the gradual development of a nodule within four weeks. The early tuberculin-like response is much weaker than the late response at four weeks (Table 5.4). Mitsuda's integral lepromin has been used all over the world to make a clinical classification of leprosy and to assess the host immune response to *M. leprae* (Table 5.5) [156].

In 1979, a WHO memorandum dictated standard safety requirements [157] for the lepromin test, whose preparation method is reported in other works [4], according to which two concentrations of bacteria, 4.0×10^7 and 1.6×10^8 bacilli/ml should be prepared [4]. Nowadays, lepromin is prepared with *M. leprae* from the armadillo in the same way as the human-derived bacillus. Mitsuda lepromin has a shelf-life of 2 years stored at 4°C. The skin dose is 0.1 ml given intradermally like tuberculin, in general on the volar region of the forearm.

The second type of lepromin that was adopted on a large scale was described by Dharmendhra [158, 159]. Instead of using whole bacteria as in the Mitsuda skin test, this lepromin employs fractionated *M. leprae*. The aim of fractionating

Table 5.4 Evaluation of the reaction to lepromin

Fernandez reaction (after 48–72 h)	Mitsuda reaction (after 3–4 weeks)
0 = infiltrate 5 mm 1+ = infiltrate 6–9 mm 2+ = infiltrate 10–14 mm 3 + = infiltrate >14 mm	0 = no reaction ± = infiltrate <3 mm 1+ = nodule 3–5 mm 2 + = nodule 6–10 mm 3+ = nodule >10 mm, with possible ulceration (3 + U)

Table 5.5 Results of the Mitsuda reaction in the various leprosy forms

LL/BL	Negative
BB	Variable: negative or faintly positive
BT	Weakly positive (1 +, 2 +)
TT	Strongly positive (3 +)
IL	Variable

LL polar lepromatous leprosy, *BL* borderline lepromatous leprosy, *BB* borderline borderline leprosy, *BT* borderline tuberculoid leprosy, *TT* polar tuberculoid leprosy, *IL* indeterminate leprosy

the bacilli is to isolate a tuberculin-like antigen that, like a soluble skin test material, would be more specific than Mitsuda lepromin because it has only a monophasic skin reaction at 48–72 h, like tuberculin [4]. This lepromin, too, is obtained from bacilli-rich skin lesions of patients with lepromatous leprosy. The bacteria are separated from the tissues by chloroform-extraction. The purified bacteria are broken by grinding and the supernatant is fractionated into protein, polysaccharide, glyceride, phosphatide and wax. Of these five antigens, in patients with tuberculoid leprosy only the protein fraction will yield a reaction at 48–72 h. The skin dose is 0.1 ml, given intradermically. This lepromin, widely used only in India, has some drawbacks, including the fact that the bacilli are only partially broken by grinding. Using *M. leprae* from armadillos, optimal methods of purification and disintegration of the bacilli have been devised. Integral lepromin, that is the most commonly used, is obtained from the liver of experimentally infected armadillo (lepromin A = armadillo, while the human type is lepromin H = human), and can be requested directly from the Leprosy Division World Health Organization, Geneva, Switzerland.

5.6 Transmission

5.6.1 Exit Portals

The exit portals of *M. leprae* are the skin and nasal mucosa. As to the skin, even if cases of lepromatous leprosy show a large number of bacilli in the derma, it seems doubtful that a sufficient number can reach the surface. Although there have been reports of resistant acid-fast bacilli in the epidermis, various authors have referred that in their experience it was not possible to find bacilli in the epidermis of patients and contacts [160], nor on the skin surface of lepromatous patients [161]. However, it is certain that in cases of lepromatous patients with skin ulcerations of nodules or other lesions, large quantities of bacilli can be eliminated. It is also likely that a minor quantity of microorganisms may be present on the skin surface owing to secretions from the sebaceous or sweat glands, as demonstrated by the recent finding of bacilli in the superficial keratin layer of lepromatous patients [162].

The importance of the nasal mucosa as the principal source of bacilli has been recognized since 1898 [163], especially in cases of ulcerated mucosa. A huge quantity of bacilli can be obtained from lesions of the nasal mucosa in subjects with lepromatous leprosy, with counts ranging from 10,000 to 10,000,000 [107, 164].

Among other sources, it is known that *M. leprae* is also present in breast milk. It has been calculated that a child breastfed by a lepromatous mother can receive up to two million bacilli from a single suckle [165]. The epidemiological significance of this source is not known, however.

5.6.2 Entry Portals

The entry portals of *M. leprae* are the skin and the upper airways. According to some authors, *M. leprae* can cross both healthy and slightly damaged skin to reach the superficial lymphatics [166], whereas others doubt that it can cross the skin via simple passive contact [167]. Instead, it is known that this passage can occur through accidental inoculation, like tattooing for instance. In any case, the evidence reported by various authors that the first lesions are always in more exposed and injury-prone body sites suggests skin contact. In 1947, Cochrane observed that lesions were common on the forehead of children with lepromatous mothers in Africa, who were in the habit of carrying them on their naked backs. By contrast, such lesions were rare in Korea, where children were also carried on their mothers' backs but with the difference that these mothers were fully clothed [168].

As regards the various routes of entry of *M. leprae*, it has been observed in studies of the mouse footpad model that the onset of leprosy, as also the various clinical types, varies according to the entry portal: while the intradermic route sensitizes the animal, the intravenous and intraperitoneal routes tend to induced tolerance, as shown by skin tests [169]. For this reason, it seems possible that tuberculoid and lepromatous leprosy result from different entry portals of the bacilli. As regards the airways, there has been evidence of experimental transmission of leprosy through aerosols containing *M. leprae* in immunosuppressed mice, and this suggests a similar possibility in humans [170]. Nevertheless, some authors doubt this possibility under natural conditions among human beings [171]. In short, there is no true conclusion about the entry portal: the respiratory route appears to be the most likely but other portals including broken skin cannot be excluded.

5.6.3 Subclinical Infection and Re-Infection

In leprosy, as in other communicable diseases, it is possible to contract a sub-clinical infection (with no clinical signs). This has been demonstrated in vitro by tests for cell-mediated immunity, such as the lymphocyte transformation test (LTT) and serological tests for detecting humoral antibodies like the fluorescent leprosy antibody absorption (FLA-ABS) test.

Godal and Negassi were the first to use the LTT in different categories or people exposed to leprosy [172]. They found that this test, that was generally positive in subjects with tuberculoid leprosy, showed a variable response among Europeans visiting Ethiopia, depending on the period of their stay there and their proximity to leprosy patients. People in contact with leprosy patients showed a high rate of response to the LTT: up to 48% after contact with tuberculoid leprosy and about 41% after contact with lepromatous leprosy.

As to the humoral response, the FLA-ABS test has been performed in different categories of people in Okinawa [173]. The test is positive not only in 100% of patients with lepromatous and borderline lepromatous leprosy, in 88% of patients with tuberculoid borderline leprosy and in 77% of those with tuberculoid leprosy, but in up to 92% of their household contacts. This same test was negative in healthy non-contacts and in patients with pulmonary tuberculosis.

The occurrence of a subclinical infection has also been demonstrated by skin tests with different lepromin preparations and with soluble antigens from *M. leprae*. Using a particularly soluble skin test antigen, in an area of Venezuela the test was positive in 19% of the general population (non-contacts), in 36% of contacts outside the household and in 48% of household contacts [174]. This variable reactivity suggests a clear correlation between exposure and a possible subclinical infection. It also points out that a higher proportion of subjects acquire the infection than those who develop the disease, although the factors that influence this proportion are not clear.

The onset of leprosy, presumably for the first time, in elderly subjects in endemic areas has also raised the possibility of a re-infection in these subjects, since it is difficult to believe that they could have remained uninfected for so long despite living in an endemic area. But this same onset could also suggest that in these elderly subjects it could really be a re-activation of an old, undetected primary disease due to age-related waning of a previously acquired immunity. Because there is no evidence of a distinct primary disease in leprosy, as there is in tuberculosis, the hypothesis of a re-infection could be important. Moreover, the occurrence of relapse in lepromatous leprosy also suggests the possibility of a re-infection, at least in some proportion of relapsed individuals [175].

5.6.4 Incubation Period

It is difficult to define the incubation period, or interval between the moment of infection and the onset of the disease, partly because of the lack of suitable immunological tools and partly due to the insidious disease onset. The minimum incubation time is a few weeks, as evinced by reports of the rare onset of the disease in children [176]. The maximum time can be up to 30 years or more, as seen in war veterans exposed for brief periods in endemic areas but who lived in non endemic areas. The onset of leprosy in US veterans exposed for brief periods occurred after an interval ranging from 2.9 to 5.3 years for tuberculoid leprosy, and 9.3 to 11.6 years for the lepromatous form

(National Communicable Disease Center, 1970) [177]. Other authors have estimated a mean incubation time of 8.4 years [178], and in South India of 4.4 years [179]. It can therefore be assumed that the incubation period of leprosy is generally quite long, albeit highly variable, but in most cases seems to be in the range of 2–5 years.

5.6.5 Scientific Investigation and Antileprosy Campaign

Already in 1847, in an illustrated book ("Om Spedalsked"), two Norwegian dermatologists, Danielssen and Boeck, had accurately described the skin and nerve manifestations of advanced leprosy. The authors also mentioned lagophthalmos and atrophy of the musculature of the hands, and divested leprosy of much of the myth and folklore that had accompanied the disease since the beginning of time. Their precise observations paved the way for subsequent studies.

About 25 years later, again in Norway, a young physician working in his Bergen laboratory observed material obtained from skin lesions from leprosy patients under the microscope. Working in a leprosy hospital, G.H. Armauer Hansen was the first to discover the leprosy bacillus in 1872, and his discovery was made official on 28 February 1873, published in 1874 [180] and ascertained to be the cause of leprosy in 1875 [181].

Many centuries would pass, therefore, before the treatment of leprosy passed from the horrific to the scientific, from bathing in the blood of infants under 2 years of age to the modern day mycobacteriostatic drugs [182]. In an earlier era, in China and in India, the oil expressed from the ripe seeds of *Hydnocarpus wightiana* was administered for leprosy. Later studies showed that while the oil may have had slight mycobacteriostatic properties it did little more than stimulate fibrosis when intradermically and intralesionally injected [182].

The treatment of leprosy continued in this state until the early 1940s. In 1908, two German chemists synthesized a compound, diaminodiphenylsulfone, that would then be adopted as chemotherapy for leprosy some three decades later [183]. In the search for a treatment, various other products were tried for a while such as gurjan oil, methylene blue, aniline dyes, diphtheria toxoid, etc.

The advent and success of sulfonamides in streptococcal infections then led to the use of sulfanilamide in leprosy patients in 1940 but with no success. One year later, a sulfone derivative (Promin) was found to be efficacious, despite some symptoms such as anemia and gastrointestinal disorders [184]. Subsequently other sulfone derivatives were shown to be efficacious and at last the era of an effective treatment of leprosy had arrived. Various authors in different parts of the world identified the correct dosage of sulfone (dapsone) as 100 mg daily for an adult, avoiding the risk of toxic side-effects. Other drugs were synthesized but did not reveal the same success. Thanks to the use of dapsone, old-style leprosy asylums began to close down and patients could be treated at home. A proven efficacy was later demonstrated, because of its anti-inflammatory actions, for clofazimine (B 663; Lamprene, Geigy), an aminofenozone introduced in the treatment of leprosy in 1962 [185].

The enthusiastic reaction to the success of monotherapy would not last long: in fact, the mouse footpad inoculation technique demonstrated the problem of the development of drug resistance, confirming some clinical suspicions. But multi-drug therapy became the treatment of choice only as from 1982, when the WHO authorized its use [186]. Luckily, a new semi-synthetic antibiotic, rifampicin, with a high mycobactericidal activity, had already made its appearance in the previous decades.

5.6.6 Inactivation of Disease and Mortality

Extreme importance should be attached to the data about the elimination of cases from the prevalence pool in places where leprosy treatment facilities existed, and succeeded in bringing about inactivation or cure of the disease. But even in the absence of treatment, some patients, especially those with tuberculoid and indeterminate leprosy, tend to recover spontaneously. In a study conducted in India over a period of 20 years, it was found that about 90% of children with the tuberculoid form achieved a spontaneous regression of the disease [175]. In a study in the Philippines, a self-healing rate in children of 77.7% was reported [187], and in another study in South India with long-term follow-up, among new cases of tuberculoid leprosy of all ages and both sexes, a rate of 10.9% of spontaneous inactivation per year emerged [188].

Leprosy is rarely the cause of immediate death, even if patients are exposed to increased mortality risks due to its indirect effects. A study in Cebu, Philippines, showed that the mortality rate among patients with lepromatous leprosy was fourfold the rate in the general population, whereas in non-lepromatous patients it was comparable to the latter rate [189]. Another study in a rural area of South India found a mortality rate among lepromatous patients that was three and a half times higher than in the general population, while the risk in non lepromatous cases was twice that in the general population. In this study, leprosy accounted for about 1% of all deaths [190].

5.7 Genetics

M. leprae is known for its limited diversity between strains from different areas [119, 191]. This near-clonal characteristic, together with the observation of a wide range of leprosy clinical phenotypes, strongly suggests that most of the disease variability, including the susceptibility to leprosy per se, depends on the genetic background of the host [192–194]. It is widely accepted today that exposure to *M. leprae* is necessary but not sufficient to trigger the onset of the disease, and that different sets of genes modify the host susceptibility to leprosy into three different stages, namely: 1. the control of the infection per se, in other words the disease in terms of the clinical manifestations; 2. once the infection has become established, the manifestation of the different clinical forms of leprosy; e 3. the risk of developing leprosy reactions (Fig. 5.3).

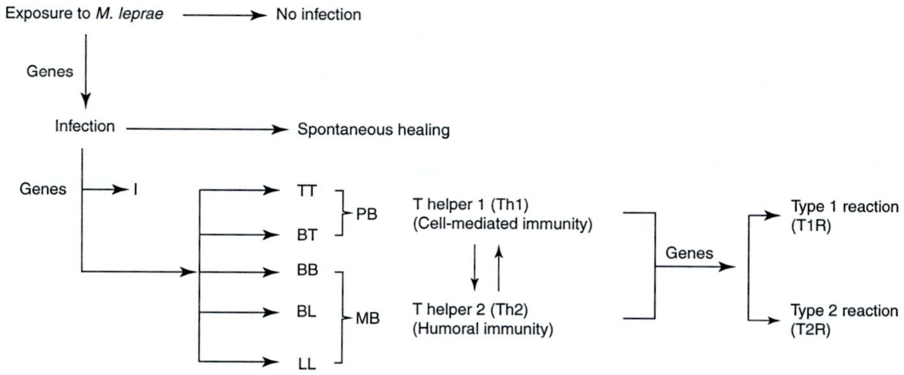

Fig. 5.3 Model of the leprosy spectrum (Modified, by [193]). *TT* polar tuberculoid, *BT* borderline tuberculoid, *BB* borderline borderline, *BL* borderline lepromatous, *LL* polar lepromatous, *I* indeterminate, *PB* paucibacillary, MB multibacillary

Various studies indicate that there is a familial component in the susceptibility to leprosy, as emerges from the concordance of the disease in itself, and of the clinical forms between monozygotic compared to dizygotic twins [195–197].

While there can be no doubt that the susceptibility to leprosy is under genetic control, there is no information as yet on the precise nature of the genetic factors involved, in other words the identity and number of genes and the variants of these genes that cause the various leprosy phenotypes [193]. For this reason, a number of studies have been conducted that demonstrated various candidate chromosomal regions and genes, such as class I and II MHC/HLA-linked genes and non-HLA genes [193].

5.7.1 Major Histocompatibility Complex Genes

The major histocompatibility complex (MHC), in man known as the leukocyte antigen complex (HLA), is a cluster of polymorphic genes, localized on chromosome 6 p21, many of which encode for proteins that are essential in the processing and binding of antigenic peptides during the immune response [198]. The HLA region includes 3 classes: HLA class I contains subclasses A, B, and C, which present antigenic peptides of intracellular origin to CD8+ T cells; HLA class II includes subclasses -DR, -DQ, -DM, and –DP, that bind peptides of extracellular origin and present them to CD4+ T cells; HLA class III contains genes coding for cytokines such as TNFA (tumor necrosis factor alpha) and LTA (lymphotoxin alpha) and for other intermediates of the immune response.

It is reasonable to suppose that HLA genes play an important role in leprosy, bearing in mind that clinical manifestations of the disease depend on the type of host immune response. Many studies have reported the involvement of HLA alleles and haplotypes in controlling the susceptibility to the disease. In particular, HLA-DR alleles are strongly associated with leprosy [199], and various HLA class I alleles (HLA-A*2,A*11,B*40, and C*7) have been detected more frequently in leprosy cases than in unaffected controls [200].

There is evidence that the class III genes TNFA and LTA are involved in the immune response against leprosy [201]. TNFA encodes TNF-α, a pro-inflammatory and immunostimulatory cytokine involved in various biological processes including the modulation of both innate and adaptive immune responses. TNF-α, secreted above all by macrophages, has a central role because it mediates the protective response to *M. leprae* invasion. Various studies indicate that TNFA variants can influence leprosy phenotypes [202, 203]. LTA, α cytokine member of the TNF super-family and produced by lymphocytes, is important in the control of intracellular bacterial infections, like *M. tuberculosis* and *M. leprae*. In leprosy, LTA seems to play an important role in patients with early onset of the disease [204]. LTA also seems to regulate granuloma formation, while TNF-α is responsible for its integrity [201, 205].

Variants of additional HLA-linked genes, such as MICA (MHC class I polypeptide-related sequence A), MICB (MHC class I polypeptide-related sequence B), and TAP (Transporter I, ATP-binding cassette, subfamily B), have been reported in association with leprosy phenotypes [206].

5.7.2 Non-HLA Genes

The IL10 gene encodes for the anti-inflammatory cytokine IL-10. Higher levels of IL-10 have been observed in multibacillary lepromatous patients as compared with paucibacillary tuberculoid patients, and a low TNF- α/IL-10 ratio is correlated to disease progression [201, 207].

Among various studies in different populations, a significant association between leprosy and the genes PARK2 (Parkinson protein 2)/PACRG (Parkin Co-Regulated Gene) has emerged [123, 208, 209]. Many other genes have been associated with susceptibility to leprosy [193, 194].

5.7.3 Genetics of Leprosy Reactions

The first evidence of an association between leprosy reactions and genetic polymorphisms was gained from studies involving Toll-like receptor (TLR) genes. TLRs are transmembrane proteins that play an important role in the inflammatory response to microbial pathogens. A study in a Nepalese population showed polymorphisms on both TLR1 and TLR2 associated with a high risk for a type 1 reaction (T1R or reversal reaction) [210, 211]. Other studies have revealed an association between variants of the IL6 gene and susceptibility to a type 2 reaction (T2R or erythema nodosum leprosum) [212].

5.8 Immunopathogenesis

Leprosy presents with different clinical manifestations, depending on the host immune responses. It is therefore an optimal human model for the study of host responses to intracellular pathogens in general. Nowadays, most researchers adopt Redley and Jopling's leprosy classification based on histological and immunological criteria [35]. This classification defines a five point leprosy spectrum with stable polar forms (TT and LL) at the ends and borderline forms (TB, BB, BL) in the middle (Figs. 5.4 and 5.5; Tables 5.6 and 5.7) [212–214].

The tuberculoid leprosy (TT) pole shows few lesions with well-defined margins and a hypoanaesthetic center and does not have acid-fast bacilli. The main histological finding is an infiltrate consisting of foci of well-developed epithelioid macrophages, with or without Langhans-type multinuclear giant cells, surrounded by a cuff of lymphocytes. The smaller nerves in the granuloma may be destroyed, and thickened peripheral nerves are palpable in the vicinity of a lesion.

The lepromatous leprosy (LL) pole shows multiple symmetrical nodular lesions with an infiltrate largely made up of macrophages with various degrees of foamy changes and few scattered lymphocytes and plasma cells. Inside and outside the macrophages there will be many bacilli, that may be clamped in globi. The nerves may show structural damage and thickening; they will undergo a slow, gradual destruction. In addition, Schwann cells, perineural cells, axons, and intraneural macrophages of dermal nerves may contain bacilli.

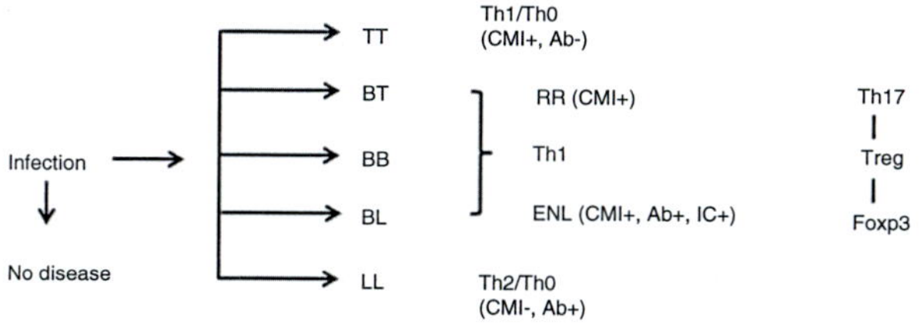

Fig. 5.4 Immunology of the leprosy spectrum and leprosy reactions (Modified, by [212]). *TT* polar tuberculoid, *BT* borderline tuberculoid, *BB* borderline borderline, *BL* borderline lepromatous, *LL* polar lepromatous, *Th1* T helper 1, *Th2* T helper 2, *Th0* T helper 0, *RR* type1/reversal reaction, *ENL* type2/erythema nodosum leprosum reaction, *Th17* T helper cell producing IL-17, *Foxp3* T cell with nuclear fork head box 3 transcription factor, *CMI* T cell mediated immunity, *Ab* antibodies, *IC* immune complex, *Treg* regulatory cells

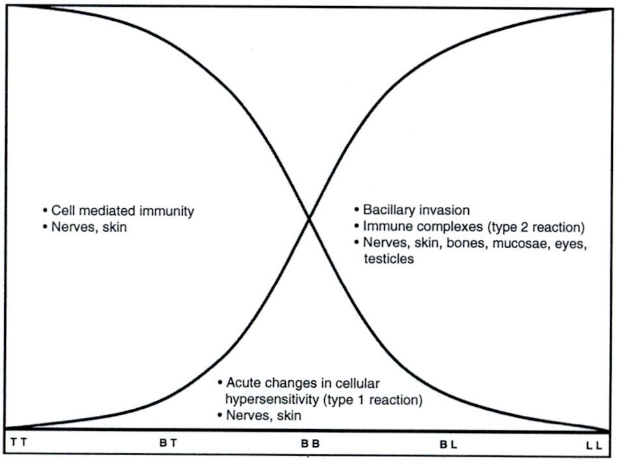

Fig. 5.5 Mechanisms of tissues damage in leprosy (Modified, by [2]). *TT* polar tuberculoid, *BT* borderline tuberculoid, *BB* borderline borderline, *BL* borderline lepromatous, *LL* polar lepromatous

Table 5.6 Bacteriological and histopathological features according to the Ridley-Jopling five group classification

	TT	BT	BB	BL	LL
Mitsuda reaction	+++	++	+	±/ –	–
Bacilli in nasal mucosa	–	–	–	+	++
Bacilli in skin lesion	0–1+	1–3+	3–4+	4–5+	5–6+
Globi	–	–	–	–	+
Epithelioid cells	+	+	+	–	–
Langhans cells	+++	++	–	–	–
Foamy cells	–	–	–	+	+++
Type 1 reaction	±	+	++	+	–
Type 2 reaction	–	–	–	–	+
Infiltration of sub-epidermis zone	+	+/±	–	–	–
Nerve destruction (skin)	+++	++	+	±	±

TT polar tuberculoid leprosy, *BT* borderline tuberculoid leprosy, *BB* borderline borderline leprosy, *BL* borderline lepromatous leprosy, *LL* polar lepromatous leprosy

Table 5.7 Immunological features in leprosy and leprosy reactions (Modified, by [212])

	TT	LL	T1R	T2R
Immunology stability	++	++		
Specific antibodies to PGL	→	→	→	→
Autoantibodies	–	↑	–	↑
T cells number in blood	→	↓	→	→
Lymphoproliferation	↑	↓	↑	↑
M. leprae specific antigens	↑	↓	↑	↑
PPD	→	→	↑	↑
IL-1	↑	↓	↑	↑
IL-2	↑	↓	↑	↑
IL-12	↑	↓	↑	↑
IL-10	↓	↑	↓	↓
IFN-γ	↑	↓	↑	↑
Th phenotype	Th 1/Th 0	Th 2/Th 0	Th 1	Th1
Th 17	↑	↓	–	↑
Foxp 3	↓	↑	–	↑/↓

TT polar tuberculoid leprosy, *LL* polar lepromatous leprosy, *T1R* type 1 reaction, *T2R* type 2 reaction, → normal, ↑ increased, ↓ decreased

Between these two polar forms are the unstable borderline forms, including borderline tuberculoid (BT), mid-borderline (BB), and borderline lepromatous (BL) leprosy, that have intermediate clinical and histopathological features as compared to the above polar forms. Patients with BT present several anaesthetic and granulomatous lesions with a cellular pattern similar to that of TT forms but that may contain few bacilli. BB patients show intermediate lesions in terms of number and size between tuberculoid and lepromatous forms, with moderate anesthesia and irregular shapes; they consist of diffuse epithelioid cells and lymphocytes, while giant cells are absent. A bacilloscopic index of 3+ or 4+ is regularly found. In BL patients, the lesions are numerous and sometimes hypoanaesthetic; the infiltrate is composed of histiocytic cells that tend to evolve to epithelioid cells, while lymphocytes are scanty. The bacilloscopic index is positive.

A significant proportion of patients, in particular those with borderline forms, will develop leprosy reactions during the disease course and even after starting multidrug therapy. These reactions are considered to be immune exacerbations, in view of the changes of lymphocytes to histiocytes, and it is thought that they should be interpreted as a lymphocytic reactivity to *M. leprae* and its antigens [215]. There are two types of such reactions: the type 1, or reversal reaction (RR), and the type 2 reaction, denominated erythema nodosum leprosum (ENL). Type 1 reactions are localized at the dermal patch and neighboring nerves, and demonstrate an acute increase in both mature and blast lymphocytes, and a specific increase of cell-mediated immunity accompanied by an excessive release of type 1 helper T cell (Th 1) cytokines into the tissue. Type 2 reactions are characterized by immune complex deposits in the vessel walls and later in tissues, and by a fluctuating T-cell immunity.

To further refine the disease spectrum of leprosy, it can be added that LL and BL lesions exhibit a characteristic infiltrate and significant numbers of macrophages, B/plasma cells and scattered T cells, especially of the CD8+ subtype, while TT and BT lesions primarily show a T cell infiltrate, mostly CD4+, with a small number of plasma cells, macrophages, or CD8+ and regulatory T cells (Treg). In addition, monoclonal antibodies against the *M. leprae* antigens can help to optimize the differential diagnosis between the various forms of leprosy. LL and BL lesions exhibit a strong expression of mycobacterial lipoarabinomannan and the *M. leprae*-specific phenolic glycolipid (PGL I) antigens, while TT and BT lesions show a much weaker staining [216]. A very important point is that in situ detection of *M. leprae* antigens seems to offer a confirmatory diagnosis even in the absence of bacilli. Moreover, the different expression of these two antigens can also distinguish reactive lesions as compared to non reactive lesions [216].

5.8.1 Innate Immune Response

The defense against pathogenic agents is mounted by the innate immune response, followed by the acquired immune response; both types of response act via the cells and soluble factors.

M. leprae can enter and take up residence within macrophages and Schwann cells according to multiple modes [213, 214]. Receptors to complement fragments of CR1, CR3 and CR4 aid phagocytosis. Phenolic glycolipid I is recognized by complement 3. As well as the complement receptors, the Toll-like receptors (TLRs) present on the macrophages are also important in the recognition of microbial pathogens. TLR2 and TLR4 recognize the leprosy bacillus, activate monocytes and release IL-12, a cytokine that induces proinflammatory cytokines and killing of the bacilli. Cytokines IFN-γ and GM-CSF enhance TLR1 expression, which leads to inflammation through the production of TNF-α. TLR1 and 2 are more strongly expressed in the skin lesions of tuberculoid leprosy [194, 217, 218].

Vitamin D can contribute to the innate immune response through the production of antimicrobial peptides, and is differentially expressed in tuberculoid leprosy as compared to lepromatous leprosy. While IL-10 induces the phagocytic pathway, IL-15 induces the vitamin D antimicrobial pathway and reduces phagocytosis [194].

5.8.2 Acquired Immune Response

The acquired immune response is triggered by dendritic cells, potent antigen-presenting cells that act as a bridge between the two arms, innate and acquired, of the immune response. Dendritic cells migrate from the site of infection and present the antigen to naïve T cells in the regional lymph nodes. Depending on their degree of maturity and signaling, dendritic cells can stimulate naïve T cells to differentiate into different effector subpopulations. CD+ T cells play a determinant role in the induction and effector phases of the immune response. After engagement of the antigen by their T-cell receptors (TCRs), they can differentiate into Th 1 cells, secreting interleukin 2 (IL-2) and interferon-γ (IFN-γ) and resulting in macrophage activation, or into Th 2 cells, secreting IL-4, IL-5, and IL-13, that stimulate the production of antibodies and inhibit the activation of macrophages [219]. Alternatively, they can differentiate into Th 17 cells that produce IL-17 and IL-22, and are involved in inflammation and autoimmunity [220]. In addition, the activities of Th 1 and Th 2 cells can be under the control of another subset of CD4+ CD25+ Foxp3+, IL-10 or transforming growth factor β+ T cells, known as regulatory T cells [221, 222].

In general, antigen-specific T cells, macrophages and dendritic cells are recruited to the site of lesions, giving rise to various types of granuloma, modulated by different cytokines in the disease course, thereby inducing the different clinical pictures in the leprosy spectrum [213, 214].

The acquired immune response also involves soluble factors such as antibodies released by B cells, that capture free microbes. In leprosy patients there is a dichotomy between the B and T cell response. Tuberculoid patients show undetectable antibodies and good T cells responses, while lepromatous patients have abundant antibodies and a poor to nil T cell response, as demonstrated by skin tests and in vitro tests [212].

5.8.3 Antibody Responses

The search for an *M. leprae*-specific dominant antigen has led to the identification of species-specific PLG-I and paved the way for the detection of anti-PGL-I antibodies in leprosy patients sera. The anti PGL-I IgM antibody is regarded as highly specific, and useful to diagnose the various leprosy forms. It is also very helpful for monitoring contacts who could be at risk of developing the disease [148–150, 223–228]. The advantage of PGL-I serology is its relatively high specificity, up to 90% in various studies [228, 229], while the major drawback is the lack of sensitivity in paucibacillary patients [228–230].

The use of anti-PGL-I serology has been simplified since the advent of a rapid immunochromatographic flow test (ML Flow test) that can be used as a single dipstick assay even using whole blood samples. This test, whose sensitivity is comparable to that of ELISA, detects more than 90% of multibacillary patients and 40% of paucibacillary patients, showing a background seropositivity in endemic controls at around 10% [198]. Moreover, in multibacillary patients it can be employed without the need for a slit-skin smear test. However, its use has gradually declined owing to the cost [230].

5.8.4 Cell-Mediated Immune Responses

An important parameter for assessing specific cell-mediated immunity in leprosy is lepromin, the Mitsuda reagent, a skin test that can discriminate between LL and TT forms. For disease classification, the use of this test can be recommended as a primary and stand-alone mode for the definitive diagnosis of suspected paucibacillary leprosy cases. A negative Mitsuda test helps in the confirmation of multibacillary forms, when patients present with acid-fast bacillus-positive lesions and enlarged nerves. The drawbacks are its relative insensitivity, the subjective nature of the interpretation, fairly delayed response, and possible contamination by material from the animal used for extraction, in addition to batch variability in terms of activity.

Other early indicators in leprosy are T cell numbers and non-proliferation of peripheral blood mononuclear cells (PBMC) to mitogens. A notable finding is that patients with LL have a unique antigen-specific unresponsiveness, as indicated by the fact that the T cell response to other antigens, such as *M. tuberculosis*, is unimpaired. In a study conducted by administering microbial antigens by intradermal injection in 106 patients, 50 with active lepromatous leprosy and 56 with non active lepromatous leprosy, a greater percentage of positive responses was obtained in untreated subjects with clinically quiescent disease: it seems that the majority of these subjects will regain their cell-mediated immune reaction potency with the improvement in their clinical conditions (Table 5.8) [231]. Another study conducted in 26 patients with lepromatous leprosy by administering intradermic injections of mycobacterial antigens showed a relatively frequent positivity to the various agents, linked to antigenic relationships among the different mycobacteria (Table 5.9) [232].

Table 5.8 Delayed hypersensitivity to microbial antigens in lepromatous leprosy patients

Clinical form	N°	Lepromin (Mitsuda)	PPD	Candidine	Antistaphylococcus vaccine	Antistreptococcus vaccine
Active LL	50	4 (8%)	9 (18%)	0	0	2 (4%)
Non active LL	56	25 (44.6%)	20 (35.7%)	3 (5.4%)	4 (7.2%)	7 (2.5%)
Controls	110	23 (20.9%)	39 (35.4%)	8 (6.2%)	19 (14.6%)	14 (10.8%)

LL lepromatous leprosy

Table 5.9 Delayed hypersensitivity to mycobacteria in lepromatous leprosy patients

Clinical form	N°	*M. avium*	*M. kansasii*	*M. intracellulare*	*M. marinum*	*M. scrofulaceum*	*M. xenopi*
Active LL	14	0	4	1	4	2	2
Non active LL	12	1	4	2	6	7	7

LL polar lepromatous leprosy

Th 1 and 2 subsets of CD4+ cells produce IFN-γ (a marker of delayed cell-mediated immune reactions) and IL-4 (which promotes antibodies), respectively. Patients with TT have the Th 1 subset, whereas the Th 2 subset is predominant in LL patients. However, some studies have shown that a Th 0 profile with both IFN-γ and IL-4 is also possible; there are no clinical differences between patients with a polarized or a Th 0 phenotype [233].

Of the two types of regulatory T cells, Th 17 cells have been reported in erythema nodosum leprosum reactions [234]. Other authors have found that Th 17 cells are more associated with TT patients in both skin lesions and antigen/induced PBMC cultures, suggesting a differential role for these cells in the leprosy clinical spectrum [234]. They have also observed a higher association of Th 17 cells with non polarized Th 0 types, demonstrating that these cells may be a third Th type in this disease: Th 17 could be a rescue pathway in patients unable to mount a Th response or when Th polarization has not set in [235].

The other type of regulatory T cells, CD4+ CD25+ T cell with Foxp3 (forkhead box protein 3) transcription factor, has yielded conflicting results: in some studies there was a higher association with TT patients and ENL subjects [221], while in others these same cells were increased in LL patients [222, 236]. In conclusion, the T cell biology involves complex interactions between effector and regulatory cells.

5.8.5 Advances for New *Mycobacterium leprae*-Specific Antigens

Since the advent of human genome sequencing, new recombinant antigens with no known homologues have emerged, offering a better diagnostic potential. Five antigens have been found to be able to recognize individuals exposed to *M. leprae,* as assessed by the IFN-γ release assay (IGRA). The sensitivity of these antigens seems to be high, as they are able to detect 71% of healthy contacts that were not identified by PGL-I IgM serology [237].

Other proteins and peptides have been tested to evaluate exposure to leprosy [238–240]. Two proteins, largely recognized by patients serum, have been inserted, by overlapping their sequences, in a chimeric fusion protein termed LID-1 (Leprosy Infectious Disease Research Institute diagnostic 1). Positive titers of antibodies against LID-1 protein were found in 87–92% of multibacillary patients and 7–48%

of paucibacillary patients in different populations [241, 242]. A very important is the fact that some individuals presented with high titers of antibodies against LID-1 1 year before the appearance of the clinical signs of leprosy, revealing a role for this protein in the monitoring of contacts.

5.8.6 Cytokine Profiles

Research has focused on the association of differential cytokine profiles with the various clinical forms. Analysis of leprosy sera indicated an increased expression of all cytokines except IL-2 in all patients, IFN-γ in LL patients, and of IL-10 in TT patients, compared with healthy controls, suggesting an activation of immune cells by *M. leprae* antigens in all leprosy patients [243]. IFN-γ and TNF were elevated in TT compared with LL patients, yielding a significant negative correlation with a bacillus-specific index [244].

Several studies have been carried out to assess the validity of measuring serum cytokines for diagnosing and monitoring the leprosy spectrum and reactions, but conflicting results were obtained [214].

5.8.7 Leprosy Reactions

In the type 1 reaction, T cell-mediated responses towards *M. leprae* are activated, triggering an inflammatory response at the level of the skin and nerve lesions. It is not clear what causes this spontaneous, natural T-cell activation. During the reaction, increased lymphoproliferation to the *M. leprae* antigens [245] and the release of proinflammatory cytokines [246].

The ENL or type 2 reaction was initially thought to be due to immune complex deposits in the vessel but these deposits are not consistently demonstrable and conventional immune complex disease is not a clinical feature of ENL. Temporary acquisition of antigen specific T-cell activation, expression, and release of IFN-γ and IL-12, as well as the presence of CD3+ CD4+ T cells in ENL lesions, have been reported [247]. One study has also shown increases in IL-4, IL-6, and IL-8, which are chemotactic for neutrophils and consistent with histologic evidence of neutrophil infiltration in ENL lesions [248].

All this reveals a transient emergence of T-cells responses in leprosy patients undergoing reactions.

5.8.8 Immunopathology of Cutaneous Lesions

Immunopathological studies have been carried out in cutaneous leprosy lesions. In tuberculoid leprosy, the granuloma shows the presence of CD4+ T-cells scattered among epithelioid cells with CD8+ T-cells in the periphery. There are few numbers of B cells also in LL patients. Langhans cells are reduced in LL patients. Tuberculoid and lepromatous granulomas show the expression of Th 1 and Th 2 cytokines, respectively.

Both reversal and ENL reactions present a distinct polarization to the Th 1 type [214]. IFN-γ is important for killing leprosy bacilli: this has also been demonstrated in patients studies, where genetically engineered IFN-γ injected in the lesions showed a faster clearance of bacilli as compared to multidrug therapy only, administered to the control group [249].

5.8.9 Nerve Damage

Immune and non immune mechanisms play a role in nerve damage in leprosy. The Schwann cell is the major target, hosts the bacilli for long periods and protects them from the killing processes. In cultures, human Schwann cells express MHC class I and II, ICAM-1 and CD8 surface molecules, that are involved in antigen presentation. The Schwann cells process and present native *M. leprae* bacilli as well as recombinant *M. leprae* proteins and peptides to T cells; the latter, after activation, lyse the infected Schwann cells [250]. TNF-α has been observed in nerve lesions in both stable and reactional states, and may contribute to the nerve damage. TLR 2 on Schwann cells may also contribute to the nerve damage [251]. The type 1 reaction and chronic ENL often lead to nerve damage.

In cultures, demyelination is induced in the absence of an immune mechanism, suggesting a non immune mechanism during the initial stage of nerve infection. Myelin-associated Schwann cells are relatively free whereas nonmyelinized Schwann cells are heavily colonized by *M. leprae*. This distinction between myelinized and nonmyelinized Schwann cells is currently controversial, because ultrastructural studies of the nerves of lepromatous patients have demonstrated the presence of bacilli even inside the Schwann cells of myelinized axons [252, 253].

5.9 Classification

The various clinical manifestations of leprosy are not due to different strains of *M. leprae* but are rather the results of the variations in the host tissue response to the bacilli in the body. Subjects who have, or develop, an absolute resistance or immunity to the bacilli destroy them and do not contract the disease. Most of the population falls into this category. In individuals who lack or do not develop this resistance, the bacilli produce signs of the disease, that vary according to the degree of specific host resistance. If it is very high, the benign, localized form of the disease will develop; on the contrary, in the absence of resistance a severe, generalized form the disease will develop. Between these extremes there is a wide spectrum of variations in resistance that is reflected in various intermediate disease forms. While the two extremes of the spectrum have been known since ancient times and there is unanimity about their terminology, difficulties and differences in opinions have arisen as regards the terminology of the intermediate forms.

For these reasons, over time various different clinical classifications of leprosy have been adopted, based each time on particular criteria [4]. Today, the most commonly accepted is the Ridley-Jopling classification, based on immunologic criteria and widely adopted all over the world, in particular for research purposes [35]. Since the various clinical types of leprosy are linked to variations in specific cell-mediated immunity of the host to the leprosy bacilli, it is obvious why the classification is based on immunological grounds. The tuberculoid forms are located at one extreme (resistant pole) and the lepromatous forms at the other (non resistant pole), while in the central part there are various subgroups called borderline (not an entirely appropriate term for the wide spectrum between the two poles, but it has been sanctified by its long use). Ridley and Jopling defined the well-known five clinical forms of leprosy (TT, BT, BB, BL, LL) on the basis of the clinical, bacteriologic, histopathologic and immunologic findings.

Because the Ridley-Jopling classification is meant only for research purposes, it was considered necessary to make a primary clinical classification for the use of all other leprosy workers who cannot rely on the specific facilities needed. In 1982, a group of WHO experts drew up a clinical-bacteriologic classification based on the probable number of *M. leprae* harbored by a subject. Subjects with a bacterial index of less than 2+ on the Ridley scale are termed "paucibacillary", while those with a bacterial index greater than or equal to 2+ are termed "multibacillary". The two groups of subjects are treated according to the recommendations [186].

Indeterminate leprosy technically falls outside the spectrum of the Ridley-Jopling classification and is included in the paucibacillary group in the 1982 WHO system. Tuberculoid leprosy falls into the WHO paucibacillary group; borderline leprosy can be either paucibacillary or multibacillary depending on the bacterial index, while lepromatous leprosy is multibacillary in the WHO system.

5.9.1 Clinical Assessment

No other infectious disease in man can boast the same variety of clinical findings as those of leprosy. These can range from an insignificant area of hypo-pigmented skin that may heal spontaneously, to widespread damage to peripheral nerves, eyes, bones, muscles and other tissues together with deformity and disability. In general leprosy involves the skin; there is also always nerve damage, even if in cases with early disease it may not be evident except at histological examination of the nerves.

As regards the clinical history it is important to ascertain any contacts with subjects affected by leprosy. In non endemic countries great prudence should be taken before formulating a diagnosis of leprosy in a subject that has never been in contact with known diseased subjects or never been in an endemic zone. Meanwhile, in endemic countries this history of contact with the disease has no value because sooner or later the entire population is bound to come in contact with *M. leprae.*

In all suspected cases the first thing to look for is subjective symptoms of involvement of the peripheral nerves: paraesthesia, nerve pain, weakening of the muscles of the limbs. As far as the onset is concerned, it should be remembered that leprosy, like all chronic diseases, can also have an acute onset, with the development of the skin and systemic picture of erythema nodosum leprosum.

The cardinal signs are anaesthetic skin lesions and enlarged peripheral nerves, and *M. leprae* should be searched for. The early lesions will be plaques or macules, or more rarely papules and nodules, with a definite loss of sensation to a light touch, pin prick or temperature change. Other possible skin alterations like color, texture and hair growth, have no diagnostic importance if there is no loss of sensitivity. Enlarged peripheral nerves are very rarely observed in other diseases (such as amyloidosis, hereditary Charcot-Marie-Tooth peripheral neuropathies, Dejerine-Sottas disease and Refsum's disease), that are rare diseases. In endemic areas, the findings of a definite enlargement of peripheral nerves is sufficient to make the diagnosis. A proper palpation to assess the nerves is essential, and must be done bilaterally. Leprosy is the only disease in which there may be massive invasion of the derma or nasal mucosa by acid-fast bacilli.

5.9.2 How to Examine the Patient

It is necessary to examine the entire skin surface under a good light. The skin must also be scrutinized very closely to avoid missing pale patches. Early lesions may be hypopigmented or erythematous or both, and can sometimes be difficult to see.

5.9.2.1 Skin

At the skin level, the type of lesions, number, distribution and symmetry, superficial appearance (color, dryness, roughness, shine) and characteristics of the margins (clear or indistinct) are important; it is also necessary to assess the presence of undamaged areas inside the lesions. Another important aspect is any modifications of sensitivity to touch, heat and pain, changes in the sweating pattern and any sign of alopecia.

5.9.2.2 Peripheral Nerves

The morbid process will involve the sensitive and vegetative nerve fibers that innervate the skin structures (glands, vessels) and those of the deeper sensitive or mixed nerve endings. Alterations of the sensitive and vegetative functions must be assessed both at the sites of lesions and of apparently undamaged skin in the districts innervated by the nerves most severely affected. Involvement of the motor fibers will develop later, with weakness, atrophy, muscle paralysis and limb deformity. The neurological symptoms will show a progressive course, with a gradual loss of sensitivity and the sweating function, up to the final phase of paralysis. The disease rarely has an acute course, unlike leproreactions.

Heat sensitivity is generally the first to go, followed by pain and touch. In paucibacillary forms the sensory branches are affected earlier and more severely than in multibacillary forms. The examination of the patient's sensitivity must be done in a quiet environment and the patient should not be able to see the examiner's hands.

Heat sensitivity is tested by using two test tubes filled with hot water (40°C) and cold (20°C). The skin zone to be tested is touched with one of the two tubes and the patient must discern the temperature difference. Pain sensitivity is checked by skin stimulation using the blunt or the sharp end of a hypodermic needle and the patient must discriminate between touch and prick. Tactile sensitivity is assessed using graded nylon bristles [254]; the bristle is fixed at the end of a handle and used as follows: after explaining the aim and method of the test, the patient is asked to close her/his eyes. The bristle is placed at right angle on the skin surface, exerting slight pressure so that it bends a little (but contact with the skin must not be prolonged). The patient is then asked to indicate the point where the bristle was pressed for a short time (1, 4).

The involvement of the vegetative fibers occurs earlier and more intensely in paucibacillary forms. It can be evinced by examining the function of the sweat glands (pilocarpine or acetylcholine test) and the integrity of the axon reflex (histamine test). These examinations must be done both on the site of the lesion and on clinically undamaged skin [1, 4].

Hypertrophy of the nerve trunks can be observed at palpation of the main reference points such as the joints, bone prominences and osteofibrous channels (Table 5.10). In these points the nerve trunks are more exposed to trauma or compression and are cooler than deeper nerve tracts, which explains why they are more prone to damage.

In paucibacillary leprosy forms, one or few nerves are affected; thickening is circumscribed and at palpation they appear fusiform or nodular (isolated or multiple "rosary" nodules). In multibacillary forms the nerve involvement is gradual, and evolves slowly and symmetrically, while the symptoms appear late. With disease progression, palpation reveals uniform thickening of the nerves. In advanced stages the nerve parenchyma is replaced by fibrous tissue, and so the nerve has a greater consistency and feels like a thick hard cord.

For diagnostic purposes, palpation is done bilaterally at the above points (Fig. 5.6) to determine the degree of damage and whether it is unilateral, symmetrical and bilateral or asymmetrical. Obviously, it is important to be able to differentiate between a thickened nerve and a tendon or blood vessel.

Table 5.10 Reference points of peripheral nerves most often affected by leprosy

Nerve	Reference points
Supraorbital	Median third of the supraciliary arch
Great auricular	Median third of the sterno-cleido-mastoid muscle
Radial	Posteriorly to the insertion of the deltoid muscle where the nerve turns around the humerus
Median	Distal involvement: immediately above the carpal tunnel Proximal involvement: high part of the forearm toward the elbow fold
Ulnar	Olecranon groove
Cutaneous branch of the radial	Styloid apophysis of the radius
Common peroneal	Point where nerve turns around the peroneal head
Posterior tibial	Posteriorly and inferiorly to the medial malleolus near the posterior tibial artery

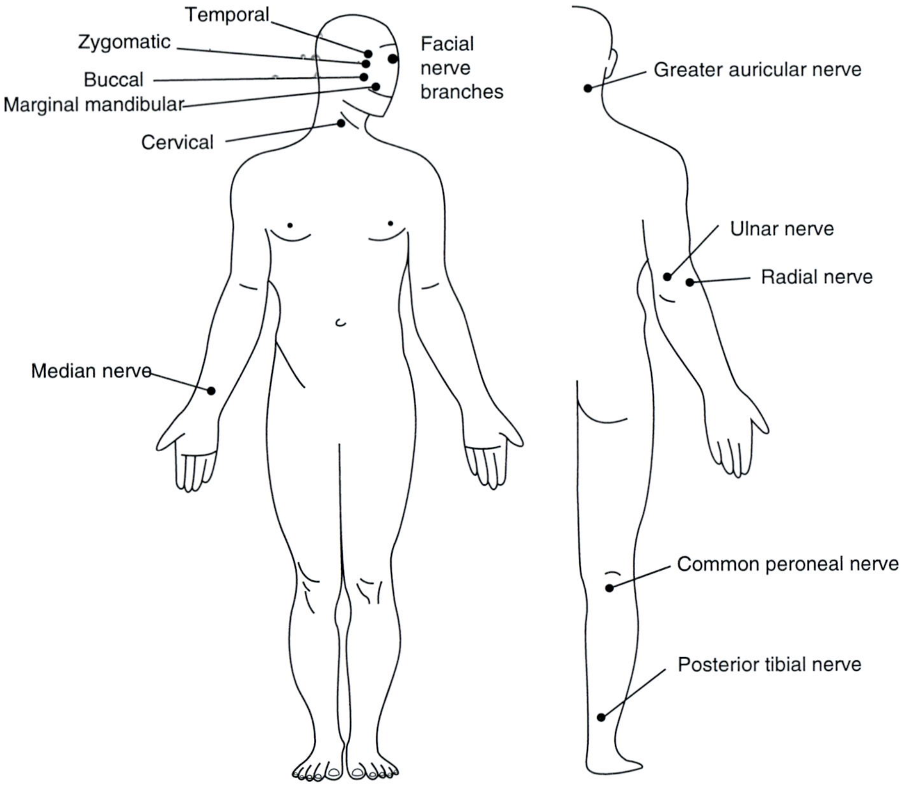

Fig. 5.6 Nerve examination sites (Modified, by [6])

5.9.2.3 Number of *Mycobacterium leprae*

The number of bacilli present in the lesion is exceedingly important in the disease classification for all patients. This is estimated by slit-skin smears and calculating the bacterial index.

5.9.2.4 Lepromin Test

This is not a diagnostic test, but it does make it possible to classify the disease along the disease spectrum. As stated above, the most commonly used lepromin test today is the integral A test (obtained from experimentally infected armadillo liver; A = armadillo), containing 40 million bacilli per ml. After 48–72 h from the intradermic injection of 0.1 ml of lepromin on the flexor face of the forearm, an early Fernandez reaction may develop, and persist for 1–2 days. After 1–2 weeks the Kensuke Mitsuda (late) reaction will appear and reach the maximum expression after 3–4 weeks. The nodule provoked by a strong reaction can ulcerate, and leave a scar. This test must be interpreted on the basis of the result of the Mitsuda reaction, whose intensity is correlated to the reactivity of the host immune reaction to *M. leprae*. The response will have a different significance according to whether the patient presents

Table 5.11 Interpretation of the Mitsuda reaction response in subjects with or without clinical signs of the disease

1. Positive response
   a. Absence of clinical signs: the subject may not develop the disease or it may manifest in a self-resolving paucibacillary form
   b. Active disease; the patient is classified in the hyperergic part of the spectrum
2. Negative response
   a. Absence of clinical signs; the subject has not been infected, or if infected is anergic and may develop a multibacillary form
   b. Active disease: the patient is classified in the anergic part of the spectrum

clinical signs of leprosy or not (Table 5.11). In patients with tuberculoid borderline leprosy evolving along the spectrum toward the anergic pole the test will gradually become negative. A type I reaction, or reversal reaction, can cause the test to be temporarily or stably positive. In patients with indeterminate leprosy the Mitsuda test may yield prognostic indications: lepromin-positive subjects will show an evolution toward spontaneous healing or toward the tuberculoid pole.

5.9.2.5 Mucosa of the Nasal Fossae

The search for bacilli in the nasal mucosa needs to be carefully interpreted. Paucibacillary disease affects skin and peripheral nerves only. *M. leprae* is found in the nasal mucosa only in the forms at the lepromatous end of the spectrum (80–87% of cases of LL, 50% of BL). During treatment, the bacilli will disappear from the nasal mucosa before the skin. However, it is also possible to observe atypical nontuberculous acid-fast bacilli in the mucosa. Searching for bacilli in nasal secretions may be useful at the beginning of the treatment to determine how contagious the patient is, since the nasal mucosa is the main pathway for bacilli spread away from the organism.

5.9.2.6 Other Examinations

Apart from histologic and serologic tests, it is necessary to check any involvement of the eyes, testicles, superficial muscles, lymph nodes, tendons and bones.

5.9.2.7 Classifications Inside the Spectrum

According to the results of the above examinations, the patient will be diagnosed with one of the various clinical forms of leprosy. Tuberculoid forms, TT and especially BT, are associated with severe large nerve damage, while the lepromatous form is associated with a chronic course and long-term complications. Near the tuberculoid pole, spontaneous healing is usual, whereas this rarely happens near the lepromatous pole. Polar forms tend to be immunologically stable, and are unlikely to change their position in the spectrum; at the two poles, type 1 reactions are non encountered. By contrast, borderline diseases are unstable, and may move up and down the spectrum. In this context, a shift in cellular immunity, "reversal" or "upgrading" in the tuberculoid pole or albeit infrequently, "downgrading" in the lepromatous pole, is often accompanied by type 1 reactions and severe nerve damage. In lepromatous leprosy type 2 reactions may develop. Multibacillary forms require longer treatment times and more drugs than paucibacillary forms.

5.10 Histopathology

The wide spectrum of different clinical pictures of leprosy is attributable to the host immune response rather than to the cytopathic effect of *M. leprae*. The histopathologic appearance also reflects the immunological situation [1, 4, 255, 256].

There are three cardinal points involved in the correct diagnosis and classification of leprosy. It is impossible to make a correct histological diagnosis with being aware of the clinical data, so the final diagnosis must always be based on a clinical-pathologic correlation. The skin biopsy must go deep (a 4 mm punch biopsy at least, including part of the subcutaneous fat) [256], and also it must be done on a representative part of the lesion. In detail, in indeterminate leprosy (IL) the center of a hypopigmented lesion must be biopsied, or better still the center of the anaesthetic area, or the margin of a ring macule. In tuberculoid (TT), borderline tuberculoid (BT), and borderline borderline leprosy (BB) it is the infiltrated margins of the lesion that are important, while in borderline lepromatous (BL) and lepromatous leprosy (LL) it is the centers of macules, plaques, or nodules that are diagnostic. In cases of a type 1 reaction the most oedematous and infiltrated area of the lesion has to be biopsied, while in cases of ENL the biopsy must include the subcutaneous fat [257].

Haematoxylin and eosin, and Fite-Faraco staining (the method of choice) allow a good assessment of the samples, which must be cut in serial sections. Immunohistochemistry of the lymphocytic infiltrate is not necessary for the diagnosis. Polymerase chain reaction (PCR) for *M. leprae* is useful only in a limited number of cases. Acid-fast bacilli on the histopathologic sections are assessed in the same way as on skin smears, according to the previously reported logarithmic indices.

To differentiate *M. leprae* from other mycobacteria, the sections can be treated with pyridine; this is also useful to check if the bacilli remain acid-fast.

Unfortunately, the Ridley-Jopling clinical classification does not always correlate with the histologic features; indeed, in some cases there is actually a discrepancy between the clinical and the histological findings [258, 259].

5.10.1 Indeterminate Leprosy

This early form of disease often poses diagnostic problems and does not reveal the patient's possible immune reactivity. The histological findings are often aspecific. Nevertheless, local lymphocytic infiltrates are frequently diagnostic; these are found selectively arranged along the course of the neurovascular fasciae and annexes (Fig. 5.7). Mast cells are found to be increased, whereas granulomas are absent. Small nerve filaments may show a modest intraneural infiltration. If this perineural inflammatory infiltrate is present, and if the history is compatible, leprosy may be suspected. However, in such cases it is necessary to search for bacilli on serial sections; even if few in number, they will generally lie parallel to the axon. It is also likely that there will be a few bacilli at the level of the papillary derma and the erector pili muscles. PCR is positive only in a small percentage of cases.

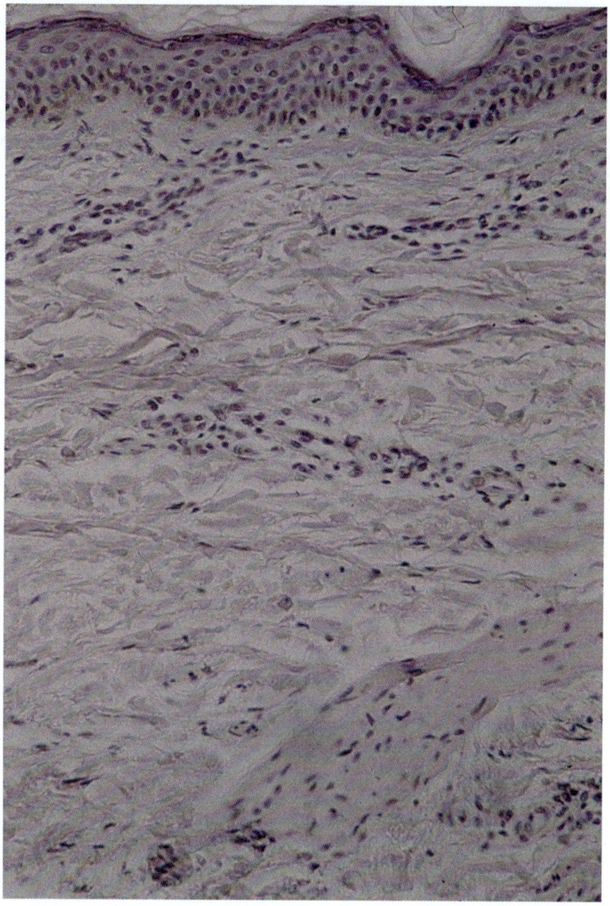

Fig. 5.7 Indeterminate leprosy. Dermal lymphocytic infiltration (Hematoxylin-eosin—×100)

5.10.2 Histological Criteria That Aid Classification

After the early or indeterminate phase of the infection, the host immune reaction will start to manifest. At tissue level the assessment must take into account the following parameters: number of bacilli, cellular composition of the granulomas, nerve alterations, and involvement of the subepidermal zone and the epidermis. A quali-quantitative crossmatch of these aspects will yield the classification of a lesion along the disease spectrum.

As we have already noted, the two forms at the poles are stable and will never evolve into one another. Instead, the borderline forms are unstable and may oscillate between one or the other pole, while borderline-borderline leprosy is extremely unstable and is therefore very rarely observed as such.

5.10.2.1 Number of Bacilli

A low number of bacilli characterizes the tuberculoid pole of the spectrum and a high number, the lepromatous pole. The number of bacilli, that helps in the sometimes difficult differentiation between borderline tuberculoid (BI: 1–2+) and borderline lepromatous forms (BI: 3–6+), can also be useful to define the type of infiltrate: in fact, the number of bacilli must be compatible with the type of infiltrate.

In mass treatments, leprosy is subdivided into only two forms, paucibacillary and multibacillary. The histopathologic findings should allow the patient to be assigned with a high degree of precision to one of the two groups.

5.10.2.2 Cellular Composition of the Infiltrate

Epithelioid cells are present in TT and BT forms, are rarer in BL, and are never present in LL.

Langhans giant cells are common in TT leprosy. They may also be found in BT, whereas they are never present in the BL form unless there is a reversal reaction in process. In LL, foreign body giant cells are often seen, containing vacuoles of lipid substances, but there could also be no giant cells present in the various forms.

Macrophages, and more properly histiocytes, are predominant in BL and LL forms. In LL the macrophages are more commonly foamy than in BL.

There are numerous lymphocytes in TT, where they surround the periphery of epithelioid cell granulomas. Variable quantities are present in BT, sometimes clumped inside the granuloma, and at others arranged on the granuloma periphery. In BL the lymphocytes may massively infiltrate the histiocytic granuloma or surround a nerve. In subpolar LL they are arranged in clumps inside the granuloma, whereas in polar LL there are few or no lymphocytes.

As to the lymphocyte subpopulations, there are abundant T helpers in the TT and BT forms, widely distributed in the granuloma, while the T suppressors are localized on the periphery. There are few T helpers in BL and LL leprosy.

5.10.2.3 Nerve Alterations

TT is characterized by marked enlargement of the deep dermal and subcutaneous nerves, while central necrosis may or may not be present. The perineurium is mildly infiltrated and separates the epithelioid cells granuloma inside the nerve from the lymphocytes outside.

BT and BL are marked by strong lymphocytic infiltration of the perineurium; in BL there is also lamellar degeneration of the perineurium. The latter is a characteristic feature of subpolar LL, together with scarse lymphocytes, while in polar LL the dermal nerves are only minimally involved.

5.10.2.4 Epidermis and Subepidermal Zone

In TT with granulomas in the superior dermis there is usually subepidermal infiltration (Grenz zone) (the infiltrate "touches the epidermis", whereas this rarely occurs in BT) and disaggregation of the epidermis. In lepromatous forms the subepidermal zone appears to lack the cellular infiltrate.

5.10.3 Tuberculoid Leprosy

In this form the intense immune response brings about a granulomatous reaction consisting of a central nucleus of epithelioid cells surrounded by lymphocytes. The granuloma, of non caseating type, may contain numerous Langhans giant cells (Figs. 5.8, 5.9, 5.10, and 5.11). The infiltrate can also involve the papillary derma and basal layer of the epidermis. The granulomas are commonly associated with the neurovascular fasciae and annexes. The cutaneous nerves are frequently damaged by the epithelioid and lymphocytic infiltrate. There will be early destruction and finally complete disappearance of these nerves. The latter finding is suggestive, but not pathognomonic of leprosy. There are few or no bacilli (0 to 1+); when present they are localized in small nerves or in nerve fragments included in the granuloma. Bacilli can also be found in the papillary derma or at the level of the erector pili muscles. PCR is negative in most cases. Differential diagnosis should be made with tuberculosis, sarcoidosis, leishmaniasis, and secondary syphilis.

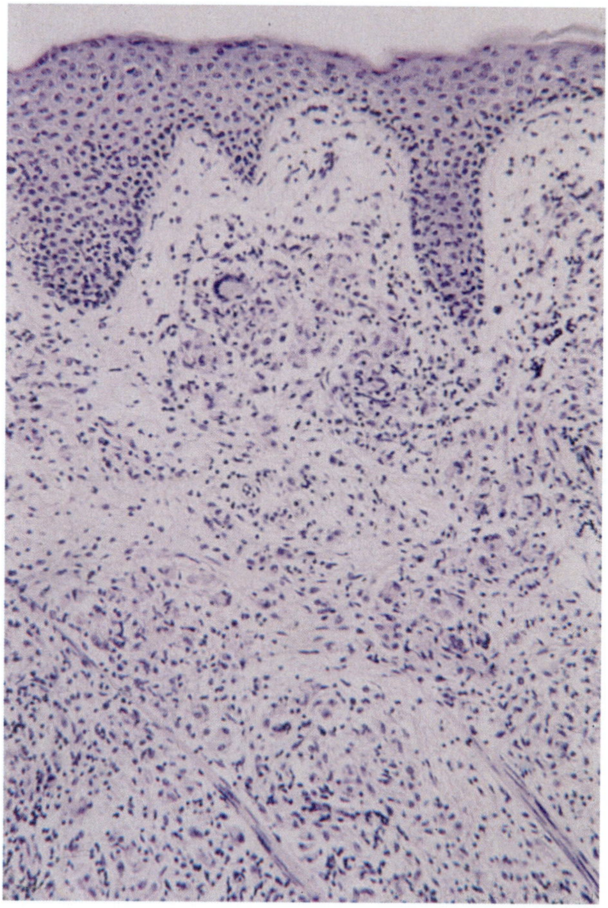

Fig. 5.8 Polar tuberculoid leprosy. Islands of epithelioid cells surrounded by lymphocytes. The infiltrate is mainly located in the superficial corium, pressing against the papillary derma. Langhans cells are present (Hematoxylin-eosin—×100)

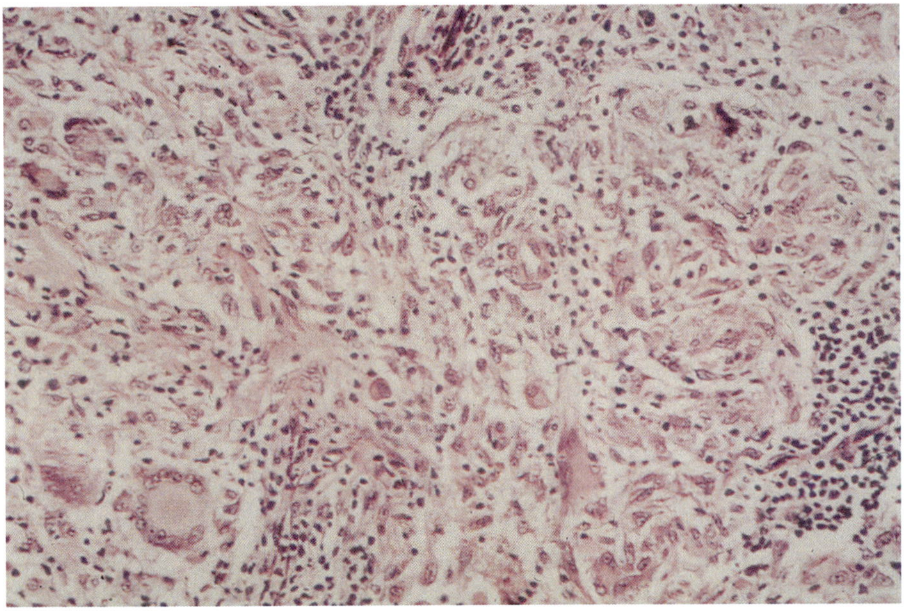

Fig. 5.9 Polar tuberculoid leprosy. Infiltrate with Langhans cells (Hematoxylin-eosin—×100)

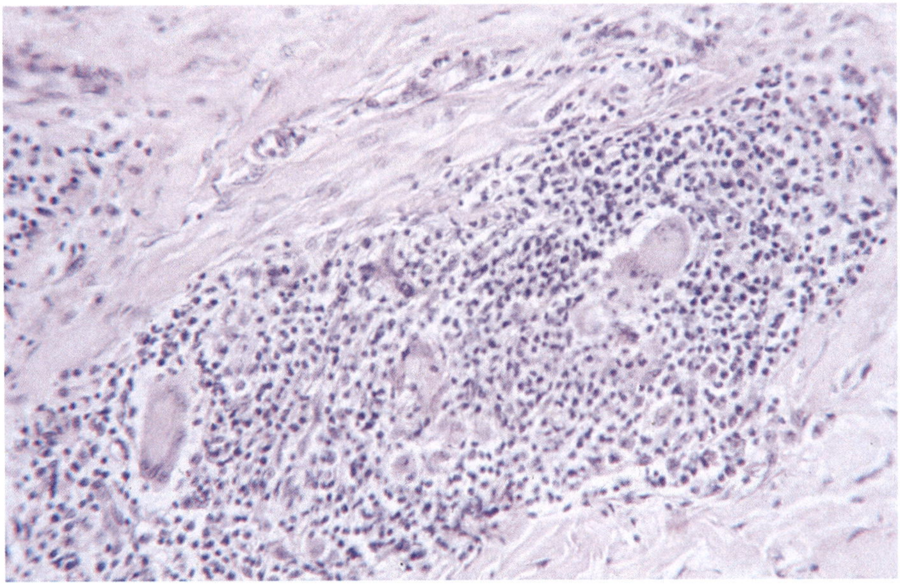

Fig. 5.10 Polar tuberculoid leprosy. Infiltrate with Langhans cells (Hematoxylin-eosin—×100)

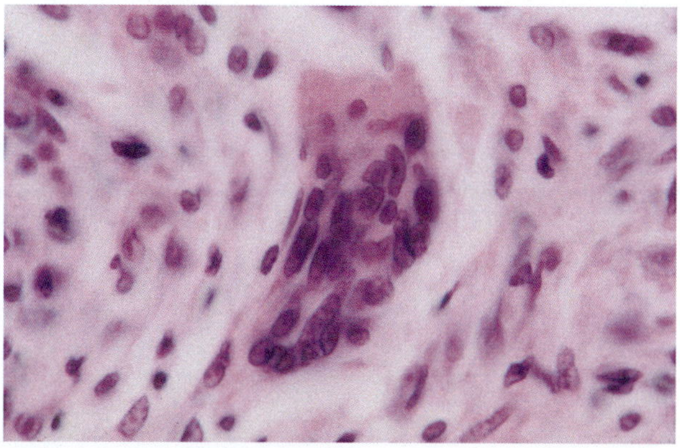

Fig. 5.11 Polar tuberculoid leprosy. Infiltrate with a giant cell (Hematoxylin-eosin—×200)

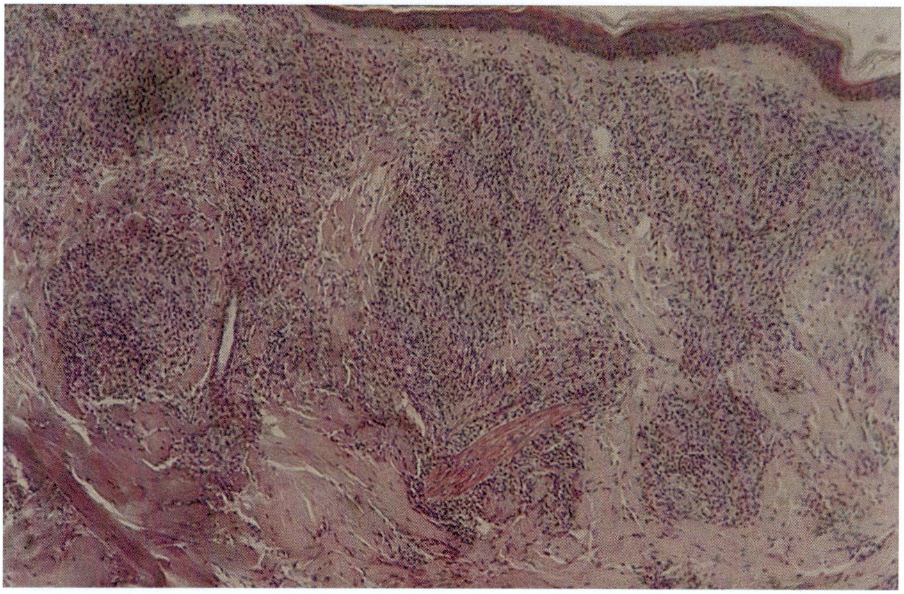

Fig. 5.12 Borderline tuberculoid leprosy. The dense dermal infiltrate is separated from the epidermis by a free zone (Hematoxylin-eosin—×40)

5.10.4 Borderline Tuberculoid Leprosy

The infiltrate is similar to that of TT; however, the epithelioid cells are less mature and the lymphocytes lie within, not only around the granuloma (Fig. 5.12). The granuloma is also less organized. Undifferentiated, medium-sized giant cells are present. The epidermis may or may not be “eroded” by the infiltrate. Nerves are mildly swollen and infiltrated. The acid-fast bacilli count is 0 to 2+. PCR is positive in about 50% of cases.

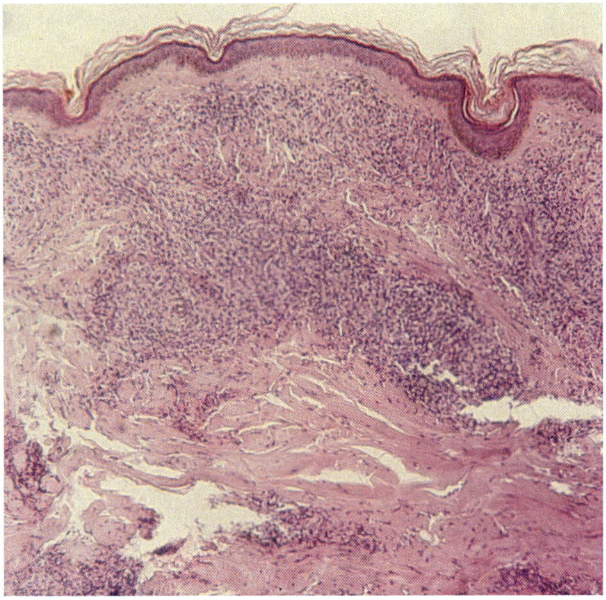

Fig. 5.13 Borderline borderline leprosy. The dermal infiltrate, which is separated from the epidermis by a free zone, consists of epithelioid cells and lymphocytes (Hematoxylin-eosin—×40)

5.10.5 Borderline Borderline Leprosy

This is characterized by the presence of immature epithelioid cells and the absence of well-defined granulomas. There are no giant cells, while there is a diffuse distribution of lymphocytes (Fig. 5.13). A large proportion of the cells are macrophages. The epidermis is atrophic but the subepidermal zone is spared. The nerves are not oedematous but they are infiltrated by lymphocytes and epithelioid cells, and partially destroyed. There may be lamination of the perineurium (reactive proliferation of perineural cells). The acid-fast bacilli count is 3 or 4+. PCR is positive in nearly all cases.

5.10.6 Borderline Lepromatous Leprosy

The infiltrate is characterized by macrophages and lymphocytes, the latter possibly being more prevalent. Some solitary clumps of epithelioid cells may be seen. The diffuse, nodular infiltrate, perivascular or around the annexes, is always separated from the epidermis by a typical narrow zone (Unna band) of collagen. The macrophages cytoplasm may show a variable degree of foaminess but there will be no large vacuoles. Plasma cells are present. The nerves show an onion-skin perineurium with lymphocytes arranged in cuffs around nerve bundles (Fig. 5.14). Acid-fast bacilli (4+ to 5+) are highly evident in the cells of the infiltrate and the erector pili muscles. PCR is positive.

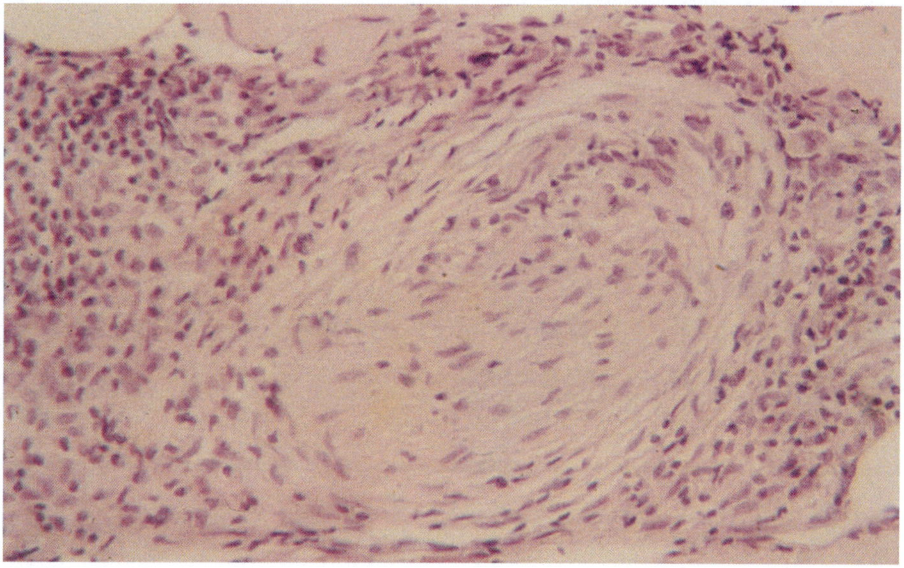

Fig. 5.14 Borderline lepromatous leprosy. A nerve surrounded by histiocytes and lymphocytes (Hematoxylin-eosin—×100)

5.10.7 Lepromatous Leprosy

In this form there are sheets of macrophages diffusely distributed in the derma or arranged in nodular formations. Lymphocytes and plasma cells are amply distributed or found in clumps. There are no epithelioid cells. The epidermis is atrophic. A clear Unna band is evident in the superficial dermis. The skin annexes, that are surrounded by macrophages, are also atrophic. The infiltrate extends down to the subcutaneous fat.

The macrophages will present a gray cytoplasm with variable degrees of foamy changes (lepra cells or Virchow cells) (Fig. 5.15), and there will be large vacuoles in more long-standing forms. The nerves are not oedematous, but are surrounded by macrophages and may show an onion-skin perineurium with no particular infiltrate. There will be very many acid-fast bacilli (5–6+) present in all the cellular elements (Fig. 5.16) and skin structures; lying in parallel array or in clusters (globi), they have a solid appearance or will be granular or fragmented during the course of treatment. PCR is positive. Differential diagnosis is made with xanthomas and xanthogranulomas, paraffinoma and, rarely, infections due to nontuberculous mycobacteria.

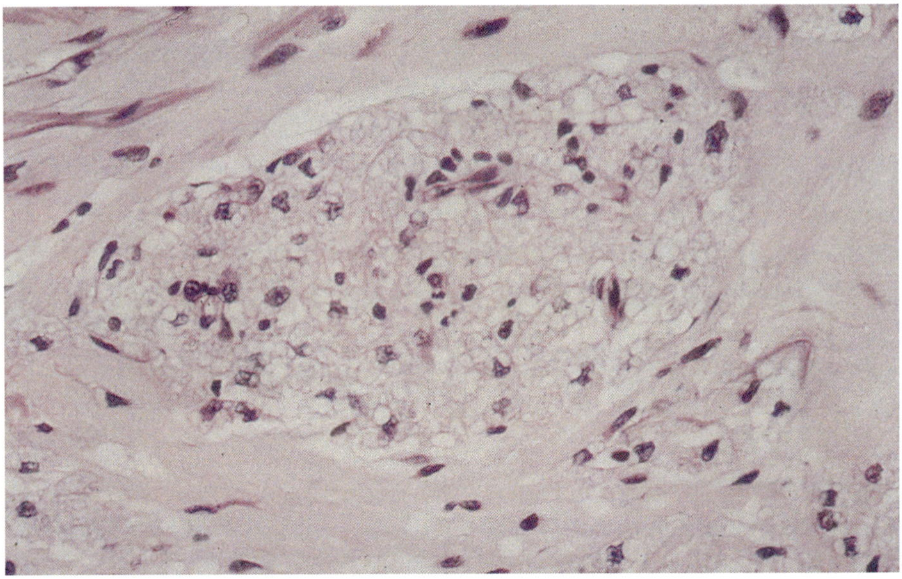

Fig. 5.15 Lepromatous leprosy. Vacuolated macrophages (Hematoxylin-eosin—×100)

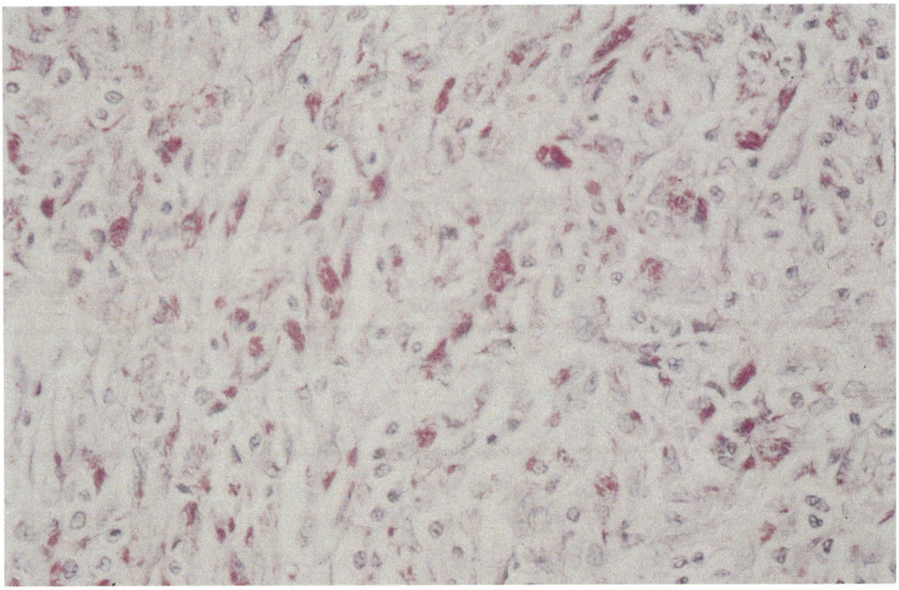

Fig. 5.16 Lepromatous leprosy. Acid-fast bacilli in vacuolated macrophages (Ziehl Neelsen—×100)

5.10.8 Leprosy Reactions

5.10.8.1 Type 1 Reaction (T1R)

T1R is observed above all in BT and BB, but sometimes also in BL patients. The superficial derma is oedematous and the granulomas are disorganized by the oedema. There will be foreign body giant cells (sometimes with vacuoles) and large Langhans giant cells. The epidermis is spongiotic. In severe forms there may be evident necrosis or ulceration, together with neutrophils. In forms in regression the oedema is reduced and the tubercles appear well-organized.

When a T1R occurs in BL, there will also be evident Virchow cells.

5.10.8.2 Type 2 Reaction (T2R)

This is observed in the course of LL and, less commonly, BL. Two variants have been described. One is named "pink node type" or classic erythema elevatum leprosum (ENL), in which the infiltrate features small granulomas in the subcutis with clusters of neutrophils around the foamy macrophages. Eosinophils, plasma cells, and mast cells are present. Vasculitic changes are seen above all in early lesions.

Necrotizing ENL (or severe ENL) is characterized by severe vasculitic changes with a neutrophilic infiltrate, hemorrhages and thrombi; these alterations can lead to collagen degeneration with necrosis of both the epidermis and dermis, and to dermal fibrosis in the resolving phase. Solid acid-fast bacilli are present in untreated patients, while granular or fragmented bacilli are evident in cases undergoing treatment.

Differential diagnosis must be made with the Lucio-Alvarado phenomenon, true erythema nodosum, erythema induratum of Bazin, Sweet syndrome, pyoderma gangrenosum, and deep mycotic infections.

5.10.9 Particular Forms of Leprosy

5.10.9.1 Histoid Leprosy

This is characterized by a circumscribed macrophage granuloma with a predominance of spindle-shaped cells or polygonal cells, and an unusually large number of acid-fast bacilli. There may also be a small number of foamy macrophages [260].

5.10.9.2 Lucio-Latapi Leprosy

This features a non nodular infiltrate similar to that of LL, with diffuse Virchow cells [261].

5.10.9.3 Lucio-Alvarado Phenomenon

There will be epidermal necrosis, ulcerations, features of diffuse LL with many acid-fast bacilli. There will also be panvasculitis of both superficial and deep vessels. Lobular panniculitis is a characteristic feature, medium-sized arteries being infiltrated by macrophages, resulting in narrowing of their lumens, occlusion and ischemic alterations [262].

5.10.10 Histopathology of the Lymph Nodes

In LL, the lymph nodes draining the skin have a thickened capsule and a macrophage infiltrate with a rich content of bacilli in the paracortical areas. This infiltrate may block the circulation of lymphocytes and contribute to the immune suppression process.

In LT the lymph nodes are invaded by epithelioid cell granulomas.

5.10.11 Histopathology of the Internal Organs

M. leprae thrives in lower temperature organs: the ear lobes, nose, upper airways mucosa (turbinates and nasal septum), anterior eye segments, testicles and superficial nerve trunks. The gastrointestinal tract, central nervous system and lower airways below the larynx are never affected.

Orchitis manifests with hyaline degeneration of the seminal tubules and a lepromatous infiltrate. The ovaries are never involved. In LL there may be signs of destructive cystic fibrosis of the bones of the hands and feet but not of other bones. In subjects with long-standing LL the liver, kidneys, spleen and adrenals are affected by amyloidosis.

5.11 Serology

Serological tests can be useful to establish the infection, and assist in the diagnosis and prognosis of the particular leprosy form [263]. For predictive purposes, these tests are strongly influenced by the disease prevalence in the geographic area investigated. In areas with a low prevalence such tests have little diagnostic utility. Serology must therefore be used to search for multibacillary cases in subjects at high risk, in order to identify the infection in preclinical stages. Serological tests can also be useful in the assessment of the response to therapy: in fact, during treatment the levels of antibodies against PGL-I will decline.

Specific anti-*M. leprae* antibodies are produced against lipoarabinomannan (LAM), the species-specific lipid phenolic glycolipid (PGL) and the protein antigens of *M. leprae*. No single antigen has been identified that could help to detect an early subclinical infection. For all three types of antigen, multibacillary patients show a prolific production of antibodies, while the response in paucibacillary patients is variable.

Evaluated in field settings, the positivity of the PGL-I test correlates with the bacterial load measured by slit-skin smears.

There are two other specific tests that reveal antibodies against *M. leprae* epitopes situated on a 35 kD protein and a 36 KD protein (with approximately 100% and 98% specificity, respectively).

Lepromatous patients also produce a range of autoantibodies, both organ-specific (directed against nerves, thyroid, testes, and gastric mucosa), and non-specific, such as rheumatoid factors, anti-DNA, cryoglobulins, and cardiolipin.

In any case, serological tests are an additional diagnostic parameter to support the essential clinical, histopathological and bacteriological tests.

5.12 Clinical Features

5.12.1 Indeterminate Leprosy

Indeterminate leprosy (IL) does not fall into the spectrum of the Ridley-Jopling classification because of the lack of correlation between the clinical and histopathological features. In this form the cell-mediated immunity picture is still not clear [264, 265].

IL, early and transitory disease form, is generally observed in endemic areas in children that come in contact with patients with untreated multibacillary leprosy forms. IL arises in individuals that have not yet developed cell-mediated immunity against *M. leprae*.

The only skin lesion present in IL is the macule, single or multiple (generally not more than 3 lesions, on one side of the body and clumped together), that will be pale red in light-skinned patients and coppery red in dark-skinned patients; it may also be hypopigmented with a uniform fading of the color (Fig. 5.17). Not more than 3–4 cm in size, the macule has a smooth surface with no scaling and will not be pruriginous. The edges are usually blurred. There will be a preserved or only mildly reduced sensory function but thermal sensation may be lost and the patient is unable to distinguish between cold and hot tub water. Sweating is normal and body hairs are present. Hyperalgesia may precede the detection of skin lesions [266–268].

The sites most frequently affected are the face, buttocks and limbs. The peripheral nerves are not involved. The search for acid-fast bacilli (slit-skin smear) is negative. The Mitsuda test will yield variable results: it may be weakly positive or negative.

A very useful diagnostic tool in light-skinned subjects is the histamine test: 1–2 min after the application of a drop of histamine (dilution 1/1000) in and around the suspected hypochromic lesion, a triphasic skin reaction will appear (triple response of Lewis). The triple reaction (first a red line due to capillary dilation at the site resulting from histamine release, then a flare around the red line due to peripheral dilation of the arterioles, and lastly a wheal due to local oedema) is observed only in normal skin or in hypochromic lesions caused by other diseases. In cases of leprosy the response will be incomplete: the stimulation will induce the capillary dilation and the wheal but not the reflex arteriolar erythema (axonic reflex), because this depends upon the integrity of sympathetic nerve fibers [268].

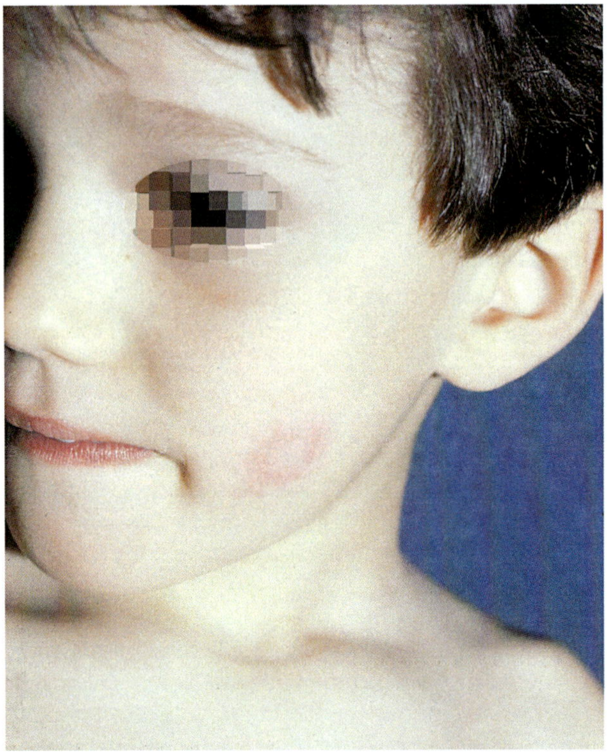

Fig. 5.17 Indeterminate leprosy. Ill-defined, slightly erythematous and hypopigmented macula on the face

Most patients with IL recover spontaneously; the remaining patients if untreated will show a disease evolution toward a "determinate" form of the spectrum. An indeterminate macule in evolution toward the tuberculoid pole will undergo the following changes: the surface becomes dry and rough due to reduced sweating; the edges appear more defined and infiltrated and there is an evident reduction of sensation. The Mitsuda test will be positive, while histology will show an increased number of lymphocytes around the nerve fibers of the derma and rare acid-fast bacilli inside the fibers.

Instead, a macule evolving toward the lepromatous pole will be bright red, while the surface remains smooth and the edges poorly defined. An infiltrate will appear at the center of the macule but there will be no changes in sensation. The Mitsuda test will continue to be negative. Histology shows numerous bacilli in the dermal nerve fibers. The changes in a macule in evolution toward the borderline forms will depend upon the classification on the spectrum of the immune cell response that the patient is developing.

From the differential diagnosis standpoint, many diseases can mimic a macule due to IL. The hypopigmentation diseases to be taken into account are pityriasis alba (featuring a variable number of hypochromic, round patches with undefined edges and rough surface on the trunk and upper limbs), a hypochromic variant of pityriasis versicolor (hypopigmented macules with superficial desquamation and a tendency to coalesce), and solar hypochromiant dermatosis (this is transient and observed after intense tanning: the lesions are irregular with a possibly rough surface). Achromic nevus, nevus anemicus, vitiligo, and postinflammatory hypopigmentation may also mimic IL.

The erythematous macules of IL must also be differentiated from those of seborrhoeic dermatitis (with squamous lesions mainly on the face and trunk). Fixed drug eruption, early-stage morphea, Lyme disease, and the herald patch of pityriasis rosea should also be considered.

The differential diagnosis of a hyperchromic macule should include residual lesions of postinflammatory hyperpigmentation, morphea, a hyperchromic lesion of pytiriasis versicolor, tinea nigra, and fixed drug eruption [269, 270].

5.12.2 Tuberculoid Leprosy

The clinical picture of the various forms in the spectrum may be monomorphous or polymorphous (Tables 5.12 and 5.13).

The disease hyperactivity at the TT pole causes a shorter incubation time and the simultaneous appearance of skin and nerve signs. The skin lesions, that will be few, have a unilateral distribution or may be asymmetrical and bilateral. The cell-mediated immune response is still able to contain the infection.

At skin level there will be macules, papules and plaques. The macules are initial lesions of early TT and generally appear immediately, being rarely derived from a transformation of indeterminate macules. The macules of TT are red in light-skinned patients and coppery in dark skinned patients; they may also be homogeneously hypopigmented. They show a dry surface and due to anhydrosis they are rough to the touch. These lesions also have rarefied body hair, and are anaesthetic: first thermal, then tactile, and finally pain sensitivity is lost. It is important to note that the lesions on the face may have normal sensitivity; in this area the rich sensory innervation compensates for the damaged nerves.

Due to the intense cell-mediated immunity, the macules may undergo a central healing process with a transformation to ring lesions (Figs. 5.18 and 5.19). In addition, papules can appear on the edges of the macules.

The TT plaque is red or coppery, has a rough dry surface, clear-cut raised margins and there is tactile hypo-anaesthesia (thermal anaesthesia develops later), and

Table 5.12 Skin lesions and leprosy forms

Lesions	IL	TT	BT	BB	BL	LL
Macules	+	+	+	+	+	+
Plaques		+	+	+	+	+
Papules		+	+	+	+	+
Nodules				+	+	+
Diffuse infiltration						+

IL indeterminate leprosy, *TT* polar tuberculoid leprosy, *BT* borderline tuberculoid leprosy, *BB* borderline borderline leprosy, *BL* borderline lepromatous leprosy, *LL* polar lepromatous leprosy

Table 5.13 Clinical, bacteriological, and immunological characteristics in the leprosy spectrum (modified, by [18])

	TT	BT	BB	BL	LL
Skin lesions	One/few (up to 5)	One/few (> than 5)	Many	Many	Very numerous
"Satellite" lesions	Absent	Present	Present	Present	–
Distribution	Localized, asymmetrical	Asymmetrical	Asymmetrical	Tendency to symmetry	Symmetrical
Hypopigmentation	Marked	Moderate	Mild	Very mild	Very mild/ absent
Edges	Well defined	Defined	Poorly defined	Rather blurred	Blurred
Surface of lesions	Dry/rough	Dry/rough	Dry/shiny	Smooth/shiny	Smooth/ shiny
Central healing	Marked	Moderate	Minor	Absent	Absent
Sensory loss	Marked	Moderate	Minor	Very minor	Very minor/ absent
Bacilli in nasal mucosa	Absent	Absent	Absent	Absent/present	Present with globi
Bacilli in skin smears	Absent/rare	1+,2+	3+,4+	5+, 6+	6+
Globi	Absent	Absent	Absent	If present, small	Frequent and large
Lepromin test (Mitsuda)	>10 mm	3–10 mm	<3 mm	Negative	Negative
Course	Regressive	Regressive	Unstable	Progressive	Progressive

TT polar tuberculoid leprosy, *BT* borderline tuberculoid leprosy, *BB* borderline borderline leprosy, *BL* borderline lepromatous leprosy, *LL* polar lepromatous leprosy

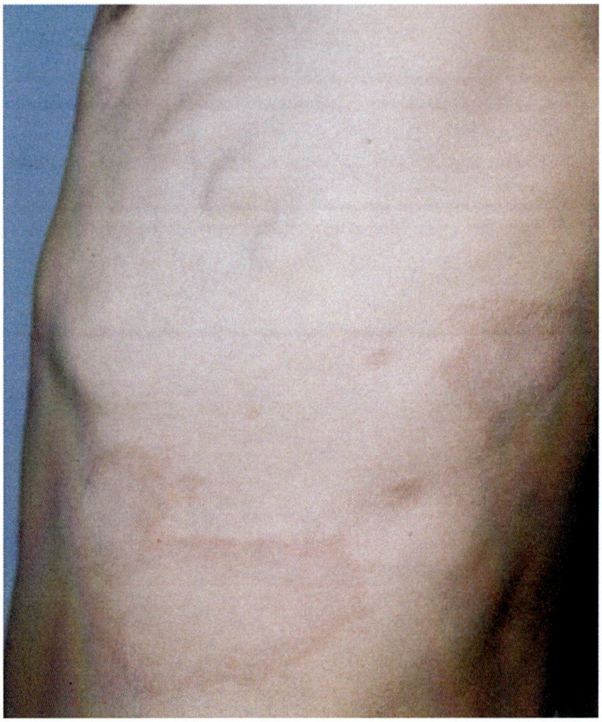

Fig. 5.18 Tuberculoid leprosy. Erythematous macules with central healing

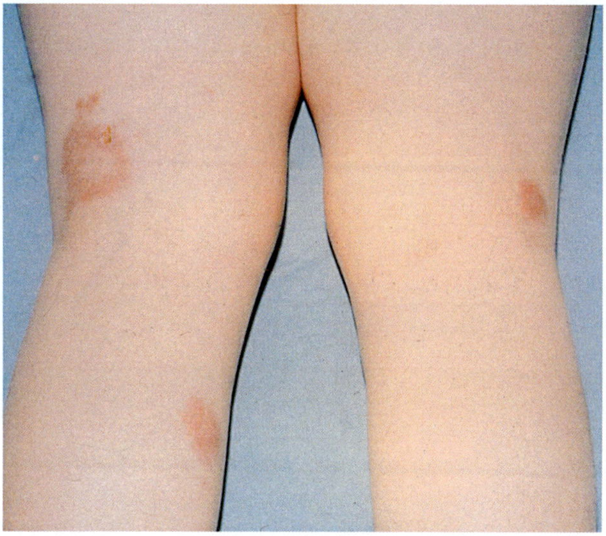

Fig. 5.19 Tuberculoid leprosy. Erythematous macules with central healing

rarefied or absent body hair. The peripheral extension and central healing transform the plaque into a ring-shaped lesion. The most common localization of such lesions is the face, buttocks and limbs [271]. Higher temperature body regions (axillary, inguinal and perineal cavities: "immune zones") are spared.

If there are more than 3 lesions and the distribution is symmetrical and bilateral, differential diagnosis must be made with the borderline tuberculoid form.

In all clinical forms of leprosy, except indeterminate, the involvement of peripheral trunk nerves may be severe and cause disabilities. In TT leprosy, peripheral nerve enlargement is unlikely and if it occurs, it is usually near the lesions. The search for bacilli on skin smears is negative; in biopsies from the margins of lesions there may be few bacilli. The Mitsuda test is strongly positive (Fig. 5.20).

In children, a particular form of leprosy characterized by nodular lesions can be observed: this form is known as infantile nodular tuberculoid leprosy. It appears only in infancy and affects children under 5 years of age. It is considered to be the most benign form of leprosy. In most cases the diagnosis is difficult, and epidemiological data and a biopsy are of the greatest importance [272–274].

Differential diagnosis must be made with various forms of dermatitis. In tinea, as in tuberculoid leprosy, there is a tendency toward central resolution; if there is pruritus and local excoriations this can help to differentiate these two diseases. Cutaneous lupus erythematosus is localized mainly on the face and other exposed sites; the lesions tend to show a spontaneous resolution with a hyperchromic and atrophic/scarring outcome; sensory tests show preservation. Secondary syphilis is generally preceded by a history of nodular-ulcerative lesions of the genitals; however, lesions on the cervix may go unnoticed, and in all cases anti-treponemal screening is necessary. In cases of an annular granuloma, whose plaques are similar to those of TT, the sensory tests are normal. In pityriasis rosea the eruption of rounded erythematous lesions with collarette desquamation is preceded by the herald patch; such lesions generally resolve in 1–2 months. Other skin complaints to be included in the differential diagnosis are seborrhoeic dermatitis, sarcoidosis, parapsoriasis, morphea, mycosis fungoides, cutaneous tuberculosis, leishmaniasis, lipidic necrobiosis.

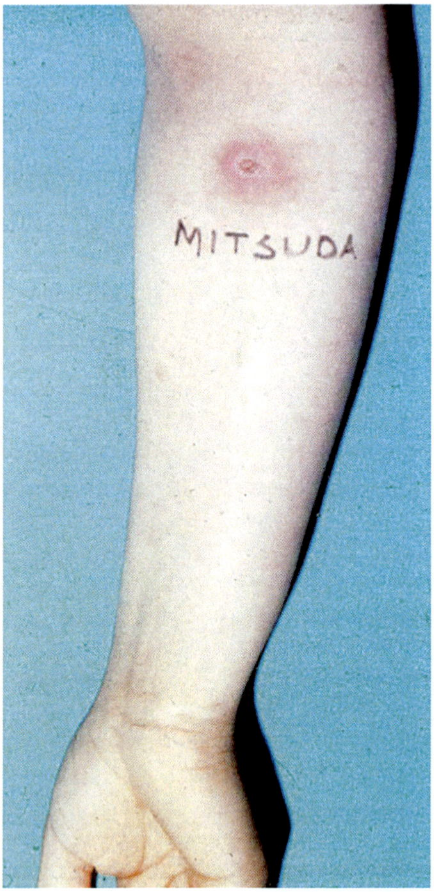

Fig. 5.20 The same patient as in Fig. 5.19. Strong positive Mitsuda reaction

5.12.3 Borderline Leprosy

It is important to make a correct classification of patients with one of the three borderline forms for prognostic and therapeutic reasons. Skin lesions will include macules, plaques, papules, and nodules. The diagnosis is based on the type and number of lesions, their size and distribution over the skin. The degree of definition of the edges and the type of surface are other important elements. An altered sensation may develop early or later and there will be sweating changes and hair loss.

The predominant characteristic of this leprosy group is its instability: if untreated, the disease may evolve toward lepromatous leprosy. During and after treatment patients may suffer reversal reactions, with worsening of skin lesions and nerves.

5.12.3.1 Borderline Tuberculoid Leprosy

The color (red, coppery or hypopigmented) and surface of the macules in this form are the same as of TL macules, while the edges may be blurred here and there, and the size of the lesions is greater than those of the tuberculoid pole (Figs. 5.21, 5.22,

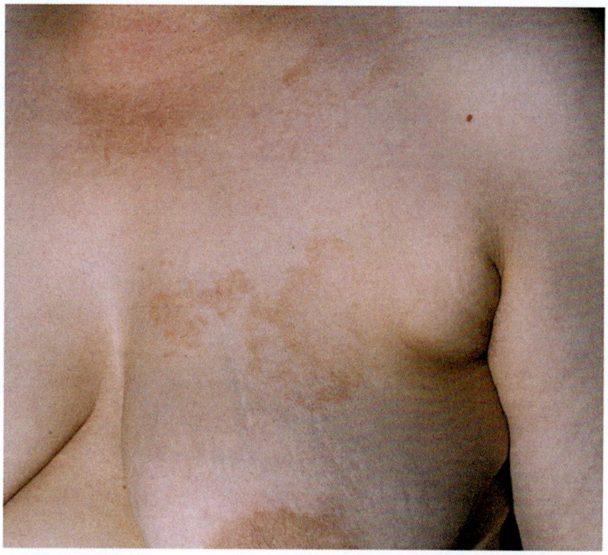

Fig. 5.21 Borderline tuberculoid leprosy. Multiple well difined annular lesions

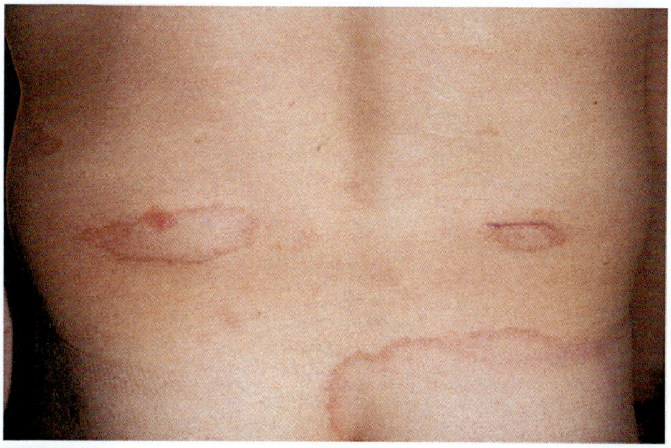

Fig. 5.22 Borderline tuberculoid leprosy. Multiple well difined annular lesions

and 5.23). The number of lesions, that is minor in the initial phase, will gradually increase to 10–20, occupying an entire skin district (Fig. 5.24). Their distribution is initially bilateral and asymmetrical but they will tend to become more symmetrical as the numbers increase.

As regards plaques, they will show clearer edges than those of TL. Around larger lesions, smaller satellite or "finger-like" lesions will often appear, sprouting out from the margins of plaques or macules. Papules will affect the margins of plaques or can also develop as satellite lesions.

In this form several nerves are affected, with a distribution that tends to be symmetrical: in the involved areas the nerves appear enlarged with a spindle or nodular shape. During reversal reactions the nerves swell and become painful; their function deteriorates rapidly and proper treatment is urgent to avoid paralysis and permanent deformity.

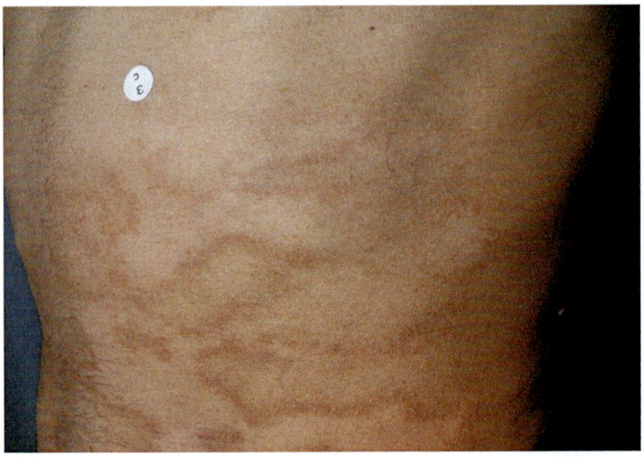

Fig. 5.23 Borderline tuberculoid leprosy. Multiple well difined annular lesions

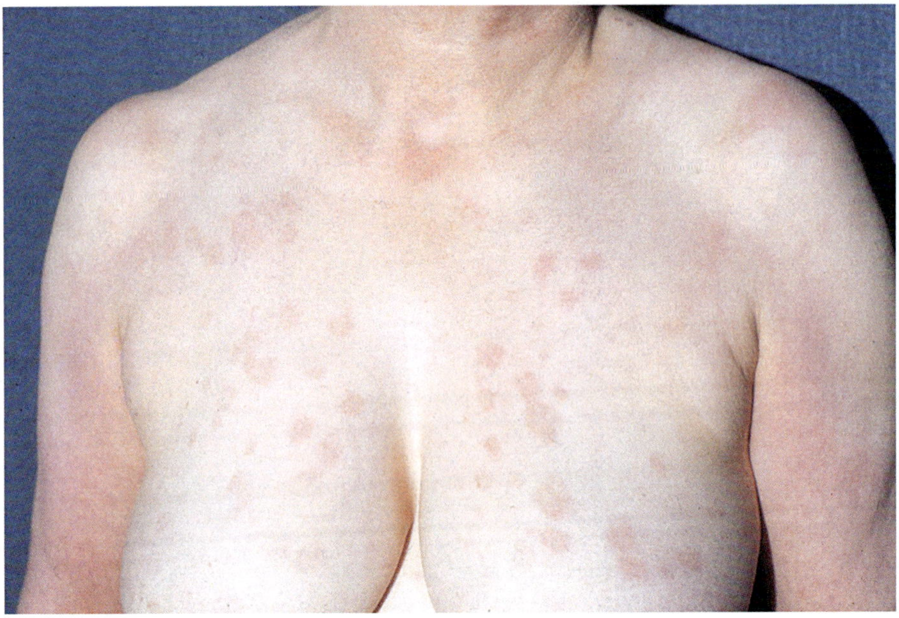

Fig. 5.24 Borderline tuberculoid leprosy. Multiple annular lesions

The BT form may evolve toward the lepromatous pole, taking on the clinical characteristics of multibacillary forms.

The bacterial index on skin smears from the margins of lesions can range from 1+ to 2+. The Mitsuda test is positive.

5.12.3.2 Mid-Borderline Leprosy

This form is highly unstable, and may upgrade under the impulse of reversal reactions toward the tuberculoid pole or downgrade toward the lepromatous pole.

The macules and plaques are of extremely variable sizes and the edges, even of the same lesion, may be blurred or clear-cut. They will be red or coppery red, while the centers are apparently spared and usually hypochromic (Figs. 5.25 and 5.26). These lesions tend to show a centrifugal extension and draw ring or map-like figured shapes: the combination of these lesions gives the "swiss cheese-like" aspect. The internal margins of ring lesions are clear while the external margins are blurred. In this form there may be red or coppery nodules.

The nerve involvement varies according to whether the disease has evolved from BT or BL. Skin smears show many scattered bacilli: the bacterial index ranges from 3+ to 4+. The Mitsuda test may be negative or weakly positive.

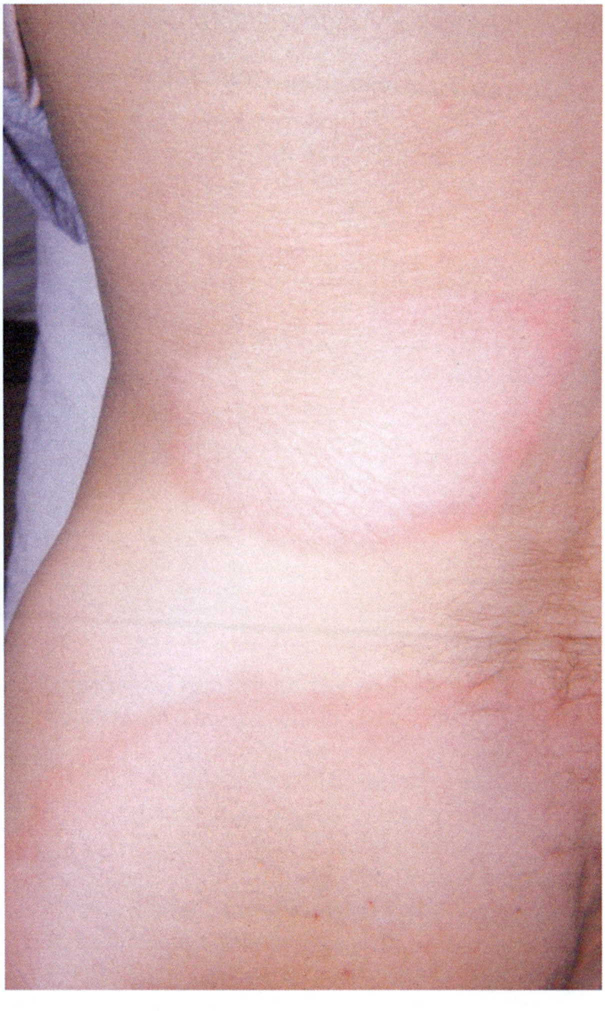

Fig. 5.25 Mid-borderline leprosy. Infiltrated lesions with hypochromic central area

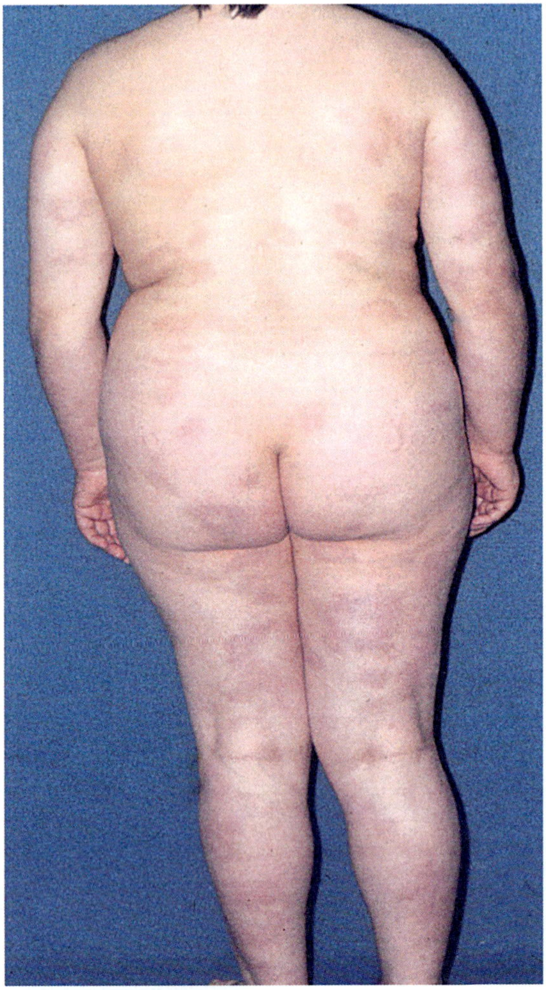

Fig. 5.26 Mid-borderline leprosy. Diffuse, bilateral and symmetric annular lesions

5.12.3.3 Borderline Lepromatous Leprosy

The skin lesions are disseminated and symmetrically distributed. The macules, that are initially hypopigmented, grow in size and become erythematous and infiltrated; they have irregular blurred edges. There will also be plaques and nodules (Figs. 5.27 and 5.28). In advanced stages there will be sparse body hair. The nerves appear enlarged in most patients but are less commonly tender than in BT. Type1 and 2 leprosy reactions are frequently observed. The bacterial index of skin smears ranges from 5+ to 6+, and the bacilli are sometimes clumped in small globi. The nasal mucus is negative in initial forms and becomes positive in advanced stages. The Mitsuda test is negative.

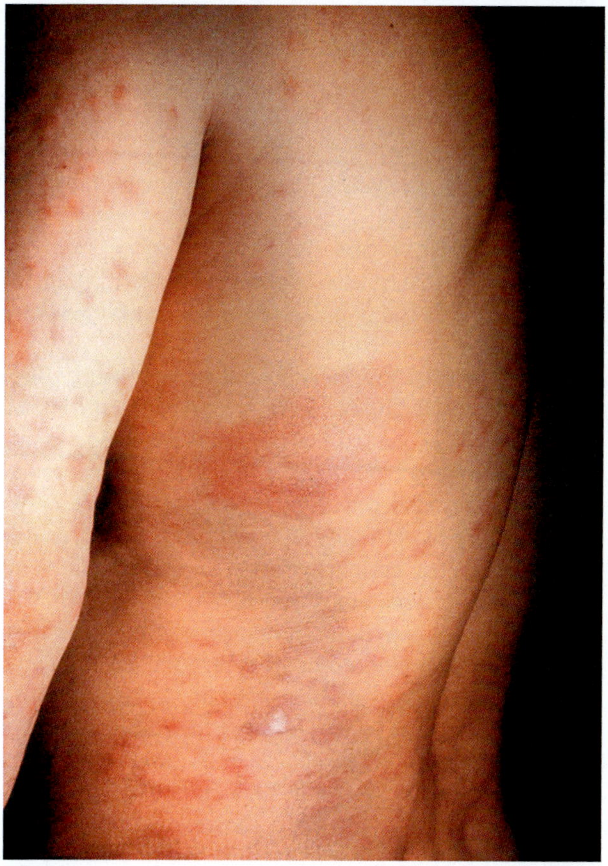

Fig. 5.27 Borderline lepromatous leprosy. Diffuse plaques and nodules

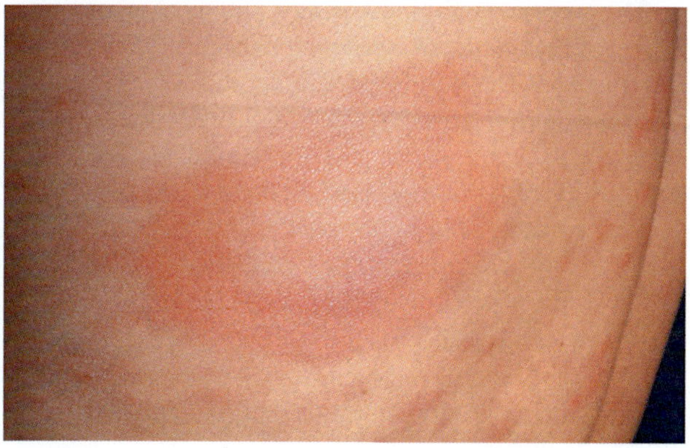

Fig. 5.28 The same patients as in Fig. 5.27. Erythematous annular plaque

5.12.4 Lepromatous Leprosy

The immunological anergy characterizing this form leads to the consequent haematogenous spread of bacilli in the skin, nerves and reticuloendothelial system. In addition, there may be bacillary invasion of the eyes, testes, bones and mucous membranes of the mouth, nose, pharynx, larynx, and trachea [275–277].

5.12.4.1 Skin Lesions

These are multiple, diffuse, small, symmetrically distributed, and include macules, plaques, papules and nodules, all of which may be present in the same patient at the same time.

The first lesions to appear are macules, non palpable, small and rounded or elliptical; they are erythematous in light skins and coppery in dark skins, sometimes with a faintly hypopigmented background. They have a smooth shiny surface and their edges are indistinct. These macules may go unnoticed because they are difficult to see and not associated with pruritus or definite anaesthesia. They are widespread all over the skin, in particular on the face, buttocks and extremities, whereas they are rare in the axillae, groin, perineum, on the external genitals and on the scalp.

Infiltrated lesions are raised above the level of the skin; their distribution and color are the same as those of macules, except than they do not appear on the palms and soles. They are raised in the centre and slope away peripherally to merge imperceptibly with the surrounding skin; they have a smooth and shiny surface and do not exhibit sensory loss, unless they are located in a skin region affected by nerve damage. Papules and nodules appear in the advanced disease stage, largely on the face, auricles and buttocks (Figs. 5.29, 5.30, 5.31, 5.32, 5.33, and 5.34). The ear lobes are thickened already in the early phases of the disease. Advanced infiltration of the nodules on the face gives rise to the "leonine facies" (Figs. 5.35, 5.36, and 5.37), in which the normal wrinkles on the forehead and cheeks turn into deep furrows.

The nodules and plaques may undergo necrosis and ulceration (Figs. 5.38 and 5.39), and large ulcers can develop on the lower legs (Figs. 5.40 and 5.41) when the infiltration of the skin is associated with chronic bilateral lymphedema (Fig. 5.42), secondary to the massive invasion of the lymphatics by bacilli. Thinning of the eyebrows is common, starting in the lateral half and progressing to complete loss of both the eyebrows and eyelashes (superciliary and ciliary madarosis).

Skin smears, even of apparently healthy skin, show extremely numerous bacilli in isolation or clumped in large globi. The bacterial index is 6+. The Mitsuda test is negative. Repeated episodes of erythema nodosum leprosum may be observed.

In cases of LL and BL the differential diagnosis includes various skin diseases. In secondary syphilis there will be a history of genital ulcer, palmoplantar erythematous papules and mucosal lesions. Drug eruptions may induce the appearance of various lesions that may resemble BL and LL leprosy. Anergic cutaneous leishmaniasis may present papules, plaques and nodules: slit-skin smears are negative, while a direct smear will be positive for amastigotes. Systemic lupus erythematosus, with the skin manifestations associated with arthralgia and madarosis, can mimic LL leprosy, also because they have various laboratory test alterations in common

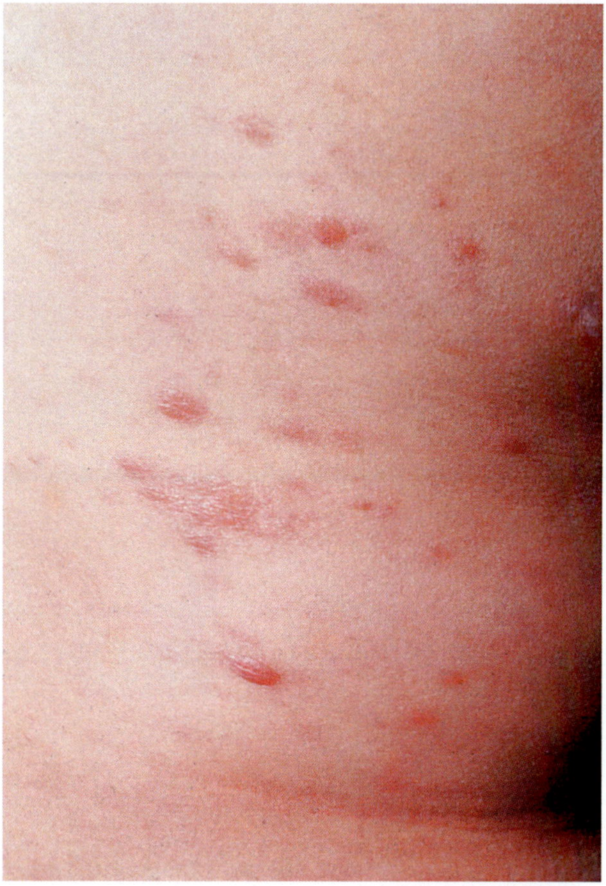

Fig. 5.29 Lepromatous leprosy. Nodular lesions

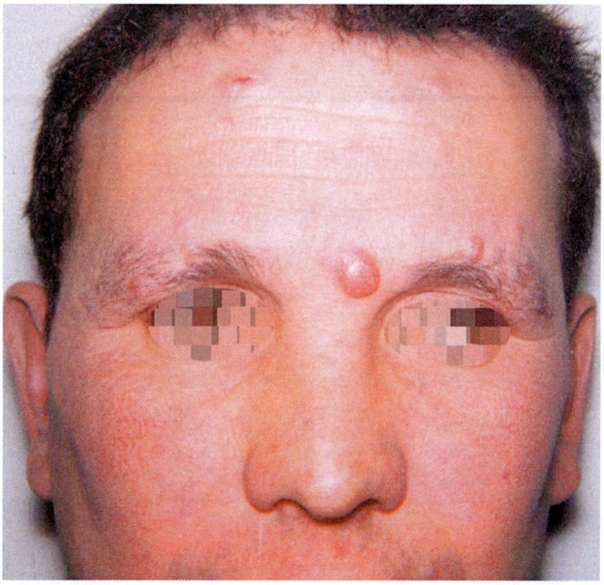

Fig. 5.30 Lepromatous leprosy. Nodular lesions and lateral loss of the eyebrow

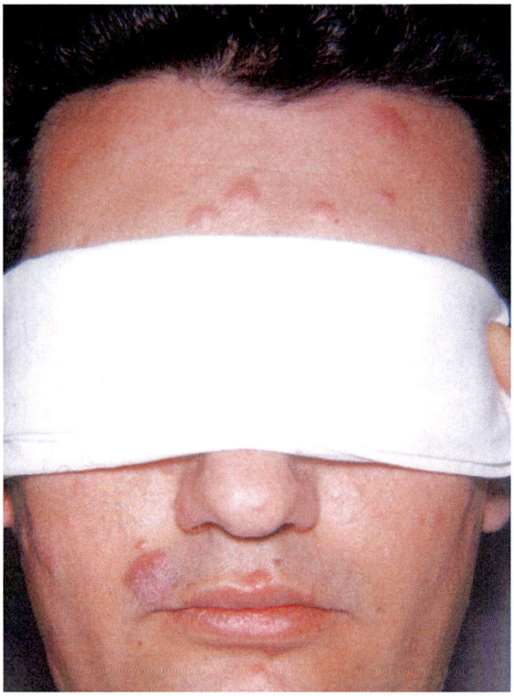

Fig. 5.31 Lepromatous leprosy. Nodular lesions

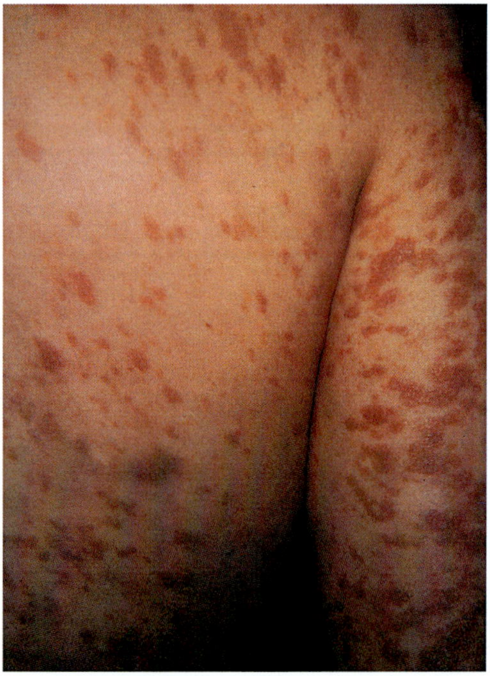

Fig. 5.32 Lepromatous leprosy. Nodular lesions

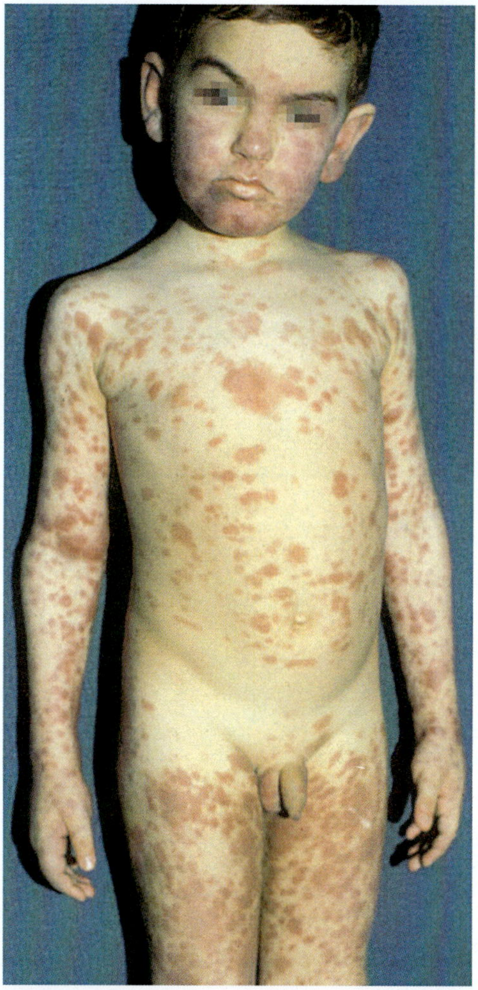

Fig. 5.33 Lepromatous leprosy in a 5-year-old child. Diffuse plaques and nodules

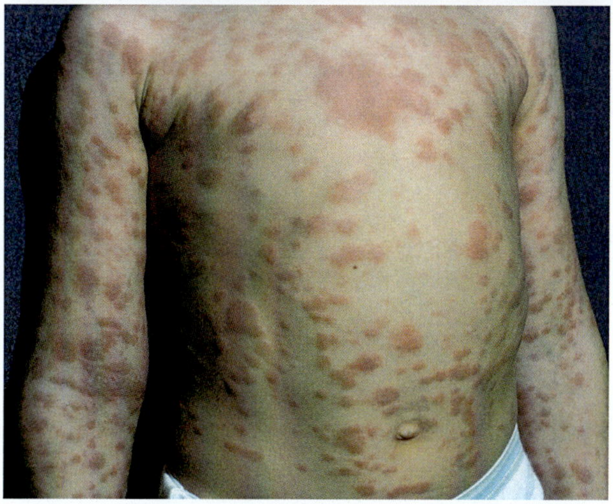

Fig. 5.34 The same patient as in Fig. 5.33

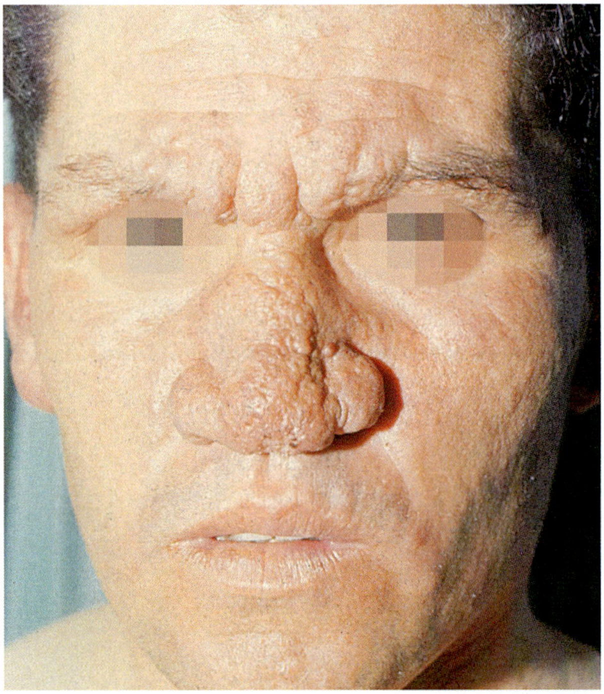

Fig. 5.35 Lepromatous leprosy. Advanced, almost diffuse disease with leonine facies

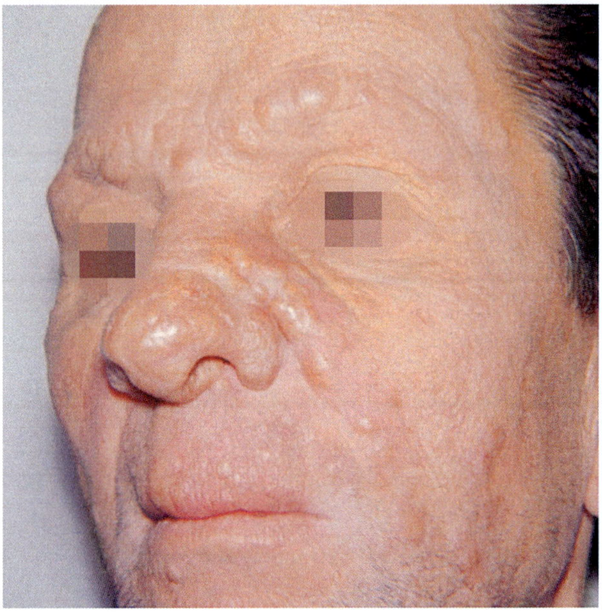

Fig. 5.36 Lepromatous leprosy. Leonine facies and loss of eyebrows and eyelashes

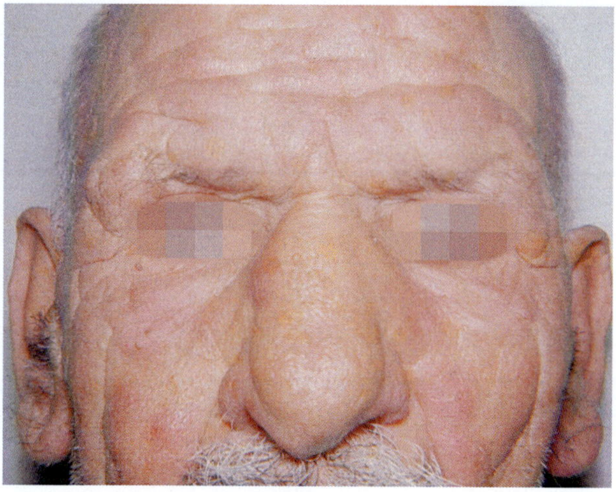

Fig. 5.37 Lepromatous leprosy. Diffuse infiltration of the skin with leonine facies

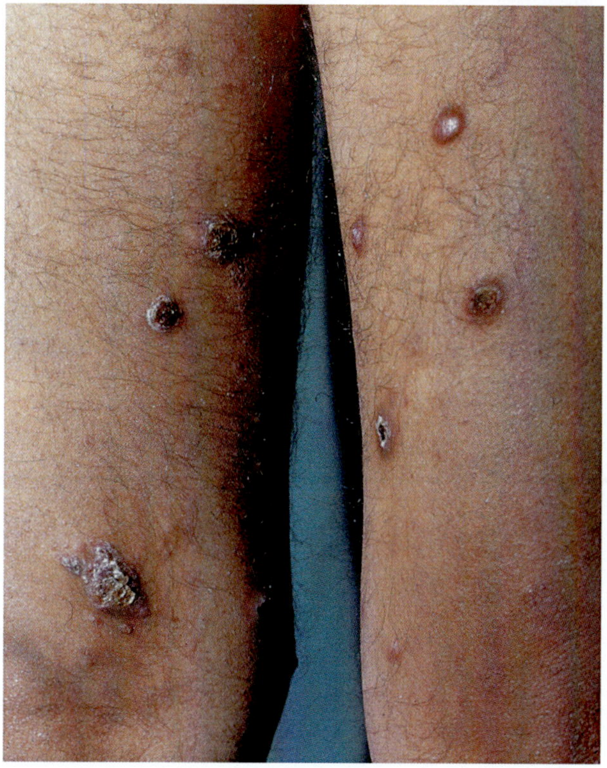

Fig. 5.38 Lepromatous leprosy. Ulcerated nodules

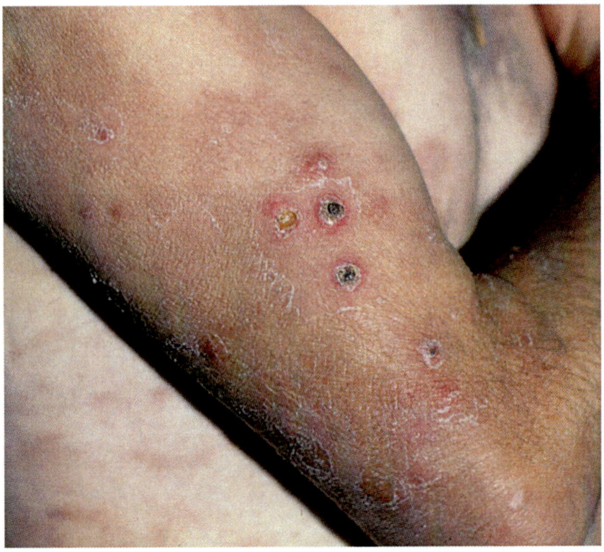

Fig. 5.39 The same patient as in Fig. 5.38

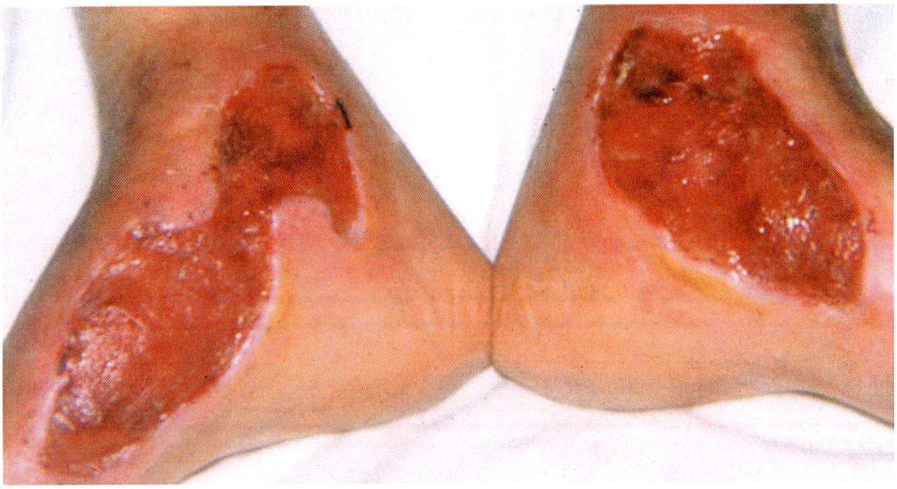

Fig. 5.40 Severe ulcers in lepromatous leprosy

(hypergammaglobulinemia, an elevated sedimentation rate, positive rheumatoid factor, LE cells and VDRL in up to 60% of LL patients). Other diseases to be considered are sarcoidosis, onchocerciasis, Kaposi's sarcoma, deep mycoses, and skin lymphoma.

5.12.4.2 Nerve Involvement

In lepromatous leprosy, nerve involvement has never been described in the absence of skin manifestations. The nerves are not affected at an early stage as in other leprosy forms, but thickening and sensory or motor dysfunction are evident as the

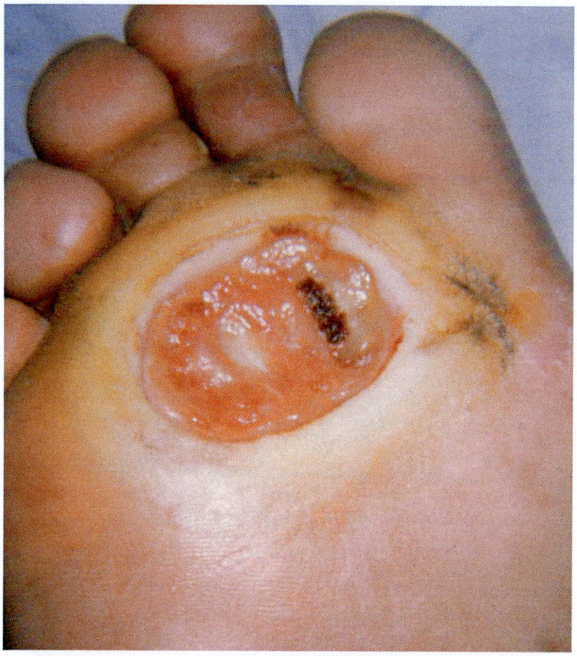

Fig. 5.41 Plantar ulcer in lepromatous leprosy

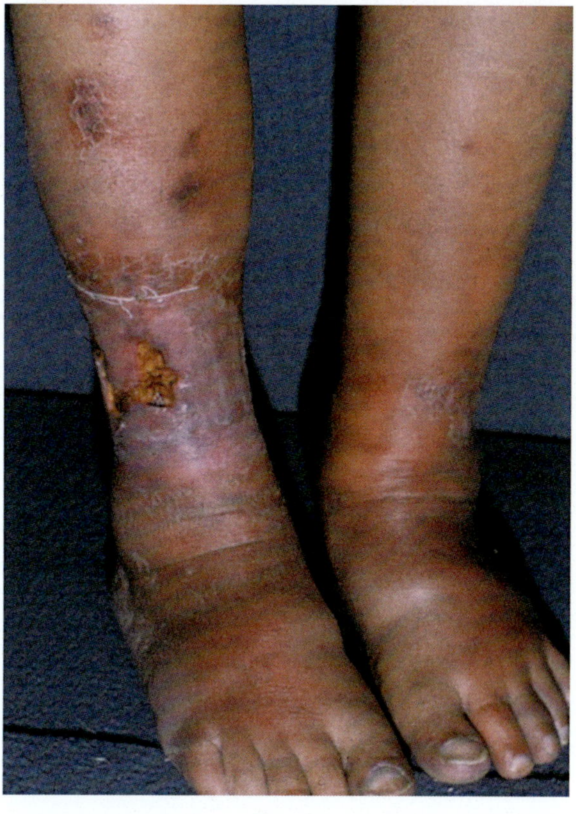

Fig. 5.42 Chronic bilateral lymphedema and ulcer in lepromatous leprosy

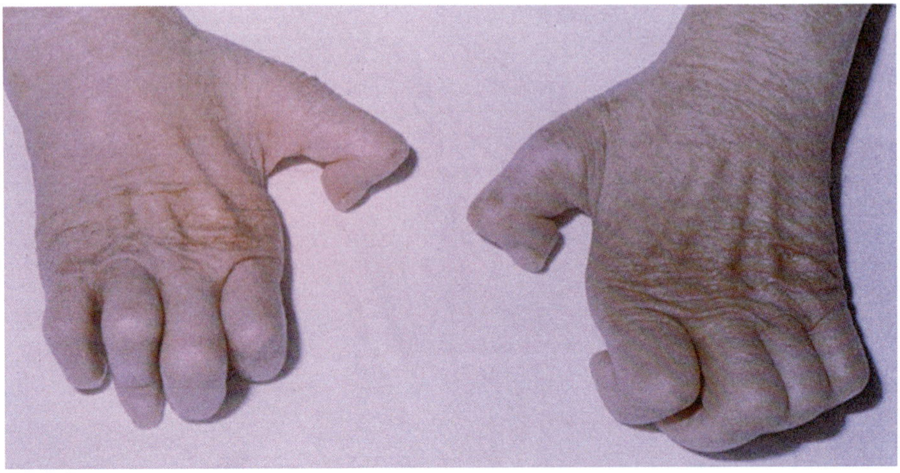

Fig. 5.43 Involvement of ulnar and median nerves with mild shortening of the fingers

disease progresses. Sensory loss is often more pronounced than muscle wasting, and severe damage may therefore occur from repeated trauma due to the insensitivity to pain. In this way the hands will become scarred from injuries and burns and trophic ulcers will develop on the soles.

The nerve thickening, like the skin lesions, tends to be bilateral and symmetrical. The superficial peripheral nerves are affected, such as the great auricular, supraclavicular, ulnar, antebrachial, radial, median, femoral, peroneal, and posterior tibial nerves.

The earliest sensory disturbances bring about paraesthesia, hyperaesthesia and hyperalgesia, followed by impaired sensation at light touch, temperature and pain. In some cases only one of these three complaints is present (dissociated anaesthesia), the ability to differentiate between hot and cold being in general the one which is lost first. Loss of position sense, vibration sense and tendon reflex are not common. Muscle wasting produces deformities such as the "claw hand" (ulnar nerve), "main-en-griffe" (ulnar and median nerves) (Fig. 5.43), "drop foot" (common peroneal nerve) and facial palsy (facial nerve). In sites with nerve damage there will be muscle weakness.

The involvement of the autonomic nerves firstly manifests in the form of slight oedema of the hands and feet, followed by vasomotor disturbances and then the skin of the hands and feet will become puffy and cyanosed.

5.12.4.3 Other Disturbances

At nasal level there will be a discharge, possibly blood-stained, and blocking of the airways. The nasal mucosa presents hyperaemia and swelling and there will be nodules and ulcers on the septum. Ulceration leads to perforation of the septum and destruction of the cartilage, and hence to the "saddle-nose" deformity (Fig. 5.44). Nodules can also grow on the lips, tongue, palate, and larynx, leading to ulceration. Laryngeal involvement gives rise to a hoarse cough, husky voice and stridor.

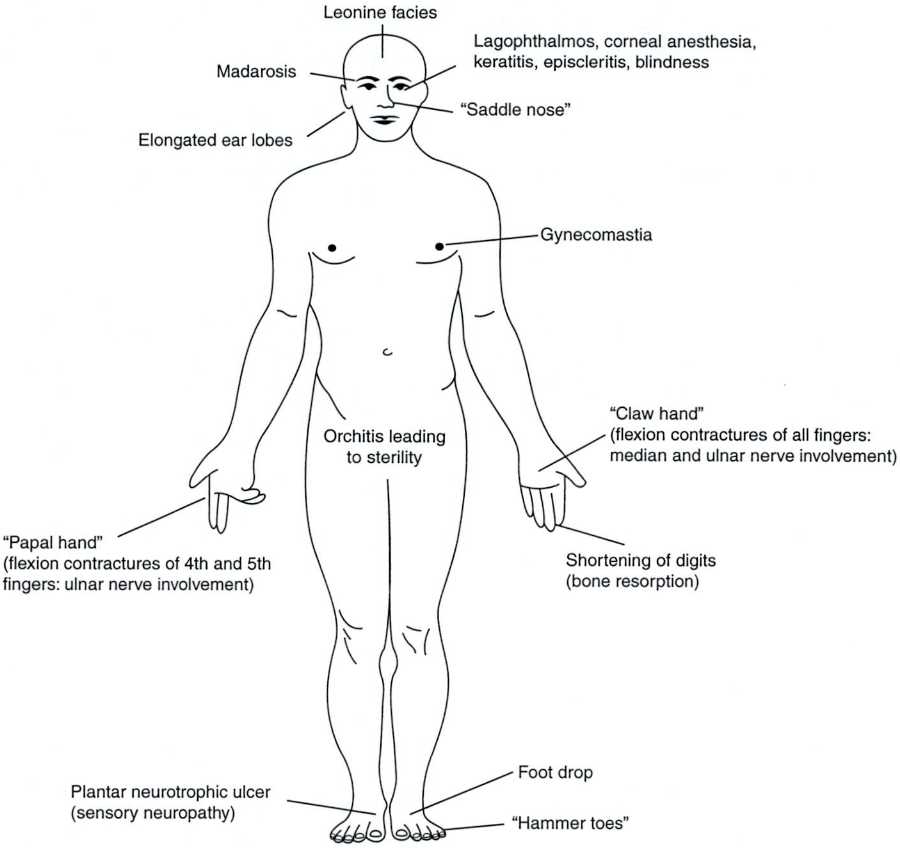

Fig. 5.44 Sequelae of leprosy (Modified, by [6])

In advanced cases there is frequently visual impairment and finally blindness. Leprosy is the third cause of blindness in the world. There are various complications that lead to blindness. At the corneal level, lagophthalmos and the reduced or absent sensation predispose to corneal ulceration and scarring. The initial stages of corneal damage manifest as punctate superficial spots. A secondary bacterial infection or foreign bodies can then cause corneal ulcer. Iris involvement may arise in an acute form, as in the case of a type 2 reaction, or in chronic disease. Acute iridocyclitis is painful and characterized by photophobia and pericorneal redness; chronic iritis presents with posterior synaechial formation and a small irregular pupil. Chronic iridocyclitis will lead over time to atrophy and a regular pinpoint pupil. Cataract can also be caused or aggravated by iridocyclitis or by the administration of systemic corticosteroids in cases of a reaction.

The onset of testicular atrophy may be observed, with consequent sterility and gynaecomastia.

Lymph nodes are enlarged but painless, and have the consistency of soft rubber. The femoral, inguinal and epitrochlear glands are particularly affected. During reaction states, several glands will become swollen and tender.

At renal level, there may be glomerulonephritis, interstitial nephritis and pyelonephritis. Renal amyloidosis, related to the severity and frequency of type 2 reactions, is observed only in some geographic areas.

5.12.4.4 Bones

The bones of the extremities and skull are affected. The involvement of the extremities will be almost exclusively confined to the hands and feet, where the lesions are linked to the invasion of bacilli, neurotrophic atrophy, repeated trauma due to the analgaesia, disuse causing paralysis and contracture, secondary infection of the trophic ulcers, and generalized osteoporosis of hormonal origin. Deposits of bacilli in the marrow cavities, periosteum and nutrient vessels give rise to bone cysts, aseptic necrosis and spindle-shaped dactylitis (simulating that of tuberculosis or syphilis). Neurotrophic atrophy affecting the hands is localized at the phalanges. Metacarpals and carpal bones are spared. On the feet, neurotrophic atrophy affects the metatarsals and phalanges, starting in the proximal phalanges or in the heads of the metatarsals. At the proximal phalanges the diaphyses become thinned owing to rarefying osteitis ("concentric bone atrophy") until only fine needles of bone remain. This may be followed by complete disappearance of the bone and the shortened toes remain connected to the foot by soft tissue only. In the metatarsals, absorption begins at the distal ends, that become thinned and pointed ("sucked candystick"). Periostitis of the tibia, fibula and ulna will develop.

Sensory loss leads to repeated injury, contributing to the bone atrophy and absorption, that can result in the development of charcot joints in the fingers, toes, wrists and ankles. Muscle paralysis causes disuse and over time, to fibrous or bony ankylosis of the interphalangeal, metacarpophalangeal and metatarsophalangeal joints. Disuse also induces osteoporosis due to a decreased osteoblastic activity. Generalized osteoporosis can ensue owing to a defective production of testosterone due to the testicular damage. Secondary infection arising from trophic ulceration of the hands and feet can give rise to pyogenic osteomyelitis.

At the level of the skull there will be atrophy of the anterior nasal spine and the maxillary alveolar process, leading to nasal collapse, loss of incisor teeth and sometimes perforation of the palate.

5.12.5 Pure Neural Leprosy

Also known as neural leprosy, this is a relatively rare form characterized by single or multiple peripheral nerve enlargement. Skin lesions are absent. It is generally agreed that cases with one or two enlarged nerves are paucibacillary and those with more than two are multibacillary leprosy [278, 279]. The symptoms include: loss of sensation, loss of muscle strength, loss of sweating, motor paralysis, trophic alterations and subjective symptoms like burning, torpor and shooting pains. Histological examination of the involved nerve is essential for the diagnosis. After months or years, some of the patients will develop skin lesions.

5.12.6 Wade's Histoid Leprosy

The term histoid leprosy (HL) was coined in 1963 by Wade to describe a picture featuring firm, reddish or skin-colored, dome-shaped or oval papules and nodules, with a regular contour and translucent, shiny and stretched overlying skin (Figs. 5.45 and 5.46) [280].

Histology demonstrates a circumscribed macrophage granuloma with a predominance of spindle-shaped cells or polygonal cells and a large number of acid-fast bacilli. Some cases may mimic a fibrohistiocytic tumor. A small number of foamy macrophages may be present [260].

The nodules may be pedunculated or umbilicated and when there are many, they will show a symmetrical distribution. The bacterial index of skin smears is 5+ or 6+. HL is a variant of multibacillary leprosy that usually arises in patients receiving long-term diaminodiphenylsulfone therapy, resulting in an initial improvement followed by relapse [260].

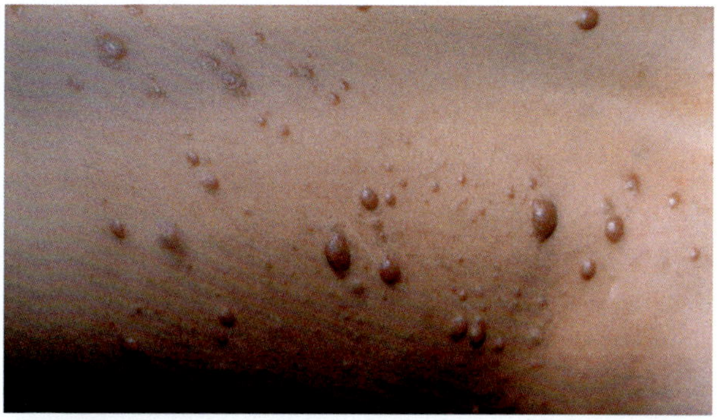

Fig. 5.45 Histoid lepromatous leprosy

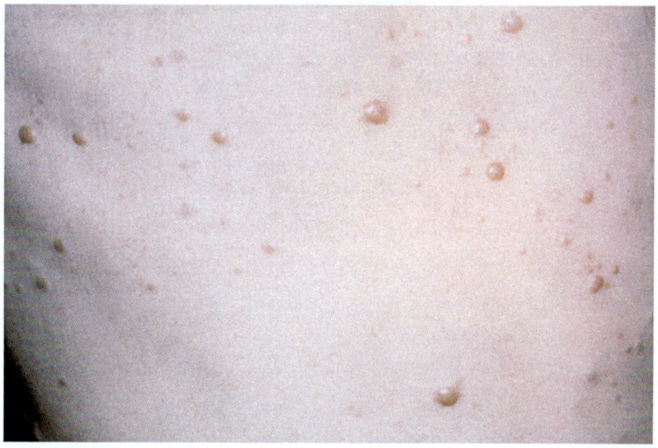

Fig. 5.46 The same patient as in Fig. 5.45

5.12.7 Lucio-Latapi Leprosy

This is a well-defined form of lepromatous leprosy, characterized by a generalized infiltration without nodules; in addition, it features a special type of lepra reaction, that corresponds at histopathological examination to necrotizing vasculitis with thrombosis, named Lucio's phenomenon or necrotizing erythema by Latapi [281–287].

This picture was described by Rafael Lucio and Alvarado in 1852 [286] and it was only many years later, in 1936, that the characteristics were better defined by Fernando Latapi [287]. Until 2011, WHO had reported 228,474 cases, mostly in India. In Latin-America, Brazil has the highest number of cases, 29,600 [288]. In Mexico, the country where the disease was first described by Lucio, there are 161 new cases, 73% of which are males of between 25 and 64 years of age.

Until 2008, *M. leprae* was considered the only aetiological agent of leprosy. Then Han and Coll from Texas published the results of a study of two Mexican immigrants who died of sepsis with cutaneous necrosis and vasculitis of internal organs: the diagnosis was diffuse lepromatous leprosy (DLL) with Lucio's phenomenon. Genetic studies of the bacilli in the two patients revealed significant differences from *M. leprae*, including a 2.1% divergence of the 16S ribosomal RNA, a highly conserved marker of bacterial evolution. Phylogenetic analysis of the genes demonstrated that the two mycobacteria evolved from a common ancestor. On the basis of this result, a new bacterial species was proposed, namely *Mycobacterium lepromatosis* [289, 290]. Since then, other cases have been reported [291], also in Ontario [292] and in Singapore [293]. However, in an editorial of 2011 Gillis and Coll pointed out that for the moment the assertion of *M. lepromatosis* as a new agent causing DLL was not proven [294]. This form, too, is thought to have airborne transmission through Flügge droplets.

5.12.7.1 Clinical features

This form may present as a diffuse variant, in which there are no circumscribed elements (nodules, macules, or plaques), but is characterized by diffuse and massive infiltration of the skin, known as diffuse lepromatous leprosy. Lucio-Latapi leprosy is usually observed in adults of both sexes, being exceptional in childhood and in the elderly.

At the beginning, the skin involvement is barely visible and may go unnoticed. The main dermatological characteristic is a diffuse non nodular infiltration. Initially, the skin appears "indurated" or myxoedema-like, especially at the level of the face and hands, thereby giving the impression of a "healthy look" and "moon face" (the so called "lepra bonita": pretty leprosy). In advanced cases there will be telangiectasiae of the trunk and face (rosaceiform aspect). The auricular pavilion are turgescent, shiny, hairless and a tanned reddish color. In particular, the hands, legs and feet look oedematous and puffy, due to the infiltration: the skin is tense, smooth, with alopecia, and the feet, above all, are purplish.

Subsequently the skin folds and becomes thinner and atrophic ("atrophic infiltration"), giving a premature aging appearance. The earlobes become stretched and saggy and the legs present xerosis with an ichthyosiform appearance. Most patients gradually develop alopecia of the eyelashes, eyebrows and body hair, while hair loss on the scalp is rare and only appears in advanced stages.

Mucosal involvement manifests with rhinitis. The nasal mucosa is firstly swollen with multiple ectasias, and then becomes pale and dry, with crusts and finally ulceration. The septum cartilage becomes affected and the nose takes on the aspect of a "crooked nose" and "saddle nose". Laryngeal involvement leads to dysphonia. At the hands there will be atrophy of the lumbricals and interosseous muscles, with minimal or no affection of the thenar and hypothenar eminences (soft hands like a "rag doll"). In all cases there is hypoesthesia, anaesthesia, and hypohydrosis. There will also be eye involvement with madarosis and exaggerated shining of the eyes ("children's eyes"). Patients may also have systemic manifestations; in particular there is diffuse infiltration of the liver and spleen with hepatosplenomegaly. Systemic involvement is common in cases of Lucio's phenomenon, being a type 2 reaction.

5.12.7.2 Histopathology

In initial forms, there is evident, modest acanthosis of the epidermis, in particular during the stage of an indurated skin appearance. In advanced stages there will be a perivascular, periannexial and perineural infiltrate in the derma, consisting of lymphocytes, histiocytes, and Virchow cells. There is thickening of the vascular walls and endothelial proliferation, together with the obliteration of small and medium vessels. The annexes are destroyed: firstly the sebaceous glands, then the hair follicles, and finally the sweat glands. Initially there is perineuritis and later the nerves will be completely destroyed [281, 295, 296].

5.12.7.3 Diagnosis

Smears from nasal mucosa and from any part of the skin reveal acid-fast bacilli (the bacteriological index is 5+ or 6+). The lepromin reaction is negative. The PCR technique is positive.

5.13 Relapse

Relapse is linked to the multiplication of bacilli in treated subjects. There are various causes: an incorrect classification of a multibacillary patient and hence inadequate treatment; inconstant taking of the drugs by the patient, and hence incomplete treatment; the onset of antibiotic resistance; a reinfection in subjects firstly affected by multibacillary forms (this is theoretically possible, but impossible to distinguish from a reactivation).

In patients with paucibacillary forms relapses manifest as a reactivation of preexisting lesions and/or the appearance of new ones. The bacteriological test is negative in most paucibacillary patients and so does not provide useful information. Thanks to the introduction of the WHO polychemotherapy treatment relapses are rarely observed.

It is fairly difficult to make a differential diagnosis between a relapse and a type 1 reaction, given the similarity of the clinical aspects. A reversal reaction usually

Table 5.14 Differential diagnosis between relapse and type 1 reaction (modified, by [18])

	Relapse	Type 1 reaction
Onset	Sudden in PL Insidious in ML	Sudden
Manifestation	After treatment	During treatment
Pre-existing lesions	Reactivation of margins in ML	Reactivation (erythema, edema, infiltration)
New lesions	Also in previously undamaged areas	Similar to preexisting ones
Ulcerative lesions	Rare	Frequent
Healing of lesions	Without desquamation	With desquamation
Systemic manifestations	Absent	Fever, arthralgia, neuralgia
Nerve involvement	Slow development	Rapid development
Antibodies	High levels in ML	–
Response to corticosteroids	None	Optimal

PL paucibacillary leprosy, *ML* multibacillary leprosy

has a more acute onset than a relapse, while histology of the reaction reveals increased lymphocytes and oedema. To differentiate, it is possible to resort to "diagnosis ex adiuvantibus": the reversal reaction responds rapidly to corticosteroid treatment whereas the relapse does not respond at all (Table 5.14).

Also in patients with multibacillary forms relapse is characterized by a reactivation of preexisting lesions and/or the appearance of new ones with a symmetrical distribution. In previously uninvolved areas these may show the clinical features of histioid leprosy. In these cases there is an increase of circulating anti-*M. leprae* antibodies (Table 5.14).

Both in paucibacillary and multibacillary forms the first manifestation of a relapse may be nerve involvement, with paraesthesia, anaesthesia and pain in affected skin areas. It is difficult to make a differential diagnosis between a type 1 reaction and a relapse in such cases. Nevertheless, a positive response to corticosteroid treatment suggests a type 1 reaction.

5.14 Leprosy in Pregnancy

First of all it should be borne in mind that all women of reproductive age are physiologically immunosuppressed for some months each year and for 10 months during pregnancy and lactation. During the menstrual cycle the immunosuppression starts with ovulation and ends at the start of menstruation. Therefore, women with leprosy need special follow-up and treatment [297–301].

During pregnancy and breast feeding, worsening of the leprosy infection, relapse and leproreactions are more frequent. Moreover, a downgrading phenomenon may occur in pregnancy, shifting the disease toward the anergic lepromatous pole. Relapses are more frequent between the second and third month of pregnancy and between the third and sixth month after delivery. In these periods it is therefore necessary to perform bacteriological controls. The onset of type 1 reactions occurs immediately after delivery, while type 2 reactions are more common in the first three months and the last trimester of pregnancy.

A prospective study of 120 term pregnancies in Ethiopian women with leprosy showed that the mean birth weight of babies was 3.075 ± 61.1 g in tuberculoid or borderline tuberculoid cases, 2.985 ± 69.9 g in borderline lepromatous leprosy and 2.558 ± 60.5 g in lepromatous leprosy, versus 3.280 ± 87.6 in babies born of healthy mothers (36 pregnancies). Respiratory problems were a significant cause of neonatal mortality in babies of LL mothers [298].

The histological examination of placentae did not reveal alterations. Acid-fast bacilli were not present at routine microscopy, but with concentration methods were found in 2 of 7 placentae of women with very active leprosy [298, 299]. The weight of children with mothers affected by leprosy appears low in the first 2 years of life as compared to the weight of children of healthy mothers (weight in healthy controls > TT and BT > BL > LL). Child mortality in the first 2 years was 22%, 12%, 10% and 10% for babies of LL, BL, BT, and TT mothers and healthy controls, respectively. Breast feeding should be continued for 2 years, with supplementary feeding introduced at 6 months [297].

M. leprae has been found on the fetal side of the placenta [300]; 5% of babies born of mothers with active LL had self-healing indeterminate leprosy under the age of 2 years and anti-*M. leprae* antibodies of the IgA, IgG and IgM classes [301]. Separation of mother and baby at birth is not advised, nor is it necessary for a nursing mother to wear a gown and mask when handling and suckling the baby. Prophylactic administration of anti-leprosy drugs to the baby is probably not necessary because the drugs generally pass the milk barrier (as also the placenta). Moreover, clofazimine would stain the baby's skin red [297].

In the event of pregnancy, antenatal care and supervision of leprosy should always be carried out. Termination of pregnancy, surgically or pharmacologically, is not effective in preventing pregnancy-associated neuritis. In the event of reactivation of the leprosy or the development of new nerve damage, a minimum of 1 year's course of multibacillary multidrug treatment should be given [297].

5.15 Leprosy and HIV Coinfection

The data on the prevalence of HIV are still on the increase in many nations where leprosy is endemic. It could therefore be expected that in geographic areas with an overlap of the two infections the number of coinfected patients would also be rising. Fortunately, global data seem to depict only a non significant increase in leprosy and HIV coinfection [69, 302].

An interesting aspect of the pathogenesis of leprosy in patients with AIDS and a low T CD4+ cell count is what is called the granuloma paradox, consisting in an apparent preservation of the ability to form granuloma among these patients, unlike what is observed in *M. tuberculosis* and HIV coinfected patients. It has been seen that the histopathological features of leprosy appear to be maintained in coinfected patients [68]. Recently, however, in contrast with the above granuloma paradox, some studies have shown a possible impact on leprosy of HIV-infection, highly active antiretroviral therapy (HAART) and multidrug therapy [303].

The most common form of leprosy in coinfected patients is BT. Most cases have been reported in association with an immunopathological phenomenon called the immune reconstitution inflammatory syndrome (IRIS). IRIS manifests in a subgroup of AIDS patients who undergo an apparent clinical deterioration despite the T CD4+ cell count improvement induced by HAART [303–308].

A particularly important point in leprosy-HIV/AIDS coinfection is to diagnose those patients with peripheral neurological manifestations. This can be confused with neuropathy associated with HIV itself, or with stavudine and other nucleoside-analogue reverse-transcriptase inhibitors. In this context, a correct interpretation of the specific tests is essential [303].

There have recently been shown to be some clinical sub-groups among patients with leprosy-HIV/AIDS coinfection: 1. true coinfection, consisting of HIV-positive patients that do not fulfill AIDS criteria and are not, therefore, taking HAART; the clinical behavior is similar to that in immune competent subjects. 2. Opportunistic leprosy disease, that includes AIDS patients not receiving HAART, and that usually presents as multibacillary leprosy; in this group the leprosy is an opportunistic mycobacteriosis, as could be expected in immunosuppressed subjects. 3. HAART-related leprosy: AIDS patients presenting all clinical forms of leprosy, related or not to IRIS, come within this group. Combined HAART and multidrug therapy might cause an upgrading shift within the leprosy clinical spectrum, that could be revealed by long-term follow-up [303].

5.16 Leprosy Reactions

Nerve damage is the worst problem in the course of leprosy, leading to impairment and permanent disability. If it were not for this damage, leprosy would actually be a "rather innocuous" skin disease [309]. The main causes of the nerve damage are the acute episodes that can arise during the chronic course of the disease, linked to changes in the host immune response to *M. leprae* antigens and denominated leproreactions.

There are two possible types of reactions: a type 1 leprosy reaction (T1R), or reversal reaction, and a type 2 leprosy reaction (T2R), or erythema nodosum leprosum (ENL). The former is observed in borderline leprosy and the latter in the lepromatous part of the spectrum (BL and LL) (Tables 5.15 and 5.16).

A third type of reaction can also occur, known as Lucio's phenomenon (or Lucio-Alvarado phenomenon), that does not generally include nerve damage and is observed in patients affected by diffuse lepromatous leprosy, or Lucio-Latapi leprosy in the lepromatous pole of the spectrum.

Table 5.15 Characteristics of type 1 reactions

1.	More common in borderline borderline and borderline lepromatous patients than in borderline tuberculoid patients
2.	Erythema and swelling of preexisting cutaneous lesions. Appearance of new lesions
3.	Worsening of neuritis with inflammation, edema, and pain Onset of neuritis
4.	Usually lesions with increase of infiltrate (lymphocytes, epithelioid and giant cells) and edema Decrease of bacterial index. Immunological response characteristic of cell-mediated immunity
5.	Increase of pro-inflammatory cytokines (IL-1, IL-2, IL-12, IFN-γ, TNF-α)
6.	The cause of the reaction is unknown

Table 5.16 Characteristics of type 2 reactions

1.	In about 20% of lepromatous and 10% of borderline lepromatous patients
2.	Painful papules and nodules. Edema of hands, feet and face
3.	Usually, neuritis is milder than in a type 1 reaction
4.	Systemic symptoms: fever, joint swelling and pain, proteinuria and malaise, myalgia, hepatosplenomegaly, orchitis, lymphadenitis, glomerulonephritis
5.	Histologically, presence of neutrophils, lymphocytes, plasma cells, and histiocytes Vasculitis is the major event, with necrotizing changes
6.	Immune complex mediated disease with some degree of cell-mediated immune response
7.	Evidence in lesion sites of chemokines, cytochines, and immune complexes
8.	The function of T cells is ill defined

5.16.1 Type 1 Reaction

In the past, various names had been used for this type of reaction but today it is called the type 1 leprosy reaction, while the term reversal reaction is discouraged.

Skin manifestations can precede, accompany or follow the nerve damage. The T1R is characterized by an exacerbated inflammatory state of the preexisting skin lesions. The macules previously slightly erythematous or hypopigmented, become red and oedematous, forming plaques and sometimes these will ulcerate. New lesions may appear and in particular in BL there may be edema of the face and the extremities (Fig. 5.47) [214, 310–312]. Patients may also complain of a burning and stinging sensation on the skin lesions, of pain at the extremities and loss of strength and/or sensory perception.

Histopathology of the lesions demonstrates all the features of the delayed-type hypersensitivity reaction. The initial lesions may present moderate edema with a minor proliferation of fibroblasts. Later, the edema will intensify and the cellular composition of the epithelioid cell granuloma will change, showing an influx of lymphocytes, mainly of the CD4+ subtype and especially of type 1 helper T cells (Th 1) class [313, 314]. Methods for detection of mRNA show increases of INF-γ, IL-2 and TNF-α, confirming the shift to the Th 1 subtype during the reaction [315, 316]. During a T1R, humoral immunity appears to be diminished, although B cells

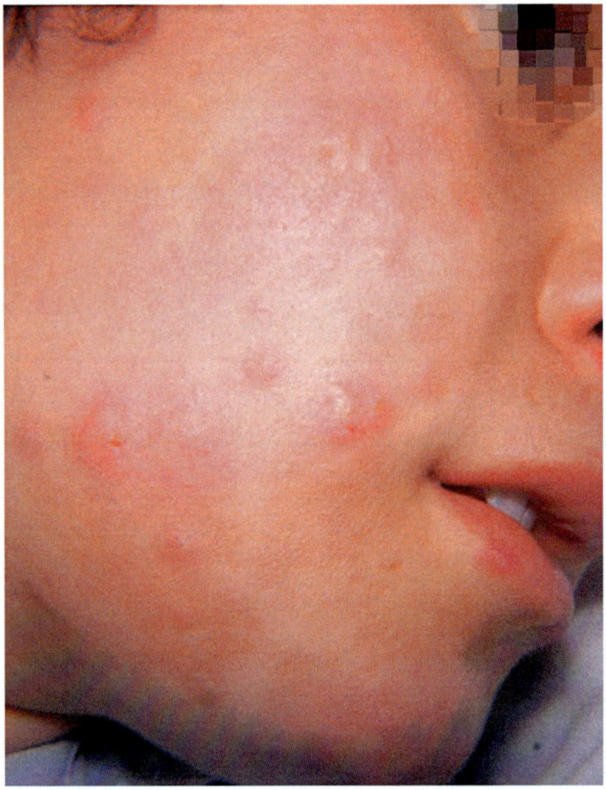

Fig. 5.47 Type 1 reaction. Edema of the face with plaques and nodules in borderline leprosy patient

are present [317]. However, a shift to Th 2 activity may occur since in some lesions there is an increase of IL-4 [315]. During the reaction or its later regression, an increased number of CD8+ (suppressor/cytotoxic) cells will be observed.

Damage to the peripheral nerves is the main consequence of a T1R, caused by the immunologic reaction and by mechanical factors. During a T1R, inflammation and edema of the nerves occurs, similar to the conditions affecting the skin. Edema is present at the level of the perineurium and endoneurium. The perineurium, that is impermeable to fluids, forms a rigid compressing tube around the expanding endoneurium: the resulting pressure rise within the nerve leads to axonal compression. As a consequence, there will be a loss of conducting nerve fibers and thus loss of muscular strength and peripheral sensation. The intra-axonal flow, which transports nutrients from the cell to the peripheral nerve ending, is interrupted and the peripheral fibers die and are destroyed [318]. At the same time, there is an increased pressure also in the vessels that cross the perineurium, and in particular in the venules. This increases the pressure in the capillaries, which leak an exudate that further exacerbates the pressure within the endoneurium. This "venous stasis" edema is self-maintaining even after the immunological factors have reduced [18, 318].

During a T1R the circulating lymphocytes show an increased immune response toward *M. leprae* antigens [318]. When the reaction subsides, the immune response also decreases. However, it is still not known which of the *M. leprae* antigens are involved in the reaction because heterogeneous findings have been recorded not only among different patients but also, in the course of time, in the same patients, when the maximum CMI response changes from one antigen to another [319].

The triggering cause of a T1R is unknown. It is thought that chemotherapy may have a role. In fact, in many cases the reaction occurs after some months of treatment, leaving the patient with more damage but with a decreased bacillary load. This is why the term "reversal" was coined. But the reaction also occurs in untreated patients and it has been noted that it is followed by an increased number of solid bacilli also in treated patients [320]. The bacilli increase disappears only after the reaction has settled, showing that this is an upgrading reaction.

The disappearance of bacilli in one reaction and not in another has given rise to the concept of upgrading and downgrading reactions. In an upgrading reaction the disease course is inverted and the disease shifts along the spectrum toward the tuberculoid pole or else may resolve. During a downgrading reaction the CMI does not determine the inversion of the disease course; the bacilli continue to multiply and the disease shifts along the spectrum toward the lepromatous pole. On this basis, the concept of protective and non protective immunity has been developed [321]. It has been suggested that during an upgrading reaction the immunity is directed against antigenic determinants that are essential for the bacterium to survive ("protective" antigens), whereas during a downgrading reaction the immunity is directed toward "non protective" antigens [322].

5.16.2 Type 2 Reaction

The term erythema nodosum leprosum usually used to indicate this reaction is referred to the most common manifestation, that is the eruption of papules and nodules. The onset of these lesions is observed during the course of a few hours, and they resolve after a few days.

The nodules are reddish-purple in fair-skinned patients and dark red in dark-skinned patients. On resolution, the lesions leave bluish desquamation areas in fair-skinned, and dark brown areas in dark-skinned patients. The nodules, that have subintrant course, can aggregate and form confluent plaques that may also ulcerate.

These lesions will particularly affect the face (Fig. 5.48), back, buttocks (Fig. 5.49) and extensor surfaces of the arms and thighs (unlike the lesions of true erythema nodosum, that electively present on the pretibial surface). The nodules, that can often be felt at palpation, are painful and have a hard consistency.

This reaction generally shows an episodic trend and has a variable duration ranging from a few days to about two weeks. It usually affects patients in treatment and only rarely untreated patients. Sometimes the lesions are recurrent for months or years, and so have a chronic trend.

Like T1R, T2R also affect the peripheral nerves, with pain and edema due to venous stasis. It also involves the lymph nodes, liver and spleen, that are enlarged and painful. There may be episodes of iridocyclitis with glaucoma and orchitis and

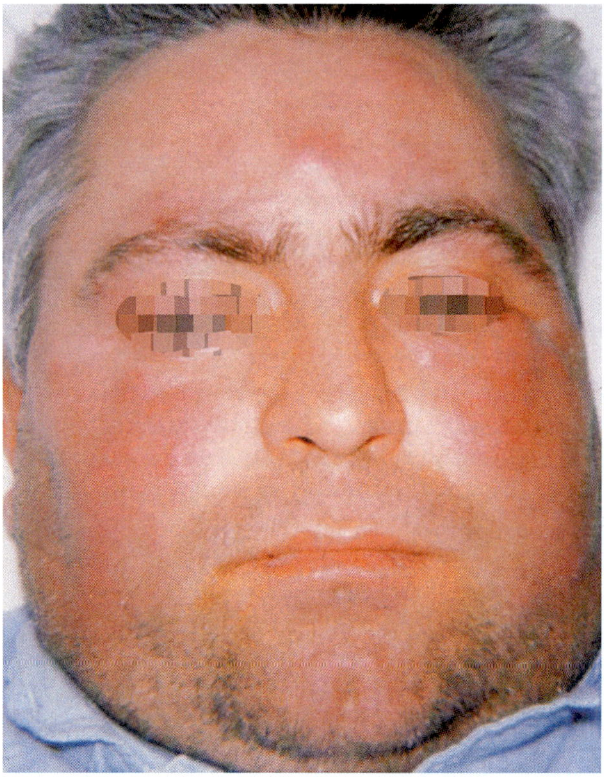

Fig. 5.48 Type 2 reaction (erythema nodosum leprosum). Nodular lesions

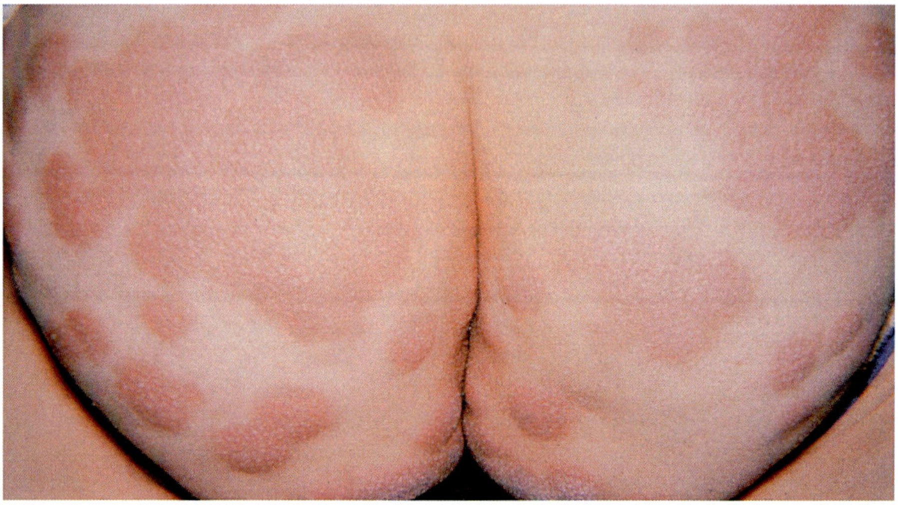

Fig. 5.49 The same patient as in Fig. 5.48

epididymitis, and possibly inflammatory phenomena of the tendons, muscles and kidneys. The patient will suffer malaise and fever and there will be leukocytosis and proteinuria.

In the initial phases of a T2R there is a modest increase in the lymphocytes, especially perivasally (unlike the histological findings in BL and LL). Most of these lymphocytes will be CD4+ (helper/inducer) cells. They will increase still further as the reaction progresses, exceeding the number of CD8+ (suppressor/cytotoxic) cells, whereas these are the majority in lepromatous lesions. The number of IL-2 receptors on immunocompetent cells increases. In the most active phase of a T2R the histological picture is dominated by neutrophils. The presence of IgG, IgM and complement, as well as *M. leprae* antigens, is demonstrable in the lesions.

The pathogenic mechanism of a T2R can be summarized as an infiltration of the tissues by Th 1 cells, stimulated in a specific or nonspecific manner (viral infections), that stimulate the B cells present in loco to produce antibodies. These antibodies precipitate, binding to the *M. leprae* antigens that are present in great quantities and thus giving rise to immune complexes. The subsequent activation of complement and granulocytic chemotaxis is what provokes the tissue damage.

In the peripheral blood the involvement of both humoral immunity (immune complexes) and cellular immunity (an in vitro increased leukocyte response to mitogenic factors) is demonstrated.

A T2R can also be triggered by various nonspecific factors such viral infections (the most common cause), stress, pregnancy or oral therapies with potassium iodide.

5.16.3 Lucio's Phenomenon

Patients with Lucio-Latapi leprosy may develop a reaction, also known as the Lucio-Alvarado phenomenon. Usually, it begins at the level of the feet and moves upward, affecting the legs, thighs, arms, trunk, and finally the face. It presents as painful erythema spots of different shapes, some angular or "stellar", and variable sizes. By 24–48 h later they appear slightly infiltrated; by the third or fourth day, they have become dark with a purpuric appearance and subsequently present central necrosis that causes them to appear as a small blister. Finally, a red dark eschar is formed, which falls off some days later, leaving a pearly-white atrophic scar. The whole process lasts about 15 days [323].

In some cases, flaccid blisters develop, especially on the legs, that evolve into ulcerations of variable sizes and depths, with well-defined borders (Figs. 5.50 and 5.51). These are followed by systemic symptoms, such as fever, shivers, arthralgia, myalgia, and general malaise [324, 325].

The histopathology shows epidermal necrosis, ulceration, and features of diffuse lepromatous leprosy in the dermis with numerous acid-fast bacilli in the endothelium and in the tunica media of the vessels [326–328]. A panvasculitis of both superficial and deep vessels is present. In particular, a lobular panniculitis is observed, the medium-sized arteries being infiltrated by macrophages resulting in narrowing of the lumens, occlusion, and ischemic changes [328].

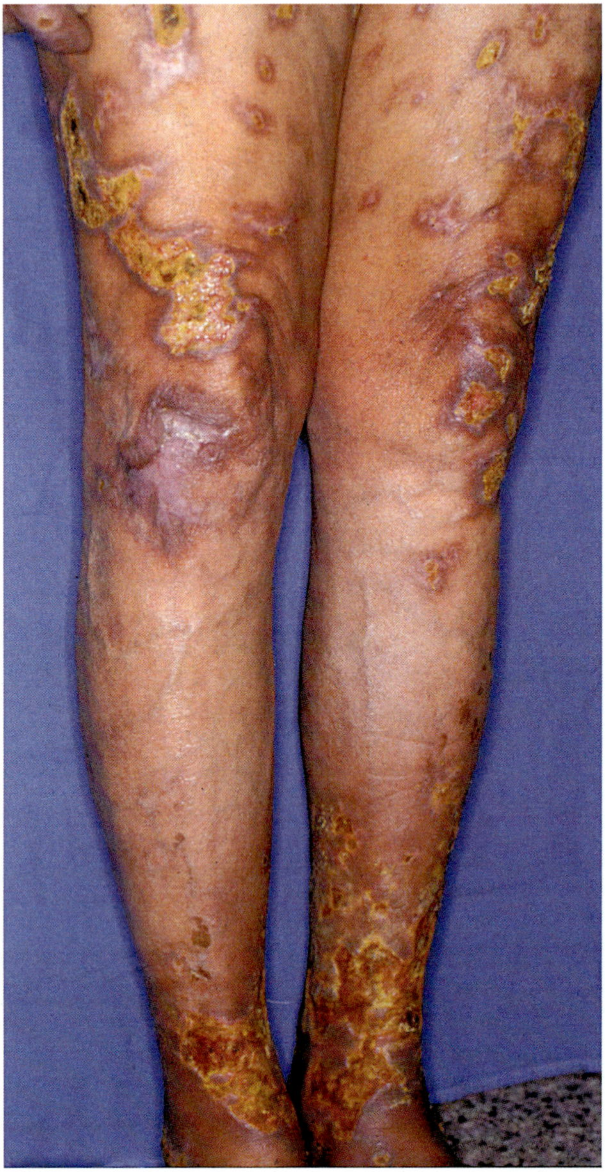

Fig. 5.50 Lucio's phenomenon with extensive ulcers

Immunopathologically, the tissue damage has been considered to be mediated by immune complexes, as proven by the deposit of these immune complexes and IgG in blood vessels [285].

Lucio's phenomenon must be differentiated from other forms of acute cutaneous necrotizing vasculitis.

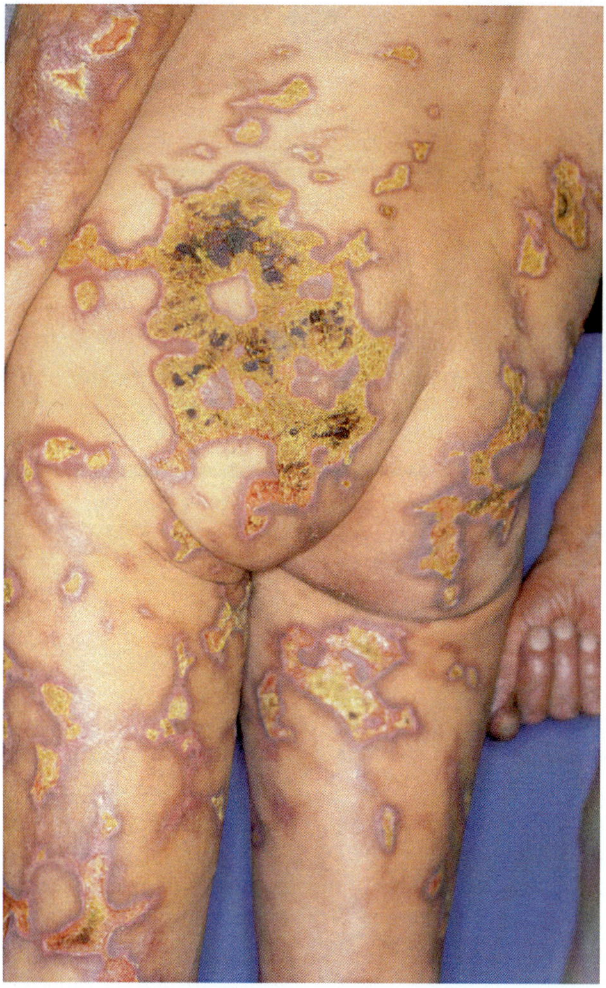

Fig. 5.51 Lucio's phenomenon with extensive necrotizing vasculitis

5.17 Nerve Damage

Leprosy is a multisystemic disease that affects tissues originating from the embryonic ectoderm, specifically the skin, mucosa and peripheral nerves. It does not affect the central nervous system [329–334].

In leprosy the neuropathy has three long-standing phases of evolution: parasitization of the Schwann cells by *M. leprae*, during which phase the clinical expression is asymptomatic or minor; this lasts from 3–5 to 10 years; the acute and subacute periods, due to type 1 and type 2 reactions, during which there are intense symptoms with sensory and motor loss and pain (lasting up to 10 years); finally, the third phase is characterized by late nerve impairment, caused mainly by the intradermal fibrosis leading to interstitial neuropathy [333].

The neuropathy affecting leprosy patients is primarily demyelinating but frequently leads to axonal loss during its evolution. The bacilli specificity to Schwann cells is well known, and is not selective of one type of fiber: the involvement of fibers is universal.

5.17.1 Pain

Neuropathic pain develops in damaged nerves and may coexist with the nociceptive pain in both types of reactions. The symptoms may appear spontaneously, and be constant or intermittent, or may be stimulus-evoked. Paraesthesia is very common. Spontaneous painful sensations include burning, stabbing, stinging, squeezing, cramp, aching, shooting, and "pins and needles"; stimulus-evoked pain includes disaesthesia, allodynia, hyperalgesia, and hyperpathia [332, 334].

It should be borne in mind that even in successfully treated patients a chronic neuropathy may develop as a delayed manifestation, that will severely affect the quality of life [335, 336].

5.17.2 Sensory Component

Sensory loss precedes motor loss in almost all patients. The sensory loss is to light touch, pain and temperature and the pattern of loss varies according to the temperature of the part, the coolest parts of the body being affected first, while the warmest are spared. On the face, the nose and ears are the first to become insensitive, then the parts overlying prominent bones, such as the chin, cheek bones, zygoma and the bone of the forehead. The lips are spared, as well as any part that is regularly covered with thick hair, but the shaven scalp loses sensation, as does the bald head.

On the hands and feet, the loss of sensation is on the dorsum first and later on the palms and soles. At the level of the limbs, the antecubital fossae and popliteal fossae are spared and will remain sensitive for a long time. In very advanced lepromatous leprosy, the whole body may be insensitive, with the exception of the axillae, perineum and under a bushy head of hair. Clothing may affect the pattern of sensory loss but only if warm clothing is worn almost all the time [4].

5.17.3 Autonomic Component

The most important autonomic manifestation is sweating loss in areas with sensory loss. The sweating loss in skin lesions is associated with loss of hair growth, of sebaceous secretions, and poor pigment formation. In advanced stages of the disease, on the skin there are also trophic changes due to capillary stasis, cyanosis and dryness, which predispose to fissuring. Cardiac denervation and postural hypotension have also been reported [332].

Autonomic function can be checked with histamine testing, that reveals the absence of secondary erythema, and pilocarpine nitrate testing, that shows the absence of blue spots [336].

5.17.4 Motor Component

Studies of this aspect have shown that the posterior tibial nerve is the most frequently affected, followed by the ulnar, median, lateral popliteal and facial nerves. Ulnar and median nerve lesions are generally low, affecting small muscles but not causing deep flexor weakness, and anaesthesia of two halves of the hand. Common peroneal nerve lesions cause difficulty in dorsiflexion and eversion of the foot and anaesthesia of the outer border of the foot, a combination that predisposes to traumatic damage and plantar ulceration. Posterior tibial nerve lesions cause paralysis and contractures of the small muscles of the foot and anaesthesia of the sole [337].

5.18 Ocular Leprosy

Compared to other bacterial infections, leprosy has the highest incidence of ocular involvement [338, 339]. Worldwide, this is estimated to be 70–75%; about 10–50% of leprosy patients suffer from severe ocular symptoms, and blindness occurs in about 5% of these patients [340]. The most common causes of blindness are corneal disease secondary to lagophthalmos and chronic iritis. Patients with borderline and lepromatous leprosy are more often affected than those whose disease is nearer to the tuberculoid pole, or with indeterminate leprosy.

M. leprae often invade the anterior segment of the eyes because it is the coldest part of the bulb. The entry of *M. leprae* into the eyes presumably occurs through the blood vessels of the ciliary body and from there, via small autonomic nerves, they invade the iris. The ciliary body nerves destruction can extend over time to the posterior ciliary nerves, beyond the posterior pole of the eyeball and laterally to the optic nerve [341].

5.18.1 Eyeball Adnexa Changes

Madarosis (loss of eyebrows and eyelashes) (Figs. 5.52 and 5.53) is due to direct *M. leprae* invasion of the hair follicles and subsequent atrophy. Madarosis occurs in 25.7% of patients and is more frequent in the multibacillary forms [342, 343]. Trichiasis (an inward misdirection of the lashes due to loss of support of the lash follicles secondary to *M. leprae* infiltration) is present in about 1–9% of patients [343]. It causes cornea irritation, punctate epithelial erosions and pannus in severe cases.

Thickened eyelids from direct infiltration of *M. leprae* is present in 5% of cases. Ptosis (an abnormally low position of the upper eyelid) is the result of

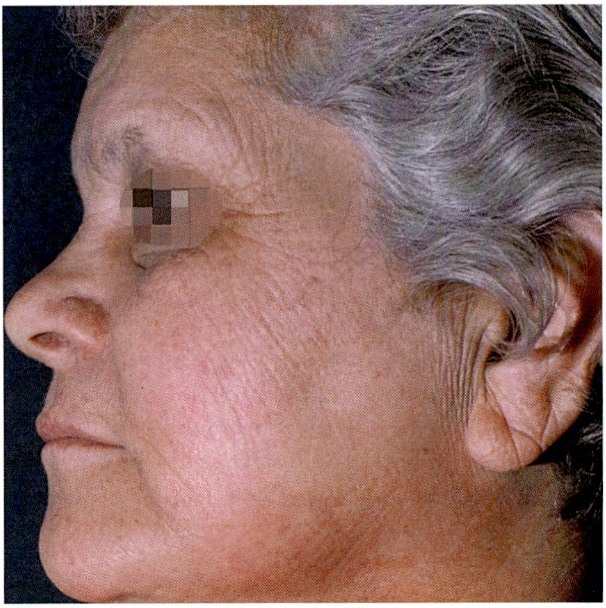

Fig. 5.52 Lateral loss of eyebrows in cured lepromatous leprosy patient

direct infiltration of the bacilli or may be due to oculomotor (third) cranial nerve involvement. Entropion (an inversion of the eyelid) is present in up to 6% of patients, while ectropion of the lower lid (an outward turning of the eyelid from the globe) is caused by facial nerve involvement, and is observed in about 0.5–6% of the cases [343].

A decreased blinking rate (hypometric blink) and lagophthalmos (inability to fully close the eye) are linked to nerve damage, as a result of orbicularis oculi muscle weakness or paralysis due to damage of the zygomatic branch of the cranial nerve in tuberculoid and borderline leprosy. An abnormal blinking pattern is present in 24.8% of patients [344]; lagophthalmos occurs in up to 20% of patients and is bilateral in 5% [345]. Paralytic lagophthalmos is a progressive condition and causes further severe complications. In tuberculoid and borderline leprosy, lagophthalmos is caused mainly by a type 1 reaction in the face. Tearing may be caused by chronic dacrocystitis or a blocked naso-lachrymal duct, and occurs in up to 2% of patients.

5.18.2 Leprosy of the Surface of the Eye

Conjunctivitis is due to direct primary *M. leprae* infection. Pterygium may also occur in up to 21% of patients. In patients on long standing multidrug therapy, as a side-effect of cumulative doses of clofazimine and a form of toxicity, conjunctival crystalline deposits occur; these deposits do not affect the vision and in both eyes look like polychromatic crystalline deposits, along with a brownish-red discoloration in the interpalpebral region of the conjunctiva [346, 347].

Corneal nerve beading results from the primary infection and is more evident at the lepromatous end than the tuberculoid end of the spectrum. Corneal hypoesthesia or anesthesia result from massive corneal nerves invasion by *M. leprae*, mainly in long standing multibacillary leprosy. The reduced corneal sensation may contribute to tear production (these patients are at risk of developing keratoconjunctivitis sicca or dry eye, observed in about 4% of cases) and to an abnormal blinking pattern and lagophthalmos. There are many risk factors for corneal ulceration. Corneal opacification and corneal scarring result from superficial exposure keratopathy. Corneal opacities, that may be mild, moderate or severe, often lead to unilateral visual impairment or blindness, rather than bilateral blindness.

5.18.3 Intraocular Changes

Iridocyclitis is more often seen in multibacillary patients compared with paucibacillary patients. It is caused by direct *M. leprae* invasion, or may be neuroparalytic or autoimmune. Leprosy iridocyclitis may present clinically as chronic or acute iridocyclitis, iris pearls, or nodular lepromata. Circumcorneal congestion, keratitic precipitates (Fig. 5.54), synechiae and pupil abnormalities are the manifestations of uveitis. Iris atrophy is very frequent in multibacillary patients, as well as myotic pupils (small, showing poor dilatation with mydriatic drugs).

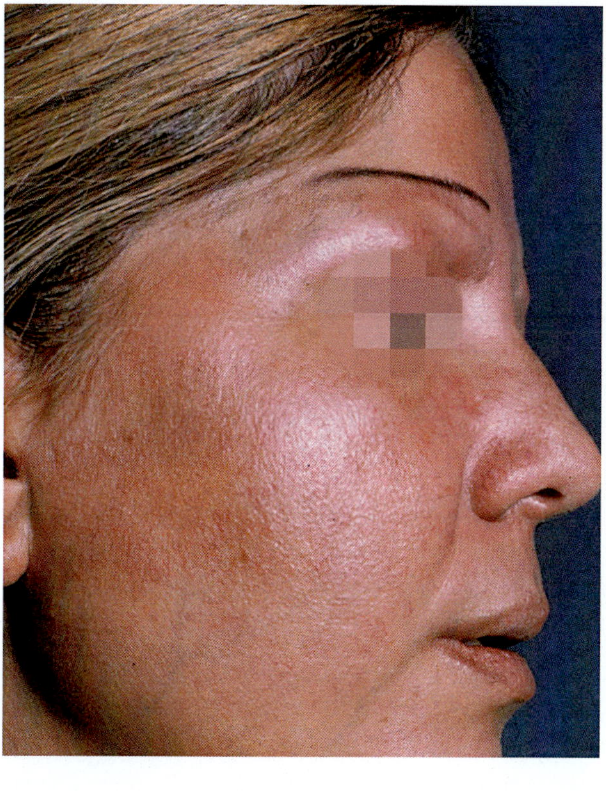

Fig. 5.53 Loss of eyebrows and eyelashes in cured lepromatous leprosy patient

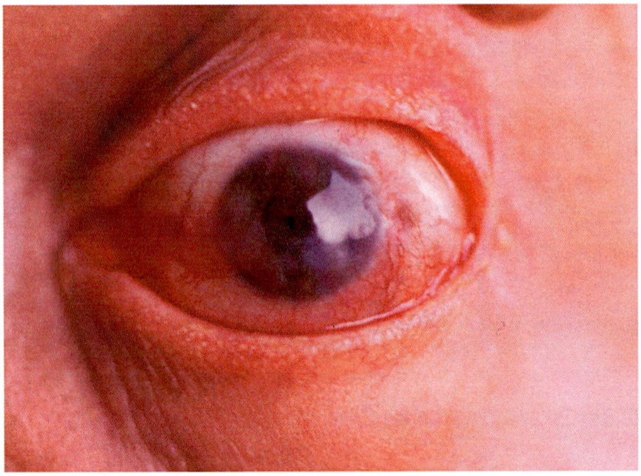

Fig. 5.54 Loss of eyelashes, conjunctivitis, and corneal pannus in lepromatous leprosy patient

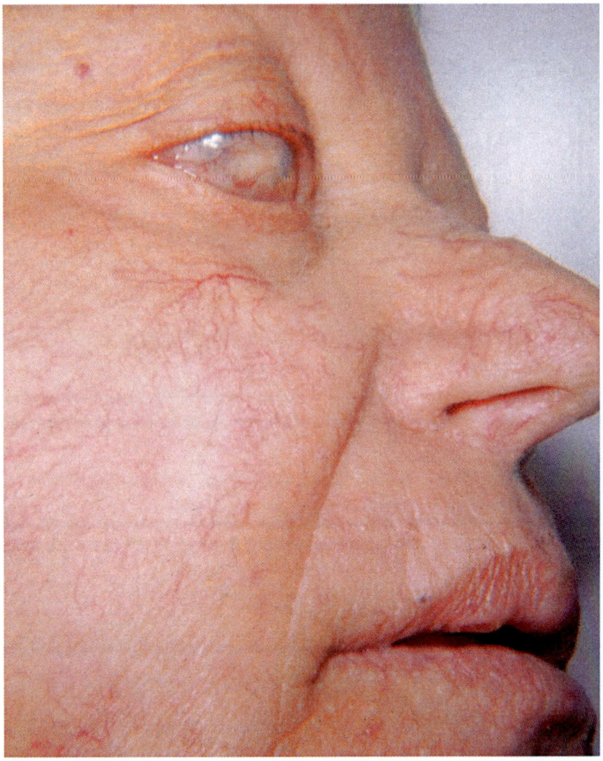

Fig. 5.55 Loss of eyebrows and eyelashes, blindness, and telangiectasiae in lepromatous leprosy patient

Cataract (lens opacification reducing the vision) is more common in multibacillary patients, and is age-related in the majority of these. Various authors have concluded that corneal disease, secondary to lagophthalmos, and chronic iritis are the most common causes of blindness (Fig. 5.55) [348]. Glaucoma is present in 10% of patients, in most cases secondary to uveitis [349].

5.19 Ear, Nose and Throat Involvement

5.19.1 The Ear

In tuberculoid and borderline cases the great auricular nerve (sensitive nerve running from the second and third branches of the cervical plexus) is large and palpable. Loss of sensation in these areas is of no great significance. Moreover, we should remember that this nerve is sometimes palpable even in healthy subjects. A more severe problem is the involvement of the facial nerves, that may lead to partial or total paralysis of the facial mimicry muscles. This damage also leads to lagophthalmos. In lepromatous leprosy the skin of the ear pavilions is commonly infiltrated. The lobe and helix are particularly at risk of bacilli infiltration due to their lower temperature (Fig. 5.56); in fact, the ear lobe is a standard sampling site for skin smears.

5.19.2 The Nose

In the borderline lepromatous form and especially the lepromatous form, the nasal cavity is always involved. Firstly there will be thickening of the mucosa, that will appear pale or yellowish; then plaques or nodules will develop, infiltrating the septum and the inferior turbinates, above all. As the process evolves, nasal obstruction will develop, and possible ulceration of the cartilage and nasal bones. In advanced stages the classic triad will be evident: saddle nose (Fig. 5.57), perforation of the septum and atrophic rhinitis with malodorous crusts. The formation of scar tissue can lead to partial or total stenosis of the upper airways.

The importance of the nose involvement has to do with the nasal secretions, in particular, because, as is well known, this is the main excretion site of bacilli. Through their nasal secretions patients release millions of bacilli into the environment every day; a 24 h collection of nasal mucus revealed a count of 1.5×10^9 bacilli [107].

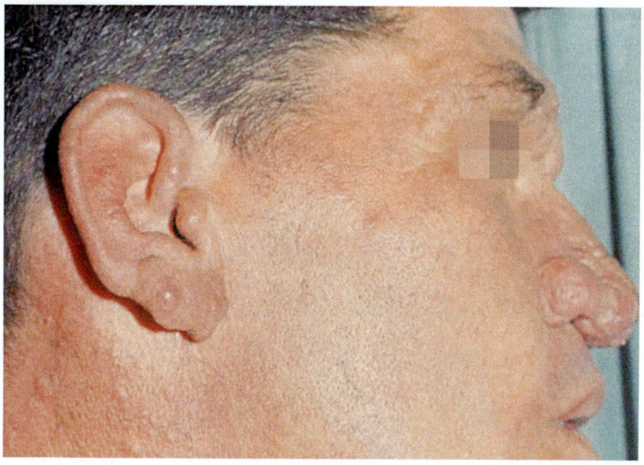

Fig. 5.56 Nodular infiltration of helix and lobe in lepromatous leprosy patient

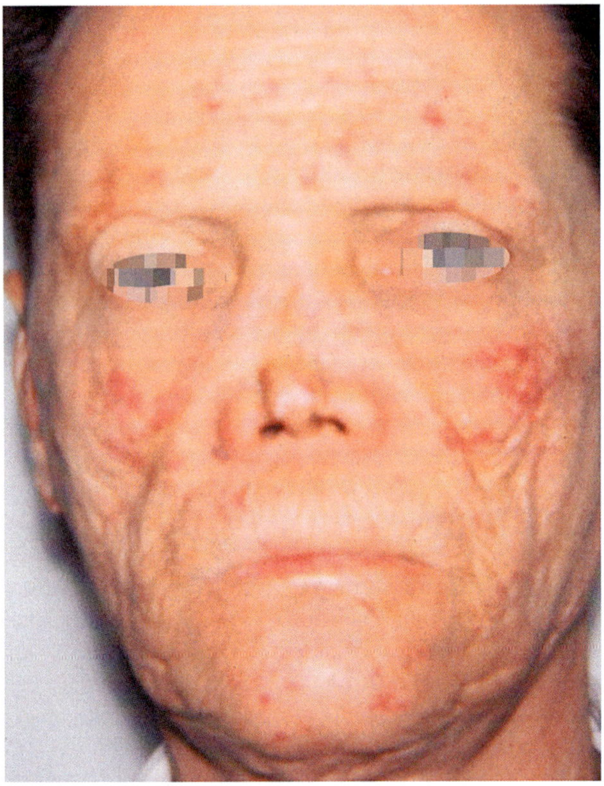

Fig. 5.57 Lepromatous leprosy. Saddle nose, loss of eyebrows and eyelashes, and telangiectasiae

5.19.3 The Throat

The oral cavity, oropharynx and larynx are not affected in the tuberculoid and borderline forms, but are infiltrated in the lepromatous form. On the hard palate, pale, opaque nodules will be evident. The uvula, soft palate and tonsils may be affected, while the tongue, lips and cheek mucosa are less commonly involved. As the process evolves there will be ulceration, periostitis, necrosis and scar formation.

The infiltration may extend to the pharynx and larynx, reducing as it descends toward the respiratory tract. The most severely affected part is the epiglottis, likely because it is more exposed to the cold air inhaled.

5.20 Systemic Involvement

Despite its predilection for the peripheral nerves and skin, *M. leprae* can also be localized in other organs, where it arrives through the lymphatic or hematic route. A visceral localization is frequent in the lepromatous pole of the spectrum: bacillaemia is present in 88% of lepromatous forms and in 50% of borderline lepromatous forms; it subsides after 2–3 months of multidrug therapy. In patients with tuberculoid leprosy the bacilli are present in particular in organs with a rich content of reticuloendothelial tissue, where they likely localize before the cell-mediated immune response has gained momentum. To date, only one case of lepromatous hepato-splenic leprosy with no skin and nerve localization of *M. leprae* has been reported [350]. In any case, visceral localizations are not useful for diagnostic purposes.

5.20.1 Lymph Nodes

After the skin and the peripheral nerves, the lymph nodes are the next most frequent localization of *M. leprae*. In indeterminate leprosy the lymph nodes are spared. In tuberculoid leprosy, in 60% of cases the lymph nodes draining the affected skin regions present granulomas consisting of epithelioid cells, Langhans cells and lymphocytes. There may also be some bacilli.

In lepromatous patients, the lymph nodes are enlarged and have a hard consistency; those most affected include the supraclavear, axillary and inguinal nodes. At histology, the granulomas consist of macrophages containing isolated bacilli or bacillar globi; foamy cells are also present. In a type 2 reaction the lymph nodes are very enlarged and painful, and have a floating consistency. The inguinal, axillary, cervical and epitrochlear lymph nodes are affected. At histology, granulomas with neutrophils and macrophages containing bacilli are observed.

5.20.2 Liver and Spleen

After the lymph nodes, the most frequent visceral localization is the liver, affected in both the tuberculoid and lepromatous forms. In one third of lepromatous patient hepatomegaly is observed, with altered functional parameters in more advanced stages. The histological picture will vary according to the clinical form of the leprosy. In general, there will be agreement of the bacterial index at the skin and liver levels.

The spleen is involved only in lepromatous patients in the advanced stage. Histology shows granulomas with macrophages containing bacilli, that generally have a granular morphology.

5.20.3 Bones

The bone marrow can be involved, prevalently in lepromatous patients. The bone alterations may be specific or nonspecific. The former, with the presence of bacilli, are relatively rare and observed in lepromatous patients with advanced disease. The small bones of the hands, feet and nose are affected. At histology, the infiltrate is seen to invade the periosteum and destroy the bone trabeculae. In fact, fractures of the hands may be observed even after no apparent trauma, that manifest with sudden edema. In advanced stage lepromatous patients, proliferative periostitis of the tibias ("saber tibia") can develop.

Most bone lesions are nonspecific. On the hands and feet, the skin appears xerotic and hypoaesthesic, and since it undergoes continual trauma because of the deformity, it is highly subject to infections and ulceration. Over time, these will involve the bone structures and contribute to the distal reabsorption of the phalanges.

5.20.4 Testicles and Other Organs

In lepromatous patients orchiepididymitis is frequent, leading to bilateral testicular atrophy. *M. leprae* reaches the testicles through the bloodstream, favored by their low temperature. In advanced stages there may be fibrosis. In the course of type 2 reactions, the testicles become edematous and painful. Acute orchiepididymitis can also be the only manifestation of this reaction.

In 8–20% of lepromatous patients in the advanced stage, gynecomastia is present. The onset is due to various factors and not only linked to testicular involvement, even if this is present in 90% of these patients. Affected subjects show a reduction of the excretion of 17-ketosteroids and increased gonadotropins.

In severe, advanced stages the adrenal glands and kidneys can also be involved. The latter will be affected in particular in the course of a type 2 reaction due to the presence of immune complexes; glomerulonephritis, with haematuria and albuminuria, is the most common cause of death linked to leprosy infection.

The central nervous system is notoriously exempt: if there is a decline or loss of deep reflexes and the appearance of pathological reflexes then the diagnosis of leprosy can be excluded.

In patients suffering from severe, repeated type 2 reactions, amyloidosis can develop, featuring amyloid deposits on the liver, kidneys, spleen and adrenal glands.

5.21 Diagnosis and Prognosis

In view of the severity of the disease from the individual standpoint, due to the disabling sequelae and social emargination, it is essential that the diagnosis be "certain" and made as early as possible.

The symptoms that most often bring the sufferer to the doctor are the skin lesions: trauma and indolent burns, as well as macules, papules, plaques, nodules with a chronic, non pruriginous evolution, that are not painful and do not respond to common treatments. In endemic nations, the skin and peripheral nerve lesions are sufficient for the diagnosis, while in nations with sporadic cases microbiological and histological investigations are necessary.

It should be remembered that the disease onset may also be in an acute form drawing the picture of a type 2 reaction, that can be triggered by pregnancy, delivery, concomitant diseases, vaccinations. In the indeterminate form there will be no lesions of the nerve trunks, and in the lepromatous form the skin lesions will precede the nerve damage. Finally, the possibility of a presentation of pure neuritic leprosy without skin lesions, as described by some Indian authors, should also be borne in mind.

The finding of acid-fast bacilli in skin lesions is not enough in itself to make a certain diagnosis of leprosy. In mycobacteriosis due to environmental nontuberculous mycobacteria, a similar histopathological picture to that of hyperergic leprosy (abundant lymphocytes and epithelioid cells) can coexist with multibacillary microbiological findings similar to those of anergic leprosy forms. This incongruence, together with the possibility of in vitro culture of the bacilli, will exclude the diagnosis of leprosy. Also the presence of acid-fast bacilli in the nasal mucosa does not have diagnostic value because in the nasal fossae there may be environmental mycobacteria. On the other hand, negative skin and nasal microbiological findings do not exclude the leprosy diagnosis.

Therefore, the diagnosis must be formulated on the basis of clinical, microbiological and histopathological criteria. It should be noted that although there are no pathognomonic skin lesions for leprosy, these must be associated with peripheral nerve damage. *M. leprae* can be inoculated in the mouse footpad, where a typical growth pattern will ensue: after a latency of about 3 months the multiplication phase will start. This test must be employed, together with other specific investigations (serological and instrumental) when the above-described three criteria are not concordant [351–353].

Diagnostic difficulties arise in particular in indeterminate leprosy (there is no involvement of peripheral nerves and the diagnosis may be suspected only in the presence of bacilli, even in limited numbers) and tuberculoid forms (microbiological tests and antibody titers are of little aid). A history of staying in a nation with endemic leprosy and of contact with leprosy patients is not a valid diagnostic criterion.

Once the diagnosis of leprosy has been made it is time to proceed with the clinical classification of the disease form. On all accounts therapeutic attempts used as "diagnosis ex adiuvantibus" are to be avoided.

From the prognostic standpoint, the specific antibacterial therapy is highly effective, with low relapse rates, although it needs to be administered for many months. In untreated patients the disease evolves toward severe forms and leaves irreversible sequelae. Borderline patients are at risk of type 1 reactions, which may result in devastating nerve damage. Patients with a borderline lepromatous form can also suffer type 2 reactions, like those with a lepromatous form. It is impossible to predict which patients will develop reactions or nerve damage.

5.22 Differential Diagnosis

Leprosy tends to be over-diagnosed in endemic countries and under-diagnosed in non-endemic countries. Among the new patients seen in the period 1995–1999 at the Hospital for Tropical Diseases in London, diagnosis had been delayed in over 80% of cases [353]. Patients had been misdiagnosed by dermatologists, neurologists, orthopedic surgeons, and rheumatologists. A delayed diagnosis has serious consequences for patients, over half of whom will develop nerve damage and disability.

The differential diagnosis with some of the skin and nerve diseases resembling leprosy is reported below.

5.22.1 Macular Lesions

Birthmarks are abnormally pigmented but otherwise physiologically normal. Vitiligo lesions are depigmented, whereas leprosy lesions are never completely depigmented. In hypopigmented lesions of pityriasis alba in children, the surface is often scaly and smears do not contain acid-fast bacilli. Pityriasis versicolor is not always scaly, but the central distribution on the trunk and the presence of minute distinct macules are quite unlike the characteristics of lepromatous macules. Tinea corporis lesions may have a vesicular edge and be itchy, while these symptoms are absent in tuberculoid patches, and scraping usually reveals the fungus.

5.22.2 Plaques and Annular Lesions

In addition to the above-mentioned ringworm, granuloma multiforme, sarcoidosis and cutaneous tuberculosis may resemble tuberculoid leprosy, having a similar immunological basis and often a comparable histological pattern. However, the lesions are not anesthetic and there is no nerve thickening except very exceptionally in sarcoidosis [354]. Granuloma annulare may simulate tuberculoid leprosy, but there is no sensory loss or nerve thickening and the histological appearance is different.

5.22.3 Nodules

Nodules are observed in cutaneous leishmaniasis, but usually they are crusted over and ulcerate after some weeks or months, and they are seldom as numerous as those of lepromatous leprosy. Slit-skin smears, appropriately stained, reveal leishmania, and the leishmanin test is positive. Lesions of the rare, diffuse form of cutaneous leishmaniasis can be confused with those of lepromatous leprosy but not after examination of slit-skin smears. Post-Kalaazar dermal leishmaniasis in India and East Africa has a similar distribution and appearance to the cutaneous lesions of lepromatous leprosy [355].

Erythema nodosum leprosum may be mistaken for other forms of erythema nodosum or for Weber-Christian syndrome, a relapsing, febrile, non-suppurative, nodular panniculitis.

5.22.4 Nerves

Peripheral nerve thickening is rarely seen except in leprosy. Hereditary sensory motor neuropathy type III is associated with palpable peripheral nerve hypertrophy. Amyloidosis, that can also complicate leprosy, presents with thickening of peripheral nerves. Peroneal muscular atrophy (Charcot-Marie-Tooth disease) is an inherited neuropathy with distal atrophy and weakness; nerve biopsy is, however, characteristic. Other polyneuropathies, such as those caused by HIV infections, diabetes, alcoholism, vasculitides, and heavy metal poisoning, should be considered in the differential diagnosis.

5.22.5 Eye Involvement

Finally, in endemic countries there are many diseases of the eye that may mimic leprosy, such as trachoma in particular, in which trichiasis and ectropion follow scarring of the lids, and onchocerciasis, which causes uveitis and its complications.

5.23 Treatment

Treatment is based on five important principles:

1. Halt the infection with chemotherapy
2. Treat reactions and reduce the risk of nerve damage
3. Teach the patient how to cope with existing nerve damage, in particular anaesthesia
4. Treat complications of the nerve damage
5. Rehabilitate the patient, both socially and psychologically

5.23.1 Chemotherapy: First-Line Drugs

In ancient times, leprosy was treated with topical agents or injections into the skin lesions. Vegetable oil preparations was used, such as hydnocarpus or chaulmoogra oil, the ripe seed of *Hydnocarpus wightiana* (family Flacourtiaciae) or *Taraktogenos kurzi* (family Bixaceae). The active ingredient of this oil, chaulmoogric acid (2-cyclopentenyltridecanoic acid: a cyclic fatty acid found among hydrolysis products of the glycerides of chaulmoogra oil) did demonstrate some antileprosy actions [356].

Nowadays, the backbone of the treatment is multidrug therapy (MDT) consisting of dapsone, clofazimine, and rifampicin [3, 357–361].

5.23.1.1 Dapsone (4,4-Diaminodiphenylsulfone, or DDS)

This was introduced in the treatment of leprosy in 1946 by Faget [361]; a bacteriostatic drug, it acts by competitive inhibition of dihydrofolate synthetase and dihydrofolate reductase, key enzymes in the folate biosynthesis pathway in *M. leprae* [362]. In patients on dapsone monotherapy, killing of bacilli occurred over a period of 3–6 months and complete clinical regression in 2–3 years. With this drug, as with all the others, the first to resolve are the mucosal lesions (resulting in clearing of nasal passages, subsidence of epistaxis and a decrease of the foul smell from the nose), and then the skin ulcers. Instead, the regression of nodules and skin thickening starts later. Nerve thickenings, sensorimotor loss, and trophic ulcers respond very slowly and often incompletely.

Despite early reports of widespread resistance, it remains a very useful drug with MDT regimens. Its role in the paucibacillary MDT regimen is to prevent the emergence of rifampicin-resistant organisms. In combination with clofazimine, as used in the multibacillary regimen, dapsone has a bactericidal efficacy, although this is not as powerful as the bactericidal activity of single-dose rifampicin. At a dosage of 100 mg daily, dapsone is used in both MDT regimens for leprosy.

Dapsone is generally well tolerated. Among side effects (Table 5.17), mild hemolytic anemias are common, and the hemolysis is dose-dependent. Severe hemolytic anemias are rare except in patients with a glucose-6-phosphate deficiency. Agranulocytosis has been reported in rare cases. At the dose of 100 mg per day, dapsone can cause methaemoglobinemia, but this is usually asymptomatic unless there is hypoxaemia secondary to lung disease. Gastrointestinal disturbances with anorexia, nausea and vomiting may occur. There have been occasional reports of delayed hypersensitivity reactions presenting as "dapsone syndrome", whose skin manifestations are similar to the Stevens-Johnson syndrome. The onset of this syndrome is usually observed 4–6 weeks after the beginning of treatment; the drug must be discontinued because it can be associated with significant morbidity and mortality. The syndrome manifests with exfoliative dermatitis, fever, generalized lymphadenopathy, and hepatosplenomegaly. Dapsone is obviously contraindicated in patients who are allergic to any of the sulfa drugs.

Dapsone is well absorbed orally and is distributed throughout body fluids. Its plasma half-life is 28 h, and there is some drug retention up to 3 weeks; 80% of dapsone is excreted as metabolites in urine: the dosage must therefore be reduced in cases with renal failure [361].

Table 5.17 Side effects of first-line drugs for leprosy

Drug	Side effects
Dapsone	Hemolytic anaemia (in G6PD deficiency)
	Hepatotoxicity
	Methaemoglobinemia
	Agranulocytosis (rare)
	"Dapsone syndrome"
	Gastric intolerance
Clofazimine	Reddish brown pigmentation of the skin (in 75–100% of cases)
	Ichthyosis and dryness (in 8–28% of cases)
	Corneal xerosis
	Erythroderma
	Acne-like eruptions
Rifampicin	Trombocytopoenia
	Hepatotoxicity
	Renal failure
	Flu-like syndrome (chills, shivering, fever, headache, bone and joint pains)
	Gastrointestinal symptoms (nausea, vomiting, diarrhea, pain)

Folic acid antagonists, such as pyrimethamine, may increase the risk of haematological reactions with dapsone, and so patients must be monitored for agranulocytosis in the second and third months of treatment. Dapsone can inhibit the anti-inflammatory effects of clofazimine. The concomitant administration of rifampicin can decrease the levels of dapsone because of an increased renal clearance [361].

5.23.1.2 Clofazimine

This is an aminophenazone brick red dye which binds to mycobacterial DNA, that both inhibits the mycobacterial growth and exerts a bacteriostatic effect on *M. leprae*. It has also anti-inflammatory properties (via the stimulation of prostaglandin E2 synthesis, inhibition of neutrophil motility, and suppression of Th 1 cells) and so it is used at higher doses (200–300 mg daily) in type 2 reactions [363], where it acts

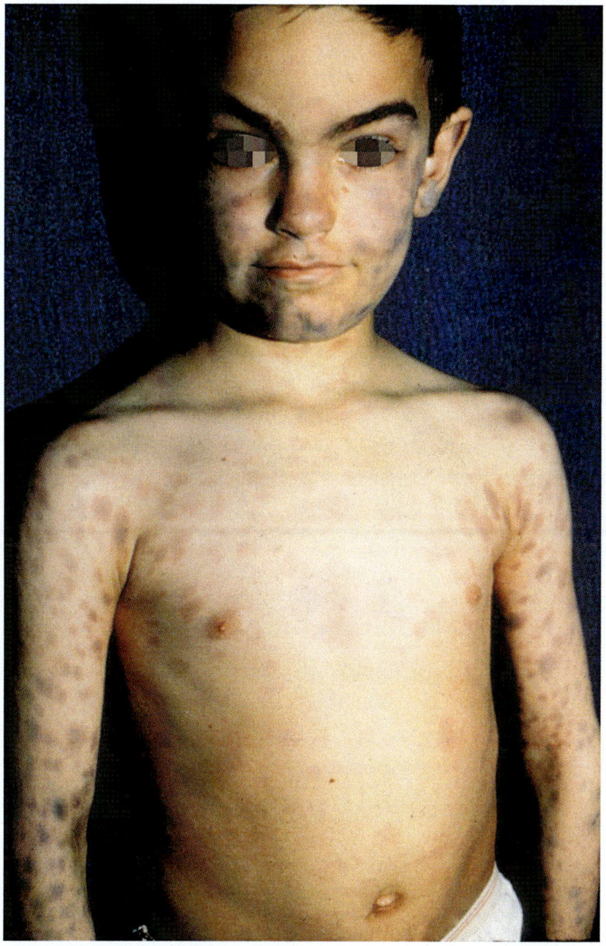

Fig. 5.58 The same patient as in Figs. 5.33 and 5.34. Hyperpigmentation due to clofazimine

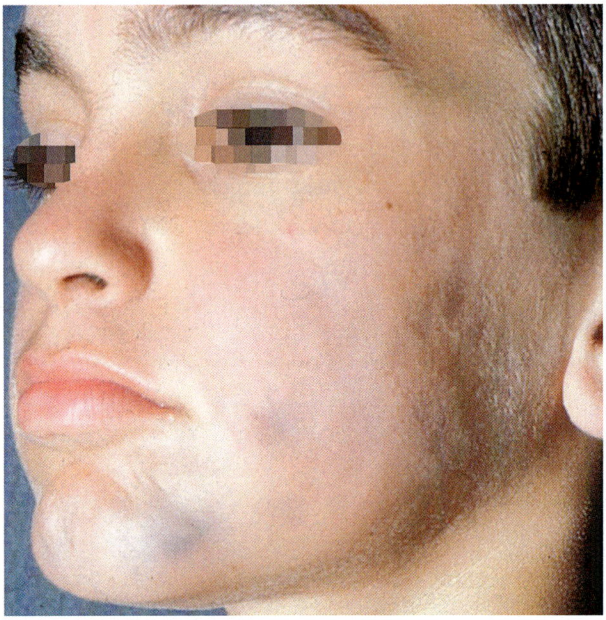

Fig. 5.59 The same patient as in Fig. 5.58

as a steroid-sparing agent, thereby permitting lower doses of steroids. Reports of resistance to clofazimine are extremely rare.

Clofazimine is very well tolerated at the normal dosages of MDT regimens, that is 300 mg monthly and 50 mg daily for adults. However, it frequently causes darkening (Figs. 5.58 and 5.59) and dryness of the skin. The conjunctiva are also affected. Darker skin colors are more susceptible to this hyperpigmentation, that develops during the third month of treatment and resolves in a period ranging from 6 to 36 months after suspension of the drug.

The accumulation of clofazimine in the macrophages possibly interferes with their capacity to process and present antigens, thereby preventing their mobilization and activation, IL-2 release, and clonal expansion [363]. Clofazimine is also excreted through breast milk and can cause mild discoloration of the infant's skin. The prolonged use of high-dose clofazimine induces strong skin pigmentation and ichthyosis, and rarely, gastrointestinal side-effects due to crystal deposits in the intestinal tract (Table 5.17).

The oral absorption of clofazimine is very variable. It has a long half-life, of approximately 70 days, and is distributed throughout the reticuloendothelial tissue. It binds to lipids and is released slowly. It is largely unmetabolized and excreted through the bile, less than 1% being passed in the urine [361].

Dapsone can inhibit the anti-inflammatory action of clofazimine. The contemporary administration of clofazimine and aluminum- or magnesium-containing antacids should be avoided because they reduce the absorption of clofazimine. Clofazimine is active against dapsone-resistant *M. leprae*.

5.23.1.3 Rifampicin

The only bactericidal component of MDT against *M. leprae*, this drug was introduced in 1970. It acts by selectively inhibiting bacterial DNA-dependent RNA polymerase and blocking RNA synthesis [364–368]. It is also effective against dapsone-resistant bacilli. A single dose of 600 mg of rifampicin is capable of killing 99.99% of the viable *M. leprae* [364]. The WHO Study Group recommended 600 mg once-monthly supervised doses for adults. This dosage has the same efficacy as the daily dose and the advantages of lower rates of adverse effects, as well as being very cost-effective for leprosy control programs. Unfortunately, these benefits were immediately superseded by the emergence of resistance caused by mutation in the *rpoB* gene, which encodes the beta subunit of RNA polymerase. Rifampicin resistance probably developed as a result of its use in monotherapy or in combination with dapsone in dapsone-resistant patients [368].

Although the protocol stipulates the monthly dose, rifampicin occasionally causes flu-like symptoms, thrombocytopenia, hepatitis and renal failure. Moreover, it characteristically produces a reddish-brown color in urine, sweat, tears, and saliva.

The drug taken by mouth is rapidly absorbed, with a peak serum concentration 2 h after the administration of 600 mg. About 80% is transported in the blood bound to plasma proteins, mainly albumin; following deacetylation in the liver, rifampicin becomes more microbiologically active. It is excreted in bile and urine, so excretion is slower in patients with an impaired liver and kidney function (Table 5.17).

Co-administration of rifampicin with isoniazid may increase the risk of hepatotoxicity. Because it induces cytochrome P450 microsomal enzymes, rifampicin may therefore decrease the efficacy of various drugs (barbiturates, benzodiazepines, beta-blockers, corticosteroids, cyclosporin, oral contraceptives) [364].

The evidence that rifampicin is acting not only as an antibiotic in leprosy, but very likely also as a biofilm dispersing agent, is of recent date [369]. Rifampicin is a potent biofilm disperser: it "pokes holes" in the biofilm, allowing other animicrobials (dapsone and clofazimine) to penetrate and kill the *M. leprae* (protected while they were in the biofilm) [369, 370]. Clofazimine, on the contrary, does not have the same biofilm-dispersing capability, and so it acts both as an antibiotic and as an anti-inflammatory agent [264, 369].

5.23.2 Drug-Resistant *Mycobacterium leprae*

As with streptomycin when it was used as monotherapy for tuberculosis, secondary dapsone resistance rapidly developed during the 1950s, because it was the only drug available [371]. Primary dapsone resistance, that is to say resistance in a patient never previously treated with dapsone, was first confirmed in Ethiopia in 1977 [372]. After the introduction of MDT, dapsone resistance gradually declined.

Rifampicin resistance is rare outside Brazil. The widespread use of ofloxacin is worrying; more cases have been reported in India than in Brazil. Ofloxacin has been used in leprosy almost always in combination with rifampicin and minocycline (so-called ROM treatment). However, the development of resistance is linked not to the employment of ROM but rather to the widespread use of ofloxacin to treat minor infections, such as respiratory and urinary tract infections.

In the past, the mouse footpad technique was carried out to monitor drug resistance. This technique is no longer used for this purpose because the results only became available after 6–9 months. Thanks to the knowledge of the *M. leprae* genome, it is now possible to identify resistance-causing mutations using molecular techniques in a matter of hours, rather than months [371]. Mutations in the *folP1* gene have been found to be responsible for dapsone resistance. Mutations in the *rpoB* gene are linked to rifampicin resistance and those in the *gyrA* gene to resistance to fluoroquinolones [373]. Owing to the fact that the mode of action of clofazimine is still unknown, no molecular method is available to detect clofazimine resistance; nevertheless, very few cases of resistance have been suspected clinically, or confirmed using the mouse footpad technique.

5.23.3 Multidrug Therapy

The introduction of MDT in 1982 approved by the WHO Expert Committee was one of the most important events in the history of the fight against leprosy. The treatment immediately became the standard of care and since 1995 it has been supplied by WHO free of charge to all endemic countries. The concept of administering the combination of several drugs is based on the estimate that a subject with lepromatous leprosy harbors about 11 logs of live organisms. Of these, the proportion of naturally occurring drug-resistant mutants is estimated to be in 1 in 7 logs for rifampicin and in 1 in 6 logs each for dapsone and clofazimine. Bacilli resistant to one drug should be susceptible to the other drugs in MDT because their mechanisms of action are different. With MDT, the probability of emergence of mutant resistance to one of the other two drugs is reduced to 1 in 13 logs, a negligible proportion [374] (Table 5.18).

Initially, the duration of treatment with MDT was very long (e.g., 24 months or until smear negativity), with the accompanying disadvantages of a decrease in compliance, and the development of resistance, and relapse. This was then changed to a fixed-duration treatment (FDT) for 12 months for multibacillary, and 6 months (FDT-12/6) for paucibacillary groups of patients. Following this scheme, the number of relapses was found to be insignificant, and so in 1997 FDT-12/6 was introduced worldwide.

Multibacillary leprosy included LL, BL and BB cases in the Riddley-Jopling classification, with a bacteriological index of 2 or more at any site in the initial skin smears. Paucibacillary leprosy included indeterminate, TT and BT cases in the same classification, with a bacteriological index of <2 at all sites in the initial skin smears.

Table 5.18 Therapeutic schemes recommended by WHO

1. *PB Leprosy*	
Adults: -Rifampicin 600 mg/month (supervised) -Dapsone 100 mg/day (unsupervised)	For 6 months
Children 10–14 years: -Rifampicin 450 mg/month (supervised) -Dapsone 50 mg/day (unsupervised)	
Children below 10 years: -Rifampicin 300 mg/month (supervised) -Dapsone 25 mg/day (unsupervised)	
2. *MB Leprosy*	
Adults: -Rifampicin 600 mg/month (supervised) -Clofazimine 300 mg/month (supervised) +50 mg/day (unsupervised) -Dapsone 100 mg/day (unsupervised)	For 12 months
Children 10–14 years: -Rifampicin 450 mg/month (supervised) -Clofazimine 150 mg/month (supervised) +50 mg alternate-daily (unsupervised) -Dapsone 50 mg/day (unsupervised)	
Children below 10 years: -Rifampicin 300 mg/month (supervised) -Clofazimine 100 mg/month (supervised) +50 mg/twice weekly (unsupervised) -Dapsone 25 mg/day (unsupervised)	

PB paucibacillary, *MB* multibacillary

Table 5.19 Clinical classification of leprosy

Symptoms	Paucibacillary leprosy	Multibacillary leprosy
Skin lesions (macules, papules, plaques, nodules)	Up to 5 lesions Hypopigmented or erythematous Asymmetrically distributed Definite loss of sensation	More than 5 lesions Symmetrical distribution Loss of sensation
Nerve damage (loss of sensation or weakness of muscles)	Only 1 nerve trunk	Many nerve trunks

In 1993, the WHO Study Group on Chemotherapy of leprosy decided that approaches based on clinical classification may be required if reliable facilities for the bacteriological examination of skin smears are not available; it also recommended that when the classification is in doubt, the patient should be treated as having multibacillary leprosy [368]. Since then, many programs have based the classification on clinical criteria: the essential feature is based on the number of lesions, especially the skin lesions. The assumption is that the protective immunity is inversely correlated to the number of lesions, and so multibacillary cases have a higher number of lesions or affected body areas than paucibacillary cases (Table 5.19).

To simplify the treatment schedule for patients, WHO in collaboration with Novartis Pharma (Switzerland) supply MDT in "blister packs". Each blister pack contains treatment for 4 weeks. The patient must visit the leprosy center monthly to collect the monthly blister pack and to swallow the monthly supervised doses in front of a leprosy worker/doctor. The patient must then observe regular self-administration of the rest of the drugs in the blister pack [359].

It is important that the standard MDT is continued unchanged during pregnancy. Through breast milk, small quantities of the antileprosy drugs are excreted; however, no adverse effects have been reported other than a mild discoloration of the infant due to clofazimine.

The information available indicates that in patients with concomitant HIV infection the standard MDT does not need to be modified. Patients affected by leprosy and tuberculosis require standard antituberculosis therapy in addition to MDT for leprosy; only rifampicin is common to the two regimens, and it must be given at the dosage required for tuberculosis.

With MDT the relapse rate is very low (0.1% per year for paucibacillary groups and 0.06% per year for multibacillary groups on average), and there is also a low frequency of side effects. Unfortunately, not all centers report good results with the MDT regimens. Most of the problems have arisen with the paucibacillary regimen due to various possible classification errors: subjects classified as paucibacillary on the basis of clinical criteria alone who were in fact multibacillary [368]. For this reason, WHO is now exploring possibilities of introducing other treatment methods.

5.23.4 Novel Drugs and Treatment Regimens

Despite the efficacy of MDT, various other antibiotics have been tested to ensure a wider choice and overcome the problem of drug resistance, as well as to address the aim of reducing the treatment duration, that is considered to be still too long [359, 375–379].

The following drugs have been considered the most efficacious: quinolones (ofloxacin, pefloxacin, sparfloxacin, and moxifloxacin), tetracyclines (minocycline), macrolides (clarithromycin), and rifampicin derivatives (rifapentine).

The use of quinolones in the treatment of leprosy was discovered two decades ago. After the failure of various regimens, now the focus is on monthly administrations of ROM (intermittent therapy) for 12 months for multibacillary and 6 months for paucibacillary leprosy:

Rifampicin 600 mg + ofloxacin 400 mg + minocycline 100 mg, once a month.

A number of other new regimens with various combinations of the above drugs have been proposed [359, 375].

Ofloxacin, one of the fluoroquinolones, has a bactericidal effect against *M. leprae*. Side effects include nausea, diarrhea and other gastrointestinal complaints, and a variety of central nervous system complaints, such as insomnia, headaches, dizziness, and nervousness. The bactericidal effect of minocycline against *M. leprae* is greater than that of clarithromycin, but much less than that of rifampicin. Its side effects include discoloration of the teeth in infants and children; occasional pigmentation of the skin and mucous membranes, and various gastrointestinal symptoms and central nervous system complaints. It should not be given to children and pregnant women. Clarithromycin displays a significant bactericidal activity; side effects include nausea, vomiting, and diarrhea.

5.23.5 Special Treatment Regimens

A single administration of ROM regimen has been shown to work in new patients classified as having single-lesion paucibacillary leprosy.

In subjects who are unable to take rifampicin due to side effects, concomitant diseases (chronic hepatitis), or resistance, the recommended WHO protocol is as follows:

Ofloxacin 400 mg/day + minocycline 100 mg/day + clofazimine 50 mg/day for 6 months and then clofazimine 50 mg/day + ofloxacin 400 mg/day or minocycline 100 mg/day for the following 18 months.

In multibacillary patients who refuse to take clofazimine because of skin discoloration, the WHO recommend the following alternative:

Rifampicin 600 mg + ofloxacin 400 mg + minocycline 100 mg (ROM) once a month for 24 months.

In patients who cannot take dapsone because of side effects, the WHO recommend the following regimens:

1. In multibacillary patients: standard MDT without dapsone (only rifampicin and clofazimine).
2. In paucibacillary patients: rifampicin 600 mg/months + clofazimine 300 mg/month + clofazimine 50 mg/day for 6 months.

5.23.6 Treatment of Leprosy Reactions

Leprosy reactions, that can occur during or after the specific treatment, must be treated as emergencies. The immunological alterations that induce these acute episodes are sometimes so violent as to provoke hypertrophic nerve damage leading to paralysis and neurotrophic deficits, that can result in severe and irreversible sequelae.

During leproreactions the appropriate leprosy MDT is continued without any interruption.

5.23.6.1 Type 1 Reaction (Reversal Reaction)

This is caused by the increased patient cell-mediated immunity against *M. laprae*. In association with neuritis, the following treatment is recommended: physical rest, immobilization of the limb (corresponding to the damaged nerve), and systemic corticosteroid therapy with prednisone at the dosage of 1 mg/kg/day. Corticosteroid therapy must continue, even when the patient is better, at the same initial dosage for

2–3 weeks. After the third week, the dosage can be very gradually tapered, by approximately 2.5 mg/week, for a total treatment period of 5–8 months. The treatment may need to be prolonged, especially in cases of BB and BL leprosy. This is, of course, a very general scheme, because each patient is an individual case.

During reactions, patient surveillance is fundamental because without adequate corticosteroid treatment, the damage caused by neuritis could be permanent. If the neuritis attack does not decrease after 5–6 days, surgical external decompression of the affected nerve is recommended.

In the presence of only skin lesions (without neurological signs), sedatives and analgesics (non steroid anti-inflammatory drugs: e.g. acetylsalicylic acid) drugs are sufficient.

5.23.6.2 Type 2 Reaction (Erythema Nodosum Leprosum)

This is due to an imbalance of humoral immunity and the formation of circulating immune complexes. In general, this type of reaction seems to be less common in patients treated with MDT than those treated with dapsone in monotherapy, likely due to the anti-inflammatory activity of clofazimine. Treatment will vary according to the severity of the reaction, its duration and the organs affected. A mild type 2 reaction can be treated with rest and analgesic or antipyretic drugs such as aspirin. Instead, severe forms, often accompanied by neuritis, must be treated with prednisone, like a type 1 reaction, or thalidomide. The latter is the drug of choice, although its teratogenicity and the difficulty in obtaining it restrict its use. Thalidomide is absolutely contraindicated in women during their fertility cycle, even if a contraceptive is used, because of the interaction between rifampicin and oestroprogestinic drugs. Thalidomide also poses other problems, the worst of which is the development of a sensory neuropathy if used for a long time. The initial dosage is 400 mg/day in two administrations. Patients improve quickly, and the dosage must be tapered when the attack is under control. Thalidomide can be used only in referral centers because it needs to be strictly controlled, and its routine use in the field is difficult. In Europe it can only be prescribed through hospital pharmacies.

Clofazimine, at the dosage of 300 mg/day, should have good effects as an anti-inflammatory drug, but it is less potent than corticosteroids and often takes 4–6 weeks to develop its full effects, so it should never be started as the sole agent in severe cases. However, clofazimine may be extremely useful in order to reduce or withdraw corticosteroids in patients with chronic or recurrent reactions. The dosage can be given in three divided daily doses to minimize the gastrointestinal side effects; the total duration of high-dose clofazimine therapy should not exceed 12 months. Obviously, skin pigmentation can limit its prescription.

5.23.6.3 Lucio's Phenomenon

There is no consensus as to the therapy for Lucio's phenomenon, and controversies as regards its management have arisen [285]. Some studies have reported no success with thalidomide, although in some cases it was administered in low doses.

Up to now, however, thalidomide has been regarded as the treatment of choice, due to its anti-TNF-α effect. It has therefore been postulated that other anti-TNF-α drugs could be useful, such as pentoxyphylline, infliximab, and etanercept, mainly in patients for whom thalidomide is contraindicated, or in countries where it is restricted due to its teratogenicity [285].

5.23.6.4 Leprosy Reactions in Pregnancy

Appropriate leprosy MDT should be continued throughout pregnancy. For the treatment of a type 2 reaction or leprosy neuritis, clofazimine 100 mg can be given three times daily: it is safe and effective, but crosses the placenta and goes into breast milk (which will be a pinkish color). After delivery, mothers should be advised that regurgitated milk may be colored pink, that this shows that the mother's clofazimine is reaching the baby via the breast milk, and that clofazimine may temporarily discolor the baby's skin [297].

5.23.7 Surgical Treatment

This is performed to address neurological complications of leprosy.

5.23.7.1 Nerve Surgery

During a type 1 reaction, if the patient does not show an improvement after 4–5 days of corticosteroid treatment and if important nerves are inflamed, surgery is strongly recommended: external decompression is possible by opening the osteofibrous canal [375]. The nerves which can be affected are the ulnar at the elbow, median in the carpal tunnel, common peroneal near the peroneal neck, and posterior tibialis in the medial retromalleolar region. The surgery is simple and can carried out anywhere by general surgeons. It must be supported by systemic corticosteroid therapy [375].

5.23.7.2 Palliative Surgery

This is aimed at restoring most movements which have been lost or limited. The claw hand deformity can be corrected with the transfer of tendons, capsule shortening, and arthrodesis. The steppage gait due to affection of a lower limb can be corrected with anterior transposition of the posterior muscles (not affected by neuropathy). Plastic surgery may be done to treat osteocartilagineous deformities of the face (nasal pyramid).

5.23.7.3 Surgery of Sequelae

Neurotrophic problems, such as chronic plantar ulcers, osteoarthritis, and phalangeal osteolysis, may be treated with amputations, suppuration cleansing, and grafts. This surgery must be carried out together with health education of the patient to prevent the relapse of plantar ulcers (daily skin care, orthopedic soles and shoes, etc.) [375, 380].

5.24 Prophylaxis

Isolation of the patients is absolutely useless. Paucibacillary patients are considered non contagious, and multibacillary patients non contagious after one dose of 600 mg rifampicin.

5.24.1 Chemoprophylaxis

Pharmacological prophylaxis in patients who live in endemic countries is not advisable [375]. The risk of infection is so small that lifelong drug administration is not recommended. In addition, some studies have failed to demonstrate the efficacy of this method, and the risk of *M. leprae* developing resistance in monotherapy is very high [42, 375].

5.24.2 Immunoprophylaxis

The hunt for a vaccine as a means of primary prevention of leprosy is still ongoing. Various drugs and biologicals attempted as immunotherapeutic and immunoprophylactic agents are based on cultivable mycobacteria, such as the Indian Cancer Research Centre bacillus, *Mycobacterium w* (*Mw*), *Mycobacterium habana*, bacillus Calmette-Guérin (BCG), *M. vaccae*, and drugs like levamisol and zinc. Of these, *Mw* and BCG have been most closely studied [359].

Theoretically, the *Mw* (renamed *Mycobacterium indicus pranii* after elucidation of the full genome) vaccine acts by mediating the release of various cytokines and chemokines involved in the stimulation of T-cell migration and natural killer cells. Given along with MDT in multibacillary patients, this vaccine results in faster clearance of dead bacilli from the body and thus may be helpful in preventing the occurrence of leprosy reactions. Unfortunately, in clinical trials the results did not live up to this expectation [381].

At an early stage, it was recognized that BCG could possibly also protect against leprosy, and several vaccine trials using BCG were carried out, often in combination with *M. leprae* or related mycobacterial vaccines [382, 383].

Meta-analyses have confirmed the protective effect of BCG against leprosy [382–385]. A recent study showed a variable protection of BCG vaccination in different study areas, ranging from 20% to 90%, and presented evidence for protection at a young age; the results are inconsistent when vaccination is carried out at an older age. BCG efficacy appeared to be significant higher among contacts of leprosy patients than among the general population: 68% versus 53% [63]. A study conducted in Brazil indicated a possible increased risk of tuberculoid leprosy in the first months [386].

The ideal vaccine, that would induce strong, long-lasting T-cell responses directed against *M. leprae* and that would both prevent disease and reduce bacterial transmission, is still lacking.

5.25 Control

The "control" of leprosy does not only mean protecting the community against the infection but also treating and rehabilitating patients, as well as providing the general population with proper, complete information about the disease.

Now that new cases are becoming ever rarer in most endemic countries, it is no longer necessary to apply intensified, population-based approaches for case detection and to target preventive interventions such as chemoprophylaxis and immunoprophylaxis to total population groups, with the possible exception of small, highly endemic pockets of leprosy [42].

Since the greatest risk of exposure to the infection is through close contacts with new untreated cases, future leprosy control strategies should be addressed to prevent these contacts. The strategy has three main objectives: case detection, case management, and contact management. The first two include early case detection, appropriate treatment, prevention of disabilities and social action to reduce stigma [387].

Contact surveys, recommended in national and international guidelines and routinely performed in the past, have long been neglected in many countries due to the lack of resources. The strategy based on early case detection and treatment with MDT is not sufficient to interrupt the transmission of *M. leprae* and significantly reduce the incidence of leprosy [42, 388]. Therefore, well-developed contact management approaches are needed, focused not only on household contacts (which, as is well known, pose an increased risk for leprosy), but also extended to neighbors and consanguineous relatives, especially in cases of multibacillary patients [389]. A contact survey, when properly performed in a control area, could probably reduce the transmission of the bacilli [390].

At the same time as the contact survey, a combined approach could be adopted, providing both chemoprophylaxis (which offers a relatively short protective window, of approximately 2 years) and immunoprophylaxis (which provides long-term protection). Bearing in mind that rifampicin and BCG containing live mycobacteria cannot be given at the same time, chemoprophylaxis could be administered during a first visit and immunization during the second visit at least 4 weeks later [42].

Another important component of contact-based preventive strategy would be reliable, valid, simple diagnostic tests to establish both the disease and type of infection.

Currently available tests based on antibody responses to *M. leprae* phenolic glycolipid I are only effective for detecting infection in multibacillary patients and do not accurately predict the development of disease in subclinical cases [391, 392]. Instead, for control purposes it is important to establish whether leprosy contacts are infected, and still more importantly, whether their organism will control the infection or develop the disease, in which case they should receive prophylactic treatment. The triad of detection of subclinical infection, treatment, and prophylaxis (scientific evidence of the efficacy of chemoprophylaxis with single-dose rifampicin and immunoprophylaxis with BCG has accumulated), when appropriately applied in household contacts of leprosy patients, should reduce the incidence of the disease in the general population [392].

Leprosy is a disease that has extremely severe effects on the social life of the patient and community. Health education is therefore an essential component of any control campaign, addressed to both patients and the community. The general population should be made aware that leprosy is a curable disease, that does not require compulsory isolation of the sufferer, who can be treated at home. It must also support the patient, who must not fear ostracism. Patients should know that deformities are not an inevitable consequence of leprosy if early diagnosis and treatment are ensured, and the drugs are taken regularly. Patients should also undergo periodical control visits, and be instructed about how to manage the disease and any complications responsibly. The age-old reaction to this disease of fear and repulsion should be eradicated because otherwise a complete control of leprosy can never be achieved.

References

1. Leiker D, Nunzi E (1985) Leprosy in the light skin: an illustrated manual. O.C.S.I., AIFO, Bologna
2. Bryceson A, Pfaltzgraff RE (1990) Leprosy, 3rd edn. Churchill Livingstone, Edinburgh
3. Canizares O, Harman R, Adriaans B (1992) Leprosy. In: Canizares O, Harman R (eds) Clinical tropical dermatology, 2nd edn. Blackwekk Scientific, Boston, p 165
4. Hastings RC (ed) (1985) Leprosy. Churchill Livingstone, Edinburgh
5. Britton W. Leprosy. In: Armstrong D, Cohen J (eds) Infectious diseases. London, Mosby, 1999:16.1.
6. Ramos-e-Silva M, Riberio de Castro MC (2003) Mycobacterial infections. In: Bolognia JL, Jorizzo JL, Rapini RP (eds) Dermatology. Mosby, London, p 1145
7. Leprosy Group, WHO (2003) Leprosy. In: Cook GC, Zumla A (eds) Manson's tropical diseases, 21st edn. WB Saundersm, London, p 1065
8. Lockwood DNJ (2010) Leprosy. In: Burns T, Breathnach S, Cox N et al (eds) Rook's textbook of dermatology, 8th edn. Wiley-Blackwell, Oxford, p 32.1
9. Lee DJ, Rea TH, Modlin RL (2012) Leprosy. In: Goldsmith LA, Katz SI, Gilchrest BA et al (eds) Fitzpatrick's dermatology in general medicine, 8th edn. McGrow Hill, New York, p 2253
10. Nunzi E, Fiallo P, Clapasson A (2013) Leprosy. In: Giannetti A, Del Forno C (eds) Textbook of dermatology & sexually transmitted diseases. Piccin Nuova Libraria S.P.A., Padova, p 515
11. Brubaker ML, Meyers WM, Bourland J (1985) Leprosy in children one year of age and under. Int J Lepr Other Mycobact Dis 53:517
12. Meyers WM (1992) Leprosy. Clin Dermatol 10:73
13. Truman RW, Singh P, Sharma R et al (2011) Probable zoonotic leprosy in the southern United States. N Engl J Med 364:1626
14. Sugita Y (1995) Leprosy. Clin Dermatol 13:235
15. Ramos-e-Silva M, PFB R (2001) Leprosy. Recognition and treatment. Am J Clin Dermatol 2:203
16. Browne SG (1989) The history of leprosy. In: Hasting RC (ed) Leprosy. Churchill Livingstone, Edinburgh, p 1
17. Robbins G, Tripathy VM, Misra VN et al (2009) Ancient skeletal evidence for leprosy in India (2000 B.C.) PLoS One 4:e5669
18. Nunzi E, Leiker L (1995) Manuale di leprologia, 2nd edn. O.C.S.I.,AIFO, Bologna
19. Grzybowski A, Nita M (2016) Leprosy in the Bible. Clin Dermatol 34:3
20. Goldman L, Moraites RS, Kitzmiller KW (1966) White spots in biblical times. Arch Dermatol 93:744

21. Baillie RA, Baillie EE, Anderson SC (1982) Biblical leprosy as compared to present-day leprosy. South Med J 75:855
22. Freilich AR (1982) Tzaraat-"biblical leprosy". J Am Acad Dermatol 6:131
23. Davies ML, Davies TA (1989) Biblical leprosy: a comedy of errors. J R Soc Med 82:622
24. Kaplan DL (1993) Biblical leprosy: an anachronism whose time has come. J Am Acad Dermatol 28:507
25. Appelboom T, Cogan E, Klastersky J (2007) Job of the Bible: leprosy or scabies? Mt Sinai J Med 74:36
26. Nunzi E, Clapasson A (2004) La lebbra oggi. Bologna, AIFO
27. Gonzalez Prendes MA (1964) Gerhard Henrik Armauer Hansen (1841–1912). Lepr Rev 35:127
28. Hansen GA (1872) Om vort Kjendskab til Spedalskhedens Aarsager og om vore Forholdsregler mod Sygdommen. Nor Mag Laegevidenskaben 2:1
29. Grzybowski A, Sak J, Pawlikowski J et al (2013) Gerhard Henrik Armauer Hansen (1841–1912)-the 100th anniversary of the death of the discoverer of *Mycobacterium leprae*. Clin Dermatol 31:653
30. Volgesang TM (1963) A serious sentence passed against the discoverer of the leprosy bacillus (Gerhard Armauer Hansen), in 1880. Med Hist 7:182
31. Vogelsang TM (1964) Hansen's first observation and publication concerning the bacillus of leprosy. Int J Lepr 32:330
32. Mitsuda K (1953) On the value of a skin reaction to a suspicious of leprous nodules. Int J Lepr Other Mycobact Dis 21:347
33. Faget GH, Johansen FA, RossH (1942) Sulfanilamide in the treatment of leprosy. Public Health Rep 57:1892
34. Shepard CC (1960) Acid-fast bacilli in nasal excretions in leprosy, and results of inoculation of mice. Am J Hyg 71:147
35. Ridley DS, Jopling WH (1966) Classification of leprosy according to immunity. A five-group system. Int J Lepr Other Mycobact Dis 34:255
36. Kirchheimer WF, Storrs EE (1971) Attempts to establish the armadillo (*Dasypus novemcinctus* Linn.) as a model for the study of leprosy. I. Report of lepromatoid leprosy in an experimentally infected armadillo. Int J Lepr Other Mycobact Dis 39:693
37. Cole ST, Eiglemeier K, Parkhill J et al (2001) Massive gene decay in the leprosy bacillus. Nature 409:1007
38. Grzybowski A, Sak J, Korecki K (2016) Misericordia and leprosy in the 20th century. Clin Dermatol 34:11
39. World Health Organization (2015) Global leprosy update, 2014: need for early case detection. Wkly Epidemiol Res 90:461
40. Schreuder PAM, Noto S, Richardus JH (2016) Epidemiologic trends of leprosy for the 21st century. Clin Dermatol 34:24
41. Declercq E (2009) Leprosy global statistics: beware of traps. Lepr Rev 80:350
42. Richardus JH, Oskam L (2015) Protecting people against leprosy: chemoprophylaxis and immunoprophylaxis. Clin Dermatol 33:19
43. Blok DJ, De Vlas SJ, Richardus JH (2015) Global elimination of leprosy by 2020: are we on track? Parasit Vectors 8:548
44. Grzybowski A, Sak J, Pawlikowski J et al (2016) Leprosy: social implications from antiquity to the present. Clin Dermatol 34:8
45. Grzybowski A, Sak J, Suchodolska E et al (2015) Lepra: various etiologies from miasma to bacteriology and genetics. Clin Dermatol 33:3
46. Glickman FS (1986) Lepra, psora, psoriasis. J Am Acad Dermatol 14:863
47. GER L (ed) (1978) Hippocratic writings. Penguin Books, London
48. Wales AE (1963) Sir Jonathan Hutchinson, 1828–1913. Br J Vener Dis 39:67
49. Hutchinson J (1906) On leprosy and fish-eating. A statement of facts and explanations. Archibald Constable & Co., Ld, London

50. Fite GL, Wade HW (1955) The contribution of Neisser to the establishment of the Hansen bacillus as the etiologic agent of leprosy and the so-called Hansen-Neisser controversy. Int J Lepr 23:418
51. Vogelsang TM (1963) The Hansen-Neisser controversy, 1879–1880. Int J Lepr 31:74
52. Jensen RW, Rivest J, Li W et al (2011) DNA fingerprinting of *Mycobacterium leprae* strains using variable number tandem repeat (VNTR)—fragment length analysis (FLA). J Vis Exp 53:e3104
53. Turankar RP, Lavania M, Singh M et al (2012) Dynamics of *Mycobacterium leprae* transmission in environmental context: deciphering the role of environment as a potential reservoir. Infect Genet Evol 12:121
54. Monot M, Honoré N, Garnier T et al (2005) On the origin of leprosy. Science 308:1040
55. Fine PEM (1982) Leprosy: the epidemiology of a slow bacterium. Epidemiol Rev 4:161
56. Bakker MI, Hatta M, Kwenang A et al (2002) Epidemiology of leprosy among five isolated islands in the Flores Sea Indonesia. Tropical Med Int Health 7:780
57. Meima A, Gupte MD, van Oortmarssen GJ et al (1999) SIMLEP: a simulation model for leprosy transmission and control. Int J Lepr Other Mycobact Dis 67:215
58. van Beers SM, Hatta M, Klatser PR (1999) Patient contact is the major determinant in incident leprosy: implications for future control. Int J Lepr Other Mycobact Dis 67:119
59. Fine PEM, Sterne JA, Pönnighaus JM et al (1997) Household and dwelling contact as risk factors for leprosy in Northern Malawi. Am J Epidemiol 146:91
60. van Beers SM, Izumi S, Madjid B et al (1994) An epidemiological study of leprosy infection by serology and polymerase chain reaction. Int J Lepr Other Mycobact Dis 62:1
61. Bakker MI, Hatta M, Kwenang A et al (2004) Population survey to determine risk factors for *Mycobacterium leprae* transmission and infection. Int J Epidemiol 33:1329
62. Moet FJ, Pahan D, Schuring RP et al (2006) Physical distance, genetic relationship, age, and leprosy classification are independent risk factors for leprosy in contacts of patients with leprosy. J Infect Dis 193:346
63. Merle CS, Cunha SS, Rodrigues LC (2010) BCG vaccination and leprosy protection: review of current evidence and status of BCG in leprosy control. Expert Rev Vaccines 9:209
64. Fine PEM, Sterne JA, Pönnighaus JM et al (1994) Delayed-type hypersensitivity, mycobacterial vaccines and protective immunity. Lancet 344:1245
65. Bray GW (1930) The story of leprosy at Nauru. Proc R Soc Med 23:1370
66. Leiker DL (1971) Some aspects of the epidemiology of leprosy. On the relationship of leprosy and other mycobacterial diseases. Int J Lepr Other Mycobact Dis 39:610
67. Feenstra SG, Nahar Q, Pahan D et al (2011) Recent food shortage is associated with leprosy disease in Bangladesh: a case-control study. PLoS Negl Trop Dis 5:e1029
68. Ustianowski AP, Lawn SD, Lockwood DN (2006) Interactions between HIV infection and leprosy: a paradox. Lancet Infect Dis 6:350
69. Massone C, Talhari C, Ribeiro-Rodrigues R et al (2011) Leprosy and HIV coinfection: a critical approach. Expert Rev Anti-Infect Ther 9:701
70. Bratschi MW, Steinmann P, Wickenden A et al (2015) Current knowledge on *Mycobacterium leprae* transmission: a systematic literature review. Lepr Rev 86:142
71. Singh G, Tutakne MA, Tiwari VD et al (1985) Inoculation leprosy developing after tattooing--a case report. Indian J Lepr 57:887
72. Ghorpade A (2002) Inoculation (tattoo) leprosy: a report of 31 cases. J Eur Acad Dermatol Venereol 16:494
73. Singh RK (2009) Tattoos and paucibacillary leprosy. Travel Med Infect Dis 7:325
74. Brandsma JW, Yoder L, MacDonald M (2005) Leprosy acquired by inoculation from a knee injury. Lepr Rev 76:175
75. Ghorpade A (2013) Post traumatic borderline tuberculoid leprosy over knee in an Indian male. Lepr Rev 84:248
76. Ghorpade A (2009) Post-traumatic inoculation tuberculoid leprosy after injury with a glass bangle. Lepr Rev 80:215

77. Sharma P, Bhardwaj M, Kar HK (2009) Inoculation leprosy and HIV co-infection: a rare case with nerve involvement preceding development of skin patch and type 1 reaction as immune reconstitution syndrome following antiretroviral therapy. Indian J Lepr 81:75
78. Marchoux PE (1934) Un cas d'inoculation accidentelle du bacille de Hansen en pays non lepreux. Int J Lepr 2:1
79. Job CK, Harris EB, Allen JL et al (1986) Thorns in armadillo ears and noses and their role in the transmission of leprosy. Arch Pathol Lab Med 110:1025
80. Sehgal VN, Rege VL, Vadiraj SN (1970) Inoculation leprosy subsequent to small-pox vaccination. Dermatologica 141:393
81. Ghorpade A (2007) Inoculation indeterminate leprosy localised to a smallpox vaccination scar. Lepr Rev 78:398
82. Bechelli LM, Garbajosa PG, Gyi MM et al (1973) Site of early skin lesions in children with leprosy. Bull World Health Organ 48:107
83. Kapur TR, Rao SM (1979) Post-traumatic tuberculoid leprosy. A case report. Lepr India 51:112
84. Gupta CM, Tutakne MA, Tiwari VD et al (1984) Inoculation leprosy subsequent to dog bite. A case report. Indian J Lepr 56:919
85. Kerr-Pontes LR, Barreto ML, Evangelista CM et al (2006) Socioeconomic, environmental, and behavioural risk factors for leprosy in Northeast Brazil: results of a case-control study. Int J Epidemiol 35:994
86. Kazda J, Irgens LM, Kolk AH (1990) Acid-fast bacilli found in sphagnum vegetation of coastal Norway containing *Mycobacterium leprae*-specific phenolic glycolipid-I. Int J Lepr Other Mycobact Dis 58:353
87. Matsuoka M, Izumi S, Budiawan T et al (1999) *Mycobacterium leprae* DNA in daily using water as a possible source of leprosy infection. Indian J Lepr 71:61
88. Truman R, Fine PEM (2010) "Environmental" sources of *Mycobacterium leprae*: issues and evidence. Lepr Rev 81:89
89. Kazda J, Ganapati R, Revankar C et al (1986) Isolation of environment-derived *Mycobacterium leprae* from soil in Bombay. Lepr Rev 57(Suppl 3):201
90. Blake LA, West BC, Lary CH et al (1987) Environmental nonhuman sources of leprosy. Rev Infect Dis 9:562
91. Lavania M, Katoch K, Katoch VM et al (2008) Detection of viable *Mycobacterium leprae* in soil samples: insights into possible sources of transmission of leprosy. Infect Genet Evol 8:627
92. Kazda J, Irgens LM, Müller K (1980) Isolation of non-cultivable acid-fast bacilli in sphagnum and moss vegetation by foot pad technique in mice. Int J Lepr Other Mycobact Dis 48:1
93. Kazda J (1981) Occurrence of non-cultivable acid-fast bacilli in the environment and their relationship to *M. leprae*. Lepr Rev 52(Suppl 1):85
94. Mostafa HM, Kazda J, Irgens LM et al (1995) Acid-fast bacilli from former leprosy regions in coastal Norway showing PCR positivity for *Mycobacterium leprae*. Int J Lepr Other Mycobact Dis 63:97
95. Lahiri R, Krahenbuhl JL (2008) The role of free-living pathogenic amoeba in the transmission of leprosy: a proof of principle. Lepr Rev 79:401
96. Saha K, Jain M, Mukherjee MK et al (1985) Viability of *Mycobacterium leprae* within the gut of *Aedes aegypti* after they feed on multibacillary lepromatous patients: a study by fluorescent and electron microscopes. Lepr Rev 56:279
97. Sreevatsa (1993) Leprosy and arthropods. Indian J Lepr 65:189
98. Couret M (1911) The behavior of bacillus leprae in cold-blooded animals. J Exp Med 13:576
99. Chaussinand R (1952) Inoculation of Hansen and Stefansky bacilli in the rainbow perch *Eupomotis gibbosus*. Int J Lepr Other Mycobact Dis 20:420
100. Gormus BJ, Xu K, Baskin GB et al (1998) Experimental leprosy in rhesus monkeys: transmission, susceptibility, clinical and immunological findings. Lepr Rev 69:235
101. Walsh GP, Meyers WM, Binford CH (1986) Naturally acquired leprosy in the nine-banded armadillo: a decade of experience 1975–1985. J Leukoc Biol 40:645

102. Truman RW, Shannon EJ, Hagstad HV et al (1986) Evaluation of the origin of *Mycobacterium leprae* infections in the wild armadillo, *Dasypus novemcinctus*. AmJTrop Med Hyg 35:588
103. Taylor CE, Elliston EP, Gideon H (1965) A symptomatic infections in leprosy. Int J Lepr Other Mycobact Dis 33:716
104. Deps PD, Alves BL, Gripp CG et al (2008) Contact with armadillos increases the risk of leprosy in Brazil: a case control study. Indian J Dermatol Venereol Leprol 74:338
105. Abide JM, Webb RM, Jones HL et al (2008) Three indigenous cases of leprosy in the Mississippi delta. South Med J 101:635
106. Sterne JA, Pönnighaus JM, Fine PEM et al (1995) Geographic determinants of leprosy in Karonga District, Northern Malawi. Int J Epidemiol 24:1211
107. Davey TF, Rees RJ (1974) The nasal dicharge in leprosy: clinical and bacteriological aspects. Lepr Rev 45:121
108. Rees RJ, Meade TW (1974) Comparison of the modes of spread and the incidence of tuberculosis and leprosy. Lancet 1:47
109. Huang CL (1980) The transmission of leprosy in man. Int J Lepr Other Mycobact Dis 48:309
110. Desikan KV (1977) Viability of *Mycobacterium leprae* outside the human body. Lepr Rev 48:231
111. Desikan KV, Sreevatsa (1995) Extended studies on the viability of *Mycobacterium leprae* outside the human body. Lepr Rev 66:287
112. Mosi L, Williamson H, Wallace JR et al (2008) Persistent association of *Mycobacterium ulcerans* with West African predaceous insects of the family Belostomatidae. Appl Environ Microbiol 74:7036
113. Leininger JR, Donham KJ, Rubino MJ et al (1980) Naturally acquired leprosy in a chimpanzee: necropsy findings and experimental transmission to other animals. Lab Investig 42:132
114. Meyers WM, Gormus BJ, Walsh GP (1992) Nonhuman sources of leprosy. Int J Lepr Other Mycobact Dis 60:477
115. Levy L, Ji B (2006) The mouse foot-pad technique for cultivation of *Mycobacterium leprae*. Lepr Rev 77:5
116. Balamayooran G, Pena M, Sharma R et al (2015) The armadillo as an animal model and reservoir host for *Mycobacterium leprae*. Clin Dermatol 33:108
117. Walsh GP, Storrs EE, Burchfield HP et al (1975) Leprosy-like disease occurring naturally in armadillos. J Reticuloendothel Soc 18:347
118. Smith JH, Folse DS, Long EG et al (1983) Leprosy in wild armadillos (*Dasypus novemcinctus*) of the Texas Gulf Coast: epidemiology and mycobacteriology. J Reticuloendothel Soc 34:75
119. Talmage RV, Buchanan CD (1954) The armadillo (*Dasypus novemcinctus*). A review of its natural history, ecology, anatomy, and reproductive physiology. The Rice Institute Pamphlet Monograph in Biology. 41(2):1–135 Rice Institute, Huston
120. Kirchheimer WF, Sanchez RM (1976) Quantitative aspects of leprosy in armadillos. Int J Lepr Other Mycobact Dis 44:84
121. Truman RW, Sanchez RM (1993) Armadillos: models for leprosy. Lab Anim 22:28
122. Truman RW (2008) Leprosy. In: Vizcaino SF, Loughry WJ (eds) The biology of Xenarthra. University Press of Florida, Gainesville, p 111
123. Mira MT, Alcaïs A, Nguyen VT et al (2004) Susceptibility to leprosy is associated with PARK2 and PACR6. Nature 427:636
124. Alter A, Grant A, Abel L et al (2011) Leprosy as a genetic disease. Mamm Genome 22:19
125. Adams LB, Pena MT, Sharma R et al (2012) Insights from animal models on the immunogenetics of leprosy: a review. Mem Inst Oswaldo Cruz 107(Suppl 1):197
126. Binford CH, Meyers WM, Walsh GP et al (1977) Naturally acquired leprosy-like disease in the nine-banded armadillo (*Dasypus novemcinctus*): histopathologic and microbiologic studies of tissues. J Reticuloendothel Soc 22:377
127. Rosa PS, Belone AF, Silva EA (2005) Mitsuda reaction in armadillo *Dasypus novemcinctus* using human and armadillo derived antigens. Hansen Int 30:180

128. Badger LF (1955) Leprosy in the United States. Public Health Rep 70:525
129. Zumarraga MJ, Resoagli EH, Cicuta ME et al (2001) PCR-restriction fragment length polymorphism analysis (PRA) of *Mycobacterium leprae* from human lepromas and from a natural case of an armadillo of Corrientes, Argentina. Int J Lepr Other Mycobact Dis 69:21
130. Deps PD, Antunes JM, Tomimori-Yamashita J (2007) Detection of *Mycobacterium leprae* infection in wild nine-banded armadillos (*Dasypus novemcinctus*) using the rapid ML Flow test. Rev Soc Bras Med Trop 40:86
131. Deps PD, Antunes JM, Faria C et al (2008) Research regarding anti-PGL-I antibodies by ELISA in wild armadillos from Brazil. Rev Soc Bras Med Trop 41(Suppl 2):73
132. Frota CC, Lima LN, Rocha Ada S et al (2012) *Mycobacterium leprae* in six-banded (*Euphractus sexcinctus*) and nine-banded armadillos (*Dasypus novemcinctus*) in Northeast Brazil. Mem Inst Oswaldo Cruz 107(Suppl 1):209
133. Cardona-Castro N, Beltrán JC, Ortiz-Bernal A et al (2009) Detection of *Mycobacterium leprae* DNA in nine-banded armadillos (*Dasypus novemcinctus*) from the Andean region of Colombia. Lepr Rev 80:424
134. Amezcua ME, Escobar-Gutiérrez A, Storrs EE et al (1984) Wild Mexican armadillo with leprosy-like infection. Int J Lepr Other Mycobact Dis 52:254
135. Colleen M, McDonough CM (2000) Social organization of nine-banded armadillos (*Dasypus novemcinctus*) in a Riparian habitat. Am Midl Nat 144:139
136. Lisa N-T, Jose Luis M, Adrian T et al (2003) Wildlife survival beyond park boundaries: the impact of slash-and-burn agriculture and hunting on mammals in Tambopata, Peru. Conserv Biol 4:1106
137. Pattyn SR, Persi A (1990) Microbiologia. In: Nunzi E, Leiker DL (eds) Manuale di leprologia. O.C.S.I., Bologna, p 7
138. Draper P (1982) The anatomy of mycobacteria. In: Rutledge C, Stanford J (eds) The biology of the mycobacteria. Academic Press, London, p 9
139. Rees RJW (1994) The microbiology of leprosy. In: Hastings RC (ed) Leprosy. Churchill Livingstone, Edinburgh, p 31
140. Nishiura M, Okada S, Izumi S et al (1969) An electron microscope study of the band structure of the leprosy bacillus and other mycobacteria. Int J Lepr Other Mycobact Dis 37:225
141. Shepard CC, McRae DH (1965) *Mycobacterium leprae* in mice: minimal infectious dose, relationship between staining quality and infectivity, and effect of cortisone. J Bacteriol 89:365
142. Levy L (1976) Studies of the mouse foot pad technique for cultivation of *Mycobacterium leprae*. 3. Doubling time during logarithmic multiplication. Lepr Rev 47:103
143. Rees RJ (1971) The impact of experimental human leprosy in the mouse on leprosy research. Int J Lepr Other Mycobact Dis 39:201
144. Storrs EE (1971) The nine-banded armadillo: a model for leprosy and other biomedical research. Int J Lepr Other Mycobact Dis 39:703
145. Shepard CC (1965) Temperature optimum of *Mycobacterium leprae* in mice. J Bacteriol 90:1271
146. Draper P (1982) Bacteriology of *Mycobacterium leprae*: state of the art paper. Ann Microbiol (Paris) 133:13
147. Brennan PJ, Barrow WW (1980) Evidence for species-specific lipid antigens in *Mycobacterium leprae*. Int J Lepr Other Mycobact Dis 48:382
148. Hunter SW, Brennan PJ (1981) A novel phenolic glycolipid from *Mycobacterium leprae* possibly involved in immunogenicity and pathogenicity. J Bacteriol 147:728
149. Payne SN, Draper P, Rees RJ (1982) Serological activity of purified glycolipid from *Mycobacterium leprae*. Int J Lepr Other Mycobact Dis 50:220
150. Brett SJ, Draper P, Payne SN et al (1983) Serological activity of a characteristic phenolic glycolipid from *Mycobacterium leprae* in sera from patients with leprosy and tuberculosis. Clin Exp Immunol 52:271

151. Draper P, Payne SN, Dobson G et al (1983) Isolation of a characteristic phthiocerol demycocerosate from *Mycobacterium leprae*. J Gen Microbiol 129:859
152. Waters MF, Rees RJ (1962) Changes in the morphology of *Mycobacterium leprae* in patients under treatment. Int J Lepr 30:266
153. Ridley DS (1971) The SFG (solid, fragmented, granular) index for bacterial morphology. Lepr Rev 42:96
154. Wheeler PR, Damiani G (1990) Biochimica del *Mycobacterium leprae*. In: Nunzi E, Leiker DL (eds) Manuale di leprologia. O.C.S.I., Bologna, p 13
155. Khanolkar SR (1982) Preliminary studies of the metabolic activity of purified suspensions of *Mycobacterium leprae*. J Gen Microbiol 128:423
156. Rees RJ (1964) The significance of the lepromin reaction in man. In: Kallós P, Waksman BH (eds) Progress in allergy. Vol. 8, Chem Immunol Allergy. Karger, Basel, p 224
157. World Health Organization Memorandum (1979) Recommended safety requirements for the preparation of lepromin. Bull WHO 13:88
158. Dharmendra (1941) The active principle of lepromin is a protein antigen of the bacillus. Lepr India 13:89
159. Dharmendra (1942) Immunological skin tests in leprosy. Indian J Med Res 30:1
160. Weddell G, Palmer E (1963) The pathogenesis of leprosy. An experimental approach. Lepr Rev 34:57
161. Pedley JC (1970) Composite skin contact smears: a method of demonstrating the non-emergence of *Mycobacterium leprae* from intact lepromatous skin. Lepr Rev 41:31
162. Job CK, Jayakumar J, Aschhoff M (1999) "Large numbers" of *Mycobacterium leprae* are discharged from the intact skin of lepromatous patients; a preliminary report. Int J Lepr Other Mycobact Dis 67:164
163. Schaffer (1898) Uber die Verbreitung der Lepra bazillen von den oberon Luftwegen aus (The spread of leprosy bacilli from the upper parts of the respiratory tract). Arch Dermatol Syphilis (Berlin) 44:159
164. Pedley JC (1973) The nasal mucus in leprosy. Lepr Rev 44:33
165. Pedley JC (1967) The presence of *M. leprae* in human milk. Lepr Rev 38:239
166. Khanolkar VR (1955) Perspectives in pathology of leprosy. Indian J Med Sci 9:1
167. Wedded AGH, Palmer E, Reas RJW et al (1963) Experimental observations related to histopathology of leprosy. In: CIBA Foundation Study Group No. 15 (ed) The pathogenesis of leprosy. J and A Churchill Ltd, London, p 3
168. Cochrane RG (1947) A practical text-book of leprosy. Oxford University Press, London
169. Shepard CC, Walker LL, Van Landingham RM et al (1982) Sensitization or tolerance to *Mycobacterium leprae* antigen by route of injection. Infect Immun 38:673
170. Rees RJ, McDougall AC (1977) Airborne infection with *Mycobacterium leprae* in mice. J Med Microbiol 10:63
171. Leiker DL (1977) On the mode of transmission of *Mycobacterium leprae*. Lepr Rev 48:9
172. Godal T, Negassi K (1973) Subclinical infection in leprosy. Br Med J 3:557
173. Abe M, Minagawa F, Yoshino Y et al (1980) Fluorescent leprosy antibody absorption (FLA-ABS) test for detecting subclinical infection with *Mycobacterium leprae*. Int J Lepr Other Mycobact Dis 48:109
174. Zuniga M, Castellazziz Z, Lambert P et al (1982) Immunoprophylaxis in contacts of leprosy endemic area. Preliminary results. Paper presented at Pan American Center for Research and Training in Leprosy and Tropical Diseases, CEPIALET, Caracas, 29–30 April 1982
175. Noordeen SK (1985) The epidemiology of leprosy. In: Hastings RC (ed) Leprosy. Churchill Livingstone, Edinburgh, p 15
176. Montestruc E, Berdonneau R (1954) Two new cases of leprosy in infants in Martinique. Bull Soc Pathol Exot Filiales 47:781
177. National Communicable Disease Center (1970) US Department of Health Education and Welfare/Public Health Service 1970 Leprosy Surveillance. January 1970, Report No 1
178. Bechelli LM (1936) O tempo de incubação da lepora. Rip Brasil Lepr 4:355

179. Prasad KUN, Ali PM (1967) Incubation period of leprosy. Indian J Med Res 55:29
180. Hansen GHA (1874) Undersogelser angraaende spedalskhedens aasager. Nor Mag Laegervidenskaben (Suppl) 4:1
181. Hansen GHA (1875) On the etiology of leprosy. Chirurg Rev 55:459
182. Bowne SG (1985) The history of leprosy. In: Hastings RC (ed) Leprosy. Churchill Livingstone, Edinburgh, p 15
183. Tram E, Liftmann J (1908) Derivate des *p*-nitrophenols. Berichte Deutsche Chemischen Gesellschaft 21:2264
184. Faget GH, Pogge RC, Johansen FA et al (1943) The Promin treatment of leprosy. Public Health Rep 58:1729
185. Browne SG, Hogerzeil LM (1962) "B 633" in the treatment of leprosy. Lepr Rev 33:6
186. World Health Organization (1982) Chemotherapy of leprosy for control programmes. World Health Organization, Technicall Report Series 675
187. Lara CB, Falasco JO (1956) Self-healing or abortive and residual forms of childhood leprosy and their probable significance. Int J Lepr 24:245
188. Noordeen SK (1975) Evolution of tuberculoid leprosy in a community. Lepr India 47:85
189. Giunto RS, Doull JA, de Guia L et al (1954) Mortality of persons with leprosy prior to sulfone therapy, Cordova and Dalisay, Cebu, Philippines. Int J Lepr 22:273
190. Noordeen SK (1972) Mortality in leprosy. Indian J Med Res 60:439
191. Monot M, Honoré N, Garnier T et al (2009) Comparative genomic and phylogeographic analysis of *Mycobacterium leprae*. Nat Genet 41:1282
192. Schurr E, Alcaïs A, de Léséleuc L et al (2006) Genetic predisposition to leprosy: a major gene reveals novel pathways of immunity to *Mycobacterium leprae*. Semin Immunol 18:404
193. Sauer ME, Salomão H, Ramos GB et al (2016) Genetics of leprosy: expected- and unexpected-developments and perspectives. Clin Dermatol 34:96
194. Mazini PS, Alves HV, Reis PG et al (2016) Gene association with leprosy: a review of published data. Front Immunol 6:658
195. Schields ED, Russel DA, Pericak-Vance MA (1987) Genetic epidemiology of the susceptibility to leprosy. Clin Invest 79:1139
196. Mohamed AP, Ramanujan K (1966) Leprosy in twins. Int J Lepr Other Mycobact Dis 34:405
197. Chakravartti MR, Vogel F (1973) A twin study on leprosy. In: Becker PE, Lenz W, Vogel F et al (eds) Topics in human genetics, vol 1. Georg Thieme Publishers, Stuttgart, p 1
198. Prado Montes de Oca E (2011) Human polymorphisms as clinical predictors in leprosy. J Trop Med 2011:923943
199. Fava VM, Mira MT (2012) Genetics of leprosy. In: Nunzi E, Massone C (eds) Leprosy: a practical guide. Springer, Milan, p 19
200. Shankarkumar U (2004) HLA associations in leprosy patients from Mumbai, India. Lepr Rev 75:79
201. Cardoso CC, Pereira AC, de Sales Marques C et al (2011) Leprosy susceptibility: genetic variations regulate innate and adaptive immunity, and disease outcome. Future Microbiol 6:533
202. Misch EA, Berrington WR, Vary JC Jr et al (2010) Leprosy and the human genome. Microbiol Mol Biol Rev 74:589
203. Cardoso CC, Pereira AC, Brito-de-Souza VN et al (2011) TNF -308G>A single nucleotide polymorphism is associated with leprosy among Brazilians: a genetic epidemiology assessment, meta-analysis, and functional study. J Infect Dis 204:1256
204. Alcaïs A, Alter A, Antoni G et al (2007) Stepwise replication identifies a low-producing lymphotoxin-alpha allele as a major risk factor for early-onset leprosy. Nat Genet 39:517
205. Hagge DA, Saunders BM, Ebenezer GJ et al (2009) Lymphotoxin-alpha and TNF have essential but independent roles in the evolution of the granulomatous response in experimental leprosy. Am J Pathol 174:1379
206. Mira MT (2006) Genetic host resistance and susceptibility to leprosy. Microbes Infect 8:1124
207. Ishida H, Hastings R, Thompson-Snipes L et al (1993) Modified immunological status of anti-IL-10 treated mice. Cell Immunol 148:371

208. Malhotra D, Darvishi K, Lohra M et al (2006) Association study of major risk single nucleotide polymorphisms in the common regulatory region of PARK2 and PACRG genes with leprosy in an Indian population. Eur J Hum Genet 14:438
209. Misch EA, Hawn TR (2008) Toll-like receptor polymorphisms and susceptibility to human disease. Clin Sci (Lond) 114:347
210. Bochud PY, Sinsimer D, Aderem A et al (2009) Polymorphisms in Toll-like receptor 4 (TLR4) are associated with protection against leprosy. Eur J Clin Microbiol Infect Dis 28:1055
211. Sousa AL, Fava VM, Sampaio LH et al (2012) Genetic and immunological evidence implicates interleukin 6 as a susceptibility gene for leprosy type 2 reaction. J Infect Dis 205:1417
212. Nath I, Saini C, Valluri VL (2015) Immunology of leprosy and diagnostic challenges. Clin Dermatol 33:90
213. de Souza VN, Iyer AM, Lammas DA et al (2016) Advances in leprosy immunology and the field application: a gap to bridge. Clin Dermatol 34:82
214. Naafs B (2000) Current views on reactions in leprosy. Indian J Lepr 72:97
215. Verhagen C, Faber W, Klatser P et al (1999) Immunohistological analysis of *in situ* expression of mycobacterial antigens in skin lesions of leprosy patients across the histopathological spectrum. Association of mycobacterial lipoarabinomannan (LAM) and *Mycobacterium leprae* phenolic glycolipid-I (PGL-I) with leprosy reactions. Am J Pathol 154:1793
216. Modlin RL (2010) The innate immune response in leprosy. Curr Opin Immunol 22:48
217. Cho SN, Yanagihara DL, Hunter SW et al (1983) Serological specificity of phenolic glycolipid-I from *Mycobacterium leprae* and use in serodiagnosis of leprosy. Infect Immun 41:1077
218. Lipscomb MF, Masten BJ (2002) Dendritic cells: immune regulators in health and disease. Physiol Rev 82:97
219. Harrington LE, Mangan PR, Weaver CT (2006) Expanding the effector CD4 T-cell repertoire: the Th17 lineage. Curr Opin Immunol 18:349
220. Attia EA, Abdallah M, Saad AA et al (2010) Circulating CD4+ CD25 high FoxP3+ T cells vary in different clinical forms of leprosy. Int J Dermatol 49:1152
221. Kumar S, Naqvi RA, Ali R et al (2013) CD4+CD25+ T regs with acetylated FoxP3 are associated with immune suppression in human leprosy. Mol Immunol 56:513
222. Bührer-Sékula S, Smits HL, Gussenhoven GC et al (2003) Simple and fast lateral flow test for classification of leprosy patients and identification of contacts with high risk of developing leprosy. J Clin Microbiol 41:1991
223. Brett SJ, Payne SN, Draper P et al (1984) Analysis of the major antigenic determinants of the characteristic phenolic glycolipid from *Mycobacterium leprae*. Clin Exp Immunol 56:89
224. Fujiwara T, Hunter SW, Cho SN et al (1984) Chemical synthesis and serology of disaccharides and trisaccharides of phenolic glycolipid antigen from the leprosy bacillus and preparation of a disaccharide protein conjugate for serodiagnosis of leprosy. Infect Immunol 43:245
225. Fujiwara T, Aspinall GO, Hunter SW et al (1987) Chemical synthesis of the trisaccharide unit of the species-specific phenolic glycolipid from *Mycobacterium leprae*. Carbohydr Res 163:41
226. Fujiwara T, Aspinall GO, Hunter SW et al (1986) Chemical synthesis of the disaccharides of the specific phenolic glycolipid antigenes from *Mycobacterium leprae* and of the related sugars. Carbohydr Res 148:287
227. Lefford MJ, Hunegnaw M, Siwik E (1991) The value of IgM antibodies to PGL-I in the diagnosis of leprosy. Int J Lepr Other Mycobact Dis 59:432
228. Smith PG (1992) The serodiagnosis of leprosy. Lepr Rev 63:97
229. Cho SN, Cellona RV, Fajardo TT Jr et al (1991) Detection of phenolic glycolipid-I antigen and antibody in sera from new and relapsed lepromatous patients treated with various drug regimens. Int J Lepr Other Mycobact Dis 59:25
230. Oskam L, Slim E, Bührer-Sékula S (2003) Serology: recent developments, strengths, limitations and prospects: a state of the art overview. Lepr Rev 74:196
231. Lospalluti M, Angelini G, Meneghini CL (1972) Observations sur les réactions cutaneés du type immunologique différé à divers allergènes dans un groupe de sujets lépromateux. Acta Leprol 135:48

232. Meneghini CL, Angelini G, Lospalluti M et al (1974) Cutaneous responses to irritants and microbial antigens in lepromatous patients. Trans St John's Hosp Derm Soc 60:91
233. Yamamura M (1992) Defining protective responses to pathogens: cytokine profiles in leprosy lesions. Science 255:12
234. Martiniuk F, Giovinazzo J, Tan AU et al (2012) Lessons of leprosy: the emergence of TH17 cytokines during type II reactions (ENL) is teaching us about T-cell plasticity. J Drugs Dermatol 11:626
235. Saini C, Ramesh V, Nath I (2013) CD4+ Th17 cells discriminate clinical types and constitute a third subset of non Th1, non Th2 T cells in human leprosy. PLoS Negl Trop Dis 7:e2338
236. Palermo ML, Pagliari C, Trindade MA et al (2012) Increased expression of regulatory T cells and down-regulatory molecules in lepromatous leprosy. Am J Trop Med Hyg 86:878
237. Geluk A, Klein MR, Franken KL et al (2005) Postgenomic approach to identify novel *Mycobacterium leprae* antigens with potential to improve immunodiagnosis of infection. Infect Immunol 73:5636
238. Geluk A, Bobosha K, van der Ploeg-van Schip JJ et al (2012) New biomarkers with relevance to leprosy diagnosis applicable in areas hyperendemic for leprosy. J Immunol 188:4782
239. Martins MV, Guimarães MM, Spencer JS et al (2012) Pathogen-specific epitopes as epidemiological tools for defining the magnitude of *Mycobacterium leprae* transmission in areas endemic for leprosy. PLoS Negl Trop Dis 6:e1616
240. Bobosha K, Tang ST, van der Ploeg-van Schip JJ et al (2012) *Mycobacterium leprae* virulence-associated peptides are indicators of exposure to *M. leprae* in Brazil, Ethiopia and Nepal. Mem Inst Oswaldo Cruz 107(Suppl 1):112
241. Duthie MS, Goto W, Ireton GC et al (2007) Use of protein antigens for early serological diagnosis of leprosy. Clin Vaccine Immunol 14:1400
242. Hungria EM, Oliveira RM, Souza AL et al (2012) Seroreactivity to new *Mycobacterium leprae* protein antigens in different leprosy-endemic regions in Brazil. Mem Inst Oswaldo Cruz 107(Suppl 1):104
243. Iyer A, Hatta M, Usman R et al (2007) Serum levels of interferon-gamma, tumour necrosis factor-alpha, soluble interleukin-6R and soluble cell activation markers for monitoring response to treatment of leprosy reactions. Clin Exp Immunol 150:210
244. Moubasher AD, Kamel NA, Zedan H et al (1998) Cytokines in leprosy. I. Serum cytokine profile in leprosy. Int J Dermatol 37:733
245. Laal S, Bhutani LK, Nath I (1985) Natural emergence of antigen-reactive T cells in lepromatous leprosy patients during erythema nodosum leprosum. Infect Immunol 50:887
246. Moraes MO, Duppre NC, Suffys PN et al (2001) Tumor necrosis factor-alpha promoter polymorphism TNF2 is associated with a stronger delayed-type hypersensitivity reaction in the skin of borderline tuberculoid leprosy patients. Immunogenetics 53:45
247. Narayanan RB, Bhutani LK, Sharma AK et al (1983) T cell subsets in leprosy lesions: *in situ* characterization using monoclonal antibodies. Clin Exp Immunol 51:421
248. Moraes MO, Sarno EN, Almeida AS et al (1999) Cytokine mRNA expression in leprosy: a possible role for interferon-gamma and interleukin-12 in reactions (RR and ENL). Scand J Immunol 50:541
249. Kaplan G, Mathur NK, Job CK et al (1989) Effect of multiple interferon gamma injections on the disposal of *Mycobacterium leprae*. Proc Natl Acad Sci U S A 86:8073
250. Spierings E, De Boer T, Zulianello L et al (2000) Novel mechanisms in the immunopathogenesis of leprosy nerve damage: the role of Schwann cells, T cells and *Mycobacterium leprae*. Immunol Cell Biol 78:349
251. Oliveira RB, Ochoa MT, Sieling PA et al (2003) Expression of Toll-like receptor 2 on human Schwann cells: a mechanism of nerve damage in leprosy. Infect Immunol 71:1427
252. Job CK (1971) Pathology of peripheral nerve lesions in lepromatous leprosy. A light and electron microscopic study. Int J Lepr Other Mycobact Dis 39:251
253. Rambukkana A (2004) *Mycobacterium leprae*-induced demyelinization: a model for early nerve degeneration. Curr Opin Immunol 16:511

254. Naafs B, Dagne T (1977) Sensory testing: a sensitive method in the follow-up of nerve involvement. Int J Lepr 45:364
255. Meyers WM (1990) Istopatologia. In: Nunzi E, Leiker DL (eds) Manuale di leprologia. O.C.S.I., Bologna, p 87
256. Massone C, Belachew WA, Schettini A (2015) Histopathology of the lepromatous skin biopsy. Clin Dermatol 33:38
257. Singh A, Weng X, Nath I (2011) Skin biopsy in leprosy. In: Khopkar U (ed) Skin biopsy—perspectives. In Tech, Rijeka, Croatia, p 73
258. Riddley DS (1977) Skin biopsy in leprosy. Ciba-Geigy, Basel, p 63
259. Massone C (2012) Histopatholgy of the skin. In: Nunzi E, Massone C (eds) Leprosy. A practical guide. Spriger, Berlin, p 115
260. Pradeep NS, Nanda KG (2013) A clinical and histopathological study of histoid leprosy. Int J Dermatol 52:580
261. Magaña M (2012) Lucio-Latapi leprosy. In: Nunzi E, Massone C (eds) Leprosy. A practical guide. Spriger, Berlin, p 111
262. Magaña M (2012) Lucio's phenomenon. In: Nunzi E, Massone C (eds) Leprosy. A practical guide. Spriger, Berlin, p 241
263. Klatser PR, Cardo PP (1990) Esami sierologici. In: Nunzi E, Leiker DL (eds) Manuale di leprologia. O.C.S.I., Bologna, p 103
264. Britton WJ, Lockwood DN (2004) Leprosy. Lancet 363:1209
265. Talhari C, Talhari S, Penna GO (2015) Clinical aspects of leprosy. Clin Dermatol 33:26
266. Pereira AC Jr, Do Nascimento LV (1982) Indeterminate Hansen's disease. Med Cutan Ibero Lat Am 10:159
267. Sehgal VN, Srivastava G (1987) Indeterminate leprosy. A passing phase in the evolution of leprosy. Lepr Rev 58:291
268. Walker SL, Lockwood DN (2007) Leprosy. Clin Dermatol 25:165
269. Schaller KF (1971) Differential diagnosis of leprosy. Int J Lepr Other Mycobact Dis 39:447
270. Mahé A (1996) Leprosy differential diagnosis in 1996. Acta Leprol 10:69
271. Meneghini CL, Angelini G (1972) Sur un cas de lèpre tuberculoïde: contagion par le conjoint attent de lèpre lepromateuse. Acta Leprol 48–49:187
272. Meneghini CL, Angelini G, Lospalluti M (1986) Hansen's disease in children. Pediatric Dermatol News 5:162
273. Bechelli LM, Pagnano PM (1990) Reflections on some aspects of leprosy among children in Brazil and in other countries. Acta Leprol 7:229
274. Cortés SL, Rodriguez G (2004) Leprosy in children: association between clinical and pathological aspects. J Trop Pediatr 50:12
275. Rollier R, Rollier B (1986) Clinical and developmental aspects of lepromatous leprosy. Acta Leprol 4:193
276. Brazin SA (1982) Leprosy (Hansen's disease). Otolaryngol Clin N Am 15:597
277. Pollack JD, Pincus RL, Lucente FE (1987) Leprosy of the head and neck. Otolaryngol Hed Neck Surg 97:93
278. Uplekar MW, Antia NH (1986) Clinical and histopathological observations on pure neuritic leprosy. Indian J Lepr 58:513
279. Gabino JA, Naafs B (2012) Primary neural leprosy. In: Nunzi E, Massone C (eds) Leprosy. A practical guide. Springer, Milan
280. Wade HW (1963) The histoid variety of lepromatous leprosy. Int J Lepr 31:129
281. Latapi F, Zamora AC (1948) The spotted leprosy of Lucio: an introduction to its clinical and histopathological study. Int J Lepr 16:421
282. Azulay-Abulafia L, Spinelli L (2005) Revisiting Lucio's leprosy and Lucio's phenomenon. Med Cutan Ibero Lat Am 33:125
283. Azulay-Abulafia L, Pereira Spinelli L et al (2006) Lucio's phenomenon. Vasculitis or occlusive vasculopathy? Hautarzt 57:1101
284. Magaña M, Fernández-Diez J, Magaña ML (2008) Lucio's phenomenon is a necrotizing panvasculitis: mostly a medium-sized granulomatous arteritis. Am J Dermopathol 30:555

285. Jurado F, Rodriguez O, Novales J et al (2015) Lucio's leprosy: a clinical and therapeutic challenge. Clin Dermatol 33:66
286. Lucio R, Alvarado I (1852) Opuscolo sobre el mal de San Lazaro o elefanciasis de los Griecos. M. Murguia y Cia, Mexico
287. Rodriguez O (1978) Lepra de Lucio. I. Historia y concepto. Dermatol Rev Mex 22:117
288. Leprosy reported by World Heart Organization. www.who.int/entity/lep/situation/latestdata/en2012
289. Han XY, Seo YH, Sizer KC et al (2008) A new mycobacterium species causing diffuse lepromatous leprosy. Am J Clin Pathol 130:856
290. Han XY, Sizer KC, Thompson EJ et al (2009) Comparative sequence analysis of *Mycobacterium leprae* and the new leprosy-causing *Mycobacterium lepromatosis*. J Bacteriol 191:6067
291. Vera-Cabrera L, Escalante-Fuentes WG, Gomez-Flores M et al (2011) Case of diffuse lepromatous leprosy associated with *Mycobacterium lepromatosis*. J Clin Microbiol 49:4366
292. Jessamine PG, Desjardins M, Gillis T et al (2012) Leprosy-like illness in a patient with *Mycobacterium lepromatosis* from Ontario. Canada J Drugs Dermatol 119:229
293. Han XY, Sizer KC, Tan HH (2012) Identification of the leprosy agent *Mycobacterium lepromatosis* in Singapore. J Drugs Dermatol 11:168
294. Gillis TP, Scolland DM, Lockwood DN (2011) What is the evidence that putative *Mycobacterium lepromatosis* species causes diffuse lepromatous leprosy? Lepr Rev 82:205
295. Novales J (1978) Lepra de Lucio. III. Aspectos histopathologicos. Dermatol Rev Mex 22:164
296. Fogaguolo L, de Sonza EM, Cintra ML et al (2007) Vasculonecrotic reactions in leprosy. Braz J Infect Dis 11:378
297. Duncan E (2012) Leprosy in pregnancy. In: Nunzi E, Massone C (eds) Leprosy. A practical guide. Springer, Milan, p 331
298. Duncan ME (1980) Babies of mothers with leprosy have small placentae, low birth weights and grow slowly. Br J Obstet Gynaecol 87:471
299. Duncan ME, Pearson JM, Rees RJ et al (1981) The association of pregnancy and leprosy. II. Pregnancy in dapsone-resistant leprosy. Lepr Rev 52:263
300. Lopez MGS, Saad MH, Sarno EN (1993) Leprosy-study of 20 placentas and the repercussion of the newborn. Int J Lepr Other Mycobact Dis 61(Suppl 122A):PA10
301. Duncan ME, Melsom R, Pearson JM et al (1983) A clinical and immunological study of four babies of mothers with lepromatous leprosy, two of whom developed leprosy in infancy. Int J Lepr Other Mycobact Dis 51:7
302. Ponnighans JM, Mwanjasi LJ, Fine PE (1991) Is HIV infection a risk factor for leprosy? Int J Other Mycobact Dis 59:221
303. Talhari C, Mira MT, Massone C et al (2010) Leprosy and HIV coinfection: a clinical, pathological, immunological, and therapeutic study of a cohort from a Brazilian referral center for infections diseases. J Infect Dis 202:345
304. Lawn SD, Wood C, Lockwood DN (2003) Borderline tuberculoid leprosy: an immune reconstitution phenomenon in a human immunodeficiency virus-infected person. Clin Infect Dis 36:e5–e6
305. Couppie P, Abel S, Voinchet H (2004) Immune reconstitution inflammatory syndrome associated with HIV and leprosy. Arch Dermatol 140:997
306. Talhari C, Machado PR, Ferreira LC et al (2007) Shifting of the clinical spectrum of leprosy in an HIV-positive patient: a manifestation of immune recostitution inflammatory syndrome? Lepr Rev 78:151
307. Talhari C, Matsuo C, Chrusciak-Talhari A et al (2009) Variations in leprosy manifestations among HIV-positive patients, Manaus Brazil. Emerg Infect Dis 15:673
308. Deps P, Lucas S, Porro AM et al (2013) Clinical and histological features of leprosy and human immunodeficiency virus co-infection in Brazil. Clin Exp Dermatol 38:470
309. Naafs B, van Hess CLM (2016) Leprosy type 1 reaction (formerly reversal reaction). Clin Dermatol 34:37
310. Walker SL, Lockwood DN (2008) Leprosy type1 (reversal) reaction and their management. Lepr Rev 79:372

311. Naafs B, Noto S (2012) Reactions in leprosy. In: Nunzi E, Massone C (eds) Leprosy. A practical guide. Springer, Milan, p 219
312. Sung SM, Kobayashi TT (2015) Diagnosis and treatment of leprosy type 1 (reversal) reaction. Cutis 95:222
313. Narayanan RB, Laal S, Sharma AK et al (1984) Differeces in predominant phenotype and distribution pattern in reactional lesions of tuberculoid and lepromatous leprosy. Clin Exp Immunol 55:623
314. Yamamura M, Uyemura K, Deaus RJ et al (1991) Definig protective responses to pathogens: cytokine profiles in leprosy lesions. Science 254:277
315. Yamamura M, Wang LH, Ohmen JD et al (1992) Cytokine patterns of immunologically mediated tissue damage. J Immunol 149:1470
316. Khanolkar-Young S, Rayment N, Brickell PM et al (1995) Tumor necrosis factor alfa (TNFα) synthesis is associated with skin and peripheral nerve pathology of leprosy reversal reaction. Clin Exp Immunol 99:196
317. Iyer AM, Mohanty KK, van Egmond D et al (2007) Leprosy-specific B-cells within cellular infiltrates in active leprosy lesions. Hum Pathol 38:1065
318. Bjune G, Barnetson RSC, Ridley DS et al (1976) Lymphocyte transformation test in leprosy. Correlation of the response with inflammation of the lesions. Clin Exp Immunol 25:85
319. Barnetson RSC, Bjune G, Pearson JMH et al (1975) Antigenic heterogeneity in patients with reactions in borderline leprosy. Br Med J 4:435
320. Shetty VP, Uplekar MW, Autia NH (1994) Immunohistological localization of mycobacterial antigens within the peripheral nerves of treated leprosy patients and their significance to nerve damage in leprosy. Acta Neuropathol 87:300
321. Youmans GP (1975) Relation between delayed type hypersensitivity and immunity in tuberculosis. Ann Rev Respir Dis 111:109
322. Naafs B (1994) Leprosy reactions: new knowledge. Trop Geogr Med 46:80
323. Souza CS, Roselino AM, Figueiredo F et al (2000) Lucio's phenomenon: clinical and therapeutic aspects. Int J Lepr Other Mycobact Dis 68:417
324. Fleury RD (2008) Diffuse lepromatous leprosy and Lucio's phenomenon: focus on new etiology. Hansen Int 33:7
325. Saul A, Novales J (1983) Lucio-Latapi leprosy and Lucio's phenomenon. Acta Leprol 1:115
326. Rea TH, Riddley DS (1979) Lucio's phenomenon. A comparative histological study. Int J Lepr 47:161
327. Rea TH, Jerskey RS (2005) Clinical and histologic variations among thirty patients with Lucio's phenomenon and pure and primitive diffuse lepromatosis (Latapi's lepromatosis). Int J Lepr Other Mycobact Dis 73:169
328. Vargas-Ocampo F (2004) Analysis of 6000 skin biopsies of the National Leprosy Central Program in Mexico. Int J Lepr Other Mycobact Dis 72:427
329. Scollard DM, Truman RW, Ebenezer GJ (2015) Mechanism of nerve injury in leprosy. Clin Dermatol 33:46
330. Raicher I, Stump PR, Baccarelli R et al (2016) Neuropatic pain in leprosy. Clin Dermatol 34:59
331. Garbino JA, Heise CO, Marques W (2016) Assessing nerves in leprosy. Clin Dermatol 34:51
332. Saunderson P (2000) The epidemiology of reactions and nerve damage. Work Shop Proceedings: Leprosy Research at the new Millennium. Lepr Rev 71(Suppl):S106
333. Wolf GI, Trivedi JR (2004) Painful peripheral neuropathy and its non-surgical treatment. Muscle Nerve 30:3
334. Hietaharju A, Croft R, Alan R et al (2000) Chronic neuropathic pain in treated leprosy. Lancet 356:1080
335. Haroun OH, Hietaharju A, Bizuneh E et al (2012) Investigation of neuropathic pain in treated leprosy patients in Ethiopia. A cross-sectional study. Pain 153:1620
336. Dabholkar VR, Gaitonde BB (1982) A study of autonomic functions in leprosy. Lepr India 54:303
337. Pearson JM, Ross WF (1975) Nerve involvement in leprosy-pathology, differential diagnosis and principles of management. Lepr Rev 46:199

338. Flytche TJ (1991) The continuining challenge of ocular leprosy. Br J Ophthalmol 75:123
339. Grzybowski A, Nita M, Virmond M (2015) Ocular leprosy. Clin Dermatol 33:79
340. Citirik M, Batman C, Asian O et al (2005) Lepromatous iridocyclitis. Ocul Immunol Inflamm 13:95
341. Ebemzer GJ, Daniel E (2004) Expression of protein gene product 9.5 in lepromatous eyes showing ciliary body nerve damage and a "dying back" phenomenon in the posterior ciliary nerves. Br J Ophthalmol 88:178
342. Mnogo CE, Bella-Hiag AL, Ellong A et al (2001) Ocular complications of leprosy in Cameroon. Acta Ophthalmol Scand 79:31
343. Singhi MK, Kacchawa D, Ghiya BC (2002) Ocular involvement in leprosy. Indian J Ophthalmol 50:355
344. Lewallen S, Tungpakom NC, Kim SH et al (2000) Progression of eye disease in "cured" leprosy patients: implications for understanding the pathophysiology of ocular disease and for addressing eye care needs. Br J Ophthalmol 84:817
345. Lavilla L, Castillo J, Dominguez AM et al (2009) Surgical treatment of bilateral paralytic lagophthalmos using scapha graft in a case of lepromatous leprosy. Lepr Rev 80:448
346. Font RL, Sobol W, Matoba A (1989) Polychromatic corneal and conjunctival crystals secondary to clofazimine therapy in leper. Ophthalmology 96:311
347. Barot RK, Viswanath V, Pattiwar MS et al (2011) Crystalline deposition in the cornea and conjunctiva secondary to longterm clofazimine therapy in a leprosy patient. Indian J Ophthalmol 59:328
348. Hogeweg M, Keunen JE (2005) Prevention of blindness in leprosy and the role of the Vision 2020 Programme. Eye 19:1099
349. Walton RC, Ball SF, Joffrion VC (1991) Glaucoma in Hansen's disease. Br J Ophthalmol 75:270
350. Azulay RD (1987) Primary visceral virchowian (lepromatous) hanseniasis. Int J Lepr 55:450
351. Clapasson A, Canata S (2012) Laboratory investigations. In: Nunzi E, Massone C (eds) Leprosy. A practical guide. Spriger, Milan, p 55
352. Nunzi E, Massone C, Noto S (2012) Diagnostic work-up. In: Nunzi E, Massone C (eds) Leprosy. A practical guide. Spriger, Milan, p 271
353. Jain S, Visser LH, Suneetha S (2016) Imaging techniques in leprosy clinics. Clin Dermatol 34:70
354. Matthews LVB (1965) Sarcoidosis of the nervous system. J Neurol Neurosurg Psychiatry 28:23
355. Mumo DD, Du Vivier A, Jopling WH (1972) Post-kala-azar dermal leishmaniasis. Br J Dermatol 87:374
356. Desai AC, Bhide MB (1977) Hydnocarpus oil as an anti-leprotic agent in mouse foot-pad technique. Lepr India 49:360
357. Grosset JH (1995) Traitement anti-bactérien dans la lèpre. In: Sansarricq H (ed) La lèpre. Ellipses, p 226
358. Talhari S, Ameen M (2012) Drugs in leprosy. In: Nunzi E, Massone C (eds) Leprosy. A practical guide. Springer, Milan, p 281
359. Kar HK, Gupta R (2015) Treatment of leprosy. Clin Dermatol 33:55
360. Noordeen SK (2016) History of chemotherapy of leprosy. Clin Dermatol 34:32
361. Faget GH (1947) Chemotherapy of leprosy. Int J Lepr 15:7
362. Colman MD (1993) Dapsone: mode of action, toxicity and possible strategies for increasing patient tolerance. Br J Dermatol 129:507
363. Anderson R (1985) Enhancement by clofazimine and inhibition by dapsone of production of prostaglandin E2 by human polymorfonuclear leucocytes *in vitro*. Antimicrob Agents Chemother 27:257
364. Campbell EA, Korzheva N, Mustaev A et al (2011) Structural mechanism for rifampicin inhibition of bacterial RNA polymerase. Cell 104:901
365. Meneghini CL, Trimigliozzi G, Angelini G et al (1970) La rifampicina nel trattamento della lebbra lepromatosa. Osservazioni su 57 casi. Simposi Scientifici Lepetit 28:169
366. Trimigliozzi G, Angelini G, Lospalluti M et al (1973) Rilievi clinico-sperimentali nella lebbra lepromatosa trattata con rifampicina. Ann It Dermatol Cl Sperim 27:261

367. Meneghini CL, Angelini G, Lospalluti M (1987) Lebbra. In: Serri F (ed) Trattato di dermatologia, Vol II, cap 36. Piccin, Padova
368. WHO Study Group (1994) Chemotherapy of leprosy. World Health Organization, Geneva, Technical Report Series no 847
369. Allen HB, Moschella SL (2017) The role of rifampin in leprosy. JAMA Dermatol 8. doi:10.1001/jamadermatol.2016.5506
370. Singh R, Ray P, Das A et al (2010) Penetration of antibiotics through *Staphylococcus aureus* and *Staphylococcus epidermidis* biofilms. J Antimicrob Chemother 65:1955
371. Saunderson PR (2016) Drug-resistant *M. leprae*. Clin Dermatol 34:79
372. Pearson J, Haile G, Rees R (1977) Primary dapsone-resistant leprosy. Lepr Rev 48:129
373. Singh P, Cole ST (2011) *Mycobacterium leprae*: genes, pseudogenes and genetic diversity. Future Mycrobiol 6:57
374. World Health Organization (1982) WHO Technical Report Series 675, Geneva
375. Bobin P (2012) Treatment and prophylaxis. In: Nunzi E, Massone C (eds) Leprosy. A practical guide. Springer, Milan, p 287
376. Grosset JH, Ji B, Guelpa-Lauras CC et al (1990) Clinical trial of pefloxacin and ofloxacin in the treatment of lepromatous leprosy. Int J Lepr 58:281
377. Ji B, Peroni EG, Petinon C et al (1996) Bactericidal activities of combination of news drugs against *M. leprae* in nude mice. Antimicrob Agents Chemother 40:393
378. Girdhar BK, Girdhar A. Short course treatment of leprosy: present status. Avaible at http://icmr.nic.in/bufeb02.pdf
379. Leprosy-new drug regimens. http://www.who.int/tdr/research/progress/9900/methods-treatment/en/index5.html
380. Brandsma JW (2016) Rehabilitation of leprosy-affected people: an overview. Clin Dermatol 34:66
381. Sharma P, Kar HK, Misra RS (2000) Reactional states and neuritis in multibacillary patients following MDT with/without immunotherapy with *Mw* anti-leprosy vaccine. Lepr Rev 71:193
382. Gupte MD, Vallishayee RS, Anantharan DS et al (1998) Comparative leprosy vaccine trial in South India. Indian J Lepr 70:369
383. Truoc LV, Ly HM, Thuy NK et al (2001) Vaccination against leprosy at Ben San Leprosy Centre, Ho Chi Minh City, Vietnam. Vaccine 19:3451
384. Setia MS, Steinmaus C, Ho CS et al (2006) The role of BCG in prevention of leprosy: a meta-analysis. Lancet Infect Dis 6:162
385. Zodpey SP (2007) Protective effect of bacillus Calmette-Guérin (BCG) vaccine in the prevention of leprosy: a meta-analysis. Indian J Dermatol Venereol Leprol 73:86
386. Duppre NC, Camacho LA, da Cunha SS et al (2008) Effectiveness of BCG vaccination among leprosy contacts: a cohort study. Trans R Soc Trop Med Hyg 102:631
387. Pannikar V (2009) Enhanced global strategy for further reducing the disease burden due to leprosy: 2011–2015. Lepr Rev 80:353
388. Smith C, Richardus JH (2008) Leprosy strategy is about control, not eradication. Lancet 371:969
389. Rodriguez LC, Lockwood DN (2011) Leprosy now: epidemiology, progress, challenges, and research gaps. Lancet Infect Dis 11:464
390. Fischer EA, de Vlas SJ, Habbema JD et al (2011) The long-term effect of current and new interventions on the new case detection of leprosy: a modeling study. PLoS Negl Trop Dis 5:e1330
391. Oskan L, Slim E, Buhrer-Sekula S (2003) Serology: recent developments, strengths, limitations and prospects: a state of the art overview. Lepr Rev 74:196
392. Moura RS, Calado KL, Oliveira ML et al (2008) Leprosy serology using PGL-I; a systemic review. Rev Soc Bras Med Trop 41(Suppl 2):11

Nontuberculous Mycobacteria and Skin Infection

6

Domenico Bonamonte, Pietro Verni, and Gianni Angelini

The current high level of interest in disease induced by nontuberculous mycobacteria (NTM) is due not only to the frequent association with AIDS, but also to the strong evidence of pulmonary and extrapulmonary diseases in the general population [1–12]. Moreover, NTM infections are emerging in previously unreported sectors, and exhibiting new clinical manifestations. Undoubtedly, the increased evidence of the disease is also attributable to methodological improvements in mycobacteriology laboratories, that have enabled the isolation and rapid, accurate identification of the various species and the clinical characteristics of some peculiar clinical pictures [7].

6.1 Taxonomy

Mycobacteria other than the *Mycobacterium tuberculosis* complex and *M. leprae*, here referred to as NTM, are rife in the environment and have been known, in part, since the discovery of the tubercle bacillus in the late 1800s. These microorganisms were previously given a variety of names, such as "atypical", "anonymous", "mycobacteria other than tuberculosis", "environmental", "environmental opportunistic", and, most commonly, "nontuberculous mycobacteria". Various species of these NTM have been associated with many diseases since the 1930s and 1940s [13, 14].

D. Bonamonte, MD, PhD (✉)
Department of Biomedical Science and Human Oncology, University of Bari "Aldo Moro", Bari, Italy
e-mail: domenico.bonamonte@uniba.it

P. Verni, MD
University of Bari "Aldo Moro", Bari, Italy

G. Angelini, MD
Professor of Dermatology, Former Professor and Chairman, University of Bari "Aldo Moro", Bari, Italy

D. Bonamonte, G. Angelini (eds.), *Mycobacterial Skin Infections*,
DOI 10.1007/978-3-319-48538-6_6

Currently, more than 170 NTM species have been cataloged: a comprehensive list of all validated NTM species can be found online at www.bacterio.net/mycobacterium.html. Thanks to the improved microbiological techniques for the isolation of NTM, and in particular to molecular techniques and the development of 16S rRNA gene sequencing in order to define new species, there has recently been a dramatic increase in the total number of mycobacteria, as well as the number of clinical significant species [7]. The American Thoracic Society and the Infections Disease Society of America issued a joint document on this topic in 2007: "An official ATS/IDSA statement: diagnosis, treatment, and prevention of nontuberculous mycobacterial diseases" [7]. Various other not-for-profit foundations have been established for further research into NTM diseases [9].

Mycobacterial taxonomy has changed since DNA sequencing became readily available: the mycobacterial 16S rRNA gene was shown to be highly conserved, and differences in the sequence by 1% or more generally indicated a new species [15, 16].

Four groups of human pathogens are recognized to belong to the *Mycobacterium* genus: the *M. tuberculosis* complex, *M. leprae*, slowly growing NTM, and rapidly growing species. NTM were classified by Runyon according to their growth rate and pigment formation (Tables 6.1 and 6.2) [17]. Types I, II, and III, slow growers, take 7 or more days to grow and are told apart by their coloration. If the pigment is produced only on exposure to light, they are photochromogens (type I); if pigment is produced even in the dark, they are scotochromogens (type II); if they are not

Table 6.1 Classification of nontuberculous mycobacteria according to Runyon (modified, by [9])

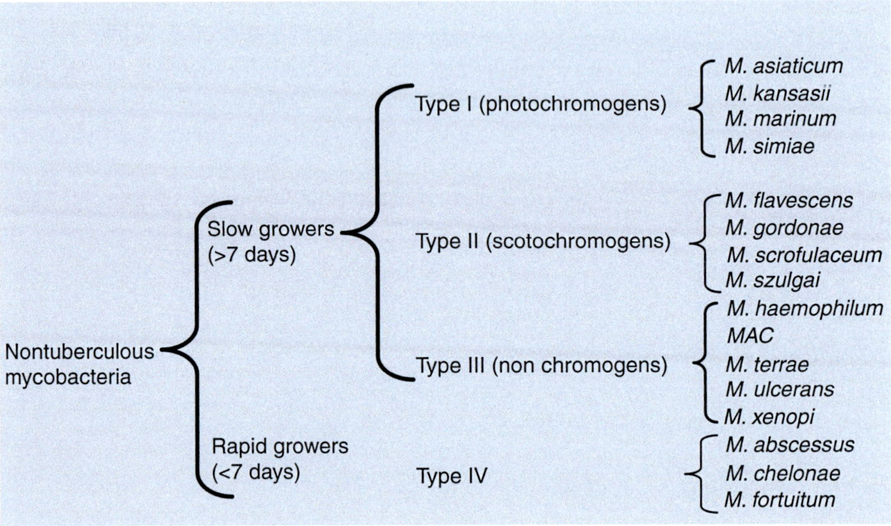

Table 6.2 Differential characteristics of some nontuberculous mycobacteria of dermatological interest

Mycobacterium	Optimal temperature (°C)	Growth speed (days)	Pigmentation light	Pigmentation dark	Pigment formation	Type
M. abscessus	28	3–7				IV
M. asiaticum	37	15–21	G	M	Photochromogen	I
M. avium complex	37	10–21	M-G	M-G	Nonchromogen	III
M. chelonae	28–35	3–7	M	M		IV
M. flavescens	37	7–10	G	G	Scotochromogen	II
M. fortuitum	28	3–7	M	M		IV
M. gordonae	37	10–25	G	G	Scotochromogen	II
M. haemophilum	30	14–28	GR	GR	Nonchromogen	III
M. kansasii	37	10–21	G	M	Photochromogen	I
M. marinum	30	5–14	G	M	Photochromogen	I
M. scrofulaceum	37	10–14	G	G	Scotochromogen	II
M. simiae	37	7–14	G	M	Photochromogen	I
M. szulgai	37	14–28	G	G	Scotochromogen	II
M. terrae	37	10–21	M	M	Nonchromogen	III
M. ulcerans	32	10–28	M	M	Nonchromogen	III
M. xenopi	42	28–40	G	G	Nonchromogen	III

M brown, *G* yellow, *GR* gray

strongly pigmented, they are nonphotochromogens (type III). Rapid grower mycobacteria (RGM) grow in less than 7 days but more slowly than most other bacteria. Species identification is of course recommended in all cases, also and above all to guide treatment selection [9].

6.2 Epidemiology

NTM are widely distributed in the environment, demonstrated by high isolation rates worldwide [18, 19]. NTM can be found in soil and water, including both natural and treated water sources. Using the same methods, environmental mycobacteria isolates have been shown to be the same in different geographic areas [18, 19]. NTM have been found in coastal swamps and adjoining streams and in forests, especially those with a lot of peat. Most recently, NTM have also been demonstrated in substantial concentrations in biofilms takes from shower-heads [20]. Health risks associated with NTM in shower-heads have still to be fully elucidated; nevertheless, some authors have suggested that shower usage may be "contraindicated in persons with compromised immune or pulmonary systems" [20]. Some NTM, such as *M. kansasii*, *M. xenopi*, and *M. simiae*, are present almost exclusively in municipal water sources and rarely, if ever, in other environmental sources [7].

There is no evidence of animal-to-human or human-to-human transmission of NTM [21–23], nor has it been observed even in subjects with cystic fibrosis, although this population is highly susceptible to opportunistic infections [24]. In man the infection is invariably contracted from the environment, even if the source is not always known [25]. NTM can induce both asymptomatic infection in humans, as demonstrated by both antibody and skin tests studies, and symptomatic infection. Skin tests studies in adults indicate that a large percentage of them had presumably contracted an asymptomatic NTM infection at an earlier date [26, 27]. Reactions to skin tests derived from NTM are not sufficiently species-specific to indicate which nontuberculous mycobacterium could be responsible for asymptomatic infections, and cross-reactivity with *M. tuberculosis* infection likely contributes to some of the reactions. In these patients, asymptomatic infection has not been shown to lead to latent infection so, unlike in tuberculosis, there is currently no evidence that NTM are associated with reactivation disease [7].

In developed countries there seems to have been an increase in NTM infections in recent years, but it is not clear where this is a true increase or just reflects better detection. In industrialized countries, the incidence of these infections ranges from 1 to 1.8 cases per 100,000 subjects [27]. The most common agent is the *M. avium* complex (MAC). The clinical manifestation most frequently observed is lung disease, although lymphatic, skin, soft tissue, and disseminated forms are also common [28, 29].

An Indian study demonstrated that the increase in NTM diseases is a worldwide phenomenon, not limited to more developed countries [30].

It has been suggested that tubercular infection and vaccination with *M. bovis* bacillus Calmette-Guérin may have a protective immunological role against NTM infections. The reduced frequency of tuberculosis is, indeed, concomitant with the increase in NTM infections. In Sweden, a marked increase in cervical lymphadenitis was observed after the law on compulsory BCG vaccination in infants was repealed [31].

6.3 Pathogenesis

In the last three decades, important discoveries have been made about the pathogenic mechanism underlying NTM infections. In patients with HIV infection, disseminated NTM infections typically occur only after the number of CD4+ T-lymphocytes drops below 50/μl: this implies that specific T-cell products or activities serve to confer resistance to mycobacteria [32, 33]. In HIV-unaffected subjects, disseminated NTM infections are associated with genetic syndromes, specific mutations in IFN-γ and IL-12 synthesis and response pathways [34, 35]. There is also an association between disseminated, often fatal NTM forms and cell-mediated immunosuppression, due for instance to chemotherapy for neoplastic disease, or to organ transplant.

Mycobacteria are phagocytized by macrophages, which respond by producing IL-12, that in turn up-regulates IFN-γ [36]. IFN-γ activates neutrophils and macrophages to kill intracellular pathogens, including mycobacteria. IFN-γ and IL-12 control mycobacteria, to a large extent through the up-regulation of TNF-α, predominantly induced by monocytes/macrophages. The major role of TNF-α in controlling intracellular infections has been clarified through the use of TNF-α blocking agents [37]. The potent TNF-α blocking antibodies infliximab and adalimumab, and the soluble receptor etanercept, are effective anti-inflammatory agents and lead to relatively high rates of development of active tuberculosis in subjects with latent infection [38, 39].

Even if the degree of risk posed by TNF-α blocking agents in predisposing to NTM infections is still not entirely clear, it is commonly believed that patients with active NTM disease should receive TNF-α blocking agents only if they are also receiving adequate therapy for the NTM disease [7].

NTM strains can enter the organism through the gastrointestinal or respiratory tract, or less commonly by inoculation. In the respiratory tract, NTM are inhaled from water, dirt, dust, or other aerosols, and in most cases are handled by innate host defenses, mainly mucociliary clearance and coughing, and so do not cause disease [40].

6.4 Diagnosis

In the last ATS/IDSA Statement on Nontuberculous Mycobacterial Disease, diagnostic criteria for NTM infections are reported [7].

Specimens for mycobacterial identification and susceptibility testing can be collected from almost all body areas. Great care must be taken to avoid potential sources of contamination, especially tap water, in which mycobacteria are often present. Specimens must be sent without fixatives in sterile, leak-proof, disposable, labeled, laboratory-approved containers. When transport to the laboratory is delayed for more than 1 h, samples must be refrigerated at 4 °C; they can also be shipped or mailed with refrigerants such as cold packs [7, 11].

Obtaining body fluids or abscess fluids by needle aspiration or surgical procedures is recommended; swabs are not because they generally yield limited culture material (they must be saturated with sample fluid) and are subject to drying out. In the case of tissues, the sample must not be wrapped in gauze or diluted in liquid material; small pieces of tissue can be immersed in sterile saline. For blood samples, various commercial mycobacterial blood culture systems are available.

For all mycobacteria, the best staining method is the fluorochrome technique; alternative less sensitive methods are Ziehl-Neelsen and the Kinyoun stain. In cases of RGM, however, the fluorochrome method may not be useful. In any case it should be borne in mind that negative smears do not necessarily mean that there are no bacilli, especially RGM, in a sample.

Mycobacteria must be cultured in both solid and broth (liquid) media for the detection and enhancement of growth. The optimal temperature for most cultures for NTM is between 28 and 37 °C. Most slowly growing mycobacteria grow well at 35–37 °C, except for *M. haemophilum* (that prefers temperatures from 28 to 30 °C) and *M. ulcerans* (it grows at 25–33°C). RGM and *M. marinum* must be incubated at 28–30 °C [7].

Samples of skin, joint fluid, and bones must be incubated at 28–30 °C and at 35–37 °C. Most NTM grow within 2–3 weeks on subculture but *M. ulcerans* takes at least 8–12 weeks in incubation. RGM generally grow in 7 days.

For clinical-therapeutic purposes, species-level identification of the NTM, not merely as groups, is important. In this regard, consultation between the clinician and the laboratory operator (of a reference laboratory) is vital: the clinician must provide the laboratory operator with indications to guide the phenotypic (growth rate, pigmentation, incubation temperatures) and above all genotypic identification (there are many commercially available molecular probes) of the NTM [7].

The role of in vitro susceptibility testing in the management of patients with NTM infections is still highly debated. For some NTM the in vitro response to susceptibility tests is confirmed in vivo in the clinical response to antimicrobial drugs but for others (MAC) there is no correspondence between the in vitro and in vivo response. It must therefore be remembered that unlike TB, some NTM infections may not be eradicated by treatment based on in vitro susceptibility results [7].

The search for bacilli in clinical samples is not always positive and will anyway be paucibacillary: microscopy shows a sensitivity ranging between 22–78% as compared with culture [3]. The histology of NTM skin infections is not peculiar, and granulomatous tubercular findings are rare whereas aspecific inflammatory signs are common. Skin tests have poor specificity: cross-reactions are very frequent (Fig. 6.1), as are false-negative responses in immunocompromised patients.

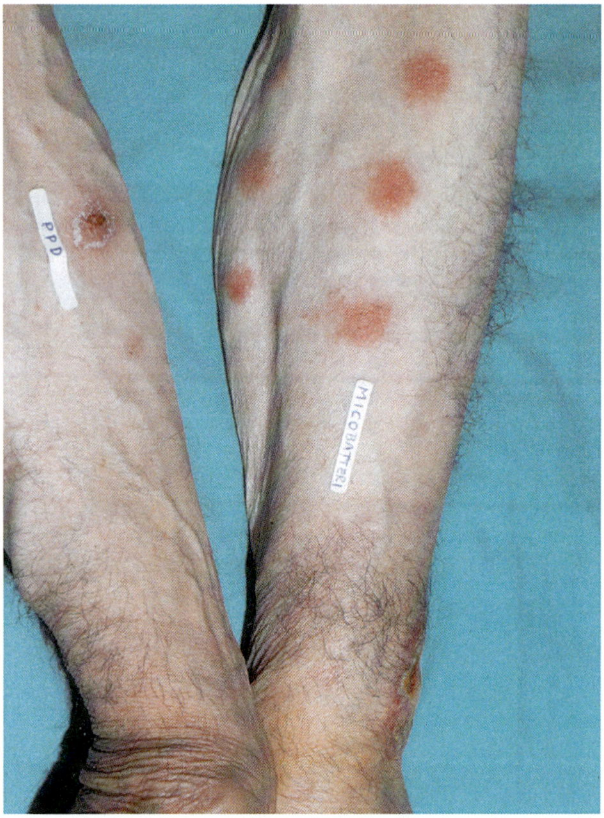

Fig. 6.1 Patient with ulcerative lupus vulgaris of the wrist (see Fig. 2.43). Strong positive PPD of *Mycobacterium tuberculosis* and positive cross-reactions to PPD of other mycobacteria

6.5 Clinical Features

Although only mildly pathogenic in man, NTM can cause a vast range of clinical pictures [2, 3, 6, 7, 11, 41–46] (Table 6.3). Pulmonary disease is the most frequent infection, followed by lymphadenitis in children [47], skin disease from *M. marinum* (particularly in fish tank enthusiasts), and other extrapulmonary or disseminated infections in immunocompromised patients [37, 48, 49]. Of the more than the reported 170 NTM species, 25 of them have been strongly associated with NTM disease; the remainder are environmental organisms rarely encountered in clinical samples.

Wagner and Young classified diseases from NTM mycobacteria in six different groups: pulmonary disease, lymphadenitis, skin and soft tissue disease, skeletal (bone, joint, tendon) infections, foreign body and central venous catheter infection, and disseminated infection [3]. Disseminated NTM infection is rare in non-HIV-infected immunocompromised patients [50] and has a decreasing incidence even in HIV-infected patients nowadays in the antiretroviral therapy era [51].

6.5.1 Lymphadenitis

The most common NTM-associated disease in children of 1–5 years of age is cervical, submandibular, submaxillary or preauricular lymphadenitis [7, 47]. The complaint usually presents without systemic signs and with non tender unilateral lymphadenopathy that may enlarge rapidly and rupture. Despite this, affected children may seem in good health, although the T cell-dependent production of type 1 cytokines may be altered [52]. Most cases of lymphadenitis are caused by MAC. In the US and Australia, most of the remaining cases are caused by *M. scrofulaceum*, whereas in parts of the northern Europe *M. malmoense* is the second most common pathogen. Other NTM species have rarely been implicated.

It is important to distinguish between tubercular and nontubercular forms of lymphadenitis. Risk factors in favor of tubercular lymphadenitis are a positive Mantoux tuberculin skin test reaction of >15 mm, exposure to an adult with tuberculosis, positive Mantoux tuberculin skin test reactions in family members, and age over 5 years. Nontubercular lymphadenitis signs are a negative tuberculin skin test reaction and the histopathology of the lymph nodes. However, cross-reactivities are possible. For a definitive diagnosis the infectious agent needs to be identified. Biopsies or incisions must be avoided, whereas fine-needle aspiration for cytology and culture is useful [53]. Instead, according to some authors, because negative culture results are often obtained after fine-needle aspiration, excisional biopsy is preferable, also in order to remove infected tissue [54].

6.5.2 Skin and Soft Tissue Disease

The clinical diagnosis of the various skin pictures is not an easy task. Apart from *M. ulcerans* infection, with its peculiar ulcerative lesions, none of the other pictures feature pathognomonic lesions. A high suspicion index is therefore important, and

Table 6.3 Clinical disease due to nontuberculous mycobacteria (modified, by [7])

Common	Uncommon
Pulmonary diseases	
M. abscessus	*M. asiaticum*
M. avium complex	*M. celatum*
M. kansasii	*M. chelonae*
M. malmoense	*M. fortuitum*
M. xenopi	*M. gordonae*
	M. haemophilum
	M. scrofulaceum
	M. shimoidei
	M. simiae
	M. smegmatis
	M. szulgai
Disseminated diseases	
M. avium complex	*M. abscessus*
M. chelonae	*M. celatum*
M. haemophilum	*M. fortuitum*
M. kansasii	*M. genavense*
	M. immunogenum
	M. malmoense
	M. marinum
	M. scrofulaceum
	M. simiae
	M. szulgai
	M. xenopi
Lymphadenitis	
M. avium complex	*M. abscessus*
M. malmoense	*M. chelonae*
M. scrofulaceum	*M. fortuitum*
	M. genavense
	M. haemophilum
	M. kansasii
	M. szulgai
Skin, soft tissue, and bone diseases	
M. abscessus	*M. avium* complex
M. chelonae	*M. haemophilum*
M. fortuitum	*M. immunogenum*
M. marinum	*M. kansasii*
M. ulcerans	*M. malmoense*
	M. nonchromogenicum
	M. scrofulaceum
	M. smegmatis
	M. szulgai
	M. terrae complex
	M. xenopi
Specimen contaminant	
M. gordonae (most common NTM contaminant)	
M. haemophilum	
M. mucogenicum	
M. nonchromogenicum	
M. terrae complex	

NTM nontuberculous mycobacteria

the conclusion must be based on assessment of both the morphological picture and the microbiological and radiological data.

Almost all NTM species have been incriminated in cutaneous diseases (Table 6.4). The most common species in the USA and Europe are *M. marinum* [52, 55, 56] and the RGM *M. abscessus*, *M. fortuitum*, and *M. chelonae*.

Table 6.4 Characteristics of some nontuberculous mycobacteria of dermatologic interest

Slowly growing mycobacteria
M. avium complex
Worldwide. Avian and mammalian pathogens. Diffuse infections common in AIDS patients. Most common NTM pathogens in USA
M. haemophilum
Difficult species for laboratory operators. Rarely isolated in pulmonary diseases. It causes multiple, purplish, soft skin nodules, often localized in the joints and legs (cooler body sites), that may develop into abscesses and ulcers. Histologically, it gives rise to suppurating granuloma. Specimen contaminant. It causes disseminated disease in AIDS and non-AIDS immunosuppressed patients. USA, Australia
M. kansasii
USA, Europe, South Africa, coal mining regions. Disseminated disease in AIDS. Rarely isolated in lymphadenitis. Often isolated from the sputum of urban patients. Rare skin lesions
M. malmoense
UK, Northern Europe (especially Scandinavia), uncommon in the USA. Disseminated disease in non-AIDS immunosuppressed patients. Possible skin, soft tissue and bone diseases
M. marinum
Worldwide. Fresh- and saltwater. Disseminated disease in AIDS. Isolated nodules and sporotrichoid pattern cutaneous disease. Tuberculoid granuloma without caseous necrosis; more often aspecific inflammatory infiltrate
M. scrofulaceum
Worldwide. Rarely isolated in pulmonary diseases (in South Africa) and disseminated diseases. Parasite of the soil. It produces cervical adenitis in children
M. smegmatis
Rarely isolated in skin, soft tissue, and bone diseases
M. szulgai
Rarely isolated in pulmonary diseases and lymphadenitis. It produces diffuse cellulitis and multiple inflammatory lesions in skin and bones in patients on corticosteroid therapy
M. terrae complex
Specimen contaminant. It produces tenosynovitis
M. ulcerans
Australia, tropics, Africa, Southeast Asia. It is limited to temperatures from 25 to 33 °C. In freshwater. It produces acute necrosis of the dermis and subcutaneous tissue with ulceration
Rapidly growing mycobacteria
M. abscessus
Worldwide. It may be found concomitant with MAC in pulmonary diseases. Rarely isolated in lymphadenitis. It produces disseminated disease in non-AIDS immunosuppressed transplant recipients. It causes circumscribed infections, post-surgical (penetrating injury) or from injections: subcutaneous abscesses, but also tuberculoid granulomas
M. chelonae
Disseminated skin lesions in non-AIDS immunosuppressed patients. Post-traumatic infection of the skin, soft tissues and bones. Most common lesions: subcutaneous nodules with sporotrichoid features, located mainly on the distal parts of limbs
M. fortuitum
Widespread in soil and water. Occasionally isolated in the sputum of healthy persons. Disseminated disease in non-AIDS immunosuppressed patients. Most common disease pattern: cutaneous abscesses from injections, sometimes with sporotrichoid pattern. Footbaths

NTM nontuberculous mycobacteria

African Buruli ulcer, or Bairnsdale ulcer as it is called in Australia, caused by *M. ulcerans*, is endemic in 33 countries in Africa, Western Pacific, Asia and South America, and is the third most common mycobacterial disease worldwide, after tuberculosis and leprosy [57, 58].

Clinical presentation of cutaneous disease consists in granulomatous or abscess formations at the site of puncture wounds. Open traumatic injuries or fractures are most often due to the RGM species [59], that can also cause nosocomial skin and soft tissue infections [60–64]. These include infections of long-term intravenous or peritoneal catheters, post-injection abscesses, infection after liposuction, surgical wound infections, infections after cardiac bypass surgery [65].

Interesting clinical data emerged from a retrospective Spanish study of 51 patients with cutaneous nontuberculous mycobacterial infections [6]. In most cases the lesions were of nodular type, followed by abscesses, plaques, papules, cellulitis, and ulcers, in that order. The number of lesions was significantly lower (1 to 5) in the group of immunocompetent subjects compared to those (>5) with immune impairment for various reasons. The lesions were localized in most cases. In 14 of 22 cases of *M. marinum* infection the clinical manifestations were lymphocutaneous sporotrichoid lesions. Sources of infection were aquagenic trauma in 23 cases (22 due to *M. marinum* and 1 to *M. chelonae*), non aquagenic trauma in seven subjects, surgical procedures in 3, internal focus in seven subjects, and unknown in 11 patients. Visceral infection was present only in two patients with AIDS [6]. Forty biopsies obtained in 38 patients showed a mixed granulomatous and suppurative inflammation, abscess, panniculitis, a diffuse histiocytic infiltrate, and an acute folliculitis. Epidermal changes, such as acanthosis, hyperkeratosis and pseudoepitheliomatous hyperplasia, were found only in cases of infection by *M. marinum*. Positive acid fast bacilli staining was found in 21% of immunocompetent and 72% of immunocompromised subjects [6].

Apart from *M. marinum*, various other NTM pathogens can induce sporotrichoid skin infections, conditions that simulate the subcutaneous linear lymphangitic form of sporotrichosis owing to the prevalently lymphatic spread of the infection [43]. Other NTM more frequently involved include *M. chelonae* [66], *M. kansasii* [67, 68], and *M. fortuitum* [69].

6.6 Prevention

Because they are ubiquitous agents whose pathophysiological characteristics are not yet entirely known, it is difficult to draw up practical, efficacious strategies to prevent NTM infections. First of all it is essential to identify the reservoir responsible, since the transmission and host susceptibility risks depend on the type. Investigations of health care-associated outbreaks have demonstrated that the most common sources of NTM infections are tap water, ice prepared from tap water, processed tap water used for dialysis, and distilled water used for preparing solutions [62, 63, 70–72]. NTM were found in municipal water supplies or treated water supplies at 95 of 115 (83%) dialysis centers in the United States [73]. *M. kansasii*,

M. xenopi, and *M. simiae* are isolated almost exclusively from municipal water sources, only rarely from other environmental sources [74]. Various NTM species, like *M. xenopi*, *M. smegmatis*, *M. simiae*, and MAC, are thermophilic and grow well at 45 °C, whereas other species such as *M. kansasii*, *M. gordonae*, *M. fortuitum*, *M. chelonae*, *M. abscessus*, and *M. mucogenicum*, do not tolerate high temperatures and are found only in cold-water systems.

Biofilms, filmy layers at the solid (pipe) and liquid (water) interface, are known to be a frequent site for mycobacterial growth [20, 75, 76]. The cell wall of mycobacteria, that has a rich content of fatty acids and wax, is impermeable and hydrophobic: this permits adherence to solid substrates (pipes and leaves) in aquatic environments, preventing them from being washed away through high flow rates [7].

Most health care-associated mycobacterial outbreaks and pseudo-outbreaks are linked to RGM, especially *M. fortuitum* and *M. abscessus*; these species are particularly hard and resistant to the action of organomercurials, chlorine, 2% concentrations of formaldehyde and alkaline glutaraldehyde, and other common disinfectants [77]. Health care-associated NTM outbreaks include cardiac surgery (sternotomy wounds), injections (contaminated biological or multidose vials), plastic surgery, liposuction, LASIK, dialysis-associated infections, long-term central intravenous catheters, and a variety of other surgical procedures [7, 77–82].

Recently, *M. fortuitum* and *M. mageritense* outbreaks of furunculosis have been associated with footbaths at nail salons. In all cases NTM were cultured from patients specimens and from the inlet suction screens of the whirlpool footbaths that contained hair and other debris [83–86].

On the basis of the above health care-associated data and of various other NTM outbreaks and pseudo-outbreaks reported in the literature [7], the recommendation for preventive purposes is to take strict care to avoid contact of catheters and other instruments with tap water, as well as the use of multidose vials, the use of benzalkonium chloride as skin disinfectant because it allows the growth of mycobacteria such as *M. abscessus*, to avoid alternative medicine practices involving injections of unknown or unapproved substances, and in the surgical field, to refrain from washing or contaminating open wounds with tap water [7].

In recent years, the increased popularity of tattoos has coincided with an increase in reports of cutaneous inoculation of NTM during the tattooing process [87–113]. *M. chelonae* is the most common pathogen causing skin NTM infection associated with tattooing; other less common pathogens include *M. immunogenum*, *M. abscessus*, *M. fortuitum*, and *M. haemophilum*. These infections are primarily associated with contamination of the inks used for tattooing, either of the ink itself or of solutions used to dilute the ink, in particular non sterile water [96, 101, 102]. Confirmation of NTM infection associated with tattoos must include culture and/or PCR data from a skin biopsy specimen. Histology shows dermal inflammatory infiltrates ranging from a sparse lymphohistiocytic infiltrate to well-formed granulomas [90, 96, 99]. Demonstration by special stains (Ziehl-Neelsen or Fite) of organisms in skin biopsy specimens may be attempted but should not be regarded as decisive for the final diagnosis. All these cases illustrate the potential importance of regulations serving to standardize tattoo ink preparation and use [101].

6.7 Transplant Recipients

NTM may cause significant disease in recipients of solid organ transplants [48]. In these individuals NTM infections generally manifest as skin and soft tissue infections, pleuropulmonary disease, musculoskeletal infections, and disseminated disease. In kidney and heart recipients, the most frequent presentation is skin and soft tissue infection [114]. The skin lesions are generally erythematous or purplish painful nodules that may ulcerate or form subcutaneous abscesses, that drain spontaneously. There may be single or multiple lesions, associated with dissemination. The skin picture may also consist of non-healing wounds occurring after accidental injury [115].

RGM and *M. marinum* are the NTM species most likely to cause skin and soft tissue infections [116], although any NTM species, including *M. avium* complex [116] and *M. kansasii*, can be responsible [117].

Although it is less common than skin and tissue infection and pleuropulmonary disease, in solid organ transplant recipients NTM can cause disseminated infection. In non-HIV patients, disseminated MAC can present as fever of unknown origin, but *M. kansasii* and RGM typically induce multiple subcutaneous nodules [7].

NTM are becoming increasingly recognized in recipients of hematopoietic stem cell transplantation (HSCT), with incidence rates ranging between 0.4 and 10% [49]. These infections are 50–600 times commoner in transplant recipients than in the general population. The time of onset of the infection ranges from 31 to 1055 days post-transplant. These infections have been reported following various forms of HSCT: risk factors are related to the underlying medical condition and its treatment, the pre-transplant conditioning therapies, and the transplant procedures and its complications [49]. Clinically, NTM may present with lymphadenopathy, osteomyelitis, skin and soft tissue infections, bacteremia, lung and gastrointestinal tract involvement. Currently, there are no guidelines for the treatment of NTM infections in recipients of stem cell transplantation; surgical debridement is generally performed and various combinations of antimicrobials are used, for 9 months after allogenic stem cell transplantation and 6 months after autologous procedures [49].

6.8 HIV-Infected Individuals

Although various NTM species have been reported in HIV-infected patients, most (>90%) of these infections are caused by MAC, more than 90% being due to *M. avium* [118–120]. What mechanism causes the acquisition of the pathogens in HIV patients is not known, although it is thought to be through ingestion from an environmental source. Apart from *M. kansasii*, very frequently reported, various other NTM can be the culprits: *M. scrofulaceum*, *M. gordonae*, *M. haemophilum*, *M. genavense*, *M. xenopi*, *M. celatum*, *M. cospicuum*, *M. fortuitum*, *M. simiae*, *M. marinum*, and *M. malmoense* [120–125].

Disseminated disease due to NTM in patients with HIV infections occurs only in severely immunocompromised subjects, as evidenced by very low CD4+ T-cell counts [119, 120]: nearly 40% of patients with less than 10 CD4+ T cell/µl develop disseminated NTM within 1 year [119]. In a series of patients with disseminated NTM, the mean CD4+ T-cell count was usually less than 25 cell/µl [119, 120]. All subjects with less than 50 CD4+ T cells/µl are at risk of disseminated NTM, and the lower the numbers of cells the higher the risk [7].

Disseminated disease is very rare with any form of immunosuppression other than advanced HIV disease. However, disseminated NTM infection has been reported in patients with renal or cardiac transplantation, chronic corticosteroid use, and leukemia. Rare genetic disorders may also be associated with disseminated infection. The pathogens most often implicated are *M. chelonae*, *M. abscessus*, *M. kansasii*, and *M. haemophilum* [126–128].

Various clinical pictures are possible, and hence confusion with various other infections. In MAC forms symptoms include fever (>80%), night sweats (>35%), and weight loss (>25%) [119], as well as abdominal pain, diarrhea, hepatosplenomegaly, and severe anemia. Disease caused by *M. kansasii*, *M. chelonae*, *M. abscessus*, and *M. haemophilum*, instead, generally presents as multiple subcutaneous nodules or abscesses with possible spontaneous drain [126–128].

6.9 Treatment

No consensus has yet been reached as regards the ideal treatment. The choice of antimicrobial therapy depends on the NTM species isolated, as well as the severity of the infection and the site of the lesions. Generally, treatment consists of the combination of several drugs administered for prolonged periods of time, thereby raising the risk of resistance, toxicity, addiction and drug interactions. While awaiting the results of susceptibility tests, drugs known to be active are started and then changed according to the results of the in vitro tests. Failure rates remain high, unfortunately, and relapses can occur [48].

Susceptibility tests are essential for most clinically significant NTM, although there is not always a correlation between the in vitro susceptibility to many antimicrobials and the in vivo response [7]: it must therefore be borne in mind that the in vitro tests may lead to treatment successes or failures.

The ATS/IDSA has published treatment guidelines for the most frequently encountered NTM [7]. Traditional anti-tuberculosis agents, like rifamycins and ethambutol, can be effective against many of the NTM but have little utility in the treatment of RGM. Fortunately, various traditional antibiotics, as well as new agents, are active against RGM. In general, combination regimens should be used, given the development of resistance on monotherapy for most isolates. When possible, in the case of transplant recipients, the immunodepression intensity should be decreased.

The combination of traditional and new antibiotics (Table 6.5) must be used for 3–4 months in localized infections, for 6 months in those involving the surrounding

Table 6.5 Traditional and new antibiotics in the treatment of nontuberculous mycobacteria infections

Traditional antibiotics	New antibiotics
Rifampicin	Cefoxitin
Rifabutin	Clarithromycin
Ethambutol	Oxazolidinone
Isoniazid	Sparfloxacin
Streptomycin	Gatifloxacin
Levofloxacin	Moxifloxacin
Ciprofloxacin	Linezolid
Amikacin	Tigecycline
Ofloxacin	Telithromycin
Imipenem	
Trimethoprim sulfamethoxazole	
Tobramycin	
Minocycline	
Doxycycline	
Azithromycin	
Pyridoxine	
Sulfonamides	
Cycloserine	
Viomycin	
Capreomycin	
Para-aminosalicylic acid	
Kanamycin	

soft tissues, and for 12 months or even their entire lifetime in immunocompromised subjects. Treatment must be prolonged for at least 2 months after clinical healing. It is wise to wait at least 1–2 months before changing the drug regimen [7].

Surgery can have an important role in the treatment of some NTM infections. Infected foreign bodies should be removed and abscesses drained. Because person-to-person transmission of NTM is not a major route of transmission, the isolation of hospitalized patients with NTM infections is not required. In any case, it is well known that nosocomial outbreaks are generally related to the contamination of medical devices or medications.

References

1. Morrone A, Fazio M (2000) Micobatteriosi atipiche. In: Veraldi S, Caputo R (eds) Dermatologia di importazione, 2nd edn, Poletto Ed, pp 82.
2. Weitzul S, Eichhorn PJ, Pandya AG (2000) Nontuberculous mycobacterial infections of the skin. Curr Ther 18:359
3. Wagner D, Young LS (2003) Nontuberculous mycobacterial infections: a clinical review. Infection 5:257
4. Ramos-e-Silva M, Ribeiro de Castro MC (2003) Mycobacterial infections. In: Bolognia JL, Jorizzo JL, Rapini RP et al (eds) Dermatology. Mosby, London, p 1145
5. Grance JM, Zumla A. (2003) Human disease due to environmental mycobacteria. In: Cook GC, Zumla A (eds) Manson's tropical diseases, 21th edn. WB Saunders, p 1053
6. Bartralot R, Garcia-Patos V, Sitjas D et al (2005) Clinical patterns of cutaneous nontuberculous mycobacterial infections. Br J Dermatol 152:727

7. Griffith DE, Aksamit T, Brown-Elliott BA et al (2007) An official ATS/IDSA Statement: diagnosis, treatment, and prevention of nontuberculous mycobacterial diseases. Am J Respir Crit Care Med 175:367
8. Yates VM (2010) Mycobacterial infections. In: Burns T, Breathnach S, Cox N et al (eds) Rook's textbook of dermatology, 8th edn. Wiley-Blackwell, Oxford, p 31.1
9. Yeager H (2011) Nontuberculous mycobacteria—introduction. In: Schlossberg D (ed) Tuberculosis and nontuberculous mycobacterial infections, 6th edn. ASM Press, Washington, DC, p 525
10. Sethi A (2012) Tuberculosis and infections with atypical mycobacteria. In: Goldsmith LA, Katz SI, Gilchrest BA et al (eds) Fitzpatrick's dermatology in general medicine, vol II, 8th edn. Mc Graw Hill, New York, p 2225
11. van Ingen J (2013) Diagnosis of nontuberculous mycobacterial infections. Semin Resp Crit Care Med 34:103
12. Ena P, Cerimele D (2013) Nontuberculous mycobacterial infections of the skin. In: Giannetti A, Del Forno C (eds) Textbook of dermatology and sexually transmitted diseases. Piccin Nuova Libreria, Padova, p 505
13. Branch A (1931) Avian tubercle bacillus infection, with special reference to mammals and to man: its reported association with Hodgkin's disease. Arch Pathol 12:253
14. Chapman JS (1977) The atypical mycobacteria and human mycobacterioses. Plenum Publishing Co., New York, NY
15. Tortoli E (2003) Impact of genotypic studies on mycobacterial taxonomy: the new mycobacteria of the 1900s. Clin Microbiol Rev 2:319
16. Mc Nabb AD, Eisler K, Adlie M et al (2004) Assessment of partial sequencing of the 65-kilodalton heat shock protein gene (*hsp65*) for routine identification of mycobacterium species isolated from clinical sources. J Clin Microbiol 42:3000
17. Runyon EH (1959) Anonymous mycobacteria in pulmonary disease. Med Clin N Am 43:273
18. Falkinhan JO (2002) Nontuberculous mycobacteria in the environment. Clin Chest Med 23:520
19. von Reyn CF, Waddell RD, Eaton T et al (1993) Isolation of *Mycobacterium avium* complex from water in the United States, Finland, Zaire, and Kenya. J Clin Microbiol 1:3227
20. Feazel LM, Baumgartner LK, Peterson KL et al (2009) Opportunistic pathogens enriched in showerhead biofilms. Proc Natl Acad Sci U S A 106:16393
21. Meissner G, Anz W (1977) Sources of *Mycobacterium avium* complex infection resulting in human disease. Am Rev Respir Dis 116:1057
22. Ahreus PS, Giese B, Klausen J et al (1995) Two markers, IS901-IS902 and p40 identified by PCR and by using monoclonal antibodies in *Mycobacterium avium* strains. J Clin Microbiol 33:1049
23. Guerrero C, Bernasconi C, Burki D et al (1995) A novel insertion element *Mycobacterium avium. IS124.5* is a specific target for analysis of strain relatedness. J Clin Microbiol 33:304
24. Olivier KN, Weber DJ, Wallace RJ Jr et al (2003) Nontuberculous mycobacteria. I: multicenter prevalence study in cystic fibrosis. Am J Respir Crit Care Med 167:828
25. von Reyn CF, Arbeit RD, Horsburgh CR Jr et al (2002) Sources of disseminated *Mycobacterium avium* infection in AIDS. J Infect 44:166
26. von Reyn CF, Horsburgh CR Jr, Olivier KN et al. Skin test reactions to *Mycobacterium tuberculosis* purified protein derivative and *Mycobacterium avium* sensitin among health care workers and medical students in the United States. Int J Tuberc Lung Dis 2001;5:1122
27. Horsburg CR Jr (1996) Epidemiology of *Mycobacterium avium.* In: Korvick JA, Benson CA (eds) *Mycobacterium avium* complex infection: progress in research and treatment. Marcel Dekker, New York, p 1
28. Good RC, Snider DE (1980) Isolation of nontuberculous mycobacteria in the United States. J Infect Dis 146:829
29. O' Brien RJ, Geiter LJ, Snider DE (1987) The epidemiology of nontuberculous mycobacterial diseases in the United States: results from a national survey. Am Rev Respir Dis 135:1007

30. Alvares-Uria G (2010) Lung disease caused by nontuberculous mycobacteria. Curr Opin Pulm Med 16:251
31. Romanus V, Hollander HO, Wahlen P et al (1995) Atypical mycobacteria in extrapulmonary disease among children. Incidence in Sweden from 1969 to 1980, related to changing BCG-vaccination coverage. Tuber Lung Dis 76:300
32. American Thoracic Society (1987) Mycobacterioses and the aquired immunodeficiency syndrome. Joint Position Paper of the American Thoracic Society and the Centers for Disease Control. Am Rev Resp Dis 136:492
33. Horsburg CR Jr (1996) Epidemiology of disease caused by nontuberculous mycobacteria. Semin Respir Infect 11:244
34. Dorman SE, Holland SM (2000) Interferon-gamma and interleukin-12 pathway defects and human disease. Cytokine Growth Factor Rev 11:321
35. Casanova JL, Abel L (2002) Genetic dissection of immunity to mycobacteria: the human model. Annu Rev Immunol 20:581
36. Fulton SA, Johnsen JM, Wolf SF et al (2533) Interleukin-12 production by human monocytes infected with *Mycobacterium tuberculosis*: role of phagocytosis. Infect Immun 1996:64
37. Winthrop KL, Chang E, Yamashita S et al (2009) Nontuberculous mycobacteria infections and anti-tumor necrosis factor-alpha therapy. Emerg Infect Dis 15:1556
38. Keane J, Gershon S, Wise RP et al (2001) Tuberculosis associated with infliximab, a tumor necrosis factor alpha-neutralizing agent. N Engl J Med 345:1098
39. Keane J (2004) Tumor necrosis factor blockers and reactivation of latent tuberculosis. Clin Infect Dis 39:300
40. Mc Garvey J, Bermudez LE (2002) Pathogenesis of nontuberculous mycobacteria infections. Clin Infect Dis 23:569
41. Stein SC (1982) Mycobacteria and the skin. Int J Dermatol 21:82
42. Grange JM (1982) Mycobacteria and the skin. Int J Dermatol 21:497
43. Glickman FS (1983) Sporotrichoid mycobacterial infections. Case report and review. J Am Acad Dermatol 8:703
44. Wallace RJ Jr (1987) Recent clinical advances in knowledge of the nonleprous environmental mycobacteria responsible for cutaneous disease. Arch Dermatol 123:337
45. Henry MT, Inamdar L, O' Riordain D et al (2004) Nontuberculous mycobacteria in non-HIV patients: epidemiology, treatment and response. Eur Respir J 23:741
46. Dodiuk-Gad R, Dyachenko P, Ziv M et al (2007) Nontuberculous mycobacterial infections of the skin: a retrospective study of 25 cases. J Am Acad Dermatol 57:413
47. Lincoln EM, Gilbert LA (1972) Disease in children due to mycobacteria other than *Mycobacterium tuberculosis*. Am Rev Respir Dis 105:683
48. Cober E, Kaul DR. Nontuberculous mycobacteria in solid organ transplant recipients. http://www.antimicrobe.org/new/t26dw.html
49. Al-Ahazi KA, Al-Jasser AM, Al-Anazi WK (2014) Infections caused by non-tuberculous mycobacteria in recipients of hematopoietic stem cell transplantation. Front Oncol 4:1
50. Wallace RJ, Glassroth J, Griffiths DE et al (1997) Diagnosis and treatment of disease caused by nontuberculous mycobacteria. Am J Respir Crit Care Med 156:s1
51. Kaplan JE, Hauson D, Dworkin MS et al (2000) Epidemiology of human immunodeficiency virus-associated opportunistic infections in the United States in the era of highly active antiretroviral therapy. Clin Infect Dis 30(Suppl 1):s5
52. Bonamonte D, Vestita M. *Mycobacterium marinum*. http://antimicrobe.org/ms05.asp
53. Chao SS, Loh KS, Tan KK et al (2002) Tuberculous and nontuberculous clinical lymphadenitis: a clinical review. Otolaryngol Head Neck Surg 126:176
54. Starke JR (2000) Management of nontuberculous mycobacterial clinical adenitis. Pediatr Infect Dis J 19:67
55. Bonamonte D, De Vito D, Vestita M et al (2013) Aquarium-borne *Mycobacterium marinum* skin infection. Report of 15 cases and review of the literature. Eur J Dermatol 23:510
56. Bonamonte D, Filoni A, Vestita M et al (2016) Cutaneous infections from aquatic environments. In: Bonamonte D, Angelini G (eds) Aquatic dermatology. Biotic, chemical and physical agents, 2nd ed, Springer, Berlin, p 185

57. Brown-Elliot BA, Griffith DE, Wallace RJ Jr (2002) Newly described or emerging human species of nontuberculous mycobacteria. Infect Dis Clin N Am 16:187
58. Asiedu K, Scherpbier R, Raviglione M (2000) Buruli ulcer. *Mycobacterium ulcerans* infection. World Health Organization Global Buruli Ulcer Initiative, Geneve
59. Wallace RJ Jr, Swenson JM, Silcox VA et al (1983) Spectrum of disease due to rapidly growing mycobacteria. Rev Infect Dis 5:657
60. Hoffman PC, Frozer DW, Rohicsek F et al (1981) Two outbreaks of sternal wound infections due to organisms of the *Mycobacterium fortuitum* complex. J Infect Dis 143:533
61. Laussucq S, Baltch AL, Smith RP et al (1988) Nosocomial *Mycobacterium fortuitum* colonization from a contaminated ice machine. Am Rev Respir Dis 132:891
62. Safranek TJ, Jarvin WT, Carson LA et al (1997) *Mycobacterium chelonae* wound infection after plastic surgery employing contaminated violet skin-marking solution. N Engl J Med 317:197
63. Wenger JD, Spika JS, Smithwick RW et al (1990) Outbreak of *Mycobacterium chelonae* infection associated with use of jet injectors. JAMA 264:373
64. Hoy JF, Ralston KV, Hopfer RL et al (1987) *Mycobacterium fortuitum* bacteremia in patients with cancer and long-term venous catheters. Am J Med 83:213
65. Wallace RJ Jr, Musser JM, Hull SI et al (1989) Diversity and sources of rapidly growing mycobacteria associated with infections following cardiac surgery. J Infec Dis 159:708
66. Greer GP, Martensen SH (1979) Sporotrichoid cutaneous infections due to *Mycobacterium chelonei*. Arch Dermatol 115:738
67. Owens DW, Mc Bride MD (1969) Sporotrichoid cutaneous infections with *Mycobacterium kansasii*. Arch Dermatol 100:54
68. Dore M, Collins JP, Mankewicz E (1979) A sporotrichoid-like *Mycobacterium kansasii* infection of the skin treated with minocycline hydrochloride. Br J Dermatol 101:75
69. Angelini G, Vena GA, De Vito D et al (1992) Micobatteriosi sporotricoide da *Mycobacterium fortuitum*. Presentazione di un caso e revisione della letteratura. G Ital Dermatol Venereol 127:507
70. Wallace RJ Jr, Zhang Y, Brown BA et al (1993) DNA large restriction fragment patterns of sporadic and epidemic nosocomial strains of *Mycobacterium chelonae* and *Mycobacterium abscessus*. J Clin Microbiol 3:2697
71. Maloney S, Welbel S, Daves B et al (1994) *Mycobacterium abscessus* pseudoinfection traced to an automated endoscopic washer: utility of epidemiologic and laboratory investigation. J Infect Dis 169:1166
72. Bolan G, Reingold AL, Carson LA et al (1985) Infections with *Mycobacterium chelonei* in patients receiving dialysis and using processed hemodialyzers. J Infect Dis 152:1013
73. Carson LA, Bland LA, Cusick LB et al (1988) Prevalence of nontuberculous mycobacteria in water supplies of hemodialysis centers. Appl Environ Microbiol 54:3122
74. Wallace RJ Jr, Brown A, Griffith DE (1998) Nosocomial outbreaks/pseudooutbreaks caused by nontuberculous mycobacteria. Annu Rev Microciol 52:453
75. Schulze-Robbecke R, Janning B, Fischeder R (1992) Occurrence of mycobacteria in biofilm samples. Tuber Lung Dis 73:141
76. Falkinham JO (2009) The biology of environmental mycobacteria. Environ Microbiol Rep 1:477
77. Zhang Y, Rajagopalan M, Brown BA et al (1997) Randomly amplified polymorphic DNA PCR for comparison of *Mycobacterium abscessus* strains from nosocomial outbreaks. J Clin Microbiol 35:3132
78. Centers for Disease Control and Prevention (1996) Infection with *Mycobacterium abscessus* associated with intramuscular injection of adrenal cortex extract: Colorado and Wyoming. MMWR Morb Mortal Wkly Rep 45:713
79. Centers for Disease Control and Prevention (2004) *Mycobacterium chelonae* infections associated with facelifts: New Jersey, 2002–2003. MMWR Morb Mortal Wkly Rep 53:192
80. Meyers H, Brown-Elliot BA, Moore D et al (2002) An outbreak of *Mycobacterium chelonae* infection following liposuction. Clin Infect Dis 34:1500
81. Freitas D, Alvarenga L, Sampaio J et al (2003) An outbreak of *Mycobacterium chelonae* infection after LASIK. Ophthalmology 110:276

82. Holmes GP, Bond GB, Fader RC et al (2002) A cluster of cases of *Mycobacterium szulgai* keratitis that occurred after laser-assisted in situ keratomileusis. Clin Infect Dis 34:1039
83. Winthrop KL, Abrams M, Yakrus M et al (2004, 1813) An outbreak of mycobacterial furunculosis associated with footbaths at a nail salon. N Engl J Med 42
84. Suiezak PJ, Graham BS, Bush HB et al (2003) Rapidly growing mycobacterium infections following pedicures. Arch Dermatol 139:629
85. Gira AK, Reisenauer H, Hammock L et al (2004) Furunculosis due to *Mycobacterium mageritense* associated with foothbaths at a nail salon. J Clin Microbiol 42:1813
86. Winthrop KL, Albridge K, South D et al (2004) The clinical management and outcome of nail salon-acquired *Mycobacterium fortuitum* skin infection. Clin Infect Dis 38, 38
87. Long GE, Rickman LS (1994) Infections complications of tattoos. Clin Infect Dis 18:610
88. Kluger N, Muller C, Gral N (2008) Atypical mycobacteria infection following tattooing: review of an outbreak in 8 patients in a French tattoo parlor. Arch Dermatol 144:941
89. Preda VA, Maley M, Sullivan JR (2009) *Mycobacterium chelonae* infection in a tattoo site. Med J Aust 190:278
90. Drage LA, Ecker PM, Orenstein R et al (2010) An outbreak of *Mycobacterium chelonae* infections in tattoos. J Am Acad Dermatol 62:501
91. Bechara C, Macheros E, Heym B et al (2010) *Mycobacterium abscessus* skin infection after tattooing: first case report and review of the literature. Dermatology 221:1
92. Ricciardo B, Weedon D, Butler G (2010) *Mycobacterium abscessus* infection complicating a professional tattoo. Australas J Dermatol 51:287
93. Hamsch C, Hartschuh W, Enk A et al (2011) Chinese tattoo paint as a vector of atypical mycobacteria-outbreak in 7 patients in Germany. Acta Derm Venereol 91:63
94. Mitchell CB, Isenstein A, Burkhart CN et al (2011) Infection with *Mycobacterium immunogenum* following a tattoo. J Am Acad Dermatol 64:e70
95. Kappel S, Cotliar J (2011) Inoculation of *Mycobacterium chelonae* from a tattoo. J Am Acad Dermatol 64:998
96. Brinić I, Jankovnić A, Ljubenović M et al (2011) *Mycobacterium chelonae* infection due to black tattoo ink dilution. Am J Clin Dermatol 12:404
97. Kay MK, Perti TR, Duchin JI (2011) Tattoo-associated *Mycobacterium haemophilum* skin infection in immunocompetent adult, 2009. Emerg Infect Dis 17:1734
98. Centers for Disease Control and Prevention (2012) Tattoo-associated nontuberculous mycobacterial skin infections-multiple States, 2011–2012. MMWR Morb Mortal Wkly Rep 61:653
99. Kennedy BS, Bedard B, Youngl M et al (2012) Outbreak of *Mycobacterium chelonae* infection associated with tattoo ink. N Engl J Med 367:1020
100. Curcó N, Prat C, Tarroch X et al (2012) Cutaneous infection in a tattoo due to *Mycobacterium chelonae*: a report of 2 cases and a review of the literature. Actas Dermosifilogr 103:840
101. Falsey RR, Kinzer MH, Hurst S et al (2013) Cutaneous inoculation of nontuberculous mycobacteria during professional tattooing: a case series and epidemiologic study. CID 57:e143
102. Reviewed P (2015) Nontuberculous mycobacterium skin infections after tattooing in healthy individuals: a systematic review of case reports. Dermatol Online J 21: http://eschlorarship.org/uc/item/8mir3r4f0
103. Rodriguez-Blanco J, Fernandez LC, Suarez-Penaranda JM et al (2011) *Mycobacterium chelonae* infection associated with tattoos. Acta Derm Venereol 91:61
104. Schwartzman WA (2012) *Mycobacterium chelonae* illnesses associated with tattoo ink. N Engl J Med 367:2356
105. Scott-Lang V, Sergeaut A, Holme A (2012) Mycobacteria introduced by tattoos. BMJ 345:e8331
106. Sergeaut A, Conaglen P, Laurenson IF et al (2013) *Mycobacterium chelonae* infection: a complication of tattooing. Clin Exp Dermatol 38:140
107. Suvanasuthi S, Wongproparut C, Pattanaprichakul P et al (2012) *Mycobacterium fortuitum* cutaneous infection from amateur tattoo. J Med Assoc Thail 95:834

108. Winthrop K, Varley C, Sullivan A et al (2012) Happy Buddha? Clin Infect Dis 54:1670
109. Wolf R, Wolf D (2003) A tattoo butterfly as a vector of atypical mycobacteria. J Am Acad Dermatol 48:s73
110. Wolliua U (2011) Nodular skin reactions in eyebrow permanent makeup: two case reports and an infection by *Mycobacterium haemophilum*. J Cosmet Dermatol 10:235
111. Philips RC, Hunter-Ellul LA, Martin JE et al (2014) *Mycobacterium fortuitum* infection arising in a new tattoo. Dermatol Online J 20 [PMID:24945647]
112. Conaglen PD, Laurenson IF, Seageaut A et al (2013) Systematic reviw of tattoo-associated skin infection with rapidly growing mycobacteria and public investigation of a cluster in Scotland, 2010. Euro Surveill 18:pii=20553
113. Ortiz AE, Alster TS (2012) Rising concern over cosmetic tattoos. Dermatol Surg 38:424
114. Doucette K, Fishman JA (2004) Nontuberculous mycobacterial infection in haemopoietic stem cell and solid organ transplant recipients. Clin Infect Dis 38:1428
115. Jil T, Matas AJ (2005) Mycobacterial infections after kidney transplant. Transplant Proc 37:937
116. Nagy GS, Rubin RH (2001) Disseminated *Mycobacterium avium-intracellulare* in a kidney transplant recipient. Transplant. Infect Dis 3:220
117. Patel R, Robert GD, Keating MR et al (1994) Infections due to nontuberculosis mycobacteria in kidney, heart and liver transplant recipients. Clin Infect Dis 19:263
118. Horsburg CR (1991) *Mycobacterium avium* complex infection in the acquired immunodeficiency syndrome. N Engl J Med 324:1332
119. Nightindale SD, Byrd CT, Southern PM et al (1992) Incidence of *Mycobacterium avium-intracellulare* complex bacteremia in human immunodeficiency virus-positive patients. J Infect Dis 165:1082
120. Horsburg CR Jr, Gettings J, Alexander LN et al (2001) Disseminated *Mycobacterium avium*-complex disease among patients infected with human immunodeficiency virus, 1985–2000. Clin Infect Dis 33:1938
121. Butler WR, O'Connor SP, Yokrus MA et al (1993) *Mycobacterium celatum* sp. Inf J Syst Bacteriol 43:539
122. Rodriguez-Barradas MC, Claridge J, Daroniche R (1992) Disseminated *Mycobacterium fortuitum* disease in an AIDS patient. Am J Med 93:473
123. Chocarra A, Gonzales Lopez A, Breznes MF et al (1994) Disseminated infection due to *Mycobacterium malmoense* in a patient infected with human immunodeficiency virus. Clin Infect Dis 19:203
124. Huminer DS, Duz Z, Samra L et al (1993) *Mycobacterium simiae* infection in Israeli patients with AIDS. Clin Infect Dis 17:508
125. Springer BE, Tortoli D, Richter R et al (1995) *Mycobacterium cospicuum* sp. now.: a new species isolated from patients with disseminated infections. J Clin Microbiol 33:2805
126. Cooper JF, Lichtenstein MJ, Graham BS et al (1989) *Mycobacterium chelonae*: a cause of nodular skin lesions with a proclivity for renal transplant recipients. Am J Med 86:173
127. Ingram CW, Tamer DC, Durock DT et al (1993) Disseminated infections with rapidly growing mycobacteria. Clin Infect Dis 16:463
128. Chetchotisakd P, Mootsikapun P, Ammatsiri S et al (2000) Disseminated infection due to rapidly growing mycobacteria in immunocompetent host presenting with chronic lymphadenopathy: a previously unrecognized clinical entity. Clin Infect Dis 30:29

Mycobacterium scrofulaceum Infection

7

Domenico Bonamonte, Pietro Verni, and Gianni Angelini

Mycobacterium scrofulaceum is a member of the Runyon class II scotochromogen acid-fast bacilli [1–3]. It is widely present in nature, but is now an infrequent human pathogen. It was first described in the 1950s [4–6] and the name likely derives from its isolation from cervical lymph nodes.

7.1 The Organism

The length of *M. scrofulaceum* varies in acid-fast bacilli staining products; it may be longer or shorter than *M. tuberculosis*, but will be thicker and more coarsely beaded. It grows slowly in Löwenstein medium, generally taking about 4–6 weeks, although strains occasionally develop colonies in about 10 days. The colonies are globular, have a smooth consistency, and are opaque [3]. The pigmentation, that is produced in the dark as well as in the light, is yellow, and turns dark orange over time. Optimal growth occurs at 37 °C, one atmosphere pressure, and under aerobic conditions; growth is slower at 25° and 35 °C and no growth occurs at 41 °C [3].

M. scrofulaceum is from the antigenic and biochemical standpoints, quite similar to *M. avium-M. intracellulare* (MAI) and for many years was classified in the

D. Bonamonte, MD, PhD (✉)
Department of Biomedical Science and Human Oncology, University of Bari "Aldo Moro", Bari, Italy
e-mail: domenico.bonamonte@uniba.it

P. Verni, MD
University of Bari "Aldo Moro", Bari, Italy

G. Angelini, MD
Professor of Dermatology, Former Professor and Chairman, University of Bari "Aldo Moro", Bari, Italy

D. Bonamonte, G. Angelini (eds.), *Mycobacterial Skin Infections*,
DOI 10.1007/978-3-319-48538-6_7

M. avium-M. intracellulare-M. scrofulaceum complex [3]. It generally yields a positive urease reaction that distinguishes it from MAI, although there are some exceptions that make this distinction difficult [7]. Base sequence analysis of the 16S ribosomal RNA has confirmed that *M. scrofulaceum* is a unique species [8]. It is this molecular methodology (DNA probes or 16S rRNA gene sequencing) that may be required to differentiate *M. scrofulaceum* from other NTM [9, 10]. Recent studies have revealed a new species, *M. parascrofulaceum*, that causes various infections that were previously attributed to *M. scrofulaceum* [9–11].

7.2 Epidemiology

M. scrofulaceum is found in raw milk and other dairy products, pool oysters, house dust, soil, and water [12–18]. In one study, the organism was isolated from raw milk but not from samples of pasteurized milk [19]. In the United states, it has been isolated from the flood plains of four eastern rivers [20]. These results have been confirmed and it has been noticed that factors favoring growth include warm temperatures, low oxygen tension, lower pH of soils, and higher water concentrations of zinc, humic acid, and fulvic acid [21].

M. scrofulaceum is an opportunistic pathogen that is uncommonly isolated from human samples. It has been associated with lymphadenitis in children, disseminated infections, pulmonary disease, and skin infections [15–18]. In a study made in 1982, *M. scrofulaceum* accounted for 2–3% of all mycobacteria isolated from clinical samples in the United States [22]. However, cases of clinical disease caused by this species were rarely disseminated except in children with cervical lymphadenopathy [23]. In the early 1980s, *M. scrofulaceum* was replaced by MAC as the most common cause of childhood cervical lymphadenitis, and even today the former is still rarely recovered in this setting [7].

In some studies, human exposure to *M. scrofulaceum* was demonstrated by analysis of skin test reactions to purified protein derivative (PPD) sensitins derived from this organism. In the Netherlands, 7.76% of army recruits had indurations measuring 10 mm or more to *M. scrofulaceum* PPD [24]. In Greece, 8507 members of the armed forces were tested with *M. scrofulaceum* PPD: those born in mountainous areas had positivity rates of 4.1% versus 7.1% for those born in seaside areas. Among those born on small Aegean islands or in inland plains near large rivers the rates exceeded 8%. According to the authors, these data supported the theory that large bodies of water serve as the principal sources of infection [25]. Of 1015 BCG scar-negative children aged between 6 and 13 years in 18 randomly selected areas in Kenya, 22.7% reacted to *M. scrofulaceum* sensitin and 6.1% reacted to PPD-RT [26]. Comparable results were obtained in 15% of 7-year-old children in two towns in rural Czechoslovakia; the reaction was greater than the one to PPD-RT performed at the same time, in about 50% of the children [27]. Although these data have various limitations, they nevertheless demonstrate that *M. scrofulaceum* is widely but unevenly distributed in nature, that humans can encounter the organism and develop an immune response, and that clinical disease is much less common than exposure [3].

7.3 Clinical Features

Although *M. scrofulaceum* may cause pulmonary disease, lymphadenitis, skin disease, and other extrapulmonary diseases are also observed.

7.3.1 Lymphadenitis

M. scrofulaceum was originally isolated from the cervical lymph nodes in children (Figs. 7.1, 7.2, 7.3, and 7.4), and this is the most commonly associated condition [28–30]. Most affected children are between 1 and 5 years old, although there have been rare observations in children over 10. The female sex seems to be more susceptible. In the majority of cases the lymphadenitis is unilateral in the upper cervical chain or just under the mandible. Bilateral cases are rare, as is involvement of other lymph nodes (axillary, inguinal, epitrochlear, or mediastinal) [3].

Affected subjects do not present systemic signs and only rarely have even local symptoms. When left untreated, the lymph nodes soften, fistulize, drain or heal spontaneously, leaving fibrosis or calcification.

The pathogenic mechanism is not well understood. The isolation of *M. scrofulaceum* in the tonsils suggests that pharyngeal lymphoid tissue is the entry portal, followed by direct drainage into the nodes [30]. In peripheral adenopathy forms, direct inoculation into the skin in the event of trauma has been demonstrated [29].

Over the course of time, the etiology of cervical lymphadenitis in children has changed. In the preantibiotic era, most cases were due to *M. tuberculosis* or *M. bovis* [31]. Today, in developed countries, where tuberculosis has become a rare disease, the NTM species predominate and *M. scrofulaceum* is the species most often isolated. Since 1970, in the United States MAI has been more frequently identified

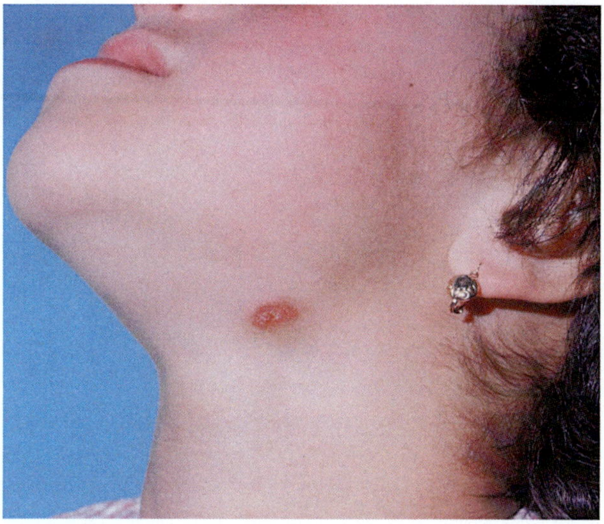

Fig. 7.1 Scrofuloderma

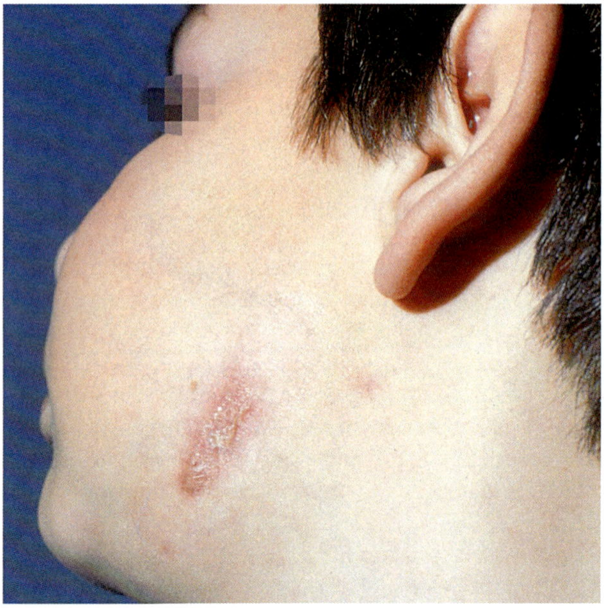

Fig. 7.2 Scrofuloderma

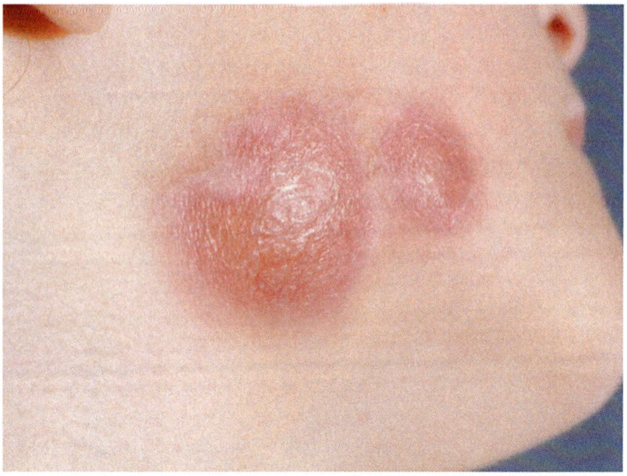

Fig. 7.3 Scrofuloderma

than *M. scrofulaceum* [29, 32]: whether this is due to a true change, to a reporting artifact, or to more reliable identification by laboratories, remains unknown [3].

Skin testing with mycobacterial antigens is useful for diagnosis. Many children with lymphadenitis evince a weak reaction to *M. tuberculosis* PPD and a stronger reaction to NTM strains sensitins [33].

Differential diagnosis must be made with infections by *M. tuberculosis*, *M. bovis*, other NTM species, and various viruses (Epstein-Barr virus, cytomegalovirus, and mumps) and deep mycoses. Other infections include brucellosis, cat scratch disease, and toxoplasmosis. Among non infectious forms, sarcoidosis, lymphoma,

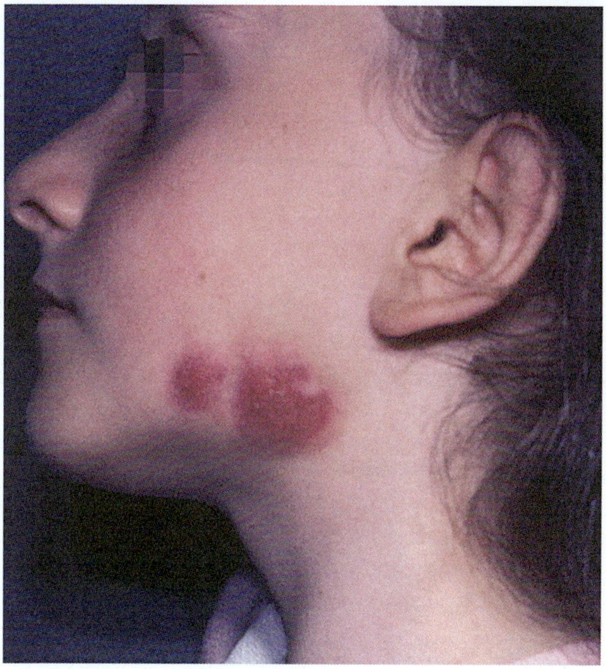

Fig. 7.4 Scrofuloderma

congenital cysts, and lipoma need to be taken into account [3]. Differentiating lymphadenitis from *M. tuberculosis* is generally easy: age (1–5 years), unilateral nodes, lack of systemic signs and symptoms, normal chest radiogram, a weak or no response to the tuberculin skin test, a nonreactive tuberculin test skin test in siblings, no history of contact with active tuberculosis, and no response to antituberculous antibodies are all factors pointing to NTM disease. To make a definitive diagnosis, isolation in culture is necessary since there are no clinical differences among the lymphadenitis forms linked to NTM [3].

A diagnostic biopsy or incisions should be avoided, but fine-needle aspiration with cytology and culture has been successfully used, with no formation of fistulas needing chronic drainage [34]. However, according to other authors fine-needle aspiration is not encouraging due to a high percentage of negative cultures. They recommend an excisional biopsy of lymph node in order to maximize the recovery of organisms, to prevent further cosmetic damage, to remove infected tissue before more extensive spread occurs, and to cure the affection [35].

7.3.2 Skin Disease

There have been various reports in literature of skin manifestations due to *M. scrofulaceum* [36–40]. One was in a man with corticosteroid-dependent systemic lupus erythematosus and multiple painful subcutaneous abscesses: skin biopsy demonstrated granulomatous inflammation and acid-fast bacilli, and culture revealed

M. scrofulaceum. The patient was afebrile, and a 9-month course of isoniazid and rifampicin healed the complaint after 5 months [37]. Positive skin lesions for *M. scrofulaceum* were reported in a kidney transplant patient on prednisone and chlorambucil therapy [38]. In a 77-year-old patient with chronic exposure to aquarium water, skin lesions with a sporotrichoid pattern were observed on both hands [39]. In another aquarium water-associated case *M. scrofulaceum* and *M. peregrinum* were isolated; the infection healed with sparfloxacin and minocycline treatment [40]. In a woman with post-autologous bone marrow transplantation for breast cancer, a post-traumatic nodular lesion of the index finger developed; azithromycin and rifampicin treatment brought about resolution [41]. In a 4-year-old girl, an asymptomatic red nodule of the cheek due to *M. scrofulaceum*, identified by biochemical and PCR testing, healed with clarithromycin (250 mg/day) treatment for 6 months [42].

7.4 Histopathology

The center of these lesions generally shows necrosis and abscess formation, and is surrounded by tuberculoid granulomas and considerable inflammatory cells. Acid-fast bacilli are usually found in lymph nodes.

7.5 Treatment

Combination chemotherapy treatment, with or without surgery, is increasingly administered. *M. scrofulaceum* is one of the most resistant of all NTM species. It is resistant to isoniazid, *para*-aminosalicylic acid, and kanamycin, but sensitive to rifampicin, rifabutin, ethambutol, streptomycin, cycloserine, amikacin, ethionamide, viomycin, and capreomycin [3].

No comparative or controlled treatment trials have yet been conducted. Various authors are in agreement that medical treatment of the lymphadenitis is difficult whereas surgical treatment is generally sufficient to bring about resolution [28, 30, 41, 43], reserving chemotherapy for young patients whose parents refuse surgery, for recurrences after surgery or in cases where surgery requires excision of a significant amount of abnormal tissue [35]. Newer macrolide and fluoroquinolones antibiotics seem to offer good promise in vitro. Treatment with 2 or more drugs shown to be active in vitro may be justified, especially in cases where surgical removal of the lesions is not feasible [3].

References

1. Weitzul S, Eichhorn PJ, Pandya AG (2000) Nontuberculous mycobacterial infections of the skin. Dermatol Clin 18:359
2. Griffith DE, Aksamit T, Brown-Elliot BA et al (2007) An official ATS/IDSA steatment: diagnosis, treatment, and prevention of nontuberculous mycobacterial diseases. Am J Respir Crit Care Med 175:367

3. Horowitz EA (2011) *Mycobacterium scrofulaceum*. In: Schlossberg D (ed) Tuberculosis and nontuberculous mycobacterial infections, 6th edn. ASM Press, Washington, DC, p 601
4. Prissick FH, Masson AM (1952) A preliminary report on a study of pigmented mycobacteria. Can J Public Health 43:34
5. Prissick FH, Masson AM (1956) Cervical lymphadenitis in children caused by chromogenic mycobacteria. Can Med Assoc J 75:798
6. Prissick FH, Masson AM (1957) Yellow pigmented pathogenic mycobacteria from cervical lymphadenitis. Can Med Assoc J 3:91
7. Good RC (1979) Isolation of nontuberculous mycobacteria in the United States. J Infect Dis 142:779
8. Rogall T, Walters T, Flohr T et al (1990) Towards the phylogeny and definition of species at the molecular level within the genus *Mycobacterium*. Int J Syst Bacteriol 40:323
9. Tortoli E (2003) Impact of genotypic studies on mycobacterial taxonomy: the new mycobacteria of the 1990's. Clin Microbiol Rev 2:319
10. Swanson DS, Pan X, Musser JM (1996) Identification and subspecific differentiation of *Mycobacterium scrofulaceum* by automated sequencing of a region of the gene (*hsp65*) encoding a 65-kilodalton heat shock protein. J Clin Microbiol 34:3151
11. Turenne CY, Cook VJ, Burdz TV et al (2004) *Mycobacterium parascrofulaceum* sp. nov., novel slowly growing scotochromogenic clinical isolate related to *Mycobacterium simiae*. Int J Syst Evol Microbiol 54:1543
12. Chapman JS, Bernard JS, Speight M (1965) Isolation of mycobacteria from raw milk. Am Rev Respir Dis 91:351
13. Hosty TS, McDurmount CI (1975) Isolation of acid-fast organisms from milk and oysters. Health Lab Sci 12:16
14. Goslee S, Walinsky E (1976) Water as a source of potentially pathogenic mycobacteria. Am Rev Respir Dis 113:287
15. Wolinsky E (1979) State of the art: nontuberculous mycobacteria and associated diseases. Am Rev Respir Dis 110:107
16. Le Mense GP, Van Bakel AB, Crumbley AJ et al (1994) *Mycobacterium scrofulaceum* infection presenting as lung nodules in a heart transplant recipient. Chest 106:1918
17. Sanders JW, Walsh AD, Snider RL et al (1995) Disseminated *Mycobacterium scrofulaceum* infection: a potentially treatable complication of AIDS. Clin Infect Dis 30:444
18. Hsueh PR, Hsine TR, Jam JT et al (1996) Disseminated infection due to *Mycobacterium scrofulaceum* in an immunocompetent host. Clin Infect Dis 22:159
19. Dunn BL, Hodgson DJ (1982) "Atypical" mycobacteria in milk. J Appl Bacteriol 52:373
20. Brooks RW, Parker BC, Gruft H et al (1984) Epidemiology of infection by nontuberculous mycobacteria. Numbers in eastern United States soil and correlation with soil characteristics. Am Rev Respir Dis 130:630
21. Kirschner RA Jr, Parker BC, Falkinham JO (1992) Epidemiology of infection by nontuberculous mycobacteria. *Mycobacterium avium*, *Mycobacterium intracellulare*, and *Mycobacterium scrofulaceum* in acid, brown-water swamps of the southern United States and their association with environmental variables. Am Rev Respir Dis 145:271
22. Good RC, Snider DE (1982) Isolation of nontuberculous mycobacteria in the United States, 1980. J Infect Dis 146:829
23. Corbett EL, Hay M, Churchyard GJ et al (1999) *Mycobacterium kansasii* and *Mycobacterium scrofulaceum* isolated from HIV-negative South African gold miners: incidence, clinical significance and radiology. Int J Tuberc Lung Dis 3:501
24. Bruins J, Gribnau JH, Bwire R (1995) Investigation into typical and atypical tuberculin sensitivity in the Royal Netherlands Army, resulting in a more rational indication for isoniazid prophylaxis. Tuber Lung Dis 76:540
25. Dascalopoulos GA, Loukas S, Costantopoulos SH (1995) Wide geographic variations of sensitivity of MOTT sensitins in Greece. Eur Respir J 8:715

26. Kwamanga DO, Swai OB, Agwanda R et al (1995) Effect of nontuberculous mycobacteria infection on tuberculin results among primary school children in Kenya. East Afr Med J 72:222
27. Svandova E, Stastna J, Kubin M (1984) Comparative testing of skin reactions to PPD mycobacterins from *Mycobacterium tuberculosis and Mycobacterium scrofulaceum* in school-age children. J Hyg Epidemiol Microbiol Immunol 29:275
28. Lincoln EM, Gilbert LA (1972) Disease in children due to mycobacteria other than *Mycobacterium tuberculosis*. Am Rev Respir Dis 105:683
29. Wolinsky E, Ryncarson TK (1968) Mycobacteria in soil and their relation to disease-associated strains. Am Rev Respir Dis 97:1032
30. Wolinsky E (1995) Mycobacterial lymphadenitis in children: a prospective study of 105 nontuberculous cases with long-term follow-up. Clin Infect Dis 20:954
31. Grzybowski S, Allen EA (1995) History and importance of scrofula. Lancet 346:1472
32. O'Brien RJ, Geiter LJ, Snider DE Jr (1987) The epidemiology of nontuberculous mycobacterial disease in the United States. Am Rev Respir Dis 135:1007
33. Margileth AM (1983) The use of purified protein derivative mycobacterial skin test antigens in children and adolescents: purified protein derivative skin test results correlated with mycobacterial isolates. Pediatr Infect Dis 2:225
34. Chao SS, Loh KS, Tan KK et al (2002) Tuberculous and nontuberculous cervical lymphadenitis: a clinical review. Otolaryngol Head Neck Surg 126:176
35. Starke JR (2000) Management of nontuberculous mycobacterial cervical adenitis. Pediatr Infect Dis 19:67
36. Gorse GJ, Fairshter RD, Friedly G et al (1983) Nontuberculous mycobacterial disease. Experience in a Southern California hospital. Arch Intern Med 143:225
37. Murray-Leisure KA, Egan N, Weitekamp MR (1987) Skin lesions caused by *Mycobacterium scrofulaceum*. Arch Dermatol 123:369
38. Abbott MR, Smith DD (1981) Mycobacteria infections in immunosuppressed patients. Med J Aust 1:351
39. Sowers WF (1972) Swimming pool granuloma due to *Mycobacterium scrofulaceum*. Arch Dermatol 105:760
40. Ishii N, Sugita Y, Sato I et al (1998) A case of mycobacterial skin disease caused by *Mycobacterium peregrinum* and *M. scrofulaceum*. Acta Derm Venereol 78:76
41. Kandyil R, Maloney D, Tarrand J et al (2002) Red nodule on the finger of an immunosuppressed woman. Arch Dermatol 128:689
42. Jang H, Jo J, Oh C et al (2005) Successful treatment of localized cutaneous infection caused by *Mycobacterium scrofulaceum* with clarithromycin. Pediatr Dermatol 22:476
43. Hautmann G, Lotti T (1995) Diseases caused by *Mycobacterium scrofulaceum*. Clin Dermatol 13:277

Rapidly Growing Mycobacteria and Skin Infection

8

Domenico Bonamonte, Angela Filoni, Pietro Verni, and Gianni Angelini

Rapidly growing mycobacteria (RGM) are among the most common nontuberculous mycobacteria (NTM) associated with cutaneous infections in industrialized countries [1–8].

8.1 Taxonomy

In the early twentieth century, the first step in the history of identification of some of the most common RGM pathogens was the isolation of *Mycobacterium chelonae* by Friedmann from the lungs of two sea turtles (hence the name *chelonae,* from the Latin chelys of the turtle) [7, 9].

M. fortuitum (formerly *M. ranae*), another RGM species, had been isolated in 1905 from frogs. In 1938, ola Costa Cruz gave the name *M. fortuitum* to a species that he believed to be new, isolated from skin abscesses following local vitamin injections [10]. It was later seen that the two organisms were the same species, that kept the name of *M. fortuitum* [11].

Another closely related RGM species, *M. abscessus*, was described in 1953, isolated from skin abscesses [12].

D. Bonamonte, MD, PhD (✉)
Department of Biomedical Science and Human Oncology, University of Bari "Aldo Moro", Bari, Italy
e-mail: domenico.bonamonte@uniba.it

A. Filoni, MD • P. Verni, MD
University of Bari "Aldo Moro", Bari, Italy

G. Angelini, MD
Professor of Dermatology, Former Professor and Chairman, University of Bari "Aldo Moro", Bari, Italy

D. Bonamonte, G. Angelini (eds.), *Mycobacterial Skin Infections*,
DOI 10.1007/978-3-319-48538-6_8

Table 8.1 Taxonomic spectrum of rapidly growing mycobacteria (RGM) (modified, by [8])

Group	Species	Species within the group
I	*M. fortuitum*	*M. fortuitum, M. boenickei, M. brisbanense, M. houstonense, M. neworleansense, M. peregrinum, M. porcinum, M. senegalense, M. septicum, M. setense*
II	*M. chelonae/ M. abscessus*	*M. chelonae, M. abscessus* subsp. *abscessus, M. abscessus* subsp. *bollettii, M. immunogenum, M. salmoniphilum*
III	*M. mucogenicum*	*M. mucogenicum, M. aubagnense, M. phocaicum*
IV	*M. smegmatis*	*M. smegmatis, M. goodii*
V	*M. mageritense/ M. wolinskyi*	*M. mageritense, M. wolinskyi*
VI	Early pigmented RGM	*M. neoaurum/aurum, M. bacteremicum, M. canariasense, M. cosmeticum, M. elephantis, M. monacense, M. novacastrense*

Recent taxonomic studies using molecular analysis with DNA-DNA hybridization and 16S ribosomal sequencing, have demonstrated that the previous classifications as "subspecies" or "biovariants" of *M. chelonae* (*M. chelonae* subsp. *chelonae* and *M. chelonae* subsp. *abscessus*) and *M. fortuitum* (*M. fortuitum* biovariant *fortuitum*, *M. fortuitum* biovariant *peregrinum*, and *M. fortuitum* third biovariant complex) actually referred to separate species, that were therefore renamed without the subgroup designation [13].

Today, the RGM are grouped into six major taxonomic groups according to pigmentation and genetic relatedness (Table 8.1) [7, 8]. An excellent in-depth review of the taxonomy of RGM has been reported by Brown-Elliot and Wallace [7]. More than 70 species of RGM are now known, accounting for nearly 50% of all the known mycobacteria species. The three most important from the clinical standpoint, and that account for more than 80% of the clinical isolates, are *M. fortuitum*, *M. chelonae*, and *M. abscessus* [14]. Among all the other species or subspecies described, some rare human pathogens have been described: *M. setense* [15], *M. canariasense*, isolated in 17 patients with suspected nosocomial infections from infected central venous catheters [16], and others [7, 17].

8.2 Epidemiology

Apart from pulmonary and extrapulmonary infections, RGM, and particularly *M. abscessus*, *M. chelonae*, and *M. fortuitum*, cause cutaneous and soft tissue infections, mostly due to direct pathogenic involvement of the skin. In cases of disseminated disease and associated skin involvement the primary focus may be respiratory.

RGM-associated skin and soft tissue infections are deep, and generally follow traumatic injuries, surgical wounds, and environmental exposure (Table 8.2). *M. fortuitum* is the most common cause of skin manifestations in young individuals, while *M. abscessus* and *M. chelonae* more often induce skin lesions in older subjects [18]. While the skin pictures due to *M. fortuitum* are generally localized and

Table 8.2 More frequent sources of cutaneous and subcutaneous infections due to rapidly growing mycobacteria (RGM) (modified, by [8])

RGM	Sources	Skin infection
M. abscessus	Acupuncture	Various lesions
	Tattoos	Tender papular lesions
	Mesotherapy	Dusky red nodules, abscesses and sinuses
	Foreign-body-associated indwelling medical devices	Tender nodules in peristomal injections
	Various conditions of immunosuppression	Multiple or disseminated erythematous nodules, papules, pustules and abscesses
	Intravenous heroin injection	Bilateral sporotrichoid infection
	Localized post-traumatic infections	Nodules and abscesses
M. chelonae	Pedicures (whirlpool footbaths and nail salons)	Lower legs recurrent furunculosis
	Tattoos	Papules, pustules and plaques
	Liposuction	Abscesses
	Various conditions of immunosuppression	Several and disseminated plaques, papules, nodules and pustules
	Localized post-traumatic infections	Nodules and abscesses
M. fortuitum	Pedicures	Furunculosis on lower legs
	Mesotherapy	Painful nodules
	Injections	Nodules and sinuses with sporotrichoid pattern
	Various conditions of immunosuppression	Multiple abscesses and nodules
	Fish handling	Fish tank granuloma with nodular lesions (rare)
	Localized posttraumatic infections	Nodules and abscesses

there may only be a single lesion, those due to *M. abscessus* and *M. chelonae* are mostly generalized, with diffuse multiple lesions [18–21].

RGM are ubiquitous in the environment [5]. Human infections have been reported in most developed areas of the world, and RGM have been isolated from 30 to 78% of soil samples from geographic regions in the United States [14, 22].

Community-acquired localized cutaneous and soft tissue diseases often ensue after traumatic injuries potentially exposing to soil contamination (e.g. stepping on a nail, a motor vehicle accident with an open fracture, etc) [7]. Various studies have documented a correlation between potable water supplies and community or health care-related infections, due to the formation of biofilms in treated water distribution mains [23]. In the health care setting, RGM grow on hard surfaces (water distribution pipes, shower fixtures, sink faucets, ice machines), and medical devices [24, 25].

Other environmental sources from which RGM have been isolated include: freshwater rivers and lakes, seawater, waste water from hospitals, and soil [26, 27]; hot drinking water distribution systems [25]; raw milk and tissue samples from livestock specimens [28]; gentian violet solutions for contaminated water [29]. Standards and guidelines for safe drinking water are supplied by municipal water treatment plants to cities. Within distribution (mains) network the water flows continuously. However, the quality of the water from the distribution system changes dramatically at the point of entrance to private buildings, due to restricted flow and so the water may stagnate [30–32]. Temperature changes also offer favorable conditions for the formation of biofilms, and disinfectant-resistant bacteria, such as RGM, may be entrapped [8, 32].

Exposure to tap water is the major risk factor for nosocomial disease [7, 14, 33]. The various water sources include water-based solutions, distilled water, ice, and ice water [34, 35]. Compared to free-living mycobacteria, those associated with biofilms, the slimy layers occurring at water-solid interfaces, are more resistant to water treatment and biofilms play a role in the development of mycobacteria resistance [36].

Sporadic health care-associated infections due to *M. fortuitum*, *M. chelonae*, and *M. abscessus* include catheter-related infections, sternal wound infections following cardiac bypass surgery, and infections following insertion of prosthetic heart valves, lens implants, artificial knees and hips [14, 37]. Various outbreaks of post-injection abscesses caused by *M. abscessus* have been reported in many countries [38–41]. One outbreak of catheter-associated bacteremia was caused by a new species, *M. phocaicum* [42].

M. chelonae, *M. fortuitum*, and *M. immunogenum* have caused infections associated with cosmetic surgery procedures, especially liposuction, breast augmentation, and mesotherapy [43–49]. Similar outbreaks linked to *M. abscessus* have been reported by United States tourists ("lipotourists") who underwent abdominoplasty in the Dominican Republic [50]. Outbreaks of RGM infections following acupuncture treatment have also been observed [14, 51]. The largest epidemic of post-video laparoscopy infections caused by *M. massiliense* was reported in Brazil [52]. Various other post-surgical outbreaks linked to RGM (including *M. massiliense* and *M. bollettii*) were reported in 63 hospitals in Brazil following laparoscopic, arthroscopic, plastic surgery, or cosmetic procedures [17, 53]. *M. abscessus* and *M. immunogenum* have induced pseudo-outbreaks due to the contamination of automated bronchoscope disinfection machines, gastric endoscopes, and other laboratory instruments [14, 54, 55].

Recently, cases of lower extremity skin infections involving *M. fortuitum*, *M. mageritense*, *M. cosmeticum*, and *M. abscessus*, associated with contaminated nail salon whirlpool footbaths, have been described [56–61]. The most common manifestations were furunculosis of the lower legs. The pathogenic mechanisms inducing the dermatitis also include microtrauma caused by shaving the legs prior to pedicures.

Tuberculosis and NTM infections associated with biological therapies that inhibit tumor necrosis factor alpha (TNF-α) have been observed. A recent review of the United States FDA Med Watch database reports identified 239 possible cases of NTM infection associated with TNF-α inhibitor use from 1999 to 2006, 105 (44%) of which met RGM disease criteria [62]. The immunosuppressive drugs implicated were infliximab, etanercept, and adalimumab. The most common underlying condition was rheumatoid arthritis (75%), and 65% and 55% of patients were taking prednisone and methotrexate, respectively. *M. avium* complex was the most frequent pathogen, while 20% of the 105 cases due to RGM were caused by *M. abscessus*, *M. chelonae*, and *M. fortuitum* [62].

Catastrophic natural events, such as Hurricanes Katrina and Rita in New Orleans (Louisiana), and the 2004 tsunami in Thailand, resulted in several skin disorders associated with contaminated water which generally carries multiple bacteria, fungal and viral pathogens. Specific examples of RGM transmission with early- or late-onset infections were reported [63, 64].

8.3 Cutaneous and Subcutaneous Clinical Infection

An RGM infection management strategy requires a careful evaluation of the case, including the clinical characteristics of the lesions, the histopathologic assessment, a computed tomography (CT) and ultrasound, culturing and appropriate speciation using molecular tools such as gene sequencing and polymerase chain reaction (PCR) restriction analyses. The choice of drug/s, dosage and duration of monotherapy or combination therapy, or combined with surgical therapy if necessary, must be based on the disease severity, localization, the patient's immune status (underlying clinical or subclinical conditions), and on the minimum inhibitory concentration (MIC) results of the RGM-specific drugs (there are laboratory-specific guidelines in this regard) [8].

Among the most common extrapulmonary infections induced by RGM are localized post-traumatic wound infections following accidental trauma [14]. After an incubation period of 3–6 weeks, local redness and swelling with spontaneous drainage occurs. Systemic symptoms like fever, chills, malaise, and fatigue are generally absent. The discharge is usually watery but can sometimes be thick and purulent, and sinus tract formations are common. The more common pathogens are *M. fortuitum*, *M. porcinum*, *M. houstonense*, and others. It should be borne in mind that these infections are polymicrobial, due to environmental contamination by more than one species of mycobacteria or a combination of bacteria and mycobacteria [7, 13, 14, 65].

Surgical wound infections, subsequent to the various surgical practices mentioned above, present in a similar fashion to accidental trauma. After an incubation of 2–8 weeks, the wound develops a serous discharge and reddens, with possible localized painful nodular lesions, that may require incision and drainage. The patient may have fever. *M. fortuitum* is the most frequent culprit in such cases [14].

RGM can induce two types of disseminated cutaneous infections. The first type features multiple non contiguous nodular draining lesions on one or more extremities. This picture is observed in subjects with chronic diseases requiring chronic corticosteroid treatments (even at doses as low as 5–10 mg of prednisone daily), the most common being rheumatoid arthritis, but also organ transplants and chronic autoimmune disorders. In general the cause is *M. chelonae* [14]. Another form of disseminated cutaneous infection is observed in patients with rapidly fatal disorders, such as poorly controlled leukemias [66] and lymphoma [14]. The entry portal of the pathogen is rarely identified, and the infection tends to be systemic. *M. abscessus* is generally implicated or, more rarely, *M. fortuitum* and *M. smegmatis* [14].

8.4 *Mycobacterium abscessus*

M. abscessus (a subset of the formerly termed *M. chelonae* complex) has been isolated from multiple environmental sites, in particular from tap water on multiple occasions as part of nosocomial outbreaks. In the management of infections linked with this pathogen, it is important to differentiate it from *M. chelonae* because the treatment of *M. abscessus* is more difficult. Like other RGM, *M. abscessus* grows at 25–40 °C in fewer than 7 days and produces arylsulfatase in fewer than 1–3 days. Unlike *M. chelonae*, *M. abscessus* grows in the presence of 5% sodium chloride but cannot use citrate as a carbon source [2].

8.4.1 Clinical Features

M. abscessus causes chronic pulmonary disease, disseminated cutaneous disease, and localized skin infections [67]. It is also commonly associated with sporadic and epidemic nosocomial infections or pseudo-outbreaks associated with bronchoscopy, various surgical procedures, post-injection abscesses, and dialysis. The prognosis of the infection is highly dependent upon the underlying immune status of the host: low CD4+ T cell counts contribute to some extent to the severity of the infection [68, 69].

M. abscessus is the third most frequently recovered nontuberculous mycobacteria respiratory pathogen in the United States and accounts for approximately 80% of RGM respiratory disease isolates [70]. Respiratory forms are often associated with disseminated skin forms [8]. Disseminated cutaneous infections occur also, and almost exclusively, in immunosuppressed subjects, hemodialysis patients, or transplant recipients [2, 8].

Localized skin infections are usually acquired after local trauma (post-traumatic wound infections which may develop into sporotrichoid-like ascending lymphadenitis) [18], surgical wound infections (resulting from mammoplasties, facial plastic surgeries, cardiac surgeries, etc.), and post-injection health care-related infections [18, 38, 70]. However, localized infections with *M. abscessus* without any history of trauma or immunosuppression have also been reported [2].

Skin infected with *M. abscessus* is usually red, warm, tender to the touch, swollen, and painful. The lesions are mostly nodules and abscesses; blisters and pustules may also be present.

In normal healthy subjects, skin piercing and tattoos can be an easy entry portal for *M. abscessus* [71]. One patient was reported who developed an *M. abscessus* infection because a tattoo artist had used tap water to turn black ink to gray [8].

Rarely, *M. abscessus* infections have been reported in fish handlers or other subjects after exposure to saltwater. The clinical manifestations are similar to those caused by *M. marinum*: therefore, dermatologists should consider *M. abscessus* alongside *M. marinum* when diagnosing and treating infections in this setting [72, 73]. A natural calamity, such as the tsunami that occurred in Thailand, resulted in soft tissues infections in some individuals, either alone or with concomitant fungi [64].

8.4.2 Histopathological Remarks

Histopathologically, most *M. abscessus* lesions consist of abscesses containing acute inflammatory cells bordered by Langhans and epithelioid cells, with necrosis and tuberculoid granulomas. Acute inflammatory cells may also be seen, similar to those observed in *M. fortuitum* and *M. chelonae* lesions [2]. In one series most biopsy specimens revealed intralesional vacuoles, that were filled with organisms in 27% of cases [74].

8.4.3 Treatment

M. abscessus is resistant to the standard antitubercular drugs. Because of the variable in vitro drug susceptibility to some agents, antibiotic susceptibility testing of all isolates is recommended. Acquired mutational resistance to clarithromycin (23S rRNA gene) and amikacin (16S rRNA gene) can occur because isolates of *M. abscessus* generally have a single copy of the gene [5].

For serious skin infections, clarithromycin 1000 mg/day or azithromycin 250 mg/day should be combined with parenteral drugs (amikacin, cefoxitin, or imipenem). Macrolides are the only oral agents reliably active in vitro against *M. abscessus* [75–77]. The most active parenteral agent is amikacin (intravenous amikacin is given at a dose of 10–15 mg/kg/day to adults with normal renal function); a lower dose (10 mg/kg) should be used in patients aged over 50 years and in patients on long-term therapy (×3 weeks). Amikacin combined with high-dose cefoxitin (up to 12 g/day given intravenously in divided doses) is recommended for the initial therapy (minimum 2 weeks), until a clinical improvement is evident [5]. Imipenem (500 mg 2–4 times daily) is an alternative to cefoxitin. For serious infections, a minimum of 4 months of treatment is necessary (Table 8.3).

Amikacin can cause major renal and auditory toxicities. The newly introduced tigecycline may be another option for therapy in serious diseases [78].

Drug monotherapy in these settings should be avoided to prevent resistance. However, clarithromycin alone for localized infections appears to carry little risk of resistance [76]. Localized skin infections in immunocompetent patients are treated for 3 or more months [77].

Table 8.3 Antibiotics recommended for the treatment of infections due to rapidly growing mycobacteria

Species	Antibiotics
M. abscessus	Oral: clarithromycin, azithromycin, linezolid
	Parenteral: amikacin, cefoxitin, imipenem, tigecycline
M. chelonae	Oral: clarithromycin, tobramycin, linezolid
	Parenteral: tobramycin, tigecycline, amikacin, imipenem
M. fortuitum	Oral: ciprofloxacin, sulfonamides, ofloxacin, clarithromycin, linezolid, doxycycline
	Parenteral: amikacin, imipenem, cefoxitin

Surgery is necessarily indicated in cases with extensive disease, abscess formation, or where drug therapy is difficult. Removal of foreign bodies, such as breast implants or percutaneous catheters, is important to assure recovery [5, 78].

The natural existence of the *erm* (erythromycin-resistant methylase) gene in *M. abscessus* suggests that this particular gene induces macrolide resistance. An interesting difference between *M. abscessus* and *M. chelonae* is the lack of the *erm* gene in the latter, which may explain its better response to macrolide-based chemotherapy [79].

8.5 *Mycobacterium chelonae*

As regards *M. chelonae* and *M. abscessus*, two subspecies now recognized as separate, acid-fast staining sensitivity is unsatisfactory in about 75% of cases [8]. However, it is important to differentiate these two species using molecular tools because the treatment is species-specific [5].

Skin, soft tissue, and bone diseases are the most important clinical manifestations of *M. chelonae* infection. In immunocompromised individuals the cutaneous infection is disseminated. Sporadic cases of keratitis associated with contact lens wear and ocular surgery have been described [80, 81]. *M. chelonae* is a less common cause of pulmonary disease than *M. abscessus* [5].

8.5.1 Clinical Features

The skin manifestations include disseminated nodular lesions, localized cellulitis, and abscesses. The most common presentation is disseminated disease, with multiple lesions (in some cases even more than 100), usually localized on a single limb or else all the extremities. These lesions are generally erythematous subcutaneous nodules, with multiple draining fistulas (Fig. 8.1); most of them exude fluid and,

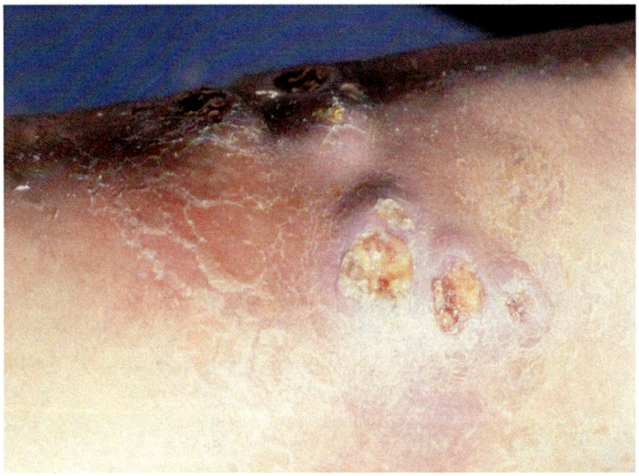

Fig. 8.1 *Mycobacterium chelonae* infection. Ulcerated nodules (reproduced with permission from Bonamonte and Coll [82])

with pressure, discharge thick necrotic material [2]. The lesions are usually non contiguous and occur in a non linear pattern, although there have been a few reports of infection by *M. chelonae* with a sporotrichoid pattern [83]. In general, systemic signs (fever, chills, weight loss) are lacking. In one report, 92% of the patients with disseminated cutaneous infections were on corticosteroid treatment for organ transplantation or autoimmune disease [84].

Contaminated water is a natural reservoir of *M. chelonae* and a source of infection in humans. Patients with poor immune responses, such as HIV/AIDS infected subjects, are more prone to *M. chelonae* infections, that can induce clinical or frequently subclinical conditions [85]. Cutaneous lesions have been observed in hemodialysis and peritoneal dialysis patients, kidney and liver transplant patients, and tattooed subjects. These infections are often localized on the upper limbs or downstream of an arteriovenous fistula. Patients with cutaneous infections due to *M. chelonae* are at risk of acquiring nosocomial infections [86–89]. Various cases of skin infections have ensued after anti-TNF therapy (adalimumab, etanercept) [88].

8.5.2 Culture and Histopathology

In culture *M. chelonae* produces rough or smooth non pigmented colonies. Optimal growth is at 28 °C and occurs within 7 days. The species may not grow at all on primary isolation at 37 °C. It produces arylsulfatase activity in 1–3 days. Unlike *M. abscessus*, *M. chelonae* uses citrate as a carbon source and does not grow in the presence of 5% sodium chloride [84].

The skin lesions are typically characterized by granulomatous reactions, identical to those due to *M. fortuitum*, although a predominance of neutrophils may be observed in cases of abscess formation [8]. In severely immunocompromised AIDS patients, skin lesions demonstrate diffuse infiltrates of histiocytes, occasionally with a foamy appearance [90].

8.5.3 Treatment

Unlike for *M. abscessus*, no *erm* gene has been identified in *M. chelonae* [8]. Isolates of *M. chelonae* are susceptible to tobramycin (100%), clarithromycin (100%), linezolid (90%), imipenem (60%), amikacin (50%), doxycycline (25%), clofazimine (25%), and ciprofloxacin (20%) [5, 84, 90–94]. Imipenem is preferred to cefoxitin because *M. chelonae* isolates are resistant to cefoxitin [81, 84, 90–94].

In some cases, *M. chelonae* appears to be susceptible only to tigecycline, clarithromycin, and tobramycin [49]. However, the in vitro susceptibility does not consistently predict the effectiveness of the treatment. Clarithromycin monotherapy may promote acquired drug resistance [95]. In another study, adult patients with disseminated cutaneous manifestations of *M. chelonae* infection were treated with 500 mg clarithromycin monotherapy twice a day for 6 months; all the patients recovered except for one patient (8%) who relapsed, with an isolate that had developed mutational resistance to the drug (Table 8.3) [96].

Optimal treatment procedures for skin infections due to *M. chelonae* have yet to be standardized. In all cases antimicrobial susceptibility tests are recommended. For serious skin disease, a minimum of 4 months of a combination drug therapy (at least initially to minimize the risk of macrolide resistance) is necessary to ensure a high likelihood of cure [5].

A 62-year-old male on long-term systemic corticosteroid therapy for unconfirmed dermatomyositis presented multiple painless cutaneous lesions at various stages of development: papules, nodules, pustules, and hemorrhagic crusts, as well as small erosions and ulcers distributed over the limbs and scalp. On the limbs, the lesions had a sporotrichoid pattern. Cutaneous biopsy showed a suppurative granulomatous infiltrate with abscess formation. Culture of a skin sample revealed *M. chelonae*. After 45 days of multidrug treatment (oral clarithromycin and ciprofloxacin and intravenous amikacin for the first 3 weeks), the patient showed a significant improvement. However, the antibiogram revealed resistance to ciprofloxacin [97].

Due to inadequate conveyance of antibiotics within abscesses, excision and drainage remains the treatment of choice for cutaneous abscesses [8].

8.6 *Mycobacterium fortuitum*

M. fortuitum, in the past denominated *M. ranae* because of its isolation in frogs in 1905 [98], owes its name to da Costa Cruz [10]. It is widely distributed in the environment: soil, dust, milk, water, marine and land animals, as well as the saliva of healthy humans [2]. The *M. fortuitum* group originally included three species/taxa: *M. fortuitum*, *M. peregrinum*, and an unnamed third biovariant complex. Recently, however, other species have been added to the group, including *M. houstonense*, *M. boenickei* and others [5].

M. fortuitum produces non pigmented smooth or rough colonies, which become visible in 1 week or less. It grows well at temperatures from 28 to 37 °C on routine bacterial media (blood and chocolate agar) as well as mycobacterial media; it does not grow at 45 °C. Apart from reducing nitrates, it uses iron, and is not pathogenic in laboratory guinea pigs.

8.6.1 Clinical Features

M. fortuitum causes a large variety of cutaneous and extracutaneous diseases, such as postoperative vasculitis, endocarditis, osteomyelitis, mediastinitis, meningitis, keratitis, hepatitis, central nervous system involvement, and disseminated infections [2, 99–101]. *M. fortuitum* skin and soft tissue infections are associated with surgery or penetrating trauma [77], whereas superficial infections most commonly result from direct inoculation of the skin after minor trauma or injections [99].

Primary cutaneous lesions are generally localized at the injured site, and can manifest as painful nodules, abscesses, ulcers, draining sinus tracts, or cellulitis, usually 4–6 weeks after injury [101]. Less commonly, skin manifestations of disseminated disease can be observed, generally in immunocompromised patients [99, 102].

Lesions in disseminated cases occur in multiple episodes and present as generalized morbilliform eruptions, nodules, or multiple abscesses, usually on the extremities [103]. Cutaneous disease generally has an indolent course, with fistula formation and scarring as healing occurs [99].

Recently, whirlpool footbaths used during pedicure procedures in nail salons have been identified as a source of both sporadic and clustered outbreaks of furunculosis associated with *M. fortuitum* and other RGM [5, 58, 61, 104]. Such furunculosis cases are usually observed in women and can persist for months.

Nodules and abscesses at the injection sites can ensue after mesotherapy [49, 105, 106]. Venous catheterization in health care settings is another source of cutaneous or subcutaneous infection by *M. fortuitum*; the organism is often isolated from blood and purulent discharge specimens [107, 108]. Infections may also occur during electromyography, or punch biopsy procedures, after face-lift procedures, or after liver transplant [109–111]. Iatrogenic wound infections are occasionally observed in health care facilities, attributable to inadequate sterilization of surgical instruments and the use of contaminated disinfectants [8].

In rare cases, skin infection by *M. fortuitum* can follow bites by animals [112]. One case of diffuse infection, without any previous trauma, has also been described in a pregnant woman [113]. Sporotrichoid cutaneous infection due to *M. fortuitum* is rare. We reported a case of a 37-year-old woman with a sporotrichoid skin infection after intralesional corticosteroid treatment administered for a preexisting neurodermatitis. The complaint spread up from the left ankle to the leg, and presented as nodular dermo-hypodermic lesions with a suppurative, ulcerative evolution (Figs. 8.2, and 8.3). Histology demonstrated an aspecific inflammatory infiltrate

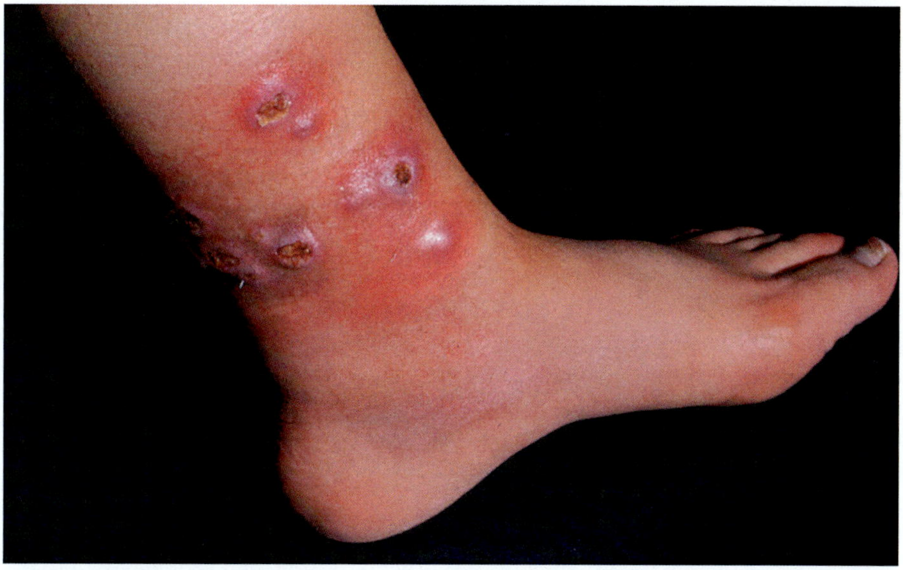

Fig. 8.2 *Mycobacterium fortuitum* infection. Dermo-hypodermic nodules with sporotrichoid pattern (reproduced with permission from Bonamonte and Coll [82])

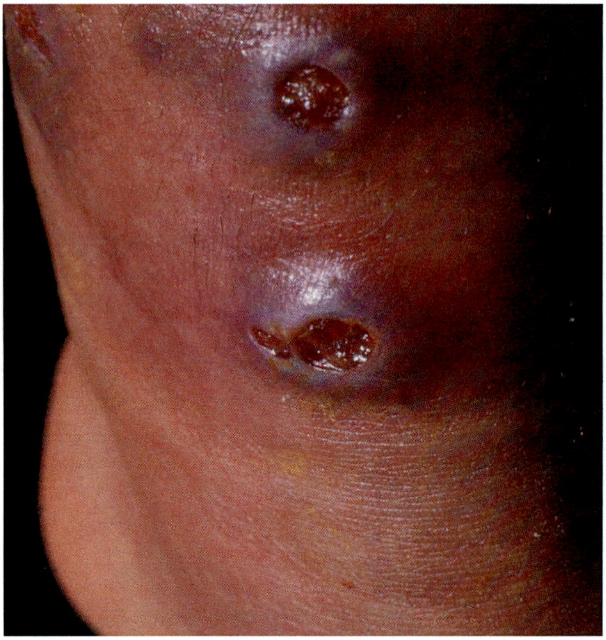

Fig. 8.3 The same patient as in Fig. 8.2

Table 8.4 Mycobacteria that may induce a sporotrichoid clinical pattern

Mycobacterium marinum
Mycobacterium chelonae
Mycobacterium fortuitum
Mycobacterium tuberculosis
Mycobacterium scrofulaceum
Mycobacterium szulgai
Mycobacterium kansasii
Mycobacterium abscessus

without the granuloma and central necrosis aspects [114]. The various blood and immunological tests were within normal limits. A mild skin reactivity to various mycobacteria antigens was elicited, likely due to cross-reactions. The sporotrichoid pattern of lesions is more frequently observed in cases of *M. marinum* [82, 115–118], but exceptional cases of other environmental mycobacterioses, due to *M. chelonae* [119, 120] and *M. kansasii* [121, 122] have also been reported. Another case of a sporotrichoid-like skin infection by *M. fortuitum* was reported in an immunocompetent subject with a history of intravenous heroin injection [123]. Because sporotrichoid mycobacterial infection is associated with several organisms, the use of molecular tools and PCR may help to distinguish *M. fortuitum* from other species (Table 8.4).

Other cases of skin infection by *M. fortuitum* have followed acupuncture procedures [124], an open fracture [125], and nipple piercing [126].

8.6.2 Histopathology

Cutaneous lesions appear as suppurative granulomas (Fig. 8.4). Caseation is not seen, and organisms are seen in extracellular sites, often associated with neutrophils (Fig. 8.5). Large, pleomorphic organisms are frequently detected on smears stained for acid-fast bacilli [99, 114].

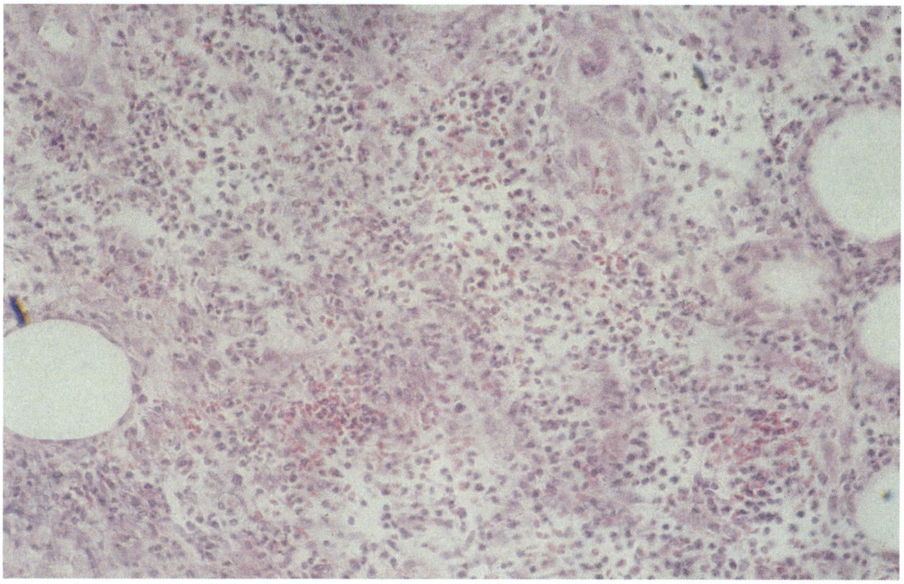

Fig. 8.4 Granulomatous suppurative infiltrate (Hematoxylin-eosin—×100)

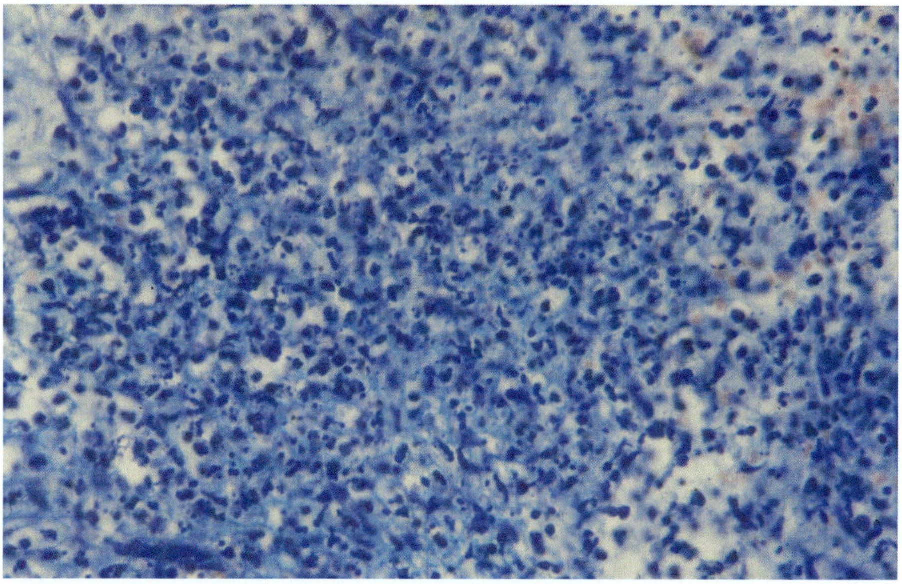

Fig. 8.5 Neutrophilic component of the infiltrate (Hematoxylin-eosin—×100)

8.6.3 Treatment

The therapeutic management of infections due to *M. fortuitum* requires in vitro drug susceptibility testing. The organism is generally susceptible to various oral antibiotics, including the newer macrolides and quinolones, doxycycline and minocycline, and sulfonamides [92, 93, 127]. Isolates are susceptible to amikacin (100%), ciprofloxacin and ofloxacin (100%), sulfonamides (100%), cefoxitin (50%), imipenem (50%), clarithromycin (80%), and doxycycline (50%) (Table 8.3). Recently, it has been shown that all isolates of *M. fortuitum* and the related species *M. smegmatis* and *M. houstonense* contain an inducible *erm* gene that confers resistance to the macrolides [8, 79]. Therefore, despite the susceptibility MICs seen in 80% of isolates for clarithromycin, macrolides should be used with caution [5].

For serious skin and soft tissue disease due to *M. fortuitum*, a minimum of 4 months of therapy with at least two agents shown to have an in vitro activity against the clinical isolates is necessary. Surgery is generally indicated in cases of extensive disease and abscess formation, or when drug therapy is ineffective.

8.7 Diagnosis

Clinical misdiagnosis of RGM infections may occur for various reasons: inadequate exposure of the physician to these specific diseases, incorrect specimen collection, inadequate communication concerning the suspected etiologic agent provided to the laboratory, and incorrect laboratory results [8].

In the differential diagnosis, it must be remembered that cutaneous infections due to *M. tuberculosis* can also present with papules and nodules with a purulent or serous-purulent discharge [8, 128], but the treatment is different. It is also important to differentiate sporotrichoid forms due to RGM from those due to *M. marinum* and to fungal species.

As regards staining and microscopic observation of the smears, there is a risk of misidentification as *Corynebacterium* when, instead, the culprit is *Mycobacterium*. Occasionally, RGM exhibit Gram-positive, long, filamentous, beaded forms that can easily be confused with the microscopic features of the *Corynebacterium* species, leading to diagnostic and treatment errors [129, 130]. There can be confusion not only with corynebacteria species but also with *Nocardia* species, which are characterized by lesions and microscopic features that resemble other RGM species [131].

The definitive diagnosis of cutaneous infections due to RGM is based on the results of the following procedures, that must always be analyzed together: cultures of organisms in drainage material, aspiration fluid; staining of tissue biopsy samples; drug susceptibility testing; histologic examination; and molecular biology methods [8].

In dermatological settings, the clinical suspicion of an infection due to RGM is very important. There are no well-established indicators yet available, but some clues may be useful: a history of exposure to various environmental and health care-related conditions; late onset of the symptoms (e.g. 2–4 months after acupuncture, trauma or surgical procedures); a chronic skin infection after an invasive procedure; an infection that does not respond to conventional antibiotics and/or with negative culture after 2 days of incubation; negative bacteriological (not mycobacteriological) cultures, and negative Gram and acid-fast staining of the specimens [8]. The diagnostic assessment should also take into account the possibility of mixed infections; a concomitant fungal infection is a primary factor. The latter can also be associated with a delayed response to therapy during the management of the RGM infection.

References

1. Wallace RJ Jr, Swenson JM, Silcox VA et al (1983) Spectrum of disease due to rapidly growing mycobacteria. Rev Infect Dis 5:657
2. Weitzul S, Eichhorn PJ, Pandya AG (2000) Nontuberculous mycobacterial infections of the skin. Dermatol Clin 18:359
3. Wagner D, Young LS (2004) Nontuberculous mycobacterial infections: a clinical review. Infection 32:257
4. Bartralot R, García-Patos V, Sitjas D et al (2005) Clinical patterns of cutaneous nontuberculous mycobacterial infections. Br J Dermatol 152:727
5. Griffith DE, Aksamit T, Brown-Elliott BA et al (2007) An official ATS/IDSA statement: diagnosis, treatment, and prevention of nontuberculous mycobacterial diseases. Am J Respir Crit Care Med 175:367
6. Cook JL (2010) Nontuberculous mycobacteria: opportunistic environmental pathogens for predisposed hosts. Br Med Bull 96:45
7. Brown-Elliot BA, Wallace RJ Jr (2011) Rapidly growing mycobacteria. In: Schlossberg D (ed) Tuberculosis and nontuberculous mycobacterial infections, 6th edn. ASM Press, Washington, DC, p 565
8. Kothavade RJ, Dhurat RS, Mishra SN et al (2013) Clinical and laboratory aspects of the diagnosis and management of cutaneous and subcutaneous infections caused by rapidly growing mycobacteria. Eur J Clin Microbiol Infect Dis 32:161
9. Cobbett L (1918) An acid-fast bacillus obtained from a pustular eruption. Br Med J 2:158
10. da Costa Cruz JC (1938) *Mycobacterium fortuitum:* un novo bacilo acido-resistente patogenico para o homen. Acta Med (Rio de Janeiro) 1:298
11. Ernest H (1972) Conservation of the specific epithet *fortuitum* in the name of the organism known as *Mycobacterium fortuitum* da Costa Cruz. Int J Syst Bacteriol 22:50
12. Moore M, Frerichs JB (1953) An unusual acid-fast infection of the knee with subcutaneous, abscess-like lesions of the gluteal region; report of a case with a study of the organism, *Mycobacterium abscessus*, nov sp. J Invest Dermatol 20:133
13. Schinsky MF, Morey RE, Steigerwalt AG et al (2004) Taxonomic variation in the *Mycobacterium fortuitum* third-biovariant complex: description of *Mycobacterium boenickei* sp. nov., *Mycobacterium houstonense* sp. nov., *Mycobacterium neworleansense* sp. nov., *Mycobacterium brisbanense* sp. nov., and recognition of *Mycobacterium porcinum* from human clinical isolates. Int J Syst Evol Microbiol 54:1653
14. Brown-Elliott BA, Wallace RJ Jr (2002) Clinical and taxonomic status of pathogenic nonpigmented or late-pigmenting rapidly growing mycobacteria. Clin Microbiol Rev 15:716
15. Lamy B, Marchandin H, Hamitouche K et al (2008) *Mycobacterium setense* sp. nov., a *Mycobacterium fortuitum*-group organism isolated from a patient with soft tissue infection and osteitis. Int J Syst Evol Microbiol 58:486
16. Jiménez MS, Campos-Herrero MI, García D et al (2004) *Mycobacterium canariasense* sp. nov. Int J Syst Evol Microbiol 54:1729

17. Leao SC, Tortoli E, Viana-Niero C et al (2009) Characterization of mycobacteria from a major Brazilian outbreak suggests that revision of the taxonomic status of members of the *Mycobacterium chelonae-M. abscessus* group is needed. J Clin Microbiol 47:2691
18. Uslan DZ, Kowalski TJ, Wengenack NL et al (2006) Skin and soft tissue infections due to rapidly growing mycobacteria: comparison of clinical features, treatment, and susceptibility. Arch Dermatol 142:1287
19. Ingram CW, Tanner DC, Durack DT et al (1993) Disseminated infection with rapidly growing mycobacteria. Clin Infect Dis 16:463
20. Wolinsky E (1992) Mycobacterial diseases other than tuberculosis. Clin Infect Dis 15(1):1
21. Lee WJ, Kang SM, Sung H et al (2010) Non-tuberculous mycobacterial infections of the skin: a retrospective study of 29 cases. J Dermatol 37:965
22. Wolinsky E (1979) Nontuberculous mycobacteria and associated diseases. Am Rev Respir Dis 119:107
23. Williams MM, Yakrus MA, Arduino MJ et al (2009) Structural analysis of biofilm formation by rapidly and slowly growing nontuberculous mycobacteria. Appl Environ Microbiol 75:2091
24. Falkinham JO (2010) Impact of human activities on the ecology of nontuberculous mycobacteria. Future Microbiol 5:951
25. Rodrigues C, Mehta A, Jha U et al (2001) Nosocomial *Mycobacterium chelonae* infection in laparoscopic surgery. Infect Control Hosp Epidemiol 22:474
26. Bland CS, Ireland JM, Lozano E et al (2005) Mycobacterial ecology of the Rio Grande. Appl Environ Microbiol 71:5719
27. Brown-Elliott BA, Wallace RJ Jr, Tichindelean C et al (2011) Five-year outbreak of community- and hospital-acquired *Mycobacterium porcinum* infections related to public water supplies. J Clin Microbiol 49:4231
28. Leite CQ, Anno IS, Leite SR et al (2003) Isolation and identification of mycobacteria from livestock specimens and milk obtained in Brazil. Mem Inst Oswaldo Cruz 98:319
29. Chen TM, Castaneda M, Wanitphakdeedecha R et al (2009) Precautions with gentian violet: skin marking made sterile, effective, and economical. Am J Infect Control 37:244
30. Kreysig D (2001) Der Biofilm. Bildung, Eigenschaften und Wirkungen, vol 24 Bioforum, GIT Verlag, Darmstadt, Germany, p 40
31. Exner M, Kramer A, Lajoie L et al (2005) Prevention and control of health care-associated waterborne infections in health care facilities. Am J Infect Control 33:S26
32. World Health Organization (2011) Water safety in buildings. WHO Press, Geneva, ISBN 978/92/4/154810/6
33. Phillips MS, von Reyn CF (2001) Nosocomial infections due to nontuberculous mycobacteria. Clin Infect Dis 33:1363
34. Gubler JG, Salfinger M, von Graevenitz A et al (1992) Pseudoepidemic of nontuberculous mycobacteria due to a contaminated bronchoscope cleaning machine. Report of an outbreak and review of the literature. Chest 101:1245
35. Tiwari TS, Ray B, Jost KC Jr et al (2003) Forty years of disinfectant failure: outbreak of postinjection *Mycobacterium abscessus* infection caused by contamination of benzalkonium chloride. Clin Infect Dis 36:954
36. Galassi L, Donato R, Tortoli E et al (2003) Nontuberculous mycobacteria in hospital water systems: application of HPLC for identification of environmental mycobacteria. J Water Health 1:133
37. Eid AJ, Berbari EF, Sia IG et al (2007) Prosthetic joint infection due to rapidly growing mycobacteria: report of 8 cases and review of the literature. Clin Infect Dis 45:687
38. Villanueva A, Calderon RV, Vargas BA et al (1997) Report on an outbreak of postinjection abscesses due to *Mycobacterium abscessus*, including management with surgery and clarithromycin therapy and comparison of strains by random amplified polymorphic DNA polymerase chain reaction. Clin Infect Dis 24:1147
39. Zhibang Y, Bixia Z, Qishan L et al (2002) Large-scale outbreak of infection with *Mycobacterium chelonae* subsp. *abscessus* after penicillin injection. J Clin Microbiol 40:2626

40. Kim HY, Yun YJ, Park CG et al (2007) Outbreak of *Mycobacterium massiliense* infection associated with intramuscular injections. J Clin Microbiol 45:3127
41. Galil K, Miller LA, Yakrus MA et al (1999) Abscesses due to *Mycobacterium abscessus* linked to injection of unapproved alternative medication. Emerg Infect Dis 5:681
42. Cooksey RC, Jhung MA, Yakrus MA et al (2008) Multiphasic approach reveals genetic diversity of environmental and patient isolates of *Mycobacterium mucogenicum* and *Mycobacterium phocaicum* associated with an outbreak of bacteremias at a Texas hospital. Appl Environ Microbiol 74:2480
43. Centers for Disease Control and Prevention (CDC) (1998) Rapidly growing mycobacterial infection following liposuction and liposculpture-Caracas, Venezuela, 1996–1998. MMWR Morb Mortal Wkly Rep 47:1065
44. Centers for Disease Control and Prevention (CDC) (2004) Nontuberculous mycobacterial infections after cosmetic surgery-Santo Domingo, Dominican Republic, 2003–2004. MMWR Morb Mortal Wkly Rep 53:509
45. Meyers H, Brown-Elliott BA, Moore D et al (2002) An outbreak of *Mycobacterium chelonae* infection following liposuction. Clin Infect Dis 34:1500
46. Sampaio JL, Chimara E, Ferrazoli L et al (2006) Application of four molecular typing methods for analysis of *Mycobacterium fortuitum* group strains causing post-mammaplasty infections. Clin Microbiol Infect 12:142
47. van Dissel JT, Kuijper EJ (2009) Rapidly growing mycobacteria: emerging pathogens in cosmetic procedures of the skin. Clin Infect Dis 49:1365
48. Del Castillo M, Palmero D, Lopez B et al (2009) Mesotherapy-associated outbreak caused by *Mycobacterium immunogenum*. Emerg Infect Dis 15:357
49. Regnier S, Cambau E, Meningaud JP et al (2009) Clinical management of rapidly growing mycobacterial cutaneous infections in patients after mesotherapy. Clin Infect Dis 49:1358
50. Furuya EY, Paez A, Srinivasan A et al (2008) Outbreak of *Mycobacterium abscessus* wound infections among "lipotourists" from the United States who underwent abdominoplasty in the Dominican Republic. Clin Infect Dis 46:1181
51. Woo PC, Leung KW, Wong SS et al (2002) Relatively alcohol-resistant mycobacteria are emerging pathogens in patients receiving acupuncture treatment. J Clin Microbiol 40:1219
52. Duarte RS, Lourenço MC, Fonseca LS et al (2009) Epidemic of postsurgical infections caused by *Mycobacterium massiliense*. J Clin Microbiol 47:2149
53. Viana-Niero C, Lima KV, Lopes ML et al (2008) Molecular characterization of *Mycobacterium massiliense* and *Mycobacterium bollettii* in isolates collected from outbreaks of infections after laparoscopic surgeries and cosmetic procedures. J Clin Microbiol 46:850
54. Lai KK, Brown BA, Westerling JA et al (1998) Long-term laboratory contamination by *Mycobacterium abscessus* resulting in two pseudo-outbreaks: recognition with use of random amplified polymorphic DNA (RAPD) polymerase chain reaction. Clin Infect Dis 27:169
55. Wilson RW, Steingrube VA, Böttger EC et al (2001) *Mycobacterium immunogenum* sp. nov., a novel species related to *Mycobacterium abscessus* and associated with clinical disease, pseudo-outbreaks and contaminated metalworking fluids: an international cooperative study on mycobacterial taxonomy. Int J Syst Evol Microbiol 51:1751
56. Cooksey RC, de Waard JH, Yakrus MA et al (2004) *Mycobacterium cosmeticum* sp. nov., a novel rapidly growing species isolated from a cosmetic infection and from a nail salon. Int J Syst Evol Microbiol 54:2385
57. Gira AK, Reisenauer AH, Hammock L et al (2004) Furunculosis due to *Mycobacterium mageritense* associated with footbaths at a nail salon. J Clin Microbiol 42:1813
58. Winthrop KL, Albridge K, South D et al (2004) The clinical management and outcome of nail salon-acquired *Mycobacterium fortuitum* skin infection. Clin Infect Dis 38:38
59. Vugia DJ, Jang Y, Zizek C et al (2005) Mycobacteria in nail salon whirlpool footbaths, California. Emerg Infect Dis 11:616
60. Redbord KP, Shearer DA, Gloster H et al (2006) Atypical *Mycobacterium furunculosis* occurring after pedicures. J Am Acad Dermatol 54:520

61. Sniezek PJ, Graham BS, Busch HB et al (2003) Rapidly growing mycobacterial infections after pedicures. Arch Dermatol 139:629
62. Winthrop KL, Chang E, Yamashita S et al (2009) Nontuberculous mycobacteria infections and anti-tumor necrosis factor-alpha therapy. Emerg Infect Dis 15:1556
63. Noe R, Cohen AL, Lederman E et al (2007) Skin disorders among construction workers following Hurricane Katrina and Hurricane Rita: an outbreak investigation in New Orleans, Louisiana. Arch Dermatol 143:1393
64. Appelgren P, Farnebo F, Dotevall L et al (2008) Late-onset posttraumatic skin and soft-tissue infections caused by rapid-growing mycobacteria in tsunami survivors. Clin Infect Dis 47:e11
65. Wallace RJ Jr, Brown-Elliott BA, Wilson RW et al (2004) Clinical and laboratory features of *Mycobacterium porcinum*. J Clin Microbiol 42:5689
66. Levendoglu-Tugal O, Munoz J, Brudnicki A et al (1998) Infections due to nontuberculous mycobacteria in children with leukemia. Clin Infect Dis 27:1227
67. Fitzgerald DA, Smith AG, Lees A et al (1995) Cutaneous infection with *Mycobacterium abscessus*. Br J Dermatol 132:800
68. Kwon YH, Lee GY, Kim WS et al (2009) A case of skin and soft tissue infection caused by *Mycobacterium abscessus*. Ann Dermatol 21:84
69. Wang H, Jin P, Wu Q (2008) Disseminated cutaneous infection with *Mycobacterium abscessus* in a patient with a low CD4+ T cell count. Eur J Dermatol 18:337
70. Griffith DE, Girard WM, Wallace RJ Jr (1993) Clinical features of pulmonary disease caused by rapidly growing mycobacteria. An analysis of 154 patients. Am Rev Respir Dis 147:1271
71. Ferringer T, Pride H, Tyler W (2008) Body piercing complicated by atypical mycobacterial infections. Pediatr Dermatol 25:219
72. Kang GC, Gan AW, Yam A et al (2010) *Mycobacterium abscessus* hand infections in immunocompetent fish handlers: case report. J Hand Surg Am 35:1142
73. Brantley JS, Readinger AL, Morris ES (2006) Cutaneous infection with *Mycobacterium abscessus* in a child. Pediatr Dermatol 23:128
74. Rodríguez G, Ortegón M, Camargo D et al (1997) Iatrogenic *Mycobacterium abscessus* infection: histopathology of 71 patients. Br J Dermatol 137:214
75. Camargo D, Saad C, Ruiz F et al (1996) Iatrogenic outbreak of *M. chelonae* skin abscesses. Epidemiol Infect 117:113
76. Wallace RJ Jr, Brown-Elliott BA, Crist CJ et al (2002) Comparison of the in vitro activity of the glycylcycline tigecycline (formerly GAR-936) with those of tetracycline, minocycline, and doxycycline against isolates of nontuberculous mycobacteria. Antimicrob Agents Chemother 46:3164
77. Wallace RJ, Glassroth J, Griffith DE et al (1997) Diagnosis and treatment of disease caused by nontuberculous mycobacteria. Am J Respir Crit Care Med 156:S1
78. Petrini B (2006) *Mycobacterium abscessus*: an emerging rapid-growing potential pathogen. APMIS 114:319
79. Nash KA, Brown-Elliott BA, Wallace RJ Jr (2009) A novel gene, *erm*(41), confers inducible macrolide resistance to clinical isolates of *Mycobacterium abscessus* but is absent from *Mycobacterium chelonae*. Antimicrob Agents Chemother 53:1367
80. Chang MA, Jain S, Azar DT (2004) Infections following laser in situ keratomileusis: an integration of the published literature. Surv Ophthalmol 49:269
81. Freitas D, Alvarenga L, Sampaio J et al (2003) An outbreak of *Mycobacterium chelonae* infection after LASIK. Ophthalmology 110:276
82. Bonamonte D, Filoni A, Vestita M et al. (2016) Cutaneous infections from aquatic environments. In: Bonamonte D, Angelini G (eds) Aquatic dermatology. Biotic, chemical and physical agents. Springer Verlag, Berlin, p 185
83. Zahid MA, Klotz SA, Goldstein E et al (1994) *Mycobacterium chelonae* (*M. chelonae* subspecies *chelonae*): report of a patient with a sporotrichoid presentation who was successfully treated with clarithromycin and ciprofloxacin. Clin Infect Dis 18:999

84. Wallace RJ Jr, Brown BA, Onyi GO (1992) Skin, soft tissue, and bone infections due to *Mycobacterium chelonae chelonae*: importance of prior corticosteroid therapy, frequency of disseminated infections, and resistance to oral antimicrobials other than clarithromycin. J Infect Dis 166:405
85. Ferreira O, Duarte AF, Baudrier T et al (2010) A cutaneous infection by *Mycobacterium chelonae* in a patient with rheumatoid arthritis. Dermatol Online J 16:3
86. Drouineau O, Rivault O, Le Roy F et al (2006) Cutaneous infection due to *Mycobacterium chelonae* in a hemodialysed patient. Nephrol Ther 2:136
87. Drage LA, Ecker PM, Orenstein R et al (2010) An outbreak of *Mycobacterium chelonae* infections in tattoos. J Am Acad Dermatol 62:501
88. Halpern J, Biswas A, Cadwgan A et al (2010) Disseminated cutaneous *Mycobacterium chelonae* infection in an immunocompetent host. Clin Exp Dermatol 35:269
89. Panossian A, Cohen MJ, Posalski I (2011) Upper extremity *Mycobacterium chelonae* cutaneous infection. Plast Reconstr Surg 127:163e
90. Bartralot R, Pujol RM, García-Patos V et al (2000) Cutaneous infections due to nontuberculous mycobacteria: histopathological review of 28 cases. Comparative study between lesions observed in immunosuppressed patients and normal hosts. J Cutan Pathol 27:124
91. Adenis-Lamarre E, Kostrzewa E, Texier-Maugein J et al (2009) Cutaneous infection due to *Mycobacterium chelonae* during anti-TNF therapy. Ann Dermatol Venereol 136:811
92. Brown BA, Wallace RJ Jr, Onyi GO et al (1992) Activities of four macrolides, including clarithromycin, against *Mycobacterium fortuitum*, *Mycobacterium chelonae*, and *M. chelonae*-like organisms. Antimicrob Agents Chemother 36:180
93. Chopra S, Matsuyama K, Hutson C et al (2011) Identification of antimicrobial activity among FDA-approved drugs for combating *Mycobacterium abscessus* and *Mycobacterium chelonae*. J Antimicrob Chemother 66:1533
94. Swenson JM, Wallace RJ Jr, Silcox VA et al (1985) Antimicrobial susceptibility of five subgroups of *Mycobacterium fortuitum* and *Mycobacterium chelonae*. Antimicrob Agents Chemother 28:807
95. Tebas P, Sultan F, Wallace RJ Jr et al (1995) Rapid development of resistance to clarithromycin following monotherapy for disseminated *Mycobacterium chelonae* infection in a heart transplant patient. Clin Infect Dis 20:443
96. Wallace RJ Jr, Tanner D, Brennan PJ et al (1993) Clinical trial of clarithromycin for cutaneous (disseminated) infection due to *Mycobacterium chelonae*. Ann Intern Med 119:482
97. Pinto-Gouveia M, Gameiro A, Ramos L et al (2015) *Mycobacterium chelonae* is an ubiquitous atypical *Mycobacterium*. Case Rep Dermatol 7:207
98. Küster E (1965) Über Kaltblüter Tuberkulose. Beinchen Mediz Wochen. Schrift 52:7
99. Hand WL, Sanford JP (1970) *Mycobacterium fortuitum*-a human pathogen. Ann Intern Med 73:971
100. Street ML, Umbert-Millet IJ, Roberts GD et al (1991) Nontuberculous mycobacterial infections of the skin. Report of fourteen cases and review of the literature. J Am Acad Dermatol 24:208
101. Rotman DA, Blauvelt A, Kerdel FA (1993) Widespread primary cutaneous infection with *Mycobacterium fortuitum*. Int J Dermatol 32:512
102. Sastry V, Brennan PJ (1995) Cutaneous infections with rapidly growing mycobacteria. Clin Dermatol 13:266
103. Hautmann G, Lotti T (1994) Atypical mycobacterial infections of the skin. Dermatol Clin 12:657
104. Winthrop KL, Abrams M, Yakrus M et al (2002) An outbreak of mycobacterial furunculosis associated with footbaths at a nail salon. N Engl J Med 346:1366
105. Nagore E, Ramos P, Botella-Estrada R et al (2001) Cutaneous infection with *Mycobacterium fortuitum* after localized microinjections (mesotherapy) treated successfully with a triple drug regimen. Acta Derm Venereol 81:291

106. Difonzo EM, Campanile GL, Vanzi L et al (2009) Mesotherapy and cutaneous *Mycobacterium fortuitum* infection. Int J Dermatol 48:645
107. Tazawa S, Maruno K, Higuchi D et al (2006) *Mycobacterium fortuitum* infection caused by the organism in subcutaneous abscess mediated by central venous catheter. Kekkaku 81:609
108. Zainal Muttakin AR, Tan AM (2006) *Mycobacterium fortuitum* catheter-related sepsis in acute leukaemia. Singap Med J 47:543
109. Buckley R, Cobb MW, Ghurani S et al (1997) *Mycobacterium fortuitum* infection occurring after a punch biopsy procedure. Pediatr Dermatol 14:290
110. Nolan CM, Hashisaki PA, Dundas DF (1991) An outbreak of soft-tissue infections due to *Mycobacterium fortuitum* associated with electromyography. J Infect Dis 163:1150
111. Angeli K, Lacour JP, Mantoux F et al (2004) *Mycobacterium fortuitum* skin infection occurring after a facelift. Ann Dermatol Venereol 131:198
112. Brock JM, Kennedy CB, Clark WH Jr (1960) Cutaneous infection with atypical *Mycobacterium*. Report of a case. Arch Dermatol 82:918
113. Katayama I, Nishioka K, Nishiyama S (1990) *Mycobacterium fortuitum* infection presenting as widespread cutaneous abscess in a pregnant woman. Int J Dermatol 29:383
114. Angelini G, Vena GA, De Vito D et al (1992) Micobatteriosi sporotricoide da *Mycobacterium fortuitum*. G Ital Dermatol Venereol 127:507
115. Angelini G, Vena GA, Grandolfo M (1995) Micobatteri e cute. Parte I. Dermotime 7(aprile-maggio):11
116. Angelini G, Vena GA, Grandolfo M (1995) Micobatteri e cute. Parte II. Dermotime 7(giugno-agosto):11
117. Bonamonte D, De Vito D, Vestita M et al (2013) Aquarium-borne *Mycobacterium marinum* skin infection. Report of 15 cases and review of the literature. Eur J Dermatol 23:510
118. Bonamonte D, Vestita M. *Mycobacterium marinum*. http://antimicrobe.org/ms05.asp
119. Greer KE, Gross GP, Martensen SH (1979) Sporotrichoid cutaneous infection due to *Mycobacterium chelonae*. Arch Dermatol 115:738
120. Bendelac A, Cambazard F, Fougerat J et al (1985) *Mycobacterium chelonae* cutaneous infections. General review apropos of a case. Ann Dermatol Venereol 112:319
121. Owens DW, McBride ME (1969) Sporotrichoid cutaneous infection with *Mycobacterium kansasii*. Arch Dermatol 100:54
122. Dore N, Collins JP, Mankiewicz E (1979) A sporotrichoid-like *Mycobacterium kansasii* infection of the skin treated with minocycline hydrochloride. Br J Dermatol 101:75
123. Régnier S, Martinez V, Veziris N et al (2008) Treatment of cutaneous infections due to *Mycobacterium fortuitum*: two cases. Ann Dermatol Venereol 135:591
124. Guevara-Patiño A, Sandoval de Mora M, Farreras A et al (2010) Soft tissue infection due to *Mycobacterium fortuitum* following acupuncture: a case report and review of the literature. J Infect Dev Ctries 4:521
125. Kwan K, Ho ST (2010) *Mycobacterium chelonae* and *Mycobacterium fortuitum* infection following open fracture: a case report and review of the literature. Indian J Med Microbiol 28:248
126. Abbass K, Adnan MK, Markert RJ et al (2014) *Mycobacterium fortuitum* breast abscess after nipple piercing. Can Fam Physician 60:51
127. Wallace RJ Jr, Brown BA, Onyi GO (1991) Susceptibilities of *Mycobacterium fortuitum* biovar. *fortuitum* and the two subgroups of *Mycobacterium chelonae* to imipenem, cefmetazole, cefoxitin, and amoxicillin-clavulanic acid. Antimicrob Agents Chemother 35:773
128. Orjuela D, Puerto G, Mejía G et al (2010) Cutaneous tuberculosis after mesotherapy: report of six cases. Biomedica 30:321
129. Williamson JC, Miano TA, Morgan MR et al (2010) Fatal *Mycobacterium abscessus* endocarditis misidentified as *Corynebacterium* spp. Scand J Infect Dis 42:222
130. Boltin D, Katzir M, Bugoslavsky V et al (2009) *Corynebacterium striatum*—a classic pathogen eluding diagnosis. Eur J Intern Med 20:e49
131. Paul J, Baigrie C, Parums DV (1992) Fatal case of disseminated infection with the turtle bacillus *Mycobacterium chelonae*. J Clin Pathol 45:528

Mycobacterium marinum Skin Infection

9

Domenico Bonamonte, Angela Filoni,
Michelangelo Vestita, and Gianni Angelini

Mycobacterium marinum lives in aquatic environments, where it causes disease in many poikilodermic fish species living in fresh or saltwater; the organism has a wide geographic distribution in the water world [1]. The first report of a mycobacterium isolated in fish (very likely *M. marinum*) is attributed to Bataillon and Coll, who isolated acid-fast bacilli, named *M. piscium*, in 1897, from a tuberculous lesion of a common carp (*Cyprinus carpio*) [2, 3]. Then in 1926 it was isolated and identified by Aronson from tubercles in various organs of marine fish found dead in the Philadelphia Aquarium [4]. Initially *M. marinum* was thought to infect fishes only and was named accordingly, but it is now known to be a ubiquitous species. The original freshwater isolate of *M. piscium* was quite possibly a variant of *M. marinum*. Other marine *Mycobacterium* species have been described in the literature, such as *M. platypoecilus*, *M. anabanti*, and *M. balnei*; however, comparative cultural, morphological, and pathogenic data suggest that they were all synonymous with *M. marinum* [5].

M. marinum was identified as a causal agent of human disease only in 1951, when it was identified from skin lesions in swimmers in a contaminated swimming pool in the city of Orebro, Sweden [6]. The term "swimming pool granuloma" was coined to denote these lesions and the causal agent was classified as *M. balnei* [7] but then, when the two mycobacteria were later seen to be identical, as *M. marinum* (Fig. 9.1).

D. Bonamonte, MD, PhD (✉)
Department of Biomedical Science and Human Oncology,
University of Bari "Aldo Moro", Bari, Italy
e-mail: domenico.bonamonte@uniba.it

A. Filoni, MD • M. Vestita, MD
University of Bari "Aldo Moro", Bari, Italy

G. Angelini, MD
Professor of Dermatology, Former Professor and Chairman, University of Bari "Aldo Moro", Bari, Italy

D. Bonamonte, G. Angelini (eds.), *Mycobacterial Skin Infections*,
DOI 10.1007/978-3-319-48538-6_9

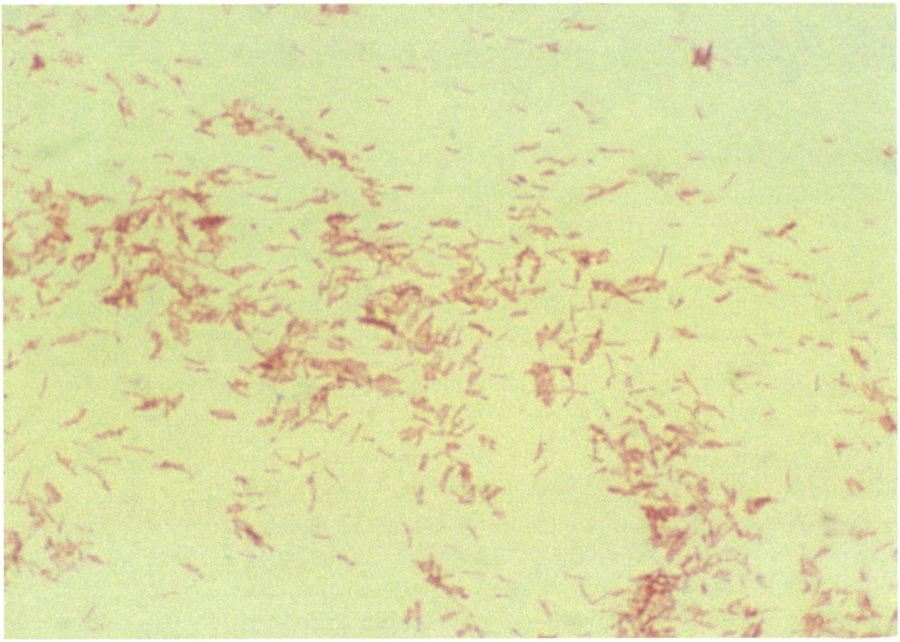

Fig. 9.1 *Mycobacterium marinum* (reproduced with permission from Bonamonte and Coll [8])

Lastly, in 1962 Swift and Cohen reported two cases of *M. marinum* infection from a tropical fish tank: the term “fish tank granuloma” was introduced at this stage [9]. Since those reports, “swimming pool granuloma” has essentially disappeared thanks to the introduction of proper chlorination of this reservoir. The terms “fish tank granuloma” and “fish handler’s disease” are used today because of the association with aquariums and water-related activities, such as skin diving [10], dolphin training [11], and a number of fishing and boating activities [12].

The recent interest in *M. marinum* is also due to its genetic relatedness with *M. tuberculosis* [13, 14] and to the fact that experimental infection of *M. marinum* in the goldfish (*Carassius auratus*) mimics the tuberculosis pathogenesis [15]. In addition, the growing interest in *M. marinum* is linked to the emergence and burden of *M. ulcerans* infection [16].

9.1 Taxonomy

M. marinum is found worldwide in saltwater and freshwater, aquariums, swimming pools, ocean beaches, rivers, lakes, natural bathing pools, and old wells. Saltwater or freshwater fish, dolphins, shrimps, and water pleas have also been reported as vectors of the disease [10–12].

This mycobacterium belongs to the first of four groups in Runyon’s classification [17]. It is photochromogenic: cultures turn yellowish-orange after photoexposure

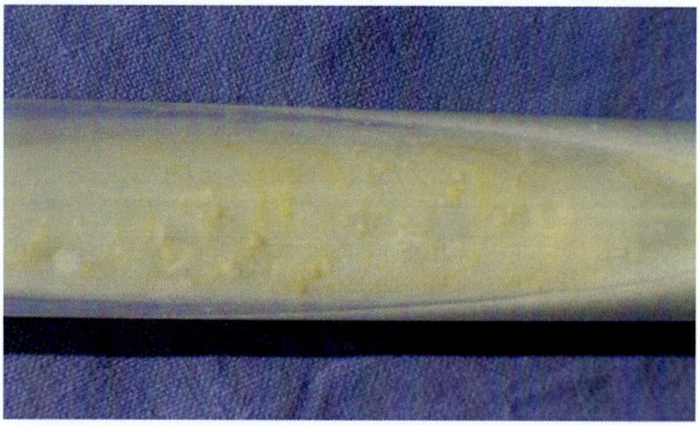

Fig. 9.2 Yellow photochromogenic colonies of *Mycobacterium marinum* in Löwenstein-Jensen culture medium (reproduced with permission from Bonamonte and Coll [8])

(Fig. 9.2). Although it can grow in fewer than 7 days, its characteristics are very different from the rapid-growing species (*M. chelonae*, *M. abscessus*, and *M. fortuitum*). Since it carries a single rRNA operon [13] and its 16S rRNA sequence contains the molecular signature of slow growing mycobacteria [18], it definitely belongs to the slow growing group of mycobacteria [3].

M. marinum, as well as its related species, *M. ulcerans*, is a pathogenic mycobacterium, unlike the other nontuberculous mycobacteria, that are opportunistic pathogens [19]. Phylogenetic analysis based on the 16S rRNA has shown that *M. marinum* lies on a branch of the genus that is close to the branch containing members of the *M. tuberculosis* complex. DNA-DNA hybridization and mycolic acid studies confirm that *M. marinum*, along with *M. ulcerans*, is closely related to the *M. tuberculosis* complex [20, 21].

9.2 Genetics

The *M. marinum* genome (strain M) is one of the major mycobacteria to have been sequenced. The length of its genome is 6.5 Mb, which is larger than that of *M. tuberculosis* (4.4 Mb), that of *M. ulcerans* (5.8 Mb), and that of *M. leprae* (3.3 Mb) [3]. Its genome is comparable to the *M. ulcerans* [22] and *M. tuberculosis* [14] genomes.

M. marinum shares a more than 98% nucleotide sequence identity with the *M. ulcerans* genome. On the basis of sequences of the genes used for identification (those coding for the ribosomal operon, RNA polymerase-*rpoB*, DNA gyrase-*gyrA* and *gyrB*, and heat shock protein 65 KDa-*hsp*), *M. marinum* cannot be differentiated from *M. ulcerans*, and the minor nucleotide differences observed in some of these genes are simply related to strain variation [14, 23, 24]. In the light of the above, *M. marinum* seems to be an ancestor of *M. ulcerans* [14, 25]. Divergence occurred along with the gain by *M. ulcerans* of genes (grouped on the virulence plasmid, pMUM001) encoding the virulence factor mycolactone [26], and of copies of the insertion sequences IS*2404* and IS*2606* [25, 27]. Besides *M. ulcerans*, other species, all closely related, are designated as mycolactone-producing mycobacteria: *M. pseudoshottsii* and *M. liflandii* are, in fact, mycolactone-producing mycobacteria described only in fishes [28]. These strains could form the *M. marinum* complex [29]. From strains of *M. marinum* that induced disease in Red Sea fishes, another mycolactone (mycolactone F) has also been isolated [30, 31].

M. marinum is less pathogenic and grows faster than *M. tuberculosis*; nevertheless, the genome of these two species is closely related. Genome sequencing shows that the region of difference 1, which contains the ESAT-6 and CFP-10 encoding genes in *M. tuberculosis*, can present also in *M. marinum* [32]. The ESAT-6-like secretion system is probably a major secretion pathway for *M. marinum*, and this system is responsible for the secretion of various proteins which are abundant in *M. marinum*. The ESX secretion system is critical for the virulence of both species and is highly conserved between the two species [14].

9.3 Microbiology

M. marinum is a 1.0–4.0 μm by 0.2–0.6 μm, non motile, true branching pleiomorphic rod, that is difficult to stain by usual methods. After Ziehl-Neelsen staining it is an acid-fast bacillus. As described for *M. tuberculosis*, the formation of microscopic cords has also been described in *M. marinum*, providing evidence of a link between cording and the virulence in both species [33, 34]. The cell wall of *M. marinum* is mainly composed of keto-mycolates and methoxy-mycolates, that are different from those of *M. tuberculosis* and other mycobacteria except *M. ulcerans* [21, 35].

M. marinum is strictly aerobic, and its carbon sources are glycerol, pyruvate, glucose, and ethanol. Its optimal growth temperature is 30 °C, whereas small colonies or no growth are observed at 37 °C. In primary culture, it grows slowly and positive cultures may be obtained after 3–4 weeks (although all cultures should be held for 6 weeks before being declared negative). In subculture, the growth rate is between 1 and 2 weeks but may be as little as 4–5 days.

M. marinum, which is less demanding than *M. tuberculosis* for growth, grows in all the mycobacteria media (egg based, broth and agar based), without any additives or with only 2–5% oxalic acid-albumin-dextrose-catalase. Although its growth is dependent upon oxygen, like other mycobacteria, the growth is improved by adding 2–5% carbon dioxide in the gas phase above the medium [3]. *M. marinum* lacks catalase and nitrate reductase activities, whereas some isolates, but not all, hydrolize Tween 80.

In view of the growth temperature of *M. marinum*, clinicians must be sure to inform the laboratory if this organism is suspected so that the specimen is incubated at the appropriate temperature in order to prevent false-negative cultures [36–38].

Phenotypically, colonies of *M. marinum* are smooth or intermediate, white or beige when the media are kept in the dark and yellowish-orange after exposure to light (photochromogenic). Their photocromogenicity is due to the active production of beta carotene mediated by the *crtB* gene, and can be inhibited by chloramphenicol [39].

PCR-based methods have been developed for the identification of *M. marinum*. Two of these methods are commercially available: INNOLIPA Mycobacteria v2

(Imunogenetics), based on the amplification of the ribosomal gene spacer (16S–23S), and Genotype mycobacteria CM/AS (Hain Lifescience), based on the amplification of a 23S rRNA gene [40, 41]. Both use PCR coupled with reverse hybridization. They cannot, therefore, differentiate *M. marinum* from *M. ulcerans*, since the rRNA sequences are similar. Specific PCR protocols for detection in fish have been described [42].

Unlike *M. ulcerans*, the *M. marinum* genotypes cannot be clearly related to the geographic origins of the isolates, and it is difficult to discriminate between recurrence and reinfection [43]. *M. marinum* isolates from humans and fish have also been genotypically compared, and in this study there were significant molecular differences between clinical isolates and fish isolates [44].

9.4 Pathogenesis

Both *M. marinum* and *M. tuberculosis* are intracellular pathogens that proliferate within macrophages in a nonacid (pH 6.1–6.5) phagosome that does not fuse with the lysosome [45]. Because both species are also genetically related, analogous molecular mechanisms are likely involved in their survival in a hostile cell environment.

M. marinum is able to survive and replicate in macrophages and even to escape from the phagosome into the cytoplasm where it can induce actin polymerization, leading to direct cell spread [46, 47]. Recently, it has been demonstrated that *M. marinum* is ejected from the cell through the ejectosome, an actin-based structure-spreading mechanism that requires a cytoskeleton regulator from the host and an intact mycobacterial ESX-1 secretion system [47, 48].

Experimental infection of zebrafish with different strains of *M. marinum* demonstrated that two different types of strains can be distinguished, based on genetic diversity and virulence. Cluster I predominantly contained strains isolated from humans with fish tank granuloma, whereas the majority of strains in cluster II contained isolates from poikilothermic species. Acute disease progression was evident with cluster I strains, whereas chronic disease was noted with cluster II strains [49].

In the last years, significant advances in the knowledge of the pathophysiology of *M. marinum* have been made. A dynamic host-pathogen interaction has been shown: metabolically active bacteria are controlled by the host immune system and products of specific bacterial genes interfere with the host's effort to eradicate the bacteria. In more detail, the ESX-55 system of the mycobacteria is responsible for the secretion of various proline-proline-glutamic acid (PPE) and proline-glutamic acid (PE)-polymorphic GC-rich repetitive sequence (PGRS) proteins. Animal model studies suggest that such proteins interact with host immune components and possibly subvert critical innate immune pathways, establishing a moderate, persistent infection [50–54]. In vitro observations on infected human macrophages further suggest that these proteins strongly modulate the human macrophage response and actively suppress T-lymphocyte receptor signaling-dependent innate immune cytokine secretion, thus allowing bacterial survival [55]. In particular the PPE38 protein, expressed on the cell-wall surface, seems to be involved in bacterial surface properties such as cord formation, sliding motility and biofilm formation, as well as in the induction of pro-inflammatory cytokines in infected macrophages [54]. Additionally, some authors have presumed that these proteins are a source of antigenic variation which allows the pathogen to evade antigenic-specific host responses [53]. Given the above data, it is easy to understand why immune system impairment is a significant factor in the establishment of *M. marinum* infection at the pathogenic level [56].

Owing to the growth temperature of *M. marinum*, the infection is primarily localized in the coolest region of the body, the skin. Less commonly it involves deeper structures, such as joints, tendons and bones [57–60].

As already pointed out, dissemination of the infection occurs more commonly in immunocompromised hosts, like transplant recipients and subjects on corticosteroid therapy [61–64]. Although there has been no reported change in the *M. marinum* infection prevalence and frequency in the developed world since the AIDS epidemic, several cases of disseminated infection in AIDS patients have been described [61, 65]. It would probably be prudent for HIV infected subjects to avoid maintenance of freshwater aquariums. Disseminated infection is rarely reported in individuals with a relatively intact immunity [66, 67].

As of recent date, *M. marinum* infection has gained a relevant role as an opportunistic infection in patients treated with anti-tumor necrosis factor (TNF)-α or other biological drugs [68–72]. However, recent reports support a safe re-exposure to anti-TNF-α therapy after elimination of the bacteria through correct antibiotic therapy [73].

9.5 Epidemiology

While endemic in fish, *M. marinum* infection in humans due to contact with contaminated water or fish is comparatively rare [4, 74–90]. In a retrospective survey carried out in 21 Spanish laboratories from 1991 to 1998, 39 bacteriologically confirmed cases were recorded [90]. Culture-confirmed *M. marinum* infection was reported in 63 patients from 1996 to 1998 in France, with an infection incidence of about 0.09 cases per 100,000 inhabitants per year [91]. The annual incidence in the United States is 0.27 confirmed cases per 100,000 inhabitants [92].

9.6 Clinical Features

9.6.1 Disease in Fish

M. marinum infection in fish is very frequent, especially in aquarium fish. The gastrointestinal tract is the primary route of infection, and the severity ranges from chronic forms associated with a low mortality to rare, acute forms with a high mortality rate [93]. Affected fishes show behavior changes, such as separating from other fish and refusing food. They show cutaneous ulcerations and pigment alterations and develop spinal curvature, together with monolateral or bilateral exophthalmia. The infection affects any organ system in fish, but especially the spleen, kidney, and liver [94].

M. marinum affects a wide range of freshwater and saltwater fish species, and is the main mycobacterium isolated from fish [95]. Mycobacteria were found in 46.8% and 29.9% of ornamental fishes imported into Italy which died, and *M. marinum* accounted for 2.4–5.3% of the isolates [96]. The organism is transmitted in fish through contaminated feed, cannibalism of infected fish, aquatic detritus, and the release of pathogens into the water from gut or skin lesions of infected fishes [94]. For this reason, infective material may be present in soil and water, in which the bacterial cells remain viable for 2 years or more [94].

M. marinum is a source of infection also in other aquatic vertebrates, such as frogs, snakes, turtles, snails, and shellfishes [94].

9.6.2 Disease in Humans

Like other nontuberculous mycobacteria infections, *M. marinum* infection is not contracted by human-to-human contagion. Before 1963, most skin *M. marinum* infections involved swimming pool-associated injuries [7, 74]. The current decline in pool-associated cases is probably linked to better water disinfection practices in recent decades: *M. marinum*, in fact, survives only briefly after exposure to free chlorine concentrations of ≥0.6 μg/ml [3].

Today, *M. marinum* cutaneous infection is often acquired during aquarium maintenance [9]. As *M. marinum* infection is an important zoonosis, *M. marinum* infection may pose an occupational hazard for various professionals, such as staff working with fish and aquatic animals, aquariums, or pet shop workers. Most infections, however, occur in fish fanciers who have an aquarium at home (hence, the name "fish fanciers' finger syndrome"). The infection may be due to direct injuries from the fish fins or to bites, but most cases are acquired during handling of the aquarium, when cleaning or changing the water [86, 97]. In one case the infection was observed in an industrial plumbing mechanic with no direct aquatic exposure [81]. Indirect infection has also been reported, through contact with a bath that was used to clean out fish tanks [91, 98]. It seems likely that the incidence of fish tank granuloma will rise with the increase in fish tank hobbyists and aquarium tourism [98].

Because the optimal *M. marinum* growth is at 30 °C, human infection is localized primarily on the skin. *M. marinum* invades the tissues through preexisting broken skin. The sites most commonly affected are the knees, elbows, arches of the feet and backs of the hands in swimming pool granulomas, and the backs of the hands in fish tank granulomas. One case of sporotrichoid infection of the face has also been reported, in a 2-year-old child, probably caught from fish in an aquarium [85].

M. marinum infection may present with various clinical features. Most commonly, in about 60% of the cases, the infection is a cutaneous disease presenting with a solitary papulonodular lesion on a finger or hand [91]. In 25% of cases, the infection spreads along the lymphatic drainage lines, producing multiple nodular lesions with a sporotrichoid pattern [92, 99]. Multiple or disseminated lesions on the trunk or limbs are rare [61, 64, 75, 78, 79, 100], except in subjects with immune deficiency.

The initial lesion presents as a reddish or reddish-blue nodule, of a soft consistency and variable diameter, that may even be as large as 5–6 cm. Ulceration or colliquation may develop and the lesion will then rupture and exude pus, or else it may remain as a verrucous surface lesion. Mild involvement of regional lymph nodes is a rare possibility (15% of cases in reference 91), while infection of the deep organs, such as the lungs, is exceptional [67].

Deep infections (tenosynovitis, the most frequent, as well as arthritis, bursitis, and osteomyelitis) are present in 20–40% of cases, due to the extension of a cutaneous infection or direct inoculation of the pathogen [57–60, 91, 99, 101–103].

The two main risk factors for *M. marinum* infection in immunocompetent subjects are exposure to *M. marinum*-infected waters and the presence of superficial cuts or abrasions. Almost half (49%) of *M. marinum* infections are aquarium-related, 27% are related to fish or shellfish injuries and 9% are related to injuries associated with saltwater or brackish water [91].

The average incubation period for *M. marinum* infection is 21 days, although it may be as long as 270 days; 35% of cases have an incubation period of 30 days [86, 91]. Since lesions may appear some time after the exposure, eliciting an appropriate history of swimming pool or seawall abrasions, barnacle scrapes, fish fin punctures or abrasions from handling tropical fish tanks is critical in making a timely and accurate diagnosis.

Usually, *M. marinum* infections are subacute or chronic. There are some rare cases of spontaneous healing, although this can take months to several years. *M. marinum* does not confer immunity, so re-infection is possible.

9.7 Diagnosis and Differential Diagnosis

Diagnosis of an infection due to *M. marinum* is based on a high suspicion index, taking an accurate exposure history, and proper laboratory examinations. Generally, because of the lack of one or more of these requirements, the diagnosis is delayed [86].

Identification of *M. marinum* on Ziehl-Neelsen staining of biopsy specimens, direct smears or a yellowish discharge is positive in only 30% of cases [3], but the number of mycobacteria is usually low [87, 102, 104]. Obviously, even when positive, smear microscopy cannot differentiate *M. marinum* from other mycobacteria.

Diagnosis is essentially made through culture; according to the literature, the positivity rate ranges from 70 to 80% of cases [3].

Generally, specimens are taken from the skin (skin biopsy specimens and aspirates of pus). Swabs should be avoided for many reasons [99]: *M. marinum* infection is a paucibacillary infection. Other specimens are obtained from articular fluids or subcutaneous tissue and exudates, often obtained at surgery. The specimen container should be sterile and should not contain any preservative or fixative. For the

Table 9.1 Differential features of some mycobacteria inducing skin lesions

Species	*M. tuberculosis*	*M. marinum*	*M. ulcerans*	*M. fortuitum*	*M. chelonae*
Growth rate	L	I	I	R	R
Optimal growth temperature	37 °C	30 °C	30 °C	37 °C	37 °C
Growth 25 °C	–	+	+	±	±
Growth 45 °C	–	–	–	–	–
Pigment	N	P	N	N	N
Niacin test	+	V	–	–	–
Reduction of nitrates	+	–	–	+	–
Tween hydrolysis (10 days)	±	+	–	+	V
Catalase 68 °C	–	+	+	+	+
Urease	+	+	–	+	V
Pirazine amidase	+	+	–	+	+
Growth NaCl 5%	–	V	–	+	V
Growth MacConkey Agar	–	–	–	+	+

Rate of growth = R (rapid: non > 7 days); I (intermediate: 8–14 days); L (slow: more than 14 days)
Pigment = *N* non photochromogenic, *P* photochromogenic, *V* variable

isolation and identification of *M. marinum*, a level 2 laboratory might be sufficient, although level 3 might be required for studies of subcultures. Skin biopsy or wound fluid specimens require a decontamination procedure. Specimens should be cultured at 30–32 °C and, because of other possible mycobacterial diagnoses, also at 37 °C (Table 9.1). Isolation of *M. marinum* has a clinical significance since it does not usually grow in the laboratory environment or uninfected human body: this very important point distinguishes *M. marinum* infection from infections due to other nontuberculous mycobacteria [105].

Molecular biology methods are limited by the above reported reasons, due to the high homology between *M. marinum* and *M. ulcerans*. Molecular identification using the analysis of 16S rRNA or another conserved gene (*gyrA*, *rpoB*, *hsp65*, 16-23S internal transcribed spacer) associated with a 7-day growth of photochromogenic colonies, can help to make an early identification of *M. marinum* [3, 23, 24, 27].

Intradermal skin tests with the purified protein derivative (PPD) of *M. marinum* need to be intensively positive to be diagnostically relevant, as PPD can cross-react with other mycobacterial PPD and especially *M. tuberculosis*, as the latter is genomically closely related to *M. marinum* [13, 14].

Gamma interferon release assays are not found useful as a diagnostic method for *M. marinum* infection because, as stated above, *M. marinum* shares the specific antigens (ESAT-6 and CFP-10) used in these tests with *M. tuberculosis* [106, 107].

As a complementary test, to confirm contamination of aquarium water, *M. marinum* can be isolated in dead fish through histological examination, direct observation or PCR analysis [108].

Differential diagnosis includes skin infections due to other nontuberculous mycobacteria, in particular *M. chelonae*, *M. fortuitum*, *M. haemophilum* and *M. tuberculosis*. *M. marinum* infection with a single verrucous plaque should be differentiated from tuberculosis verrucosa due to *M. tuberculosis* or *M. bovis*. Other noninfectious diseases to be taken into account are sarcoidosis, skin tumors, and foreign body reactions. The forms with sporotrichoid pattern must be differentiated from sporotrichosis.

9.8 Histopathology

It is widely known that a histological diagnosis of *M. marinum* infection can be difficult [109] because various aspects tend to vary according to the age of the lesion. In particular, a nonspecific inflammatory infiltrate may be observed in the first 6 months; after this period, a granuloma with epithelioid and multinucleated Langhans giant cells is much more likely [86, 103]. Various patterns can be observed: sarcoid-like granuloma, granuloma annulare, or rheumatoid-like nodules are frequent pictures [110–113]. Epidermal changes (hyperkeratosis, acanthosis, pseudo-epitheliomatous hyperplasia, intradermal neutrophilic abscesses and ulcerations), as well as dermal fibrosis (in chronic lesions) and small vessels proliferation are important findings that are generally present in such cases [109, 113]. In histological preparations, alcohol-acid-resistant bacilli can be identified using Ziehl-Neelsen staining.

9.9 Treatment

The permeability of the *M. marinum* cell wall is not known, but has been demonstrated to vary at least tenfold among mycobacterial species, that of *M. tuberculosis* being tenfold more permeable than that of *M. chelonae* [114]. Taking into account the natural *M. marinum* multidrug resistance, the permeability of its cell wall could be close to that of *M. chelonae*. Probably, this low permeability allows survival of the organism in unfavorable environments [3]. In the genome, various genes encoding antibiotic resistance mechanisms have been observed: for beta-lactams (*blaC*), aminoglycosides (*aac2'*), and chloramphenicol (*cph*) [3].

As concerns susceptibility tests in vitro and in vivo, rifampicin and rifabutin are the most active drugs against *M. marinum,* with a typical MIC90 for these agents of ≤0.5 and 0.6 mg/ml, respectively. The MIC90 (the MIC that inhibits 90% of isolates) for older or traditional agents include ethambutol 2.0–4.0 mg/ml, sulfamethoxazole 8.0 mg/ml, doxycycline 16.0 mg/ml, minocycline 4.0 mg/ml, amikacin 4.0 mg/ml, and imipenem 8.0 mg/ml [115, 116]. *M. marinum* isolates have a moderately high MIC90, above the concentrations usually obtained in tissues, for isoniazid (8.0 mg/ml), ciprofloxacin, ofloxacin, levofloxacin and streptomycin. *M. marinum* isolates are resistant to pyrazinamide [116, 117]. A number of newer agents have shown some activity against *M. marinum* including clarithromycin (MIC 90 4.0 mg/ml) and the 8-methoxyquinolones gatifloxacin and moxifloxacin (MIC90 of 1.0–2.0 mg/ml). Preliminary data suggest that the new oxazolidinone, linezolid, is also active against *M. marinum* in vitro [117].

Because MICs or fixed concentration susceptibilities show little strain to strain variation, susceptibility tests are rarely indicated for treatment of *M. marinum* infections. Acquired mutational resistance with definite changes in drug susceptibility to *M. marinum* has not been reported. Recently (December 2000), the National Committee for Clinical Laboratory Standards (NCCLS) published tentative guidelines for susceptibility testing of *M. marinum* isolates [118]. The Committee recommended that routine in vitro susceptibility testing should not be done. When testing was deemed clinically necessary, no specific test method was recommended. Drugs to be tested included clarithromycin, minocycline/doxycycline, rifampicin, ethambutol, trimethoprim/sulfamethoxazole or a sulfonamide alone, and amikacin [118].

There is currently no consensus as to the optimal treatment of *M. marinum* infection. Therapy is usually pharmacological, although adjunctive surgical procedures, cryotherapy and electrodessication may be needed to control resistant or deeper infections. Therapy duration varies widely in the literature: most authors recommend extended treatment for 1–2 months following clinical resolution, ranging from 2 to 12 months overall, given the absence of substantial dose-related and time-dependent side effects when using the recommended drugs. Spontaneous resolution is possible but rare; complete regression can take up to 2 years [99]. Various antibiotics have been reported as effective options; in agreement with other authors, however, the final choice is primarily based on the clinician's experience [69, 91, 119]. Moreover, randomized controlled trials comparing different antibiotic regimens are currently lacking. Widely used molecules include tetracyclines (mostly minocycline and doxycycline), sulfamethoxazole plus trimethoprim, rifampicin and ethambutol. Less common alternatives include clarithromycin, levofloxacin and amikacin [37, 56, 91, 102, 119–124]. Other drugs, such as new macrolides and fluoroquinolones, are also feasible solutions [91] (Table 9.2). Both success and failure have been reported for each of the listed molecules.

Table 9.2 Drugs most widely used in the treatment of *Mycobacterium marinum* cutaneous infection according to the literature

Antimycobacterial agent	Dosage[a]	Duration
Minocycline	50–100 mg/2/day	2–6 months
Doxycycline	50–100 mg/2/day	4–5 months
Clarithromycin	250–500 mg/2/day	3–6 months
Ofloxacin	200–300 mg/2/day	1–2 months
Ciprofloxacin	250–500 mg/2/day	2–3 months
Levofloxacin	250–500 mg/2/day	2–3 months
Amikacin	15 mg/kg/day—max 1 gr im	2–5 months
Rifampicin	600–900 mg/day	2–5 months
Rifamycin	250 mg im/2/day	2–5 months
Rifabutin	450–600 mg/day	2 months
Sulfamethoxazole + trimethoprim	400 mg + 80 mg/2/day	3–4 months
Ethambutol hydrochloride	15–25 mg/kg/day	2–6 months

[a]If unspecified, administration is per os

Monotherapy with minocycline, doxycycline and clarithromycin has proven successful in most cases, especially in superficial cutaneous infections [37]. Combination therapy, often with clarithromycin plus rifampicin and/or ethambutol, is preferred in severe forms characterized by deep tissues involvement, although the use of ethambutol adds to the complexity of treatment as monitoring for color vision and visual acuity must be performed [125]. There is limited published experience with clarithromycin [104, 126] but its in vitro activity against *M. marinum* suggests that it would be quite effective. Rifampicin alone has also been recommended, but there is little experience with this regimen [127].

Some authors strongly advocate combination therapy in every case, since antibiotic susceptibility tests in *M. marinum* are often inaccurate, and also to avoid the selection of resistant strains. The latter, however, has yet to be observed, as no single antibiotic has a potent activity against *M. marinum* confirmed by in vitro susceptibility tests [91, 97, 128].

Each regimen should be administered for a minimum of 3 months. The rate of clinical response is generally low with any regimen; therefore, a minimum of 4–6 weeks of therapy should be given before considering the patient as a non-responder (Tables 9.2 and 9.3).

As of today, published observations on disseminated *M. marinum* disease in AIDS patients, or other immunocompromised individuals, are limited. Hanau and Coll described a patient with AIDS and sporotrichoid *M. marinum* infection who responded well to 6 months of rifampicin and ethambutol, although recurrence was noted soon after therapy discontinuation [129]. Bonnet and Coll described an AIDS patient with fluctuant nodules due to *M. marinum* who failed 5 months treatment of ofloxacin and minocycline [130]. The patient was then shifted to rifampicin, ciprofloxacin and amikacin, but did not show a favorable clinical response until clarithromycin was added. Therefore, it seems prudent to treat immunocompromised hosts with *M. marinum* infection with at least two agents, including clarithromycin [131]. Duration of therapy in this setting is far from being standardized, but should be 6 months at least, and possibly lifelong in cases of severe, worsening immunosuppression (Table 9.3).

Table 9.3 Duration of the therapy in various pathological conditions

Localized cutaneous disease in immunocompetent host	Disseminated disease, including patients with AIDS	Adjuvant surgical treatment
Monotherapy with one of the following agents: clarithromycin, minocycline, doxycycline, sulfamethoxazole + trimethoprim, rifampicin + ethambutol Administration for 1–2 months after symptom resolution. Total duration of therapy 3–4 months	Multidrug regimen with 2 or more active agents Clarithromycin is recommended Optimal duration of therapy unknown, at least 6–12 months	In case of involvement of the closed spaces of the hands In cases of poor response to treatment

As regards the use of antibiograms for targeted therapy, antibiotic susceptibility testing is currently not recommended on a routine basis, except in patients failing treatment after several months [37]. This is mainly because in vitro results do not necessarily relate to in vivo effectiveness, *M. marinum* is particularly susceptible to many commonly used antimicrobials, and the risk of acquired resistance to such drugs is negligible [98, 132].

9.10 Surgery

This is a controversial issue. Some authors recommend surgical debridement along with antimicrobial therapy [99], whereas for others surgical debridement should be limited to those cases associated with a poor prognosis after several months of antibiotic treatment, and persistent gain [125]. Most of the infections spreading to deeper structures need surgery [36].

Other treatments, such as cryotherapy, X-ray therapy, and electrodessication have been reported but have yet to be properly evaluated [102].

9.11 Prevention

The use of adequate concentrations of free chlorine in swimming pools, spas and hot tub water is advisable, as recommended by the Center for Disease Control and prevention: the concentration of free chlorine in swimming pool water should be kept between 0.4 and 1 mg/liter and in spas and hot tub water between 2 and 5 mg/liter [133, 134].

Sanitation, disinfection, and the destruction of carrier fishes are the primary control methods of *M. marinum* infection in fish [3]. Antimicrobial treatment is not able to eliminate *M. marinum* from affected fish [135]. As for imported ornamental fish, a great variety of attitudes is observed: France, for example, requires an EU Directive 2003/858/E health certificate-derived template for all imported live fish, including tropical ornamental fish [136].

In fish tank-related activities, infections may be prevented by the use of waterproof gloves during maintenance and by appropriate care of potential upper limb skin lesions [137]. Concerning the latter, however, chlorine derivatives show a limited activity against mycobacteria, whereas phenol formaldehyde and glutaraldehyde derivatives are effective [138]. Fish tank water sterilization by UV germicide lamps, which easily inactivate mycobacteria, has been introduced on the market [139, 140] and a vaccine against *M. marinum* infection in fish has also been designed [6].

Exposed populations, including fish salesmen, should be trained to recognize signs of *M. marinum* infection in humans and fish in order to expedite the diagnosis [3]. Not installing ornamental aquariums in hospital units is also recommended, in particular in units intended to house immunocompromised patients [3].

9.12 Personal Data

From 1987 to 2015 we observed 18 patients with cutaneous *M. marinum* infection, 15 males (83.3%) and 3 females (16.7%; male to female ratio 5:1), of ages ranging from 15 to 55 years (mean: 34.7). The infection was occupational in 14 subjects (3 of them worked at institutional aquariums, 10 in shops selling aquariums and 1 was a fisherman) and extra-occupational in four patients (all of whom tended home aquariums). One of the latter four patients was in the 8th month of pregnancy at the time of observation. Each patient had a documented history of former minor trauma, such as an abrasion or a superficial wound acquired while handling fish, shellfish, or alternatively caused by infected foreign bodies within the aquarium, like wood splinters or stones. The median incubation time after the traumatic inoculation was relatively long, ranging from 3 to 24 weeks (mean: 6.3). The interval between the lesion onset and our observation was in the range of 1–6 months (average 4.2 months) [8, 82–84, 88, 89, 108, 141, 142].

Four patients (22.2%) presented with a single papulo-verrucous plaque (Figs. 9.3, 9.4, 9.5, and 9.6) and 14 (77.8%) had a sporotrichoid distribution of nodular lesions (Figs. 9.7, 9.8, 9.9, 9.10, 9.11, 9.12, 9.13, 9.14, 9.15, 9.16, and 9.17) (Table 9.4). The anatomic distribution was typically on the upper limbs, first involving the hand, fingers and dorsum (right hand in 15 cases, left hand in 3 cases), in 14 cases later spreading centripetally up the whole arm, trailing up lymphatic vessels. In 3 of these 14 sporotrichoid cases, the first observed lesions were ulcerated nodules that caused mild pain, whereas in the remaining cases the infection was painless. Associated systemic symptoms, localized adenopathy, deep structures involvement like tenosynovitis, bursitis, and arthritis, were not present in any of the 18 cases. All patients were immunocompetent and referred no history of transplantation or immunosuppressive therapy.

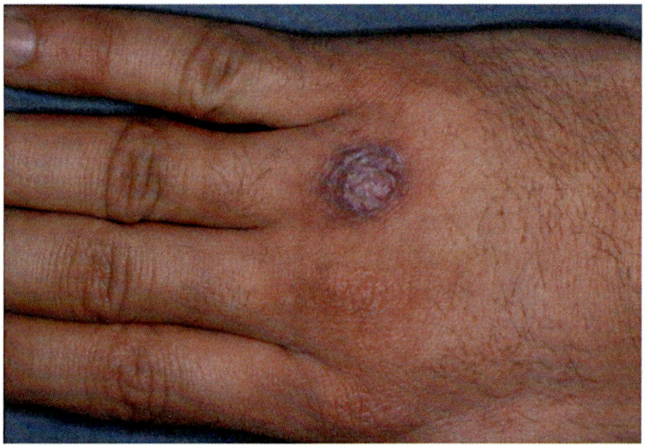

Fig. 9.3 Fish tank granuloma (reproduced with permission from Bonamonte and Coll [8])

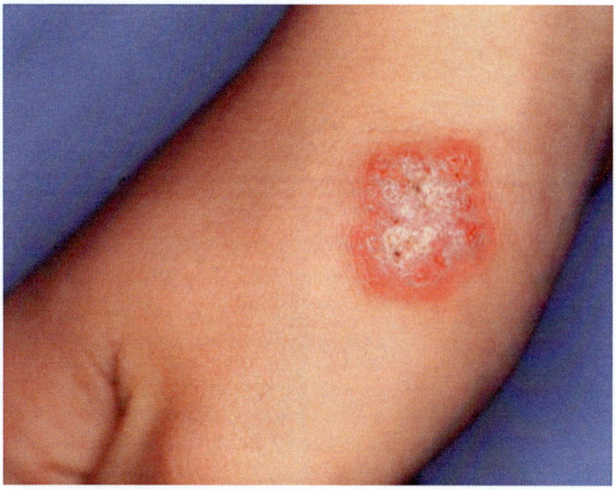

Fig. 9.4 Fish tank granuloma (reproduced with permission from Bonamonte and Coll [8])

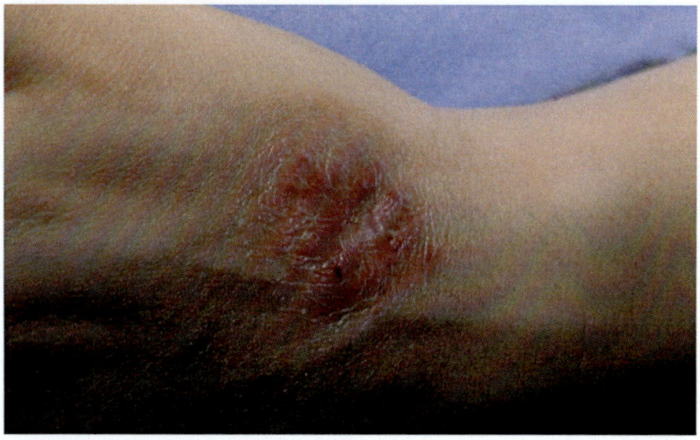

Fig. 9.5 Fish tank granuloma (reproduced with permission from Bonamonte and Coll [8])

An interesting finding emerged from the history of the 14 sporotrichoid pattern cases: nodular lesions, arranged in rosary-like chains, appeared one after the other at regular 1–2 week intervals. Moreover, each lesion firstly involved the cutis deep structures, presenting as a prominence covered by healthy skin, and then later the overlapping epidermis was affected.

Culture tests of skin biopsy fragments in Löwenstein-Jensen at 30 °C indicated *M. marinum* growth in 16 of our 18 cases (88.9%); according to the literature, positive rates of cultures range from 70 to 80%. However, in the two culture-negative cases, the history, intradermal skin tests with PPD of *M. marinum* and PCR tests were positive, lesions were classic sporotrichoid, and minocycline therapy was efficacious. Culture in Löwenstein-Jensen at 37 °C yielded negative results in each case. In all cases PPD skin tests resulted strongly positive for *M. marinum*

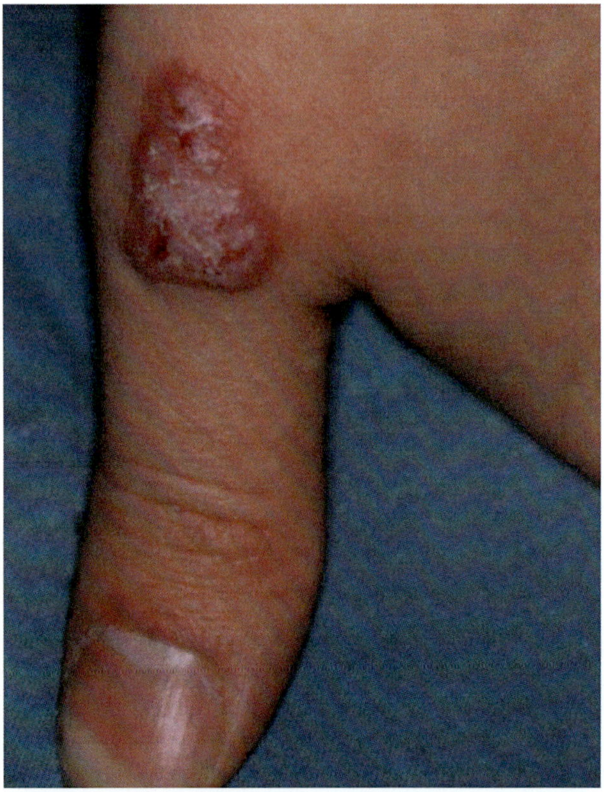

Fig. 9.6 Fish tank granuloma (reproduced with permission from Bonamonte and Angelini [88])

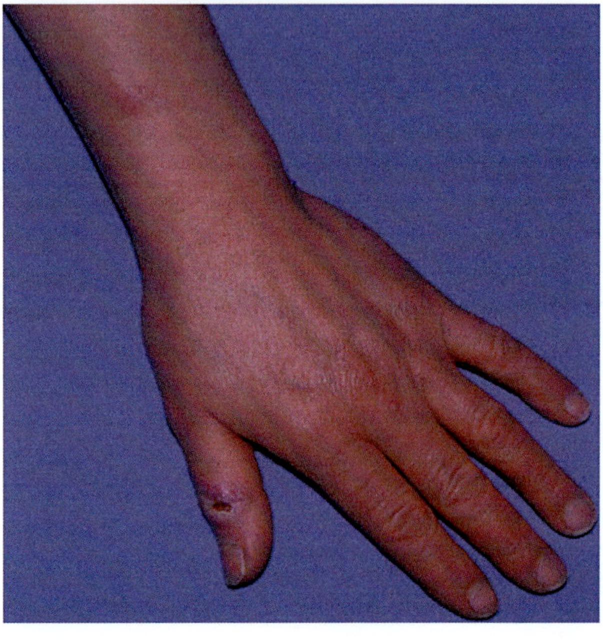

Fig. 9.7 Sporotrichoid fish tank granuloma (reproduced with permission from Bonamonte and Coll [8])

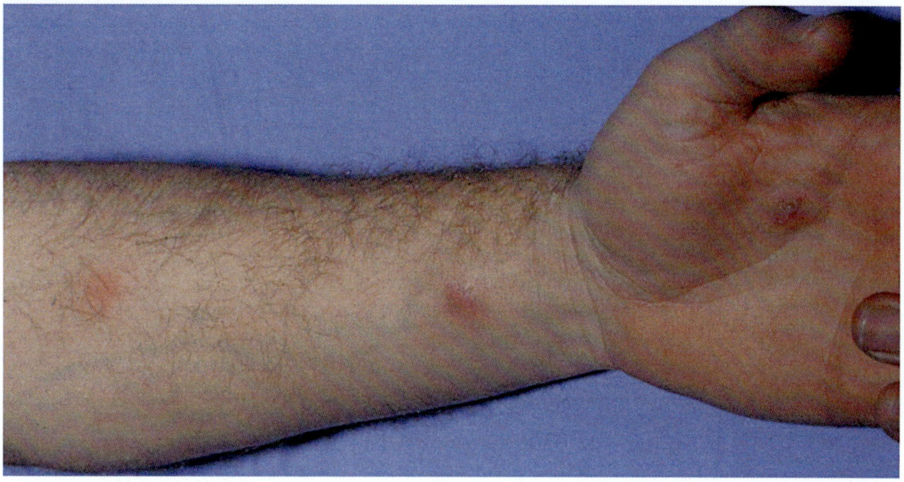

Fig. 9.8 Sporotrichoid fish tank granuloma (reproduced with permission from Bonamonte and Coll [8])

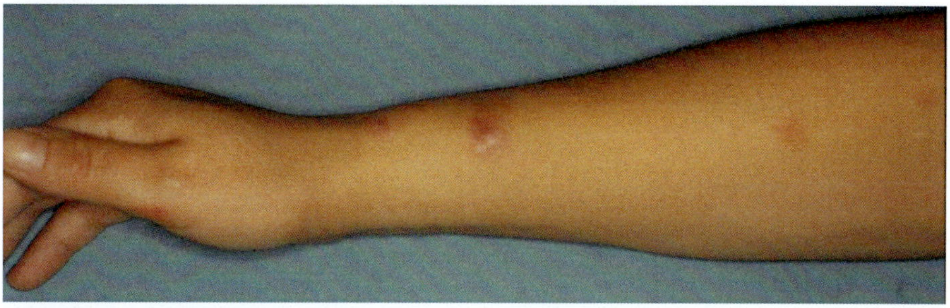

Fig. 9.9 Sporotrichoid fish tank granuloma (reproduced with permission from Bonamonte and Coll [8])

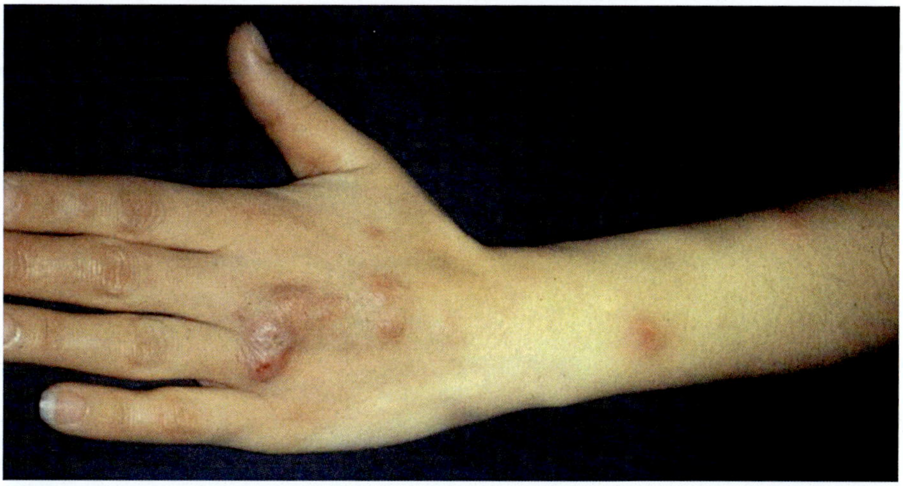

Fig. 9.10 Sporotrichoid fish tank granuloma (reproduced with permission from Bonamonte and Coll [8])

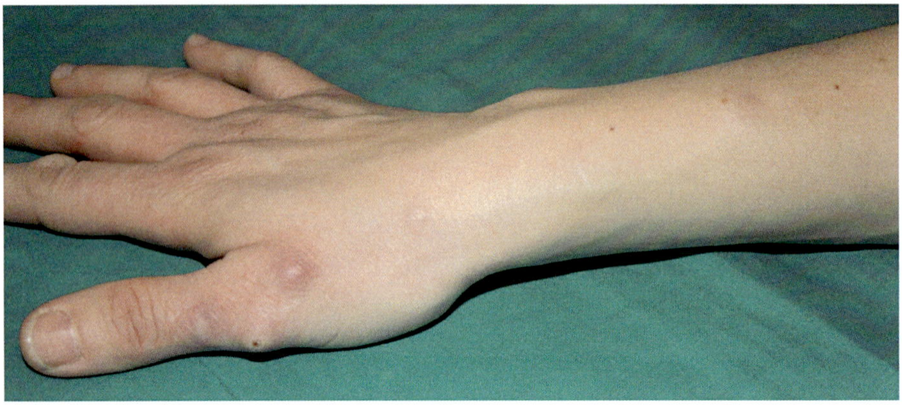

Fig. 9.11 Sporotrichoid fish tank granuloma (reproduced with permission from Bonamonte and Coll [8])

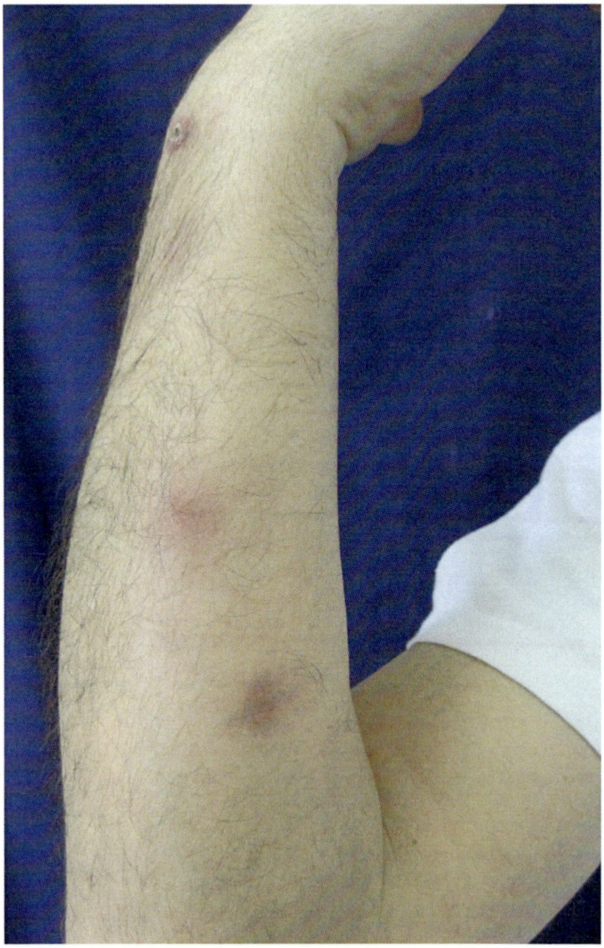

Fig. 9.12 Sporotrichoid fish tank granuloma (reproduced with permission from Bonamonte and Coll [8])

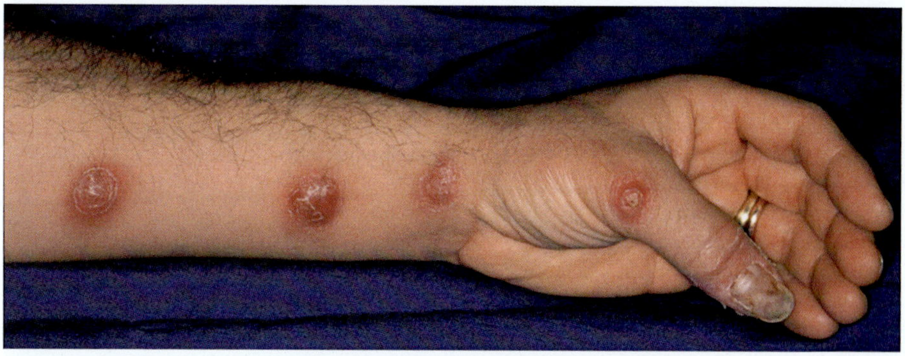

Fig. 9.13 Sporotrichoid fish tank granuloma (reproduced with permission from Bonamonte and Angelini [88])

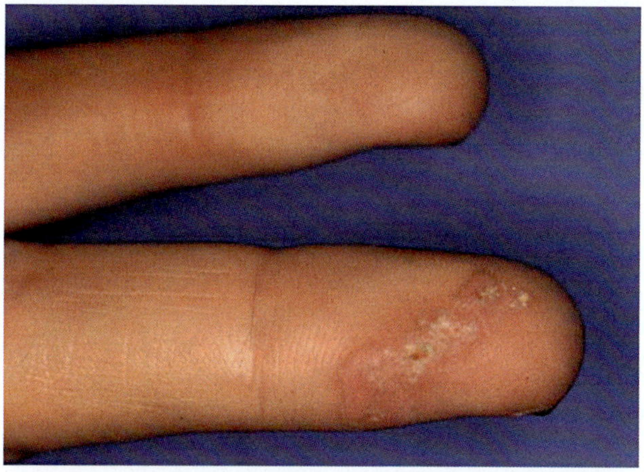

Fig. 9.14 Fish tank wound (reproduced with permission from Bonamonte and Coll [8])

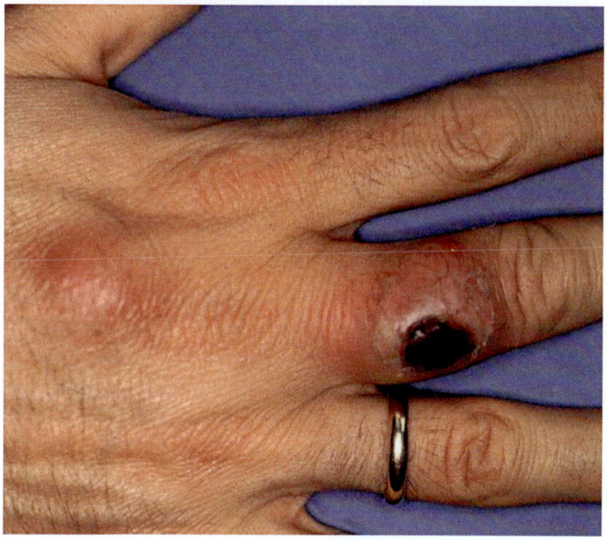

Fig. 9.15 The same case as in Fig. 9.14. Sporotrichoid fish tank granulomas, one of which with ulcerative evolution (reproduced with permission from Bonamonte and Angelini [89])

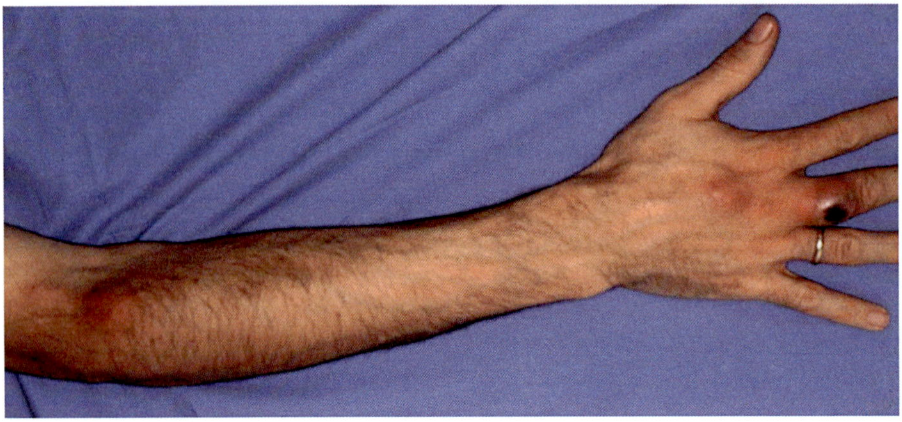

Fig. 9.16 The same case as in Fig. 9.14 with sporotricoid granulomas (reproduced with permission from Bonamonte and Coll [8])

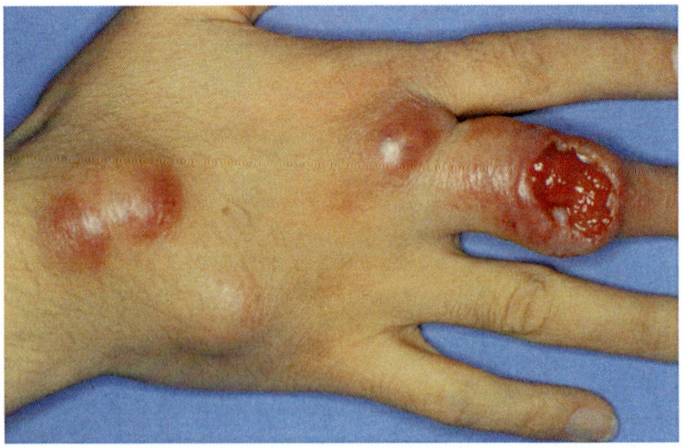

Fig. 9.17 Sporotrichoid fish tank granulomas with ulcerative evolution (reproduced with permission from Bonamonte and Coll [8])

(Fig. 9.18); the lesions featured an induration area measuring 10–15 mm in diameter, and were moderately positive for *M. tuberculosis* (Fig. 9.19). Even if none of our patients had a history of a positive tuberculin skin test result, the positive PPD results could be interpreted as cross-reactivity, consistent with studies showing a close genome relatedness between *M. marinum* and *M. tuberculosis* [13]. Deep tissue involvement was not revealed in any of our cases, likely because of the brief time lag between the disease onset and the clinical diagnosis. In 10 of the 18 patients the PCR test was performed, yielding positive results in each instance.

Biopsies were taken in all subjects. Epidermal changes were present in 46.6% of cases and included hyperkeratosis (three cases), acanthosis (seven cases) pseudo-epitheliomatous papillomatosis (four cases) and lymphocyte exocytosis (two cases). We demonstrated superficial and/or deep dermal involvement in every case. A tuberculoid granuloma, with lymphocytes, histiocytes, neutrophils, giant cells but no sign of central caseation (Figs. 9.20 and 9.21), was found in one case (5.6%), in

Table 9.4 Clinical and laboratory characteristics of 18 patients with "fish tank granuloma"

Patient number, age (years), gender	Exposure/ year	Distribution	Clinical appearance	Incubation period (weeks)	Evolution time (months)	Symptoms	*M. marinum* PPD	*M. tuberculosis* PPD	Acid-fast bacilli stain	*M. marinum* culture	Histology	PCR	Therapeutic agent, dosage and duration
1. 15 M	Aquarium 1987	Right hand dorsum	Single papulo-verrucous plaque	24	2	None	+++	+±	Negative	Positive	Nonspecific inflammation	NA	Minocycline (200 mg/ die/2 months)
2. 32 M	Aquarium 1988	Right hand III finger and forearm	Sporotrichoid, focally ulcerated nodules	3	6	Pain	+++	+±	Negative	Positive	Nonspecific inflammation	NA	Isoniazid (600 mg/die) and rifampicin (900 mg/die) for 2 months
3. 35 M	Aquarium 1990	Right hand dorsum	Single papulo-verrucous plaque	16	3	None	+++	+±	Negative	Positive	Nonspecific inflammation	NA	Minocycline (200 mg/ die/2 months)
4. 27 M	Aquarium 1991	Right hand dorsum	Single papulo-verrucous plaque	8	2	None	+++	+	Negative	Positive	Nonspecific inflammation	NA	Minocycline (200 mg/ die/2 months)
5. 30 F	Aquarium 1992	Right hand dorsum and forearm	Sporotrichoid nodules	4	4	None	+++	+±	Negative	Positive	Nonspecific inflammation	NA	Minocycline (200 mg/ die/3 months)
6. 51 M	Aquarium 1992	Left hand III finger and forearm	Sporotrichoid nodules	4	4	None	+++	+	Negative	Positive	Nonspecific inflammation	NA	Minocycline (200 mg/ die/3 months)
7. 40 M	Aquarium 1995	Right hand I finger and forearm	Sporotrichoid nodules	4	5	None	+++	+±	Negative	Positive	Nonspecific inflammation	NA	Minocycline (200 mg/ die/3 months)
8. 55 M	Aquarium 1997	Right hand dorsum and forearm	Sporotrichoid nodules	8	4	None	+++	+±	Negative	Positive	Nonspecific inflammation	NA	Minocycline (200 mg/ die/3 months)
9. 37 M	Aquarium 2000	Right thumb and forearm	Sporotrichoid nodules	3	4	None	+++	+	Negative	Positive	Nonspecific inflammation	Positive	Minocycline (200 mg/ die/2 months)

(continued)

Table 9.4 (continued)

Patient number, age (years), gender	Exposure/ year	Distribution	Clinical appearance	Incubation period (weeks)	Evolution time (months)	Symptoms	*M. marinum* PPD	*M. tuberculosis* PPD	Acid-fast bacilli stain	*M. marinum* culture	Histology	PCR	Therapeutic agent, dosage and duration
10. 35 F	Aquarium 2001	Right hand dorsum and forearm	Sporotrichoid, focally ulcerated nodules	4	6	Pain	+++	+±	Negative	Negative	Nonspecific inflammation	Positive	Minocycline (200 mg/ die/3 months)
11. 37 M	Aquarium 2003	Left hand III finger and forearm	Sporotrichoid, focally ulcerated nodules	5	5	Pain	+++	+	Negative	Positive	Nonspecific inflammation	Positive	Minocycline (200 mg/ die/3 months)
12. 28 M	Aquarium 2008	Right hand dorsum and forearm	Sporotrichoid nodules	4	5	None	+++	+±	Negative	Positive	Nonspecific inflammation	Positive	Minocycline (200 mg/ die/3 months)
13. 30 M	Aquarium 2010	Right hand dorsum and forearm	Sporotrichoid nodules	4	4	None	+++	+	Negative	Positive	Nonspecific inflammation	Positive	Minocycline (200 mg/ die/3 months)
14. 36 F	Aquarium 2011	Right hand dorsum and forearm	Sporotrichoid nodules	4	5	None	+++	+	Positive	Positive	Tuberculoid granuloma	Positive	Spontaneous regression in 3 months
15. 31 M	Aquarium 2011	Right hand dorsum and forearm	Sporotrichoid nodules	5	6	None	+++	+±	Negative	Negative	Nonspecific inflammation	Positive	Minocycline (200 mg/ die/3 months)
16. 28 M	Aquarium 2011	Left hand dorsum	Single plaque	6	5	None	+++	+±	Negative	Positive	Nonspecific inflammation	Positive	Minocycline (200 mg/ die/3 months)
17. 35 M	Aquarium 2013	Right hand dorsum and forearm	Sporotrichoid nodules	4	5	None	+++	+	Negative	Positive	Nonspecific inflammation	Positive	Minocycline (200 mg/ die/4 months)
18. 42 M	Fish 2015	Right hand dorsum	Sporotrichoid focally ulcerated nodules	3	4	None	+++	+±	Negative	Positive	Nonspecific inflammation	Positive	Minocycline (200 mg/ die/4 months)

NA not available

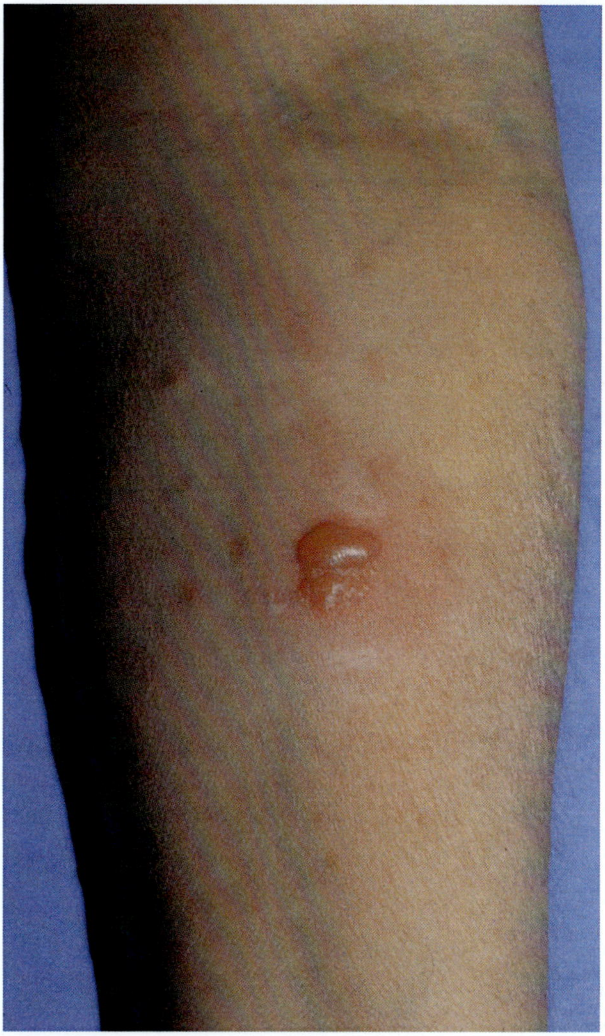

Fig. 9.18 Strongly positive reaction to PPD from *Mycobacterium marinum* (reproduced with permission from Bonamonte and Coll [8])

which the sampled lesion was 5 months old. In the remaining 17 cases, whose lesions were 3–12 weeks old, at histology a nonspecific dermic and/or hypodermic mononuclear-cell (lymphocytes, histiocytes, plasma cells) infiltrate was evidenced, showing little or no tendency to evolve to a tubercular-like granuloma formation (Fig. 9.22). Other observed features included dermal fibrosis (one case) and mild blood vessels proliferation (three cases). Ziehl-Neelsen staining highlighted acid-fast bacilli only in the histologically demonstrated tuberculoid granuloma case (5.6%). Additional laboratory tests, done for differential diagnosis purposes in particular with other mycobacteria, fell into the normal or negative range in every case.

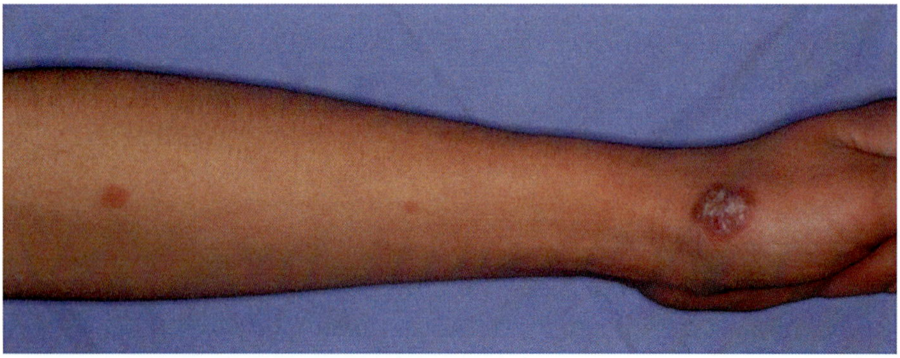

Fig. 9.19 Fish tank granuloma with intensely positive PPD to *Mycobacterium marinum* and weakly positive PPD to *Mycobacterium tuberculosis* (reproduced with permission from Bonamonte and Coll [8])

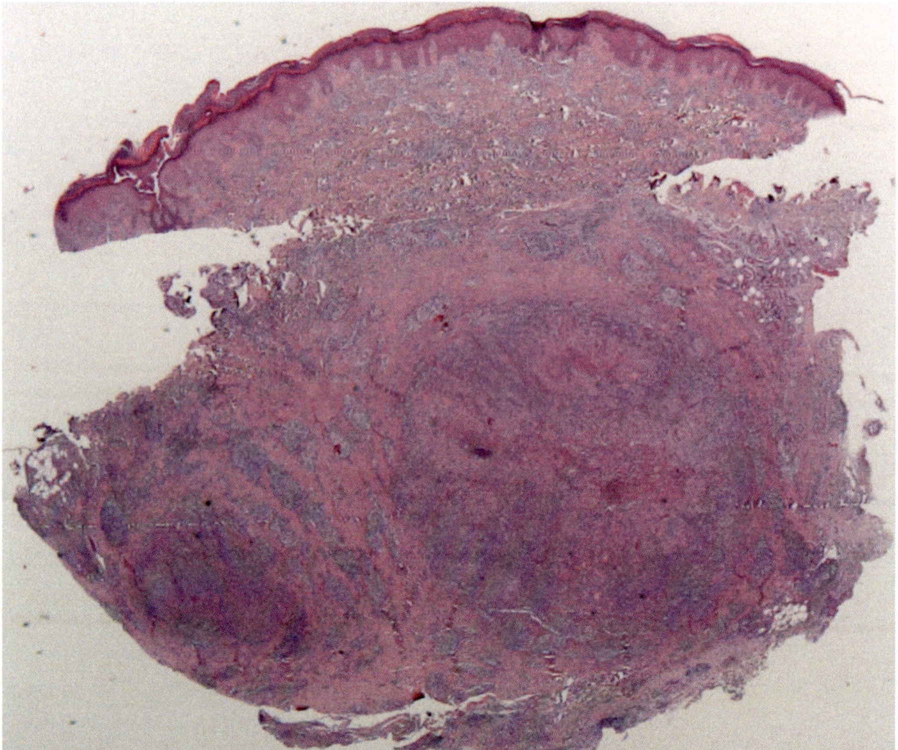

Fig. 9.20 Granulomatous inflammation of deep dermis and subcutaneous tissue (Hematoxylin-eosin—×10) (reproduced with permission from Bonamonte and Coll [108])

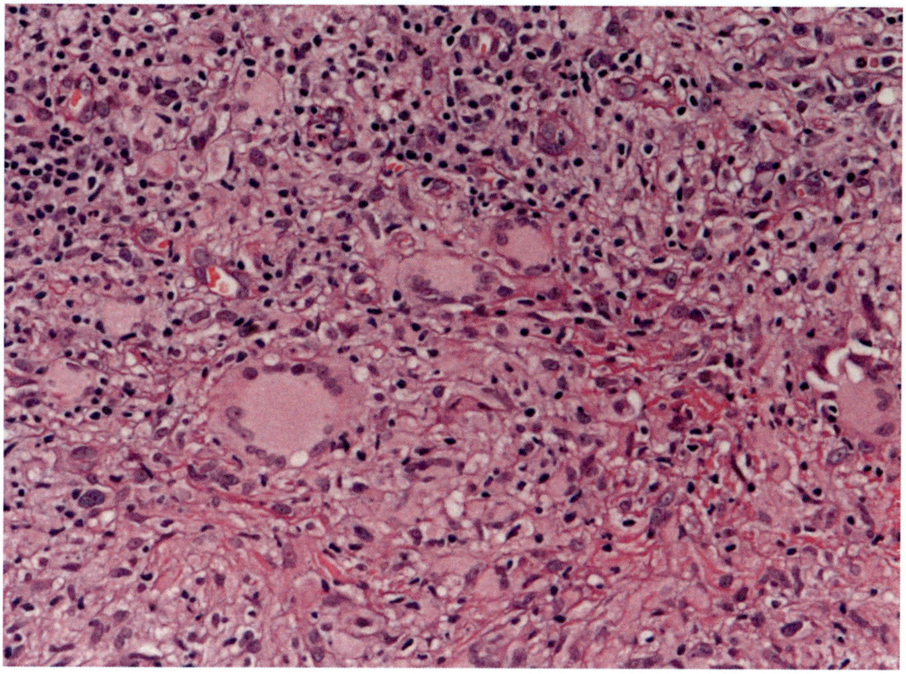

Fig. 9.21 Tuberculoid granulomatous infiltrate with lymphocytes, hystiocytes, and giant cells (Hematoxylin-eosin—×40) (reproduced with permission from Bonamonte and Coll [108])

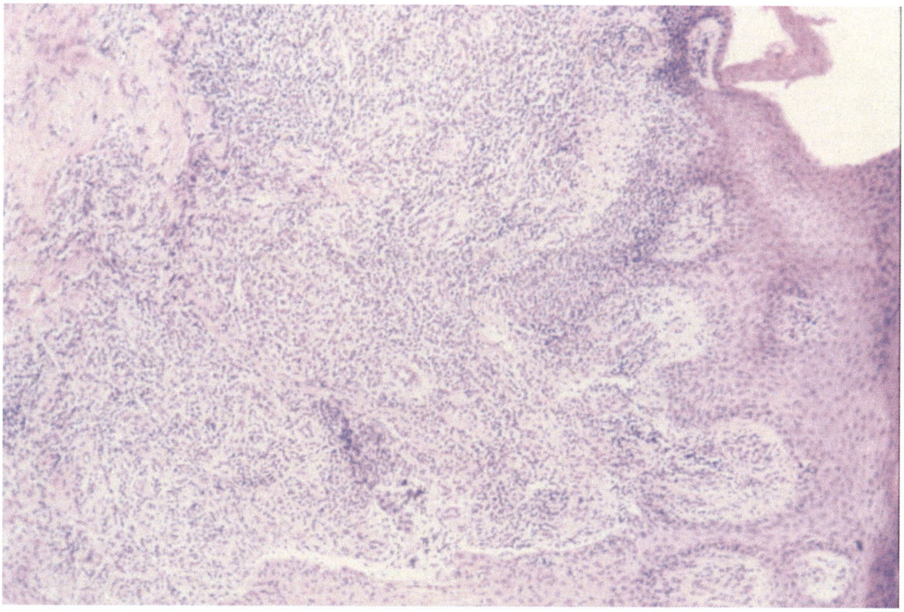

Fig. 9.22 Aspecific granulomatous infiltrate (Hematoxylin-eosin—×100) (reproduced with permission from Bonamonte and Coll [8])

We collected two dead aquarium fishes for testing purposes: notably, acid-fast bacilli were present in Ziehl-Neelsen stained sections from the two examined aquarium fishes and PCR was also positive in the single fish tested.

As to treatment, 16 patients responded completely to minocycline monotherapy 100 mg twice daily in 2–4 months. In one patient, who had already been treated with sulfamethoxazole plus trimethoprim for 30 days with no apparent benefit, the infection finally resolved after a switch to isoniazid (600 mg/die) and rifampicin (900 mg/die) for 2 months. Mean duration of treatment was 2.8 months. It should be noted that therapy, that was antibiogram-guided in all patients, was continued for at least a month after lesions clearance. None of the patients required surgical debridement. In the 8th months' pregnant patient, regardless of the antibiogram sensitivity to tetracyclines, we did not administer the drug, given the well-known contraindications. Other viable options were either ineffective, as per antibiogram, or unfit for use during pregnancy. However, a spontaneous regression of the infection was observed during weekly follow-up, and complete resolution 1 month post-partum. The duration of follow-up in all the patients ranged from 12 months to 3 years and did not reveal relapse in any case.

9.13 *Mycobacterium marinum* and Sea-Urchin Granulomas

Sea-urchins can produce two types of cutaneous reactions, immediate and delayed reactions [88, 89, 141, 143–148]. *Paracentrotus lividus*, the most common sea-urchin in Mediterranean Sea and Atlantic coastal waters, is the main culprit in the reported cases of sea-urchin granuloma [88, 89, 141, 143, 149, 150]. Generally classified as an allergic foreign-body type granuloma, it is considered as a delayed-type reaction due to an as yet identified antigen. To date, however, no causative agents have been demonstrated, and calcium carbonate, that is the main constituent of sea-urchin spines, is considered immunologically inert. Therefore, it is postulated that a proteinaceous compound produced by the spine epithelium, a substance produced by the sea-urchin pedicellaria or adherent to the spine (sand, slime, algae, etc.), could be the agent responsible for the reaction [143, 151].

In one description of a sea-urchin granuloma there was a suggestion of a histological tuberculoid infiltrate [152]. In 1968, authors researched mycobacterial infections, and detected acid-fast bacilli in only one case; in this study, the authors proposed that echinoderm granuloma could be a new mycobacterial infection [153].

In 2001, De La Torre and Coll carried out a systematic search for mycobacteria in sea-urchin granulomas [151]. The study cohort consisted of 35 patients (31 male and 4 female; median age 35 years, range 14–60) with sea-urchin granulomas. The median latency time from the injury was 7.5 months. Half of the patients affected were involved in fishing activities. Fifty biopsies specimens were available for histological study, and several inflammatory patterns were shown, mainly of sarcoidal (26%) or foreign-body type (20%). Acid-fast bacilli were not identified with Ziehl-Neelsen staining. Skin biopsies were cultured in 11 instances, none of which yielded positive isolates of mycobacteria. A PCR-amplified DNA fragment of 924 bp, encoding mycobacterial 16S rRNA, was obtained in eight biopsies from seven patients. Digestion yielded three fragments (677 bp, 132 bp, and 115 bp) specific for *M. marinum* in three of the samples. The remaining patterns, with two fragments (792 bp and 132 bp) were not specific for *M. marinum*, suggesting the possibility of mutations, subspecies or other non-identified acid-fast species [151].

The authors stated that as *M. marinum* is not a commensal and contamination is unlikely, its identification suggests a pathogenic role in some cases of sea-urchin granulomas. The spines of sea-urchins may harbor *M. marinum*, that is probably one of the various etiopathogenic agents implicated [151].

9.14 Piscine and Aquarium Mycobacteriosis

Mycobacterial infections in fish are reported as piscine mycobacteriosis. The disease, subacute to chronic in nature, affects fish in freshwater, saltwater, and brackish water. To date, piscine mycobacteriosis has been mainly attributable to three pathogens: *M. marinum*, *M. fortuitum*, and *M. chelonae* [94].

Mycobacteriosis can affect a wide range of fish species (more than 150 species), suggesting a ubiquitous distribution [135, 154]. It is generally accompanied by emaciation and death over a period of months to years. Granulomas are formed both externally and scattered throughout the internal organs. Treatment is in most cases unsatisfactory and the recommendation is usually to destroy the diseased stock [94], particularly since the pathogens can affect man as well as fish. Fish handlers and aquarium hobbyists are most commonly infected, and the disease, that presents with nodular lesions, is mostly confined to the extremities [8].

There have been ample studies of the presence of mycobacteria in aquarium fish, whereas the presence and distribution of mycobacteria in clinically healthy aquarium fish and their environment have not been adequately explored. Beran and Coll carried out a study in which the occurrence of mycobacteria in a decorative aquarium and in 5 aquariums belonging to a professional fish breeder in Moravia (Czech Republic) was analyzed [155]. After Ziehl-Neelsen staining, acid-fast rods were observed in 6 (14.3%) and mycobacteria were detected by culture in 18 (42.9%) of the 42 tissue samples from 19 fish. Sixty-five samples of the aqueous environment in 6 aquariums were examined; acid-fast bacilli were found in 16 (24.6%) and mycobacteria were detected by culture in 49 (75.4%) samples. Forty-one (70.7%) of 58 selected mycobacterial isolates were biochemically identified as follows: *M. fortuitum*, *M. flavescens*, *M. chelonae*, *M. gordonae*, *M. terrae*, *M. triviale*, *M. diernhoferi*, *M. celatum*, *M. kansasii*, and *M. intracellulare*. The clinically important species for fish and humans, *M. marinum*, was not isolated [155]. According to the authors, mycobacterial species from aquarium environments may be useful as a possible predictable source of infection for both aquarium fish and immunocompetent and immunocompromised fish handlers.

The answer to how mycobacteria get into aquarium environments is not known. However, the literature shows a high incidence of mycobacteria in drinking water distribution systems and in surface water [156, 157], so their transmission from water sources is likely. Mycobacteria can also spread into aquariums with exotic fish [158].

References

1. Petrini B (2006) *Mycobacterium marinum*: ubiquitous agent of waterborne granulomatous skin infections. Eur J Clin Microbiol Infect Dis 25:609
2. Bataillon E, Moeller A, Terre L (1902) Über die identitat des Bacillus des Karpfens und des Bacillus der Blindsschleuche. Zentralbl Tuberc 3:467
3. Cambau E, Aubry A (2011) *Mycobacterium marinum*. In: Schlossberg D (ed) Tuberculosis and nontuberculous mycobacterial infections, 6th edn. ASM Press, Washington, DC, p 586
4. Aronson JD (1926) Spontaneous tuberculosis in saltwater fish. J Infect Dis 39:315
5. Baker J, Hagan W (1942) Tuberculosis of the Mexican platyfish (*Platypoecilus maculatus*). J Infect Dis 70:248
6. Norden A, Linell F (1951) A new type of pathogenic mycobacterium. Nature 168:286
7. Linell F, Norden A (1954) *Mycobacterium balnei*, a new acid-fast bacillus occurring in swimming pools and capable of producing skin lesion in humans. Acta Tuberc Scand Suppl 33:1
8. Bonamonte D, Filoni A, Vestita M et al (2016) Cutaneous infections from aquatic environments. In: Bonamonte D, Angelini G (eds) Aquatic dermatology. Biotic, chemical and physical agents, 2nd edn. Springer, Berlin, p 185
9. Swift S, Cohen H (1962) Granulomas of the skin due to *Mycobacterium marinum* after abrasion from a fish tank. N Engl J Med 267:1244
10. Walker H, Shinn MF, Higaki M et al (1962) Some characteristics of "swimming pool" disease in Hawaii. Hawaii Med J 21:403
11. Flowers DJ (1970) Human infection due to *Mycobacterium marinum* after a dolphin bite. J Clin Pathol 23:475
12. Zeligman I (1972) *Mycobacterium marinum* granuloma. A disease acquired in the tributaries of Chesapeake Bay. Arch Dermatol 106:26
13. Helguera-Repetto C, Cox RA, Muñoz Sànchez JL et al (2004) The pathogen *Mycobacterium marinum*, a faster growing close relative of *Mycobacterium tuberculosis*, has a single rRNA operon per genome. FEMS Microbiol Lett 235:281
14. Stinear TP, Seeman T, Harrison PF et al (2008) Insights from the complete genome sequence of *Mycobacterium marinum* on the evolution of *Mycobacterium tuberculosis*. Genome Res 18:729
15. Ruley KM, Ansede JH, Pritchett CL et al (2004) Identification of *Mycobacterium marinum* virulence genes using signature-tagged mutagenesis and the goldfish model of mycobacterial pathogenesis. FEMS Microbiol Lett 232:75
16. Stinear T, Johnson PDR (2007) From marinum to ulcerans: a mycobacterial human pathogen emerges. Microbe 2:187
17. Runyon E (1959) Anonymous mycobacteria in pulmonary disease. Med Clin North Am 43:273
18. Stahl DA, Urbance JW (1990) The division between fast- and slow-growing species corresponds to natural relationships among the mycobacteria. J Bacteriol 172:116
19. Wolinsky E (1992) Mycobacterial diseases other than tuberculosis. Clin Infect Dis 15(1)
20. Rogall T, Wolters J, Flohr T et al (1990) Towards a phylogeny and definition of species at the molecular level within the genus *Mycobacterium*. Int J Syst Bacteriol 40:323
21. Tønjum T, Welty DB, Jantzen E et al (1998) Differentiation of *Mycobacterium ulcerans*, *M. marinum*, and *M. haemophilum*: mapping of their relationships to *M. tuberculosis* by fatty acid profile analysis, DNA-DNA hybridization, and 16S rRNA gene sequence analysis. J Clin Microbiol 36:918
22. Stinear TP, Seemann T, Pidot S et al (2007) Reductive evolution and niche adaptation inferred from the genome of *Mycobacterium ulcerans*, the causative agent of Buruli ulcer. Genome Res 17:192
23. Kim BJ, Lee SH, Lyu MA et al (1999) Identification of mycobacterial species by comparative sequence analysis of the RNA polymerase gene (rpoB). J Clin Microbiol 37:1714
24. Dauendorffer JN, Guillemin I, Aubry A et al (2003) Identification of mycobacterial species by PCR sequencing of quinolone resistance-determining regions of DNA gyrase genes. J Clin Microbiol 41:1311

25. Stinear TP, Jenkin GA, Johnson PD et al (2000) Comparative genetic analysis of *Mycobacterium ulcerans* and *Mycobacterium marinum* reveals evidence of recent divergence. J Bacteriol 182:6322
26. Stinear TP, Mve-Obiang A, Small PL et al (2004) Giant plasmid-encoded polyketide synthases produce the macrolide toxin of *Mycobacterium ulcerans*. Proc Natl Acad Sci U S A 101:1345
27. Chemlal K, Huys G, Fonteyne PA et al (2001) Evaluation of PCR-restriction profile analysis and IS2404 restriction fragment length polymorphism and amplified fragment length polymorphism fingerprinting for identification and typing of *Mycobacterium ulcerans* and *M. marinum*. J Clin Microbiol 39:3272
28. Stragier P, Hermans K, Stinear TP et al (2008) First report of a mycolactone-producing *Mycobacterium* infection in fish agriculture in Belgium. FEMS Microbiol Lett 286:93
29. Yip MJ, Porter JL, Fyfe JA et al (2007) Evolution of *Mycobacterium ulcerans* and other mycolactone-producing mycobacteria from a common *Mycobacterium marinum* progenitor. J Bacteriol 189:2021
30. Ucko M, Colorni A, Kvitt H et al (2002) Strain variation in *Mycobacterium marinum* fish isolates. Appl Environ Microbiol 68:5281
31. Ranger BS, Mahrous EA, Mosi L et al (2006) Globally distributed mycobacterial fish pathogens produce a novel plasmid-encoded toxic macrolide, mycolactone F. Infect Immunol 74:6037
32. van Ingen J, de Zwaan R, Dekhuijzen R et al (2009) Region of difference 1 in nontuberculous *Mycobacterium* species adds a phylogenetic and taxonomical character. J Bacteriol 191:5865
33. Julián E, Roldán M, Sánchez-Chardi A et al (2010) Microscopic cords, a virulence-related characteristic of *Mycobacterium tuberculosis*, are also present in nonpathogenic mycobacteria. J Bacteriol 192:1751
34. Glickman MS (2008) Cording, cord factors, and trehalose dimycolate. In: Daffe M, Reyrat J (eds) The mycobacterial cell envelope. ASM Press, Washington, DC, p 63
35. Daffé M, Lanéelle MA, Lacave C (1991) Structure and stereochemistry of mycolic acids of *Mycobacterium marinum* and *Mycobacterium ulcerans*. Res Microbiol 142:397
36. Bhatty MA, Turner DP, Chamberlain ST (2000) *Mycobacterium marinum* hand infection: case reports and review of literature. Br J Plast Surg 53:161
37. Griffith DE, Aksamit T, Brown-Elliott BA et al (2007) An official ATS/IDSA statement: diagnosis, treatment, and prevention of nontuberculous mycobacterial diseases. Am J Respir Crit Care Med 175:367
38. van Ingen J (2013) Diagnosis of nontuberculous mycobacterial infections. Semin Respir Crit Care Med 34:103
39. Ramakrishnan L, Tran HT, Federspiel NA et al (1997) A crtB homolog essential for photochromogenicity in *Mycobacterium marinum*: isolation, characterization, and gene disruption via homologous recombination. J Bacteriol 179:5862
40. Tortoli E, Nanetti A, Piersimoni C et al (2001) Performance assessment of new multiplex probe assay for identification of mycobacteria. J Clin Microbiol 39:1079
41. Russo C, Tortoli E, Menichella D (2006) Evaluation of the new GenoType *Mycobacterium* assay for identification of mycobacterial species. J Clin Microbiol 44:334
42. Salati F, Meloni M, Fenza A et al (2010) A sensitive FRET probe assay for the selective detection of *Mycobacterium marinum* in fish. J Fish Dis 33:47
43. Stragier P, Ablordey A, Meyers WM et al (2005) Genotyping *Mycobacterium ulcerans* and *Mycobacterium marinum* by using mycobacterial interspersed repetitive units. J Bacteriol 187:1639
44. Ucko M, Colorni A (2005) *Mycobacterium marinum* infections in fish and humans in Israel. J Clin Microbiol 43:892
45. Barker LP, George KM, Falkow S et al (1997) Differential trafficking of live and dead *Mycobacterium marinum* organisms in macrophages. Infect Immunol 65:1497
46. Barker LP, Brooks DM, Small PL (1998) The identification of *Mycobacterium marinum* genes differentially expressed in macrophage phagosomes using promoter fusions to green fluorescent protein. Mol Microbiol 29:1167

47. Stamm LM, Morisaki JH, Gao LY et al (2003) *Mycobacterium marinum* escapes from phagosomes and is propelled by actin-based motility. J Exp Med 198:1361
48. Hagedorn M, Rohde KH, Russell DG et al (2009) Infection by tubercular mycobacteria is spread by nonlytic ejection from their amoeba hosts. Science 323:1729
49. van der Sar AM, Abdallah AM, Sparrius M et al (2004) *Mycobacterium marinum* strains can be divided into two distinct types based on genetic diversity and virulence. Infect Immunol 72:6306
50. Chan K, Knaak T, Satkamp L et al (2002) Complex pattern of *Mycobacterium marinum* gene expression during long-term granulomatous infection. Proc Natl Acad Sci U S A 99:3920
51. Hodgkinson JW, Ge JQ, Grayfer L et al (2012) Analysis of the immune response in infections of the goldfish (*Carassius auratus* L.) with *Mycobacterium marinum*. Dev Comp Immunol 38:456
52. van der Sar AM, Spaink HP, Zakrzewska A et al (2009) Specificity of the zebrafish host transcriptome response to acute and chronic mycobacterial infection and the role of innate and adaptive immune components. Mol Immunol 46:2317
53. Dong D, Wang D, Li M et al (2012) PPE38 modulates the innate immune response and is required for *Mycobacterium marinum* virulence. Infect Immunol 80:43
54. Weerdenburg EM, Abdallah AM, Mitra S et al (2012) ESX-5-deficient *Mycobacterium marinum* is hypervirulent in adult zebrafish. Cell Microbiol 14:728
55. Abdallah AM, Savage ND, van Zon M et al (2008) The ESX-5 secretion system of *Mycobacterium marinum* modulates the macrophage response. J Immunol 181:7166
56. Rallis E, Koumantaki-Mathioudaki E (2007) Treatment of *Mycobacterium marinum* cutaneous infections. Expert Opin Pharmacother 8:2965
57. Barton A, Bernstein RM, Struthers JK et al (1997) *Mycobacterium marinum* infection causing septic arthritis and osteomyelitis. Br J Rheumatol 36:1207
58. Saadatmand B, Poulton JK, Kauffman CL (1999) *Mycobacterium marinum* with associated bursitis. J Cutan Med Surg 3:218
59. Powers R, Fisher M (2004) Tenosynovitis due to *Mycobacterium marinum*. N Engl J Med 351:911
60. Tsai HC, Lee SS, Wann SR et al (2006) *Mycobacterium marinum* tenosynovitis: three case reports and review of the literature. Jpn J Infect Dis 59:337
61. Tchornobay AM, Claudy AL, Perrot JL et al (1992) Fatal disseminated *Mycobacterium marinum* infection. Int J Dermatol 31:286
62. Ekerot L, Jacobsson L, Forsgren A (1998) *Mycobacterium marinum* wrist arthritis: local and systematic dissemination caused by concomitant immunosuppressive therapy. Scand J Infect Dis 30:84
63. Ho PL, Ho P, Fung BK et al (2001) A case of disseminated *Mycobacterium marinum* infection following systemic steroid therapy. Scand J Infect Dis 33:232
64. Streit M, Böhlen LM, Hunziker T et al (2006) Disseminated *Mycobacterium marinum* infection with extensive cutaneous eruption and bacteremia in an immunocompromised patient. Eur J Dermatol 16:79
65. Lambertus MW, Mathisen GE (1988) *Mycobacterium marinum* infection in a patient with cryptosporidiosis and the acquired immunodeficiency syndrome. Cutis 41:38
66. Vazquez JA, Sobel JD (1992) A case of disseminated *Mycobacterium marinum* infection in an immunocompetent patient. Eur J Clin Microbiol Infect Dis 11:908
67. Lai CC, Lee LN, Chang YL et al (2005) Pulmonary infection due to *Mycobacterium marinum* in an immunocompetent patient. Clin Infect Dis 40:206
68. Chopra N, Kirschenbaum AE, Widman D (2002) *Mycobacterium marinum* tenosynovitis in a patient on etanercept therapy for rheumatoid arthritis. J Clin Rheumatol 8:265
69. Rallis E, Koumantaki-Mathioudaki E, Frangoulis E et al (2007) Severe sporotrichoid fish tank granuloma following infliximab therapy. Am J Clin Dermatol 8:385
70. Alkhawaja S, Tammam N, Khalifa N (2010) *Mycobacterium marinum* infection after infliximab therapy. Iran J Allergy Asthma Immunol 9:255

71. Caron J, Michot C, Fabre S et al (2011) Aggressive cutaneous infection with *Mycobacterium marinum* in two patients receiving anti-tumor necrosis factor-alpha agents. J Am Acad Dermatol 65:1060
72. Kump PK, Högenauer C, Wenzl HH et al. A case of opportunistic skin infection with *Mycobacterium marinum* during adalimumab treatment in a patient with Crohn's disease. J Crohns Colitis 2013;7:e15.
73. Garzoni C, Adler S, Boller C et al (2010) Possible role of anti-TNF monoclonal antibodies in the treatment of *Mycobacterium marinum* infection. Rheumatology 49:1991
74. Philpott JA Jr, Woodburne AR, Philpott OS et al (1963) Swimming pool granuloma. A study of 290 cases. Arch Dermatol 88:158
75. Gould WM, McMeekin DR, Bright RD (1968) *Mycobacterium marinum* (balnei) infection. Report of a case with cutaneous and laryngeal lesions. Arch Dermatol 97:159
76. Reznikov M (1970) Atypical mycobacteria. Their classification, identification, and aetiological significance. Med J Aust 1:553
77. Alessi E, Finzi AF, Prandi G (1976) Infezioni cutanee da *Mycobacterium marinum.* Considerazioni su due casi clinici. G Ital Min Dermatol 111:185
78. King AJ, Fairley JA, Rasmussen JE (1983) Disseminated cutaneous *Mycobacterium marinum* infection. Arch Dermatol 119:268
79. Blank AA, Schnyder VW (1985) Aquariumgranulom vom kutan-disseminierten Typ. Hautarzt 86:48
80. Huminer D, Pitlik SD, Block C et al (1986) Aquarium-borne *Mycobacterium marinum* skin infection. Report of a case and review of the literature. Arch Dermatol 122:698
81. Cole GW (1987) *Mycobacterium marinum* infection in a mechanic. Contact Dermatitis 16:283
82. Angelini G, Filotico R, De Vito D et al (1990) Infezioni cutanee professionali da *Mycobacterium marinum.* Boll Dermatol Allergol Profes 5:165
83. Angelini G, Vena GA, Grandolfo M (1995) Micobatteri e cute. Dermotime 7:11
84. Angelini G, Vena GA (1997) Dermatologia professionale e ambientale, vol I. ISED, Brescia, p 202
85. Brady RC, Sheth A, Mayer T et al (1997) Facial sporotrichoid infection with *Mycobacterium marinum.* J Pediatr 130:324
86. Jernigan JA, Farr BM (2000) Incubation period and sources of exposure for cutaneous *Mycobacterium marinum* infection: case report and review of the literature. Clin Infect Dis 31:439
87. Ang P, Rattana-Apiromyakij N, Goh CL (2000) Retrospective study of *Mycobacterium marinum* skin infections. Int J Dermatol 39:343
88. Bonamonte D, Angelini G (2009) Aquatic dermatology. In: Hall JC, Hall BJ (eds) Skin infections. Diagnosis and treatment. Cambridge University Press, New York, p 167
89. Bonamonte D, Angelini G (2013) Aquagenic dermatology. In: Giannetti A, Del Forno C (eds) Textbook of dermatology and sexually transmitted diseases. Piccin Nuova Libraria S.P.A, Padova, p 783
90. Casal M, Casal MM (2001) Spanish Group of Mycobacteriology. Multicenter study of incidence of *Mycobacterium marinum* in humans in Spain. Int J Tuberc Lung Dis 5:197
91. Aubry A, Chosidow O, Caumes E et al (2002) Sixty-three cases of *Mycobacterium marinum* infection. Clinical features, treatment, and antibiotic susceptibility of causative isolates. Arch Intern Med 162:1746
92. Kirby JS, Elston DE Dermatologic manifestations of *Mycobacterium marinum* infection of the skin. http://emedicine.com/derm/topic281.htm. Updated 25 July 2011.
93. Harriff MJ, Bermudez LE, Kent ML (2007) Experimental exposure of zebrafish, *Danio rerio* (Hamilton), to *Mycobacterium marinum* and *Mycobacterium peregrinum* reveals the gastrointestinal tract as the primary route of infection: a potential model for environmental mycobacterial infection. J Fish Dis 30:587
94. Decostere A, Hermans K, Haesebrouck F (2004) Piscine mycobacteriosis: a literature review covering the agent and the disease it causes in fish and humans. Vet Microbiol 99:159

95. Heckert RA, Elankumaran S, Milani A et al (2001) Detection of a new *Mycobacterium* species in wild striped bass in the Chesapeake Bay. J Clin Microbiol 39:710
96. Zanoni RG, Florio D, Fioravanti ML et al (2008) Occurrence of *Mycobacterium* spp. in ornamental fish in Italy. J Fish Dis 31:433
97. Lewis FM, Marsh BJ, von Reyn CF (2003) Fish tank exposure and cutaneous infections due to *Mycobacterium marinum*: tuberculin skin testing, treatment, and prevention. Clin Infect Dis 37:390
98. Gluckman SJ (1995) *Mycobacterium marinum*. Clin Dermatol 13:273
99. Dobos KM, Quinn FD, Ashford DA et al (1999) Emergence of a unique group of necrotizing mycobacterial diseases. Emerg Infect Dis 5:367
100. Lacaille F, Blanche S, Bodemer C et al (1990) Persistent *Mycobacterium marinum* infection in a child with probable visceral involvement. Pediatr Infect Dis J 9:58
101. Clark RB, Spector H, Friedman DM et al (1990) Osteomyelitis and synovitis produced by *Mycobacterium marinum* in a fisherman. J Clin Microbiol 28:2570
102. Edelstein H (1994) *Mycobacterium marinum* skin infections. Report of 31 cases and review of the literature. Arch Intern Med 154:1359
103. Zenone T, Boibieux A, Tigaud S et al (1999) Non-tuberculous mycobacterial tenosynovitis: a review. Scand J Infect Dis 31:221
104. Collins CH, Grange JM, Noble WC et al (1985) *Mycobacterium marinum* infections in man. J Hyg (Lond) 94:135
105. Wallace R, Glassroth J, Griffith D et al (1997) Diagnosis and treatment of disease caused by nontuberculous mycobacteria. Am J Respir Crit Care Med 156:S1
106. Arend SM, van Meijgaarden KE, de Boer K et al (2002) Tuberculin skin testing and in vitro T cell responses to ESAT-6 and culture filtrate protein 10 after infection with *Mycobacterium marinum* or *M. kansasii*. J Infect Dis 186:1797
107. Kobashi Y, Mouri K, Yagi S et al (2009) Clinical evaluation of the QuantiFERON-TB Gold test in patients with non-tuberculous mycobacterial disease. Int J Tuberc Lung Dis 13:1422
108. Bonamonte D, De Vito D, Vestita M et al (2013) Aquarium-borne *Mycobacterium marinum* skin infection. Report of 15 cases and review of the literature. Eur J Dermatol 23:510
109. Cribier B, Aubry A, Caumes E et al (2011) Aspects histopathologiques de l'infection à *Mycobacterium marinum*. Ann Dermatol Vénéréol 138:17
110. Travis WD, Travis LB, Roberts GD et al (1985) The histopathologic spectrum in *Mycobacterium marinum* infection. Arch Pathol Lab Med 109:1109
111. Barr KL, Lowe L, Su LD (2003) *Mycobacterium marinum* infection simulating interstitial granuloma annulare: a report of two cases. Am J Dermatopathol 25:148
112. Dodiuk-Gad R, Dyachenko P, Ziv M et al (2007) Nontuberculous mycobacterial infections of the skin: a retrospective study of 25 cases. J Am Acad Dermatol 57:413
113. Abbas O, Marrouch N, Kattar MM et al (2011) Cutaneous non-tuberculous mycobacterial infections: a clinical and histopathological study of 17 cases from Lebanon. J Eur Acad Dermatol Venereol 25:33
114. Nikaido H (2003) Molecular basis of bacterial outer membrane permeability revisited. Microbiol Mol Biol Rev 67:593
115. Brown BA, Wallace RJ Jr, Onyi GO (1992) Activities of clarithromycin against eight slowly growing species of nontuberculous mycobacteria, determined by using a broth microdilution MIC system. Antimicrob Agents Chemother 36:1987
116. Wallace RJ Jr, Nash DR, Steele LC et al (1986) Susceptibility testing of slowly growing mycobacteria by a microdilution MIC method with 7H9 broth. J Clin Microbiol 24:976
117. Brown-Elliott BA, Wallace RJ Jr, Crist CJ et al (2003) In vitro activity of linezolid against slowly growing nontuberculous mycobacteria. Antimicrobe Agents Chemother 47:1736
118. National Committee for Clinical Laboratory Standards (NCCLS) (2000) Susceptibility testing of Mycobacteria, Nocardia and other aerobic Actinomycetes; Tenative Standard-Second Edition. NCCLS document M24-T2. NCCLS, Wayne, PA
119. Dautzenberg B, Breux JP, Febyre M et al (1992) Clarithromycin containing regimens for mycobacterial infections in 55 non AIDS patients. Am Rev Respir Dis 145:A809

120. Black MM, Eykyn S (1986) The successful treatment of tropical fish tank granuloma (*Mycobacterium marinum* infections). Arch Inter Med 146:902
121. Cober E, Kaul DR. Non-tuberculous mycobacteria in solid organ transplant recipients. http://www.antimicrobe.org/new/t26.asp
122. Esteban J, Ortiz-Pérez A (2009) Current treatment of atypical mycobacteriosis. Expert Opin Pharmacother 10:2787
123. Kaplan D (1988) *Mycobacterium marinum* cutaneous infections. Inf Med 5:257
124. Kim R (1974) Tetracycline therapy for atypical mycobacterial granuloma. Arch Dermatol 110:299
125. Chow SP, Ip FK, Lau JH et al (1987) *Mycobacterium marinum* infection of the hand and wrist. J Bone Joint Surg Am 69:1161
126. Sands M, Rosenthal E, Chavan A et al (1996) *Mycobacterium marinum* tenosynovitis treated with clarithromycin and ethambutol. Infect Dis Clin Practice 5:509
127. Donta ST, Smith PW, Levitz RE et al (1986) Therapy of *Mycobacterium marinum* infections. Arch Intern Med 146:902
128. Aubry A, Jarlier V, Escolano S et al (2000) Antibiotic susceptibility pattern of *Mycobacterium marinum*. Antimicrob Agents Chemother 44:3133
129. Hanau LH, Leaf A, Soeiro R et al (1994) *Mycobacterium marinum* infection in a patient with the acquired immunodeficiency syndrome. Cutis 54:103
130. Bonnet E, Debat-Zoguereh D, Petit N et al (1994) Clarithromycin: a potent agent against infections due to *Mycobacterium marinum*. Clin Infect Dis 18:664
131. Parent LJ, Salam MM, Appelbaum PC et al (1995) Disseminated *Mycobacterium marinum* infection and bacteremia in a child with severe combined immunodeficiency. Clin Infect Dis 21:1325
132. Woods GL (2000) Susceptibility testing for mycobacteria. Clin Infect Dis 31:1209
133. Centers for Disease Control and Prevention, US Department of Health and Human Services (DHHS) (1976) Swimming pools: safety and disease control through proper design and operation. DHHS, Washington, DC, p 61 (DHHS Publication Number CDC-88-8319)
134. Centers for Disease Control and Prevention, US Department of Health and Human Services (DHHS) (1985) Suggested health and safety guidelines for public spa and hot tubs. DHHS, Washington, DC, p 15 (DHHS Publication Number CDC-99-960)
135. Astrofsky KM, Schrenzel MD, Bullis RA et al (2000) Diagnosis and management of atypical *Mycobacterium* spp. infections in established laboratory zebrafish (*Brachydanio rerio*) facilities. Comp Med 50:666
136. Passantino A, Macrì D, Coluccio P et al (2008) Importation of mycobacteriosis with ornamental fish: medico-legal implications. Travel Med Infect Dis 6:240
137. Schmoor P, Descamps V, Bouscarat F et al (2003) Les connaissances et le comportement des vendeurs de poissons exotiques concernant la "maladie des aquariums". Ann Dermatol Vénéréol 130:425
138. Berth-Jones J (2010) Topical therapy. In: Burns T, Breathnach S, Cox N et al (eds) Rook's textbook of dermatology, 8th edn, vol 73. Wiley-Blackwell Scientific Publications, Oxford, p 1
139. Dailloux M, Laurain C, Weber M (1999) Water and nontuberculous mycobacteria. Water Res 33:2219
140. Murdoch LE, Maclean M, Endarko E et al (2012) Bactericidal effects of 405 nm light exposure demonstrated by inactivation of Escherichia, Salmonella, Shigella, Listeria, and *mycobacterium* species in liquid suspensions and on exposed surfaces. Scientific World J 137805:2012
141. Angelini G, Bonamonte D (1997) Dermatoses aquatiques méditerranéennes. Les Nouvelles Dermatologiques 16:280
142. Bonamonte D, Vestita M *Mycobacterium marinum*. http://antimicrobe-org/ms05.asp
143. Bonamonte D, Verni P, Filoni A et al (2016) Dermatitis caused by echinoderms. In: Bonamonte D, Angelini G (eds) Aquatic dermatology. Biotic, chemical and physical agents, 2nd edn, Springer, Berlin, p 89
144. Rocha G, Fraga S (1962) Seaurchin granuloma of the skin. Arch Dermatol 85:146

145. Fisher AA, Orris WL (1973) Aquatic contact dermatitis. Cutis 12:687
146. Warin AP (1977) Seaurchin granuloma. Clin Exp Dermatol 2:405
147. Haneke E (1980) Kölsch I.[Sea urchin granulomas]. Hautarzt 31:159
148. Baden HP (1987) Injuries from sea urchins. Clin Dermatol 5:112
149. Kinmont PDC (1965) Sea-urchin sarcoidal granuloma. Br J Dermatol 77:335
150. Cooper P, Wakefield MC (1974) A sarcoid reaction to injury by sea urchin spines. J Pathol 112:33
151. De La Torre C, Vega A, Carracedo A et al (2001) Identification of *Mycobacterium marinum* in sea-urchin granulomas. Br J Dermatol 145:114
152. Gaté J, Cuilleret P, Chanial G et al (1936) Lésions papulo-nécrotiques à réaction histologique tuberculoïde dues à l'ínclusion d' épines d'oursins. Bull Soc Fr Dermatol Syphiligr 43:937
153. Moynahan EJ, Montgomery PR (1968) Echinoderm granuloma: a skin lesion resulting from injury by the spines of sea-urchins inhabiting temperate waters. A new mycobacterial infection. Br J Clin Pract 22:265
154. Bruno DW, Griffiths J, Mitchell CG et al (1998) Pathology attributed to *Mycobacterium chelonae* infection among farmed and laboratory-infected Atlantic salmon *Salmo salar*. Dis Aquat Org 33:101
155. Beran V, Matlova L, Dvorska L et al (2006) Distribution of mycobacteria in clinically healthy ornamental fish and their aquarium environment. J Fish Dis 29:383
156. Fischeder R, Schulze-Röbbecke R, Weber A (1991) Occurrence of mycobacteria in drinking water samples. Zentralbl Hyg Umweltmed 192:154
157. Falkinham JO, Norton CD, LeChevallier MW (2001) Factors influencing numbers of *Mycobacterium avium*, *Mycobacterium intracellulare*, and other mycobacteria in drinking water distribution systems. Appl Environ Microbiol 67:1225
158. Novotny L, Halouzka R, Matlova L et al (2010) Morphology and distribution of granulomatous inflammation in freshwater ornamental fish infected with mycobacteria. J Fish Dis 33:947

Mycobacterium ulcerans Infection

10

Domenico Bonamonte, Angela Filoni, and Gianni Angelini

Mycobacterium ulcerans is the causative agent of a new emerging infectious disease, which has been reported in at least 33 countries worldwide with tropical, subtropical and temperate climates (Table 10.1) [1–8].

Classified by the WHO as one of the 17 neglected tropical diseases [6, 9], *M. ulcerans* infection is the third most common mycobacterial disease in the world, after tuberculosis and leprosy. In East Africa, where it is endemic and thousands of cases are observed annually, the infection is the second most important mycobacterial disease after tuberculosis [10].

Buruli ulcer disease (the name adopted for this infection worldwide) is often referred to as the "mysterious disease" because the mode of transmission remains unclear, although several hypotheses have been proposed [9]. It is a serious necrotizing infection due to a toxin, mycolactone, produced by the bacilli, that necrotizes the subcutaneous tissue leading to deep ulceration. This is the most severe form of the disease. Early detection before ulceration is therefore the key to prompt cure; otherwise, if diagnosed late, the infection may leave patients with disabling sequelae, such as scarring contractures and possible bone destruction requiring amputation.

D. Bonamonte, MD, PhD (✉)
Department of Biomedical Science and Human Oncology,
University of Bari "Aldo Moro", Bari, Italy
e-mail: domenico.bonamonte@uniba.it

A. Filoni, MD
University of Bari "Aldo Moro", Bari, Italy

G. Angelini, MD
Professor of Dermatology, Former Professor and Chairman, University of Bari "Aldo Moro",
Bari, Italy

D. Bonamonte, G. Angelini (eds.), *Mycobacterial Skin Infections*,
DOI 10.1007/978-3-319-48538-6_10

Table 10.1 Geographic distribution of *Mycobacterium ulcerans* infection

West Africa	Angola, Benin, Burkina Faso, Cameroon, Congo, Côte d'Ivoire, Equatorial Guinea, Gabon, Ghana, Guinea, Liberia, Mali, Nigeria, Sierra Leone, Togo
Other African countries	Democratic Republic of Congo, Malawi, Uganda, Sudan
Western Pacific	Australia, Kiribati, Papua New Guinea
Central and South America	Brazil, French Guyana, Mexico, Peru, Suriname
Southeast Asia	China, India, Indonesia, Japan, Malaysia, Sri Lanka

10.1 History

In his book "A walk across Africa" (1864), James Augustus Grant described how his leg became grossly swollen and stiff, and later developed a copious discharge. This is the first known description of the infection, and almost certainly refers to the severe, edematous form. In 1897, Buruli ulcer disease was identified by Sir Albert Ruskin Cook, a British physician, at Mengo Hospital in Kampala, Uganda [11].

Since 1937, the disease had been recognized as a particular entity in South-East Australia, at Bairnsdale in the State of Victoria, by two physicians, Alsop and Searls. The infection, that followed catastrophic rainfall in the State of Victoria in 1935, was confirmed by an epidemic that occurred in 1939 [1]. The first detailed description of the disease dates back to 1948, made by MacCallum and Coll, who were treating patients from the Bairnsdale district (hence "Bairnsdale ulcer", the other famous name for this disease), near Melbourne [12]. The authors observed six Australian patients with a single ulcerative lesion on an arm or a leg. The edges of the ulcers were undermined, and one patient had a positive tuberculin skin test result, although no evidence of tuberculosis was found. Acid-fast bacilli were present in histological specimens. Inoculated into animals, the *Mycobacterium* species present in the subcutaneous lesions of the patients caused ulceration. Isolation of the bacterium was at first unsuccessful but then it was noted that lesions in rats were found to be most prominent on the scrotum, limbs and tails. Culture at a lower temperature was therefore attempted, and isolation proved successful on three different occasions. The mycobacterium was provisionally named the "Bairnsdale bacillus", after the region where 5 of the 6 patients lived (the sixth patient came from Colac, 300 kilometers away); it was subsequently renamed *M. ulcerans* in 1948 [1, 2, 12, 13].

In 1950, van Oye and Ballion reported the case of a 6-year-old American expatriate boy from Zaïre (now Democratic Republic of Congo) who presented with an undermined ulcer on the dorsal aspect of the left foot. Acid-fast bacilli were present in histological specimens [14]. Many other reports from Zaïre followed; by 1974, 430 patients had been reported [15].

In 1961, the first African focus of *M. ulcerans* infection was reported by Clancey and Coll in Uganda, in a region near the Nile River called Buruli (now Nakasongola District) [16]. This epidemic, that had struck Ruandan refugees living on the banks of the lower Nile Victoria, occurred after the great flooding of the Uganda lakes.

Nevertheless, as stated above, the disease had already been described in Ugandan patients by Sir Albert Cook [17]. Following other African outbreaks, in 1972 Clancey proposed the name "Buruli ulcer" [1].

The first reports from West Africa were in Nigeria, followed by Angola, Benin, Burkina Faso, Cameroon, Congo, Côte d'Ivoire, Equatorial Guinea, Gabon, Liberia, Mali and Togo [18–26]. Cases have been reported in Southeast Asia (Malaysia, Japan, Indonesia, India, Sri Lanka, and China in the province of Shandong) [11, 27–29], in Central and South America (Brazil, French Guyana, Mexico, Peru, Suriname) [1, 30–35], and in Oceania (Papua New Guinea) [36]. Other African countries where the infection has been reported are the Democratic Republic of Congo, Malawi, Uganda and Sudan [1].

The recent Australian recrudescence of the 1996 infection in Phillip Island (Victoria) was associated with road rebuilding, that provoked the formation of marshes above an estuary that was divided in half by the road. Again in Australia, an increased number of cases was recorded between 1991 and 1994 following the use of recycled water to irrigate a golf course [37].

Hayman noted that all reported infections occurring in three different continents were closely linked to the Jurassic era, and that the distribution of the plant family Proteaceae coincided with this pattern [38].

In Table 10.2 some of the eponyms used to describe this infection in different countries are listed: some have a geographic origin, others are based on folklore, linked to cultural, ethnic or magic-religious elements, while yet authors pay homage to the Australian physician who was the first to describe the disease (Searls' ulcer) [39–41]. In this regard, in their original 1948 work [12] MacCallum and Coll acknowledged assistance from Doctors Alsop, Clay, and Searls (listed in alphabetical order). When they sent material to Melbourne University for examination, the doctors of the Bairnsdale Clinic provided a description of the ulcers. JR Searls, after whom the ulcer was originally named, was regarded as an excellent general practitioner [42, 43].

Table 10.2 Some clinical designations given to *Mycobacterium ulcerans* infection

Buruli ulcer (Uganda and worldwide)
Bairnsdale ulcer (Australia)
Searls' ulcer (Australia)
Daintree ulcer
Kasongo ulcer (Democratic Republic of Congo)
Kakerifu ulcer (Democratic Republic of Congo)
Kumusu ulcer (Papua New Guinea)
Sik belong Sepik (Papua New Guinea)
Simiki River ulcer (Papua New Guinea)
Juwe Okoro
Bile Okoro
Tora ulcer
Mexican ulcer (Yucatan)
Tefoun-Tefoun (Benin)
Atom (Cameroon)
Akinolinga (Cameroon)

On the subject of eponyms, that are anyway fairly common in Dermatology, the *M. ulcerans* infection has been reported in many different areas, and each new outbreak has tended to give rise to a new name (Table 10.2). Of all these, perhaps the most colorful is "Sik belong Sepik", referred to the infection occurring along the Sepik River in Papua New Guinea [44]. Generally, medical eponyms refer to diseases that are poorly understood or have unknown causes. For various different reasons, many authors believe the name "Buruli ulcer" should no longer be used and the disease should everywhere be called "*M. ulcerans* infection" [40]. Others, instead, think that, for better or worse, the name "Buruli ulcer" belongs in the annals of medical history [44]. Indeed, in 1998, the WHO launched the Global Buruli Ulcer Initiative [45]. These last authors therefore propose that the term "Buruli ulcer" should be internationally adopted for *M. ulcerans* infection, also because the main endemic areas in Australia (where the disease continues to be called "Bairnsdale ulcer") are now the Bellarine and Mornington Peninsulas near Melbourne [46], whereas in Uganda the Buruli District has been renamed and is now known as the Nakasongola District [47].

10.2 Epidemiology

The environmental origin of this mycobacteriosis is becoming ever more evident on the basis of epidemiological and molecular biology data [47].

Since 1980, there has been an ample increase in the detection rate of the infection, thanks to an increase in public and scientific awareness. For a long period, *M. ulcerans* infection had gone largely unnoticed, likely because it occurs in remote rural communities that are poorly covered by national health surveillance systems. Additionally, many of the affected populations do not seek health care because of financial constraints, beliefs that the treatment is not successful, fear of surgery and anesthesia, or reasons of superstition and stigma [4, 48, 49]. Some authors, however, believe that the emergence of the disease is due not only to detection bias, but also to an increased exposure of affected populations [26, 50].

The infection is observed in geographically circumscribed endemic foci, always near to a water source (rivers, natural or artificial lakes, marshes, irrigation systems) and related to environmental changes (deforestation, agriculture, and hydraulic installations) involving surface water [1, 51].

Data in literature show that this mycobacteriosis has been reported in 33 countries, mostly in tropical and subtropical regions of Africa (West and Central Africa), including Benin, Cameroon, Côte d'Ivoire, the Democratic Republic of Congo, and Ghana. Cases have also been reported in Central and South America Countries, Papua New Guinea, and in some countries with temperate climates, such as Australia and Japan. Recent studies have identified different subspecies/strains of *M. ulcerans* in the different continents [28, 29, 52, 53].

WHO data demonstrate that in 2014, in total 2251 cases were detected, 1600 cases of which (71%) were in the three West African countries with the highest incidence of the disease: Côte d'Ivoire, Ghana and Benin. Globally, a gradual decrease in cases of infection has been observed [6, 8]. However, there are limits to the data collected by the WHO, mainly for the following reasons: the data refer to only 17 of the 33 countries where the disease has been reported; health care and reporting systems to national level in zones where the infection is most endemic are lacking; there are large areas with limited or no control activities to stem the infection, causing an underestimation of the true distribution; lack of awareness and limited knowledge about *M. ulcerans* infection among community members but also among health practitioners [6, 54]. For example, in Japan an increased reporting has recently been noted, due to increased awareness of the infection among dermatologists [29]. The above data demonstrate that the incidence of *M. ulcerans* infection is probably grossly underestimated.

In West Africa, the peak age for the disease is in children aged between 5 and 15 years [21, 22, 55] but it can affect subjects in any age group. In Australia and in Japan, people aged 40 years and over are more often affected, but cases in children are not rare [29, 56]. There are no gender differences in the distribution of cases among children. Among adults, some studies report higher rates among women than males [55]. No racial or socio-economic group is exempt from the disease.

By contrast, cases of *M. ulcerans* infection are rare in some countries: apart from French Guyana (where a few 100 cases have been observed) [1, 35], in Central and South America the diseases is considered rare [31, 33, 57]. However, it should be borne in mind that cases can occur among immigrants from an endemic nation for *M. ulcerans* infection, the disease having been acquired in the country of origin, and even in travelers from a country where the infection is not endemic [58–60]. Cases such as the latter, reported in countries where the infection is present, serve as a reminder that everywhere, practitioners should possess an adequate knowledge of the disease.

Like for all environmental mycobacterioses, person-to-person transmission has rarely been reported. One case was of a surgeon who developed a Buruli ulcer lesion on his hand after performing plastic surgery in a patient with the disease in Ghana (just one example of occupational disease contraction) [61].

10.3 The Organism

M. ulcerans is a microaerophilic, slender and slightly curved, non chromogenic, non capsulated, non sporulating, immobile, catalase-, nitrate reductase- and urease-negative mycobacterium. It belongs to a group of slowly growing mycobacteria, and is an acid-fast and alcohol-fast microorganism that is best cultured in egg-yolk-enriched Löwenstein-Jensen medium at 28–33 °C (ph 5.4–7.4, pO2 < 2.5 kPa). Colony growth can be observed both on liquid and solid media. *M. ulcerans* colonies are yellowish, rough and clearly distinguishable from one another. The yellow pigmentation can also be observed in the dark [1, 2, 6, 62–64]. It may not grow when incubated at 37 °C and may require a long incubation period, from 6 to 12 weeks before growth is seen. Many conventional methods can render the organism non viable.

Attempts to culture the microorganism from clinical specimens fail in more than half of all cases. Standard techniques for isolation and identification are very time-consuming but if carbon-14 is added to the culture medium, a radiometric assay (BACTEC system) may detect growth much more quickly [65]. DNA specific sequences have been amplified by means of PCR [66, 67]. Two different target sequences have been used for the detection of *M. ulcerans* in clinical isolates and in environmental samples, notably *IS2404* and *IS2606* [2]. Restriction-fragment length polymorphism analysis has been used to "fingerprint" the different genetic strains of M. *ulcerans*. Three different patterns have been identified from Africa, America, and Australia. These data, that may or may not also show differences in virulence, could help to select appropriate tests to study the prevalence of the pathogen in specific areas of the world [2].

M. ulcerans falls into a group of closed related mycobacterial pathogens that comprise the *M. marinum* complex. This complex, that contains pathogenic species for aquatic vertebrates, includes *M. marinum* (fish), *M. pseudoshottsii* (fish), and *M. liflandii* (frogs) [9, 68–71]. From a genomic standpoint, the species in the *M. marinum* complex may be regarded as a single species based on the fact that they share over 97% identity in the 16SRNA gene sequence [72]; practical considerations, however, led to separate names based on differences in host tropism. Genomic analysis suggests that *M. ulcerans* evolved from the same ancestor as *M. marinum* [9, 73, 74]. *M. ulcerans* has two unique characteristics that distinguish it from *M. marinum*: it has a large pathogenic plasmid called pMUM001 that produces mycolactone (this plasmid does not exist in *M. marinum* or any other nontuberculous mycobacterium); additionally, it has multiple copies of *IS2404* in the genome, over 200 copies, that again is not observed in any other mycobacteria [72]. In short, during its evolution *M. ulcerans* gained pMUM001 and IS; simultaneously, it lost the functions of a number of genes because the expansion of *IS2404* disrupted coding regions and/or promoter regions. As a result, it has more than 700 pseudogenes, compared with less than 100 in *M. marinum* [75]. Furthermore, the *M. ulcerans* genome strain lacks both nitrate and fumarate reductase systems, suggesting that its ability to grow under low oxygen conditions may be handicapped as compared with *M. marinum* [9]. A mutation in *crtI*, a key gene in the pathway for carotenoid synthesis, has been suggested to compromise the ability of *M. ulcerans* to survive in direct sunlight [76].

An important phenotypic characteristic of *M. ulcerans* is the low optimal growth temperature and extremely restricted growth temperature range. *M. marinum* exhibits its growth between 25–35 °C (the optimal growth temperature is 30–35 °C) [77] and many *M. marinum* isolates are capable of growth at 37 °C. By contrast, growth of the *M. ulcerans* strains is characterized by a temperature range between 28–34 °C and optimal growth of most strains occurs between 30–33 °C [78]. This restricted growth temperature may play an important role in the pathogenesis of *M. ulcerans* infection by limiting infection to the skin. The organism has never, in fact, been isolated from internal organs of human patients or from bones in cases of osteomyelitis, or from internal organs or the blood of experimentally infected animals [74, 79–81]. Many isolates of *M. ulcerans* have been reported to survive at 37 °C for

13 days, although numbers decline after the first few days; no isolated or derived strains have been found capable of growth at 37 °C [82].

Comparative analysis of the whole genome sequences of *M. ulcerans* and other mycolactone-producing mycobacteria has revealed that *M. ulcerans* split into two lineages during its evolution, namely "classical" and "ancestral" [11, 83–85]. Isolates from Africa and Australia are included in the classical lineage, while isolates from China, French Guyana, Japan, Mexico and Suriname are included in the ancestral lineage. These data are consistent with the intercontinental differences of isolate strains [86, 87].

The characteristic clinical picture of *M. ulcerans* infection is mediated by a polyketide-derived macrolide exotoxin called mycolactone, which has cytotoxic and immunosuppressive actions [74, 88, 89].

10.4 Ecology and Route of Transmission

A great step forward was made after the development of the first PCR probes for *M. ulcerans* based on the detection of *IS2404* [9, 90]. This technique has been adopted in various environmental samples to identify *M. ulcerans* DNA: detritus soil, biofilms, water filtrates, fish, frogs, snails, insects and other invertebrates [91–96]. Although *IS2404* PCR has become the gold standard for the diagnosis of *M. ulcerans* infection, it has various limitations. In fact, PCR detects DNA and not intact organisms. The death of infected organisms causes the release of *M. ulcerans* DNA into the various substrates in the environment. In various regions, small quantities of DNA have been found in water filtration samples; the significance of this finding is difficult to assess [95]. PCR methodology detects DNA, but does not provide definitive proof of the presence of intact bacteria in a matrix.

Almost all epidemiologic studies have found an association between infection outbreaks and living in villages in close proximity to disturbed aquatic habitats, including both still water bodies and those in movement [97, 98]. Increased *M. ulcerans* infection has been reported in association with [9]: unprecedented flooding of lakes and rivers during heavy rainfall [99–101]; the damming of streams and rivers to create impoundments and wetlands [92, 100, 102]; resorts where the wetlands have been modified [99, 100]; deforestation and increased agricultural processes leading to increased flooding [91, 92, 100, 102]; the construction of agricultural irrigation systems [100–102]; rice cultivation [102]; alluvial, pit and sand mining operations [92, 100, 103]; and population expansion, resettlement and migration closer to water bodies [22, 92, 99, 100].

It is well known that many water bodies associated with increased sedimentation and eutrophication have low concentrations of dissolved oxygen that may enhance the growth of *M. ulcerans* [104]. Hayman postulated that *M. ulcerans* is washed into aquatic environments where particular conditions foster growth and proliferation, much like an algal bloom [105]. The way the bacillus could be washed down into these aquatic habitats has still to be fully explained. It has been assumed that deforestation, leading to lost riparian cover, favors an increase in water temperatures, thus fostering optimal bacilli growth at 30–33 °C [91]. The water sedimentation and associated turbidity also attenuates ultraviolet light: ultraviolet light is known to lower *M. ulcerans* cell viability [76]. Thus, deforestation and high-impact agriculture may promote increased nutrients in the water, higher temperatures, ultraviolet light attenuation and lower dissolved oxygen, all conditions that promote growth of the bacillus [9].

The infection is rare in the West African savanna and arid zones of Australia. Moreover, it is still not known why the disease is present in some settlements lying near certain water bodies and absent along others [95, 96, 100].

Various risk factors are associated with *M. ulcerans* infection, including age, poor wound care, failure to wear protective clothing, exposure to water (wading, swimming, fishing, bathing, farming, mining) [55, 56, 97, 98, 106–109]. In an Australian case-control study, the use of insect repellent was associated with a reduced risk, while the reporting of mosquito bites on the forearms and lower legs was associated with an increased risk [56]. These studies show that transmission of *M. ulcerans* could occur via direct inoculation of bacilli into the skin as a result of contact with environmental sources, insect bites or trauma, but of course further studies are needed to confirm this [106].

While some studies have reported a seasonal distribution of the infection [110, 111], no correlation was found in others [112]. Bearing in mind the variations among different regions, the problem could probably best be studied at the local level. However, the uncertainty surrounding the duration of the incubation period, that ranges from 2 weeks to 7 months, contributes to complicate the evaluation of possible seasonal factors [15, 46]. According to some authors the incidence of the infection increases during dry periods [102, 113], whereas others have observed an increase after flooding events [36, 99].

Direct human to human transmission of *M. ulcerans* is rare. There is one report of a case following a human bite [114] but it was hypothesized that the patient's skin surface was contaminated by *M. ulcerans* picked up from an environmental source, and the bite then drove it into the skin.

The infection has never been reported in Africa in wild and domesticated animals. In 1999 it was suggested that aquatic bugs (Hemiptera) could be reservoirs of *M. ulcerans* in nature [67], and the bacillus has recently been isolated from water striders (Hemiptera; Gerridae, *Gerris* sp.) in Benin [94]. Other studies based on the detection of *M. ulcerans* DNA in aquatic insects (Hemiptera, water bugs; Odonata, dragonfly larvae; Coleoptera, beetle larvae) collected from infection endemic African swamps confirmed the early findings, and suggested that small fish might also contain the bacillus [115–118]. In view of these and subsequent studies [119–121], it was concluded that biting water bugs belonging to the families Naucoridae (creeping water bugs) and Belostomatidae (giant water bugs) could be considered reservoirs, and could serve as vectors in the transmission of the infection to humans.

Growing evidence of a role of other, non-insect aquatic invertebrates as intermediate hosts or reservoirs for *M. ulcerans* is accumulating: aquatic snails could be colonized after feeding on *M. ulcerans*-containing aquatic plant biofilm [95, 96, 122]. However, it should be remembered that these bugs do not actively search for humans, they do not require a blood meal or protein source, and so their bites are a purely defensive reaction [9].

The situation in Australia is different from in Africa. More than 80% of cases of *M. ulcerans* infection in the past 15 years have been reported in the temperate south-eastern state of Victoria [46], where, unlike in West Africa, people have less direct contact with the environment. In two outbreaks, a high percentage of residents developed the infection: 1.2 and 6.0% respectively [92, 123]. Visitors can also be at risk: in one case staying in the city for just 1 day was enough to cause the onset of the infection 7 months later [92]. Two models have been proposed to explain this pattern of limited environmental contact, brief exposure and high incidence. On the occasion of one outbreak, in East Cowes, Phillip Island, following contact with a newly created wetland and a golf course (on the golf course a mixture of ground water and recycled water was used for irrigation, and the run-off from the golf course likely drained down to the new wetland), Hayman proposed the possibility of transmission by drifting aerosols from contaminated irrigation water [105, 124]. *IS2404* PCR was used and positive results were obtained from the wetland and golf course irrigation system. Moreover, no evidence of the presence of *IS2404* in other environmental mycobacteria has yet been reported, unlike in Africa [9]. During the same period, several possums (Australian native marsupials) with Buruli ulcer were identified at Phillip Island [91].

In 2002, another outbreak was observed in Point Lonsdale, a small town on the Bellarine Peninsula about 60 km to the west of Phillip Island, and also in coastal Victoria, southeastern Australia [92]. In 2004, intense local mosquito activity seemed to be associated with the new cases of infection, which featured lesions on the ankles and elbows and on the back; in short, on uncovered zones. These observations suggest a possible role for mosquitoes in the transmission of the disease. Many mosquito species present in the zone, and in particular *Aedes camptorhynchus*, yielded positive results in *IS2404* PCR [92]. Later, in 38% of ringtail possums (*Pseudocheirus peregrinus*) and 24% of brushtail possums (*Trichosurus vulpecula*) captured at Point Lonsdale *M. ulcerans* was confirmed in skin lesions and/or feces [125].

In conclusion, on the basis of studies conducted in Africa e Australia it can be argued that various routes of transmission are possible, that depend on the epidemiological setting and geographic region. As reservoirs and as vectors of *M. ulcerans*, aquatic insects, adult mosquitoes or other biting arthropods may play an important role (Table 10.3) [6, 9]. Nevertheless, the precise mode of transmission has still to be completely clarified.

Table 10.3 Possible reservoirs or vectors of *Mycobacterium ulcerans* (modified, from [6])

Environmental water	Swamp, golf course irrigation
Insects	Mosquitoes (*Aedes camptorhynchus*, *Aedes aegypti*), *Naucoris cimicoides*, *Belostomatidae*, *Nepidae*, *Culicidae*, *Protoneuridae*, *Araneae*, *Hydrophilidae*, *Libellulidae*
Fish and shellfish	Freshwater crayfish (*Cambaroides japonicus*), *Pomacea canaliculata*, *Planorbis planorbis*, *Bulinus senegalensis*, *Sarotherodon galilaeus*, *Lissemys punctata punctata* (turtle)
Land animals	Possums (*Pseudocheirus peregrinus*, *Trichosurus vulpecula*), horse (*Equus caballus*), long-footed potoroo (*Potorous longipes*), koala (*Phascolarctos cinereus*)

10.5 Pathogenesis

Unlike other mycobacteria, that are elective intracellular macrophage pathogens, *M. ulcerans* is found distributed in extracellular clusters in areas of coagulative necrosis that are far from the site of bacterial colonization [126]. This observation has prompted the idea that *M. ulcerans* may secrete an exotoxin [127]. In 1999 a cytotoxic molecule was isolated from the acetone soluble fraction of lipid extracts. This lipid toxin, named mycolactone, has been shown to have a cytopathic action on cultured L929 murine fibroblasts; moreover, intradermic injection of purified toxin into guinea pigs produces a lesion that is histologically similar to *M. ulcerans* infection necrosis of the subcutaneous fat [88]. Mycolactone is now known to cause immunosuppression and tissue necrosis in *M. ulcerans* disease, as well as the painlessness of the ulcerative lesions which is the reason why patients are slow to seek treatment [128].

Mycolactone is a polyketide composed of an invariant 12-member lactone ring to which two polyketide-derived, highly unsaturated acyl side chains are attached. The upper "northern" chain is invariant, while variations in the "southern" chain give rise to different congeners of mycolactone (formula: $C_{44}H_{70}O_9Na$, corresponding to the sodium adduct) [129]. Variants of congeners of mycolactone differ as regards the positions of hydroxyl groups in the "southern" chain, and exhibit differences in biological activity depending on the origin of strains of *M. ulcerans*. Pathogenic human strains from Africa, Australia and China predominantly produce mycolactone A/B (m/z 765), C (m/z 749) and D (m/z 779), respectively; each strain, however, also produces minor quantities of the other two congeners [130]. The most cytotoxic congener in vitro is mycolactone A/B. It is noteworthy that other genetically related organisms with a pathogenic action in fish and frogs can also produce variants of mycolactone E (m/z 737) and F (m/z 723) [70, 131].

Mycolactone is present in the lesions [132]. Cytotoxicity assays yielded positive results in 92% of tested patients (mycolactone concentrations ranged from 0.3 to 6 μg/punch biopsy), and mass spectrometry in 77% of the same patients (mycolactone concentrations ranged from 10 ng to 2 μg/punch biopsy) [133]. In addition, mycolactone was detected in peripheral blood mononuclear cells of mice after inducing subcutaneous infection [134] and in the sera of patients with the infection [135], proving that it can migrate from the infection region.

Standard antibiotic therapy for *M. ulcerans* infection (daily oral rifampicin and intramuscular streptomycin for 8 weeks) induces a decrease in mycolactone detected in skin biopsies [133], even if in some cases it can still be detected in culture-negative samples. This suggests that mycolactone may remain in tissue for some time after the killing of the pathogens, or else that viable organisms may still be present in tissue despite negative cultures. Culture is positive in 40–60% of untreated patients [136], whereas mycolactone is detectable in 77–92%. This discrepancy has implications on the duration of treatment: mycolactone is therefore a potential tool for monitoring the results of therapy.

Various direct molecular targets of mycolactone have been described in recent years [129]. A specific target may explain the painlessness of the cutaneous lesions [137]. It has been shown, in fact, that mycolactone activates the type 2 angiotensin II receptor, resulting in hypoesthesia through potassium-dependent hyperpolarization of murine neurons [137]. It will be necessary, of course, to study this mechanism also in man.

The other major functions of mycolactone are cytotoxicity, immunosuppression and inhibition of protein synthesis [129]. Cell cycle arrest, necrosis and apoptosis are induced, depending on cell types [88, 138–141]. Many studies have been focused on the effects of mycolactone on immune cells, with the aim of gaining a better understanding of the immunosuppression mechanism, which affects both innate and adaptive immune responses. In mycolactone-negative strains of *M. ulcerans* [142] and during antibiotic therapy of patients [143], for instance, infection is associated with granulomas, that are begun by macrophages. However, lack of inflammatory cell infiltration in active ulcerative lesions is one of the most striking features of histopathological evidence, and this is presumably due to the actions of mycolactone [6, 129]. Mycolactone affects the function of monocytes and macrophages, dendritic cells, T-cells, neutrophils, and skin resident non-immune cells (fibroblasts, adipocytes, endothelial cells, and keratinocytes); the various mechanisms involved have been described in detail by Sarfo and Coll [129]. For these immunosuppressive effects, very low concentrations (1/10th) of mycolactone are needed, compared with the concentrations required for its cytotoxic effect [144]. As a result, various cytokines, chemokines and cell surface receptors needed for leukocyte migration and/or immune activation are down-regulated [140, 144]. A mycolactone-induced reduction of protein synthesis appears therefore to be crucial for necrosis and immune suppression to occur in this disease [6, 129].

10.6 Clinical Manifestations

The clinical and epidemiological aspects of cases vary remarkably within and across different countries and settings [8]. In Africa, about 48% of patients are children under 15 years, whereas in Australia only 10% are children under 15 years. There are no significant differences between the rates in males and females. The lesions frequently affect the limbs: 35% on the arms, 55% on the legs, and 10% on the other parts of the body [8].

After an incubation of 6–12 weeks, cold subcutaneous nodules appear, with clearcut margins and not adherent to the deep planes; they are indolent and sometimes mildly itchy. The disease can also manifest as a diffuse, ill-defined, indolent non-pitting edema (the so-called fulminant form). The lesions are hot and hard and affect the entire limb. Being resistant to anti-inflammatory drugs and antibiotics, these forms are quite severe.

In Australia, the initial lesion is more often a papule, like an insect bite. Both papules and nodules can evolve to plaques. In children, the complaint can affect the face and trunk.

Without treatment, but sometimes even during treatment, the nodules, plaques and the edema extend slowly, fluctuate and ulcerate within 4–6 weeks. The ulceration (attributable to necrosis of the dermis and subcutaneous adipose tissue) is characteristic, featuring polycyclic or rounded margins and an adherent

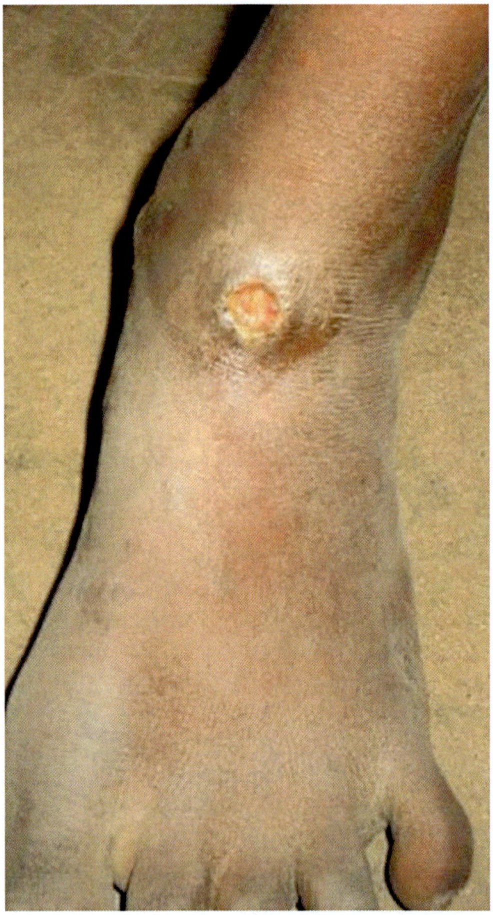

Fig. 10.1 Ulceration with rounded margins and adherent grayish-yellow base (courtesy of Prof. Giorgio Leigheb, Dermatological Clinic, University of Novara, Italy)

grayish-yellow or gelatinous base (Figs. 10.1 and 10.2). When washed, the base appears reddened and granulomatous (Figs. 10.3, 10.4, and 10.5). The margins of the ulcer are thickened and irregular, and undermined (Fig. 10.6) by wide detached areas that are often communicant with adjacent areas. There is generally a single ulcer but satellite ulcers communicating with the original lesion are possible. It will extend above all in a horizontal direction, and lay bare the affected limb, but also penetrate in depth to the muscles and tendons. Paradoxically, the patient's general health conditions remain good, with no locoregional adenopathy or fever, although there may be mild fever in edematous forms. The evolution of *M. ulcerans* infection classically follows three phases: 1. the above-described extension phase, that lasts several months; 2. a non uniform stabilization phase; 3. a scarring phase that starts at the borders of the ulcer and continues centripetally (Figs. 10.7 and 10.8). During the course of the disease, a superimposed infection may occur, and the risk of tetanus is not negligible.

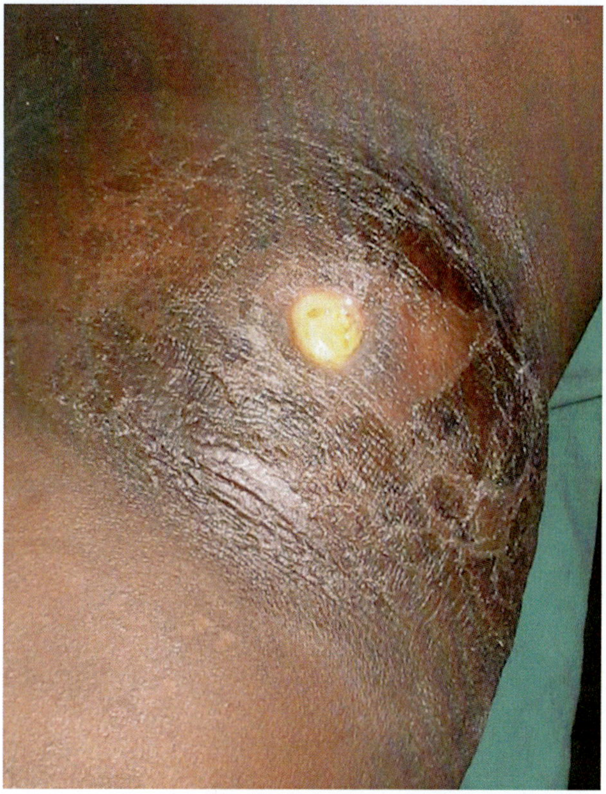

Fig. 10.2 Ulceration with rounded margins and adherent grayish-yellow base (courtesy of Prof. Giorgio Leigheb, Dermatological Clinic, University of Novara, Italy)

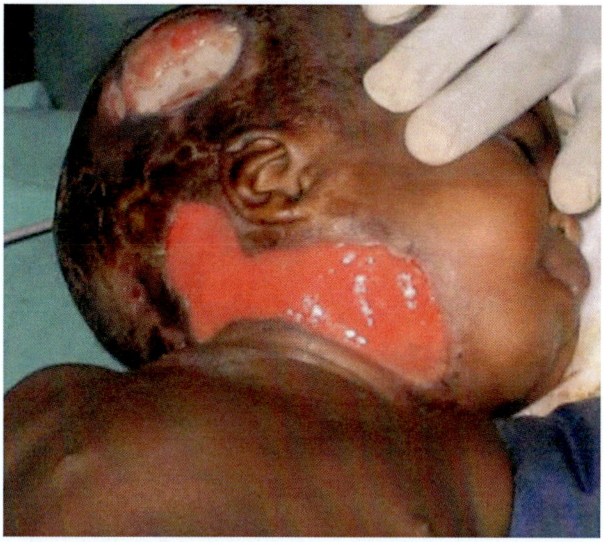

Fig. 10.3 Ulcerations with reddened and granulomatous base (courtesy of Prof. Giorgio Leigheb, Dermatological Clinic, University of Novara, Italy)

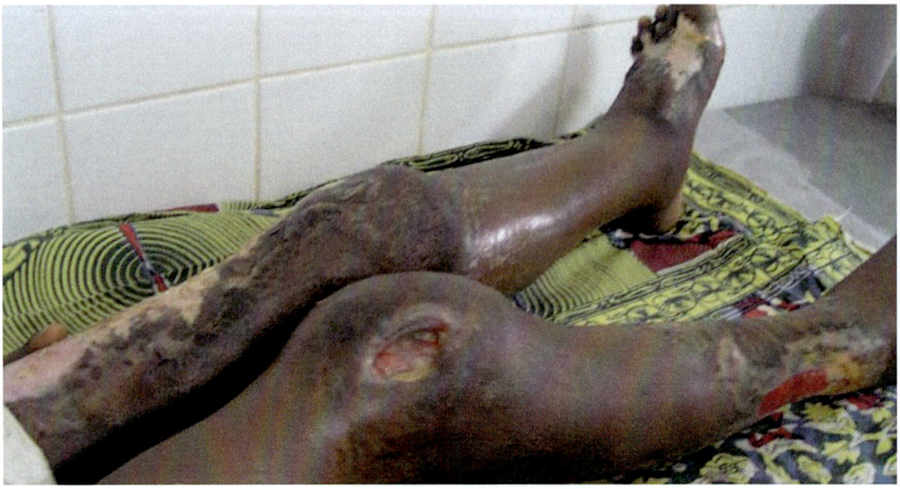

Fig. 10.4 Ulceration with thickened and undermined margins and scarring sequelae (courtesy of Prof. Giorgio Leigheb, Dermatological Clinic, University of Novara, Italy)

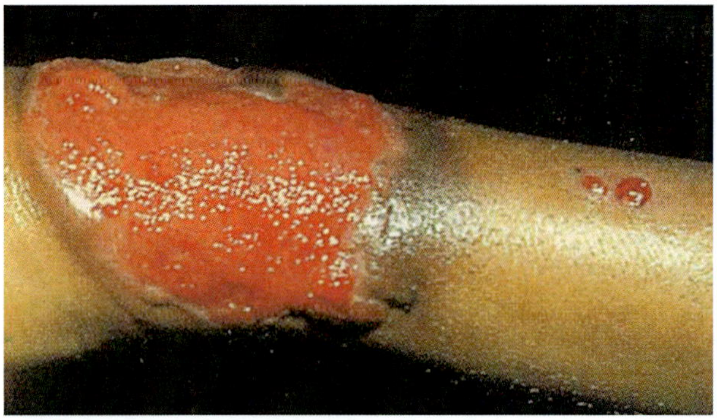

Fig. 10.5 Ulceration of the wrist with thickened margins and granulomatous base (courtesy of Prof. Roger Pradinaud, Dermatological Service Unit, Hospital of Cayenne Andrée Rosemon, Cayenne, French Guyana)

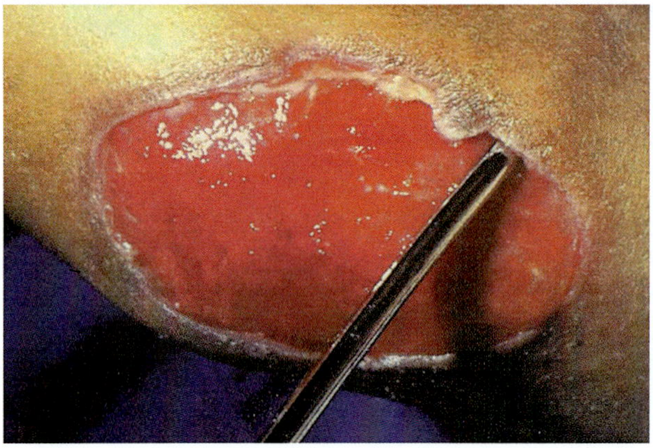

Fig. 10.6 Ulceration with undermined margins (courtesy of Prof. Roger Pradinaud, Dermatological Service Unit, Hospital of Cayenne Andrée Rosemon, Cayenne, French Guyana)

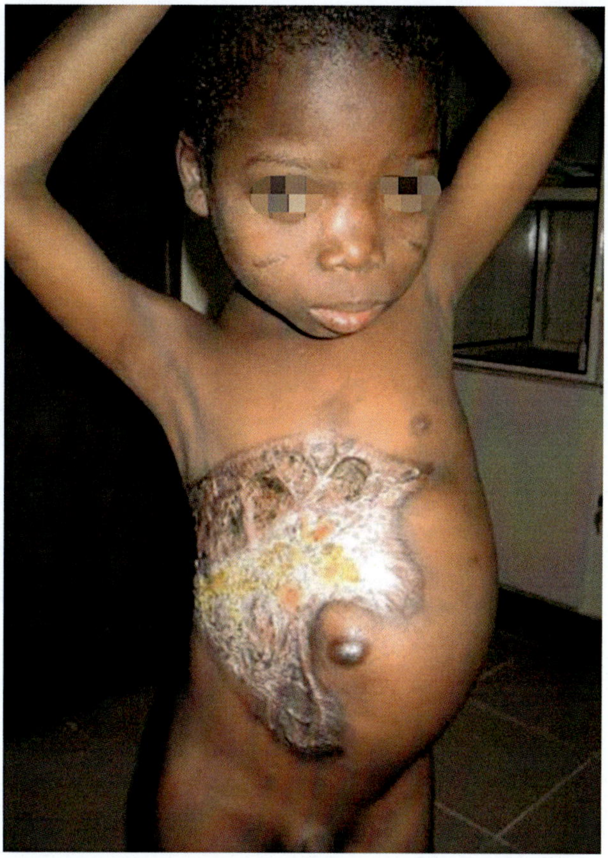

Fig. 10.7 Vast scarring sequela (courtesy of Prof. Giorgio Leigheb, Dermatological Clinic, University of Novara, Italy)

The disease has been subdivided by the WHO into three categories of severity: category I features a single small lesion (32% of cases); category II includes non-ulcerative and ulcerative lesions and edematous forms (35% of cases); and category III disseminated and mixed forms, such as osteitis, osteomyelitis, joint involvement (33% of cases). In Australia and Japan, most lesions (>90%) are diagnosed in category I [8]. In other countries, at least 70% of all cases are diagnosed in the ulcerative stage [8].

Even if it is not fatal, the affection causes permanent disabling infirmity, with tendon retraction, contracture, ankylosis, post-cicatricial lymphedema, that may even dictate amputation of the limb.

In some zones, such as Kasongo and Benin, in up to 14% of cases the skin infection may be associated with bone involvement [144, 145]. The clinical picture is that of osteomyelitis, with coexistent alcohol-acid fast bacilli and germs from a secondary infection. The bones contiguous to the subcutaneous foci are affected, but the infection may possibly spread also through the bloodstream, since distant metastases can be observed, far from the cutaneous focus. The long bones are those most commonly affected, and may undergo total necrosis.

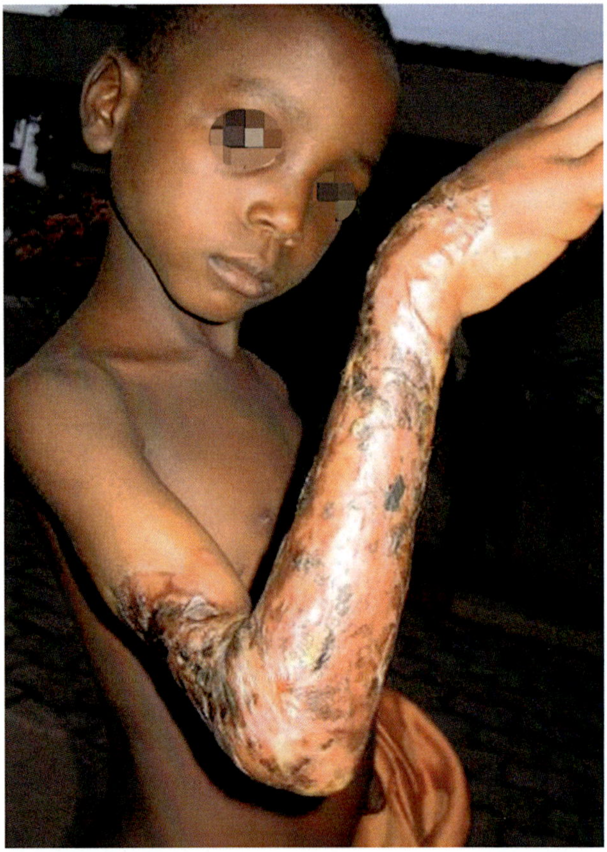

Fig. 10.8 Vast scarring sequela (courtesy of Prof. Giorgio Leigheb, Dermatological Clinic, University of Novara, Italy)

Unlike in Africa, where the infection occurs mainly in children [144, 145], in Australia it occurs mainly in adults, with a large proportion of cases aged >50 years [146]. Reported rates of infection in Australia are up to 7 times higher in subjects ≥55 years of age [147]. The clinical presentation of the disease, as well as the effectiveness of therapy, may differ in the elderly compared with younger populations. It is known that immune function reduces with aging, and this may give rise to an increased severity of the disease. In the elderly ulcerations of the lower limbs of a different nature can be observed (in particular venous disease), and this may result in misdiagnosis. Moreover, the problem of comorbidities in elderly patients can adversely affect immune function and also lead to increased drug interactions. All these aspects can cause delays in diagnosis and an increased disease severity. A retrospective analysis performed from 1998 to 2014 on an observational cohort of 327 patients confirmed *M. ulcerans* cases at Barwon Health (Victoria, Australia) revealed that 131 (40%) patients were aged ≥65 years of age [148]. In addition, significant differences between the age groups were demonstrated. Patients in the ≥65 years age-group were more likely to exhibit multiple lesions, classified as WHO category 3 severity. Especially among males, there was a higher proportion of edematous lesions, an increased incidence of antibiotic complications, and a significantly higher incidence of antibiotic-associated paradoxical reactions [148].

10.7 Histopathology

Preulcerative and ulcerative lesions are characterized by distinctive histological features [1, 6]. Preulcerative lesions (papules, nodules, plaques, and edematous forms) are observed as circumscribed areas of eosinophilic necrosis of ischemic type, localized between the deep derma and the subcutaneous adipose tissue; sometimes, the lesions may extend to the fascia. Granulomas or epithelioid cells are rarely observed. Fat cells enlarge, die and lose their nuclei but retain cell membranes ("fat-cell ghosts"). Interlobular septae of the subcutaneous tissue become thickened and necrotic. Around the necrosis there is edema with few inflammatory cells. Occlusion of small and medium-sized vessels, sometimes with marked vasculitis, can also develop.

In the ulcerative forms, the hyperplasic epidermis tends to undergo invagination, limiting the progression of the necrosis to the surface. A lymphohistiocytic infiltrate is present in the derma, with capillary congestion, while massive eosinophilic necrosis occurs in the hypoderma with arteriovenous thrombosis. In this stage, bacilli, prevalently grouped in clusters, are found at the center of the necrotic zone.

In the chronic stage granulomatous foci develop, with epithelioid cells and giant cells. The presence of bacilli fluctuates. Fibrohyalinosis progressively replaces the hypodermic necrosis as resolution proceeds.

10.8 Laboratory Tests

The least invasive method for obtaining specimens for laboratory tests from non-ulcerative lesions is by fine-needle aspiration. In cases of ulcerative lesions, swabs from the undermined edges can be taken, before scar formation. In guaranteed sterile conditions, a skin biopsy from the border of the ulcer is recommended; the biopsy must comprise epidermis, derma and subcutaneous adipose tissue.

Obviously, all specimens must be collected before starting treatment. When the analyses cannot be performed within a few days, the specimens should be kept in liquid or semisolid transport media [149, 150]. Specimens for PCR or mycolactone analysis should be placed in 30–70% (v/v) ethanol, prepared using distilled water, or 100% ethanol, respectively [151].

Bacilli can be sought in the various specimens after staining with Ziehl-Neelsen, Kinyoun or auramine. However, this test has low sensitivity, ranging from 30 to 65%, depending on the stage of the disease. The sensitivity seems to be increased if the test is done on biopsy specimens (mycobacteria are found at the center and deep within the ulcer).

Culture test is possible only in well-equipped laboratories [83]. Specimens must be obtained from bacilli-rich zones (the base and margins of the ulcer). Because skin tissue can contain contaminating microorganisms, the first step is to apply acid or alkali pretreatment of the specimen for decontamination. The specimen must be kept at +4 °C in a sterile tube and transported in suitable medium (BACTEC). Experiences in the tropics have demonstrated that *M. ulcerans* is very sensitive to high temperatures: an environmental temperature of 41 °C kills more than 90% of bacilli. Liquid and solid media are employed for tests: examples of liquid media are the BBL mycobacteria growth indicator tube (MIGIT; Becton Dickinson, Franklin Lakes, NJ, USA) and Middlebrook 7H12B medium; examples of solid media include Löwenstein-Jensen medium, Ogawa medium, Middlebrook 7H11 medium, and Brown and Buckle medium [6]. The culture media must be incubated at a temperature of 28–33 °C. Additionally, moist conditions, with 5% CO_2 (*M. ulcerans* is microaerophilic) and a dark environment can promote growth. *M. ulcerans* forms yellowish, rough colonies on solid medium. Culture test is the only reliable method to distinguish viable from non-viable bacilli. However, it takes at least 6–12 weeks (often more) to achieve colonization and sensitivity is low, being approximately 50% [152, 153]. It must be borne in mind that in vitro culture is important for monitoring patient response to treatment.

Polymerase chain reaction is the most suitable method to obtain definitive diagnostic results in 1–2 weeks. Good sample sources for this test are fresh specimens, formalin-fixed paraffin embedded biopsy samples, and culture isolates. The most common way to detect *M. ulcerans* DNA is by using gel-based visualization of PCR products [6]. PCR sensitivity and specificity are high (>90%) when *IS2404* is used as a target sequence [153–155]. Among the various protocols describing gel-based PCR targeting *IS2404*, a gene fragment of over 300 bp is usually used; however, shorter targets are better especially on formalin-fixed paraffin-embedded samples. For extensive analysis, quantitative real-time PCR is now used for differential diagnosis and also to test environmental samples [93, 156].

Mycolactone is the cause of the tissue necrosis, the impaired clearance of *M. ulcerans* infection and the painlessness of the ulcers. The recent development of techniques for the detection and quantification of mycolactone within host tissue has opened new vistas for the use of this toxic macrolide as a diagnostic and prognostic biomarker in the management of the disease [129].

10.9 Diagnosis

Clinical diagnosis is generally reliable when made by trained health professionals in endemic areas and when a patient from an endemic area presents with an atypical painless ulcer characterized by undermined edges. However, in areas where *M. ulcerans* infection is rare or unknown, the chances of making a clinical diagnosis are very low [6]. Most lesions are on the limbs, although they can also be present on the trunk or face. In this infection there is no clinically detectable lymphadenitis, and there are no systemic symptoms, such as fever and malaise, which would suggest a staphylococcal or streptococcal pyogenic infection.

Early nodular lesions must be differentiated from boils, lipomas, lymph node tuberculosis, onchocerciasis nodules, or other subcutaneous infections, such as fungal infections. In Australia, papular lesions may initially be mistaken for insect bites. Depending on the patient's age and the geographic area, as well as the localization of the lesions and whether they are painful or not, ulcerative lesions must be differentiated from tropical phagedenic ulcers, chronic lower leg ulcers due to insufficient arterial or venous flow (often in elderly populations), diabetic ulcers, cutaneous leishmaniasis, extensive ulcerative yaws, pyoderma gangrenosum, and ulcer due to *Haemophilus ducreyi* [8, 157]. Cellulitis may resemble edema due to *M. ulcerans* but in cases of cellulitis the lesions are painful and the patient is ill and febrile.

Due to international travel, cases may appear in non-endemic areas [58, 59, 158, 159]. Reports from Europe, Canada, America, and Australia have described travelers in endemic areas who manifested the infection upon return to a non-endemic area [59]. Thus, in non-endemic countries, where health care professionals are generally not familiar with the condition and its causal organism, *M. ulcerans* infection may be diagnosed late, or not diagnosed at all. Delayed diagnosis often leads to severe disabilities [159].

Four standard laboratory methods can be used to confirm the diagnosis: *IS2404* PCR, direct microscopy, histopathology, and culture [155]. Evidence of acid-fast bacilli can be an appropriate, helpful guide but a negative test result cannot rule out the diagnosis. Culture is difficult and expensive, and generally not available in all endemic regions, and may yield false-negative results when used for routine diagnostic purposes. The use of PCR is limited to research settings and reference laboratories [2]. Some authors recommend the use of Ziehl-Neelsen staining of biopsy specimens in routine practice to detect the bacilli, followed by PCR in cases of negative results only, in order to minimize costs; histology and culture remain important as quality control tests, particularly in studies of the efficacy of therapy [160].

10.10 HIV Infection and *Mycobacterium ulcerans* Infection

The role of human immunodeficiency virus (HIV) in the onset and clinical manifestations of *M. ulcerans* infection needs further studies. Two case-control studies, conducted in low HIV prevalence settings, addressed the role of HIV as a risk factor for *M. ulcerans* infection. In both studies a higher HIV prevalence was observed among *M. ulcerans* disease cases compared with controls [109, 161]. In an analysis of 73 cases of disease-associated osteomyelitis, HIV was one of the four significant factors predictive of bone involvement [162]. Immunity plays an important role in clinical manifestations [163], and strongly immunosuppressed HIV-infected subjects with disseminated *M. ulcerans* disease have been described [164, 165].

In a retrospective study of data collected in a hospital in Cameroon from 2002 to 2013, HIV prevalence among *M. ulcerans* disease patients was significantly higher than the estimated regional HIV prevalence, both in children and adults. HIV positive subjects had a more severe form of *M. ulcerans* infection, and the higher the level of immunosuppression the greater the severity. Low CD4+ cell count was significantly associated with a larger main lesion. The time-to-healing of the disease caused by *M. ulcerans* was more than double in patients with a CD4+ cell count below 500 cell/mm^3 [166]. These data confirm that HIV+ patients are at higher risk for *M. ulcerans* infection, and that HIV-induced immunosuppression seems to have an impact on the clinical presentation and evolution of *M. ulcerans* disease [166].

According to the WHO, in co-endemic countries HIV infection complicates the management of *M. ulcerans* patients [167].

10.11 Treatment

Therapy is based on a combination of antibiotics and complementary treatments. In 2004, the WHO published treatment guidance for health workers [167], and currently recommends multidrug therapy with a combination of oral rifampicin (10 mg/kg once daily) and i.m. streptomycin (15 mg/kg once daily) for 8 weeks. However, despite its effectiveness, long term streptomycin toxicity (hearing impairment, nephrotoxicity) must be taken into account, especially in children [168]. Moreover, streptomycin is contraindicated in pregnancy; according to the WHO, in this condition a combination of rifampicin and clarithromycin (7.5 mg/kg twice daily) or a combination of rifampicin and moxifloxacin (400 mg once daily) are safer options. There are also some concerns about using streptomycin, as regards both patient compliance and availability.

Several options are now being tested. The WHO recommends a combination of rifampicin and clarithromycin [167]. In 2014, the Australian Buruli Ulcer Expert Working Group published their guidelines: they recommend oral rifampicin, with either clarithromycin or fluoroquinolone (moxifloxacin or ciprofloxacin) [169]. In Japan, triple therapy with rifampicin, levofloxacin and clarithromycin is currently recommended [170].

As topical treatment, the use of nitrogen oxides 6% [171, 172] and phenytoin powder has been suggested [173]: they appear promising as a means of accelerating the healing process of ulcerative lesions.

In advanced cases, an important treatment role is played by surgical procedures such as debridement and skin grafting. There are no guidelines for this treatment but there is a consensus that it should be performed after at least 4 weeks of antibiotics [174]. It is important to perform surgical debridement with wide margins to avoid disease relapse: if possible, a mapping biopsy procedure may be a practical option for determining the extent of debridement [169].

Recently, a paradoxical phenomenon has been reported during antibiotic treatment or even long after [175–177]. This is a painful inflammatory reaction against *M. ulcerans*, with pus. Usually, culture and acid-fast bacilli research are negative, while in some cases PCR can be positive. A new lesion may sometimes develop on a different part of the body. In these cases of paradoxical reactions, treatment is necessarily corticosteroids.

The temperature sensitivity of *M. ulcerans* has long been recognized [178]. The positive effect of heat was first recognized a long time ago, when some African populations started applying hot ash [179]. The efficacy of local hyperthermia has been demonstrated in two pilot studies, one of which used commercially available cheap silicone bags filled with sodium acetate trihydrate (phase-change material) ($C_2H_3NaO_2 \bullet 3H_20$) as an easily rechargeable heat source [179–181]. In a recent work, this method was used in 53 patients in Cameroon, 51 of whom had ulcerative disease [182]. Heat was applied for up to 8 weeks and excellent results were still evident after 24 months' follow-up. The treatment was well tolerated; adverse events were limited to mild, short-lasting local skin reactions. The authors considered thermotherapy highly effective, easy to apply, cheap and well tolerated [182].

10.12 Prevention

Due to the significant reduction in quality of life for patients with extensive tissue scarring, and bearing in mind that a large percentage of the subjects are children, an anti-*M. ulcerans* disease vaccine would be of great benefit to the community. *M. bovis* bacillus Calmette-Guérin vaccination has been shown to confer some protective effects [183–187]. However, further studies are needed to evaluate the effects of implementation of this vaccine or other chemoprophylaxis for protection against *M. ulcerans* [6, 187, 188].

Daily prophylaxis has shown some protective efficacy against the disease; in fact, considering the risk factors (walking, swimming and fishing in the river or marsh, domestic use of river water, agricultural works in the paddy or near the river, and mosquito bites or injuries of the lower limbs), wearing cover-up clothing, especially long pants, and using mosquito nets and insect repellents may reduce the risk [6].

Research support to identify new drugs, new diagnostic methods and vaccines is urgently needed for *M. ulcerans* infection, as it is for all the other neglected tropical diseases (estimated to cause more than 500,000 deaths per year) [189–191].

References

1. Pradinaud R, Couppié P, Versapuech J (2003) Mycobactérioses cutanées environmentales dont l'infection à *Mycobacterium ulcerans* ("ulcère de Buruli"). Encycl Méd Chir (Editions Scientifiques et Médicales Elsevier SAS, Paris), Maladies Infectieuses, 8-038-F-15
2. van der Werf TS, van der Graaf WTA, Tappero JW et al (1999) *Mycobacterium ulcerans* infection. Lancet 354:1013
3. Centers for Disease Control and Prevention (CDC) (2015) Buruli ulcer. https://www.cdc.gov/buruli-ulcer
4. Sizaire V, Nackers F, Comte E et al (2006) *Mycobacterium ulcerans* infection: control, diagnosis, and treatment. Lancet Infect Dis 6:288
5. Sears AV, Hay RJ (2015) Buruli ulcer—a rapidly changing scene. Acta Derm Venereol 95:387
6. Yotsu RR, Murase C, Sugawara M et al (2015) Revisiting Buruli ulcer. J Dermatol 42:1033

7. World Health Organization (2015) Buruli ulcer (*Mycobacterium ulcerans* infection). http://www.who.int/mediacentre/factsheets/fs199/en/updatedfebruary2015
8. World Health Organization (2016) Buruli ulcer (*Mycobacterium ulcerans* infection). http://www.who.int/mediacentre/factsheets/fs199/en/updatedfebruary2016
9. Merritt RW, Walker ED, Small PL et al (2010) Ecology and transmission of Buruli ulcer disease: a systematic review. PLoS Negl Trop Dis 4:e911
10. World Health Organization (2013) Buruli ulcer (*Mycobacterium ulcerans* infection). Fact sheet No 199. Retrivied 23 Feb 2014
11. Nakanaga K, Yotsu RR, Hoshino Y et al (2013) Buruli ulcer and mycolactone-producing mycobacteria. Jpn J Infect Dis 66:83
12. MacCallum P, Tolhurst JC, Buckle G et al (1948) A new mycobacterial infection in man. J Pathol Bacteriol 60:93
13. Buckle G, Tolhurst JC (1948) A new mycobacterial infection in man; cultivation of the new mycobacterial infection in man; cultivation of the new mycobacterium. J Pathol Bacteriol 60:116
14. van Oye E, Ballion M (1950) Is it necessary to take into account a new infection from acid-resistant bacilli in Africa? Preliminary note. Ann Soc Belg Med Trop 30:619
15. Meyers WM, Shelly WM, Connor DH et al (1974) Human *Mycobacterium ulcerans* infections developing at sites of trauma to skin. Am J Trop Med Hyg 23:919
16. Clancey JK, Dodge OG, Lunn HF et al (1961) Mycobacterial skin ulcers in Uganda. Lancet 2:951
17. Anonymous (1970) Buruli ulcer. Br Med J 2:378
18. Gray HH, Kingma S, Kok SH (1967) Mycobacterial skin ulcers in Nigeria. Trans R Soc Trop Med Hyg 61:712
19. Oluwasanmi JO, Solankee TF, Olurin EO et al (1976) *Mycobacterium ulcerans* (Buruli) skin ulceration in Nigeria. Am J Trop Med Hyg 25:122
20. Ouoba K, Sano D, Traoré A et al (1998) Buruli ulcers in Burkina Faso: apropos of 6 cases. Tunis Med 76:46
21. van der Werf TS, van der Graaf WT, Groothuis DG et al (1989) *Mycobacterium ulcerans* infection in Ashanti region, Ghana. Trans R Soc Trop Med Hyg 83:410
22. Marston BJ, Diallo MO, Horsburgh CR Jr et al (1995) Emergence of Buruli ulcer disease in the Daloa region of Côte d'Ivoire. Am J Trop Med Hyg 52:219
23. Aguiar J, Steunou C (1997) Buruli ulcers in rural areas of Benin: management of 635 cases. Med Trop (Mars) 57:83
24. Bessis D, Kempf M, Marsollier L (2015) *Mycobacterium ulcerans* disease (Buruli ulcer) in Mali: a new potential African endemic country. Acta Derm Venereol 95:489
25. Ezzedine K, Pistone T, Guir V et al (2010) Painful Buruli ulcer in a Malian visitor to France. Acta Derm Venereol 90:424
26. Kanga JM, Kacou ED (2001) Epidemiological aspects of Buruli ulcer in Côte d'Ivoire: results of a national survey. Bull Soc Pathol Exot 94:46
27. Faber WR, Arias-Bouda LM, Zeegelaar JE et al (2000) First reported case of *Mycobacterium ulcerans* infection in a patient from China. Trans R Soc Trop Med Hyg 94:277
28. Nakanaga K, Hoshino Y, Yotsu RR et al (2011) Nineteen cases of Buruli ulcer diagnosed in Japan from 1980 to 2010. J Clin Microbiol 49:3829
29. Yotsou RR, Nakanaga K, Hoshino Y et al (2012) Buruli ulcer and current situation in Japan: a new emerging cutaneous *Mycobacterium* infection. J Dermatol 39:587
30. Aguilar PL, Iturribarria FM, Middlebrook G (1953) A case of human infection by *Mycobacterium ulcerans* in the western hemisphere; preliminary note. Int J Lepr 21:469
31. Guerra H, Palomino JC, Falconí E et al (2008) *Mycobacterium ulcerans* disease, Peru. Emerg Infect Dis 14:373
32. Soldaña-Patiño J (1988) First findings of Buruli ulcer in Peru. Acta Med Hosp Militar Central 5:55
33. dos Santos VM, Noronha FL, Vicentina EC et al (2007) *Mycobacterium ulcerans* infection in Brazil. Med J Aust 187:63

34. Pradinaud R, Basset A, Grosshans E (1974) Vingt cas de mycobactérioses cutaneés en Guyane Française. Castellania 2:273
35. Prévot G, Marsallier L, Carbonelle B et al (2004) Diagnostic de l'infection à *Mycobacterium ulcerans* en Guyane Française. Presse Méd 33:1520
36. Radforf AJ (1974) *Mycobacterium ulcerans*: a review. I. Epidemiology. Papua New Guinea Med J 17:129
37. Flood P, Street A, O'Brien P et al (1994) *Mycobacterium ulcerans* infection on Phillip Island, Victoria. Med J Aust 160:160
38. Hayman J (1984) *Mycobacterium ulcerans*: an infection from Jurassic time? Lancet 2:1015
39. Pradinaud R (2005) The mycobacterium infection cannot be called "Buruli ulcer" any longer. Bull Soc Pathol Exot 98:26
40. Pradinaud R (2007) L'infection à *Mycobacterium ulcerans* ne doit plus être restreinte à l'impropre appellation "ulcère de Buruli". Ann Dermatol Venereol 134:1523
41. Buruli ulcer (2017) Wikipedia https://it.wikipedia.org/wiki/Ulcera_del_Buruli
42. Meyers DH (2007) *Mycobacterium ulcerans* infection: an eponymous ulcer (Letter). Med J Aust 187:63
43. Alsop D (1972) The Bairnsdale ulcer. Aust N Z J Surg 41:317
44. Johnson PDR, Hayman JA (2007) Comment to the letter of Meyers: reference No 42. Med J Aust 187:63
45. World Health Organization. Buruli ulcer. Global Buruli ulcer initiative (2017). http://www.who.int/buruli/en/
46. Johnson DPR, Hayman JA, Quck TY et al (2007) Consensus recommendations for the diagnosis, treatment and control of *Mycobacterium ulcerans* infection (Bairnsdale or Buruli ulcer) in Victoria, Australia. Med J Aust 184:64.s
47. Chemlal K, De Ridder K, Fonteyne PA et al (2001) The use of IS2404 restriction fragment length polymorphisms suggests the diversity of *Mycobacterium ulcerans* from different geographical areas. Am J Trop Med Hyg 64:270
48. Stienstra Y, van der Graaf WT, Asamoa K et al (2002) Beliefs and attitudes toward Buruli ulcer in Ghana. Am J Trop Med Hyg 67:207
49. Aujoulat I, Johnson C, Zinsou C et al (2003) Psychosocial aspects of health seeking behaviours of patients with Buruli ulcer in southern Benin. Tropical Med Int Health 8:750
50. Debacker M, Aguiar J, Steunou C et al (2004) *Mycobacterium ulcerans* disease (Buruli ulcer) in rural hospital, Southern Benin, 1997–2001. Emerg Infect Dis 10:1391
51. World Health Organization (2002) Buruli ulcer disease. *Mycobacterium ulcerans* infection. Wkly Epidemiol Rec 77:271
52. Qi W, Käser M, Röltgen K et al. Genomic diversity and evolution of *Mycobacterium ulcerans* revealed by next-generation sequencing. PLoS Pathog 2009;5:e1000580.
53. Ortiz RH, Leon DA, Estevez HO et al (2009) Differences in virulence and immune response induced in a murine model by isolates of *Mycobacterium ulcerans* from different geographic areas. Clin Exp Immunol:157–271
54. World Health Organization (2015) Global Health Observatory (GHO) data: Buruli ulcer. http://www.who.int/gho/regkected.diseases/buruli_ulcer/en-. Accessed 4 Apr 2015
55. Debacker M, Aguiar J, Steunou C et al (2004) *Mycobacterium ulcerans* disease: role of age and gender in incidence and morbidity. Tropical Med Int Health 9:1297
56. Quek TY, Athan E, Henry MJ et al (2007) Risk factors for *Mycobacterium ulcerans* infection, southeastern Australia. Emerg Infect Dis 13:1661
57. Coloma JN, Navarrete-Franco G, Iribe P et al (2005) Ulcerative cutaneous mycobacteriosis due to *Mycobacterium ulcerans*: report of two Mexican cases. Int J Lepr Other Mycobact Dis 73:5
58. McGann H, Stragier P, Portaels F et al (2009) Buruli ulcer in United Kingdom tourist returning from Latin America. Emerg Infect Dis 15:1827
59. Portaels F, Debacker M, Anyo G et al (2008) Buruli ulcer is an imported and exported disease. WHO Annual meeting on Buruli ulcer: March 31–2 April 2008 Abstracts, The Organization, Geneva, p 125

60. World Health Organization (2004) Buruli ulcer disease. *Mycobacterium ulcerans* infection. Corrigendum to No 15, 2004, Weekly Epidem Record, No 20, p 194
61. Exner K, Lemperle G (1987) Buruli ulcer—necrotizing infection of the hand of a plastic surgeon. Handchir Mikrochir Plast Chir 19:230
62. Weitzul S, Eichhorn PJ, Pandya AG (2000) Nontuberculous mycobacterial infections of the skin. Dermatol Clin 18:359
63. Griffith DE, Aksamit T, Brown-Elliott BA et al (2007) An official ATS/IDSA statement: diagnosis, treatment, and prevention of nontuberculous mycobacterial diseases. Am J Respir Crit Care Med 175:367
64. Bonamonte D, Filoni A, Vestita M et al (2016) Cutaneous infection from aquatic environments. In: Bonamonte D, Angelini G (eds) Aquatic dermatology. Biotic, chemical and physical agents. Springer Verlag, Berlin, p 185
65. Palomino JC, Portaels F (1998) Effects of decontamination methods and culture conditions on viability of *Mycobacterium ulcerans* in the BACTEC system. J Clin Microbiol 36:402
66. Portaels F, Agular J, Fissette K et al (1997) Direct detection and identification of *Mycobacterium ulcerans* in clinical specimens by PCR and oligonucleotide-specific capture plate hybridization. J Clin Microbiol 35:1097
67. Portaels F, Elsen P, Guimaraes-Peres A et al (1999) Insects in the transmission of *Mycobacterium ulcerans* infection. Lancet 353:986
68. Mve-Obiang A, Lee RE, Umstot ES et al (2005) A newly discovered mycobacterial pathogen isolated from laboratory colonies of *Xenopus* species with lethal infections produces a novel form of mycolactone, the *Mycobacterium ulcerans* macrolide toxin. Infect Immun 73:3307
69. Rhodes MW, Kator H, McNabb A et al (2005) *Mycobacterium pseudoshottsii* sp. nov., a slowly growing chromogenic species isolated from Chesapeake Bay striped bass (*Morone saxatilis*). Int J Syst Evol Microbiol 55:1139
70. Ranger BS, Mahrous EA, Mosi L et al (2006) Globally distributed mycobacterial fish pathogens produce a novel plasmid-encoded toxic macrolide, mycolactone F. Infect Immun 74:6037
71. Käser M, Hauser J, Small P et al (2009) Large sequence polymorphisms unveil the phylogenetic relationship of environmental and pathogenic mycobacteria related to *Mycobacterium ulcerans*. Appl Environ Microbiol 75:5667
72. Stinear TP, Seemann T, Pidot S et al (2007) Reductive evolution and niche adaptation inferred from the genome of *Mycobacterium ulcerans*, the causative agent of Buruli ulcer. Genome Res 17:192
73. Stinear TP, Johnson PDR (2007) From marinum to ulcerans: a mycobacterial human pathogen emerges. Microbe 2:187
74. Demangel C, Stinear TP, Cole ST (2009) Buruli ulcer: reductive evolution enhances pathogenicity of *Mycobacterium ulcerans*. Nat Rev Microbiol 7:50
75. Stinear TP, Seemann T, Harrison PF et al (2008) Insights from the complete genome sequence of *Mycobacterium marinum* on the evolution of *Mycobacterium tuberculosis*. Genome Res 18:729
76. Stinear TP, Mve-Obiang A, Small PL et al (2004) Giant plasmid-encoded polyketide synthases produce the macrolide toxin of *Mycobacterium ulcerans*. Proc Natl Acad Sci U S A 101:1345
77. Kent ML, Watral V, Wu M et al (2006) *In vivo* and *in vitro* growth of *Mycobacterium marinum* at homoeothermic temperatures. FEMS Microbiol Lett 257:69
78. Boisvert H, Schreder KH (1977) Skin ulcer caused by *Mycobacterium ulcerans* in Cameroon. II. Bacteriologic study. Bull Soc Pathol Exot Filiales 70:125
79. Fenner F (1956) The pathogenic behavior of *Mycobacterium ulcerans* and *Mycobacterium balnei* in the mouse and the developing chick embryo. Am Rev Tuberc 73:650
80. Hong H, Coutanceau E, Leclerc M et al (2008) Mycolactone diffuses from *Mycobacterium ulcerans*-infected tissues and targets mononuclear cells in peripheral blood and lymphoid organs. PLoS Negl Trop Dis 2:e325
81. Vandelannoote K, Durnez L, Amissah D et al (2010) Application of real-time PCR in Ghana, a Buruli ulcer-endemic country, confirms the presence of *Mycobacterium ulcerans* in the environment. FEMS Microbiol Lett 304:191

82. Eddyani M, Portaels F (2007) Survival of *Mycobacterium ulcerans* at 37 degrees C. Clin Microbiol Infect 13:1033
83. Käser M, Rondini S, Naegeli M et al (2007) Evolution of two distinct phylogenetic lineages of the emerging human pathogen *Mycobacterium ulcerans*. BMC Evol Biol 7:177
84. Yip MJ, Porter JL, Fyfe JA et al (2007) Evolution of *Mycobacterium ulcerans* and other mycolactone-producing mycobacteria from a common *Mycobacterium marinum* progenitor. J Bacteriol 189:2021
85. Röltgen K, Stinear TP, Pluschke G (2012) The genome, evolution and diversity of *Mycobacterium ulcerans*. Infect Genet Evol 12:522
86. Stragier P, Ablordey A, Bayonne LM et al (2006) Heterogeneity among *Mycobacterium ulcerans* isolates from Africa. Emerg Infect Dis 12:844
87. Doig KD, Holt KE, Fyfe JA et al (2012) On the origin of *Mycobacterium ulcerans*, the causative agent of Buruli ulcer. BMC Genomics 13:258
88. George KM, Chatterjee D, Gunawardana G et al (1999) Mycolactone: a polyketide toxin from *Mycobacterium ulcerans* required for virulence. Science 283:854
89. Gunawardana G, Chatterjee D, George KM et al (1999) Mycolactone A and B: toxins of *Mycobacterium ulcerans*. J Am Chem Soc 121:6092
90. Ross BC, Marino L, Oppedisano F et al (1997) Development of a PCR assay for rapid diagnosis of *Mycobacterium ulcerans* infection. J Clin Microbiol 35:1696
91. Portaels F, Chemlal K, Elsen P et al (2001) *Mycobacterium ulcerans* in wild animals. Rev Sci Tech Off Int Epiz 20:252
92. Johnson PD, Azuolas J, Lavender CJ et al (2007) *Mycobacterium ulcerans* in mosquitoes captured during outbreak of Buruli ulcer, southeastern Australia. Emerg Infect Dis 13:1653
93. Fyfe JA, Lavender CJ, Johnson PD et al (2007) Development and application of two multiplex real-time PCR assays for the detection of *Mycobacterium ulcerans* in clinical and environmental samples. Appl Environ Microbiol 73:4733
94. Portaels F, Meyers WM, Ablordey A et al (2008) First cultivation and characterization of *Mycobacterium ulcerans* from the environment. PLoS Negl Trop Dis 2:e178
95. Williamson HR, Benbow ME, Nyuyen KD et al (2008) Distribution of *Mycobacterium ulcerans* in Buruli ulcer endemic and non-endemi aquatic sites in Ghana. PLoS Negl Trop Dis 2:e205
96. Benbow ME, Williamson H, Kimbirauskas R et al (2008) Aquatic invertebrates as unlikely vectors of Buruli ulcer disease. Emerg Infect Dis 14:1247
97. Aiga H, Amano T, Cairncross S et al (2004) Assessing water-related risk factors for Buruli ulcer: a case-control study in Ghana. Am J Trop Med Hyg 71:387
98. Raghunathan PL, Whitney EA, Asamoa K et al (2005) Risk factors for Buruli ulcer disease (*Mycobacterium ulcerans* infection): results from a case-control study in Ghana. Clin Infect Dis 40:1445
99. Meyers WM, Tignokpa N, Priuli GB et al (1996) *Mycobacterium ulcerans* infection (Buruli ulcer): first reported patients in Togo. Br J Dermatol 134:1116
100. Merrit RW, Benbow ME, Small PCL (2005) Unraveling an emerging disease associated with disturbed aquatic environments: the case of Buruli ulcer. Front Ecol Environ 3:323
101. Wagner T, Benbow ME, Brenden T et al (2008) Buruli ulcer disease prevalence in Benin, West Africa: association with land use/cover and the identification of disease clusters. Int J Health Geogr 7:25
102. Duker AA, Portaels F, Hale M (2006) Pathway of *Mycobacterium ulcerans* infection: a review. Environ Int 32:567
103. Kibadi K, Panda M, Tamfum JJ et al (2008) New foci of Buruli ulcer, Angola and Democratic Republic of Congo. Emerg Infect Dis 14:1790
104. Palomino JC, Obiang AM, Realini L et al (1998) Effect of oxygen on growth of *Mycobacterium ulcerans* in the BACTEC system. J Clin Microbiol 36:3420
105. Hayman J (1991) Postulated epidemiology of *Mycobacterium ulcerans* infection. Int J Epidemiol 20:1093
106. Jacobsen KH, Padgett JJ (2010) Risk factors for *Mycobacterium ulcerans* infection. Int J Infect Dis 14:e677

107. Duker AA, Carranza EJ, Hale M (2004) Spatial dependency of Buruli ulcer prevalence on arsenic-enriched domains in Amansie West District, Ghana: implications for arsenic mediation in *Mycobacterium ulcerans* infection. Int J Health Geogr 3:19
108. Debacker M, Portaels F, Aguiar J et al (2006) Risk factors for Buruli ulcer, Benin. Emerg Infect Dis 12:1325
109. Pouillot R, Matias G, Wondje CM et al (2007) Risk factors for Buruli ulcer: a case control study in Cameroon. PLoS Negl Trop Dis 1:e101
110. Revill WDL, Barker DJP (1972) Seasonal distribution of mycobacterial skin ulcers. Br J Prev Soc Med 26:23
111. Quek TY, Henry MJ, Pasco JA et al (2007) *Mycobacterium ulcerans* infection: factors influencing diagnostic delay. Med J Aust 187:561
112. Sopoh GE, Johnson RC, Chauty A et al (2007) Buruli ulcer surveillance, Benin, 2003–2005. Emerg Infect Dis 13:1374
113. Marion E, Eyangoh S, Yeramian E et al (2010) Seasonal and regional dynamics of *M. ulcerans* transmission in environmental context: deciphering the role of water bugs as hosts and vectors. PLoS Negl Trop Dis 4:e731
114. Debacker M, Zinsou C, Aguiar J et al (2003) First case of *Mycobacterium ulcerans* disease (Buruli ulcer) following a human bite. Clin Infect Dis 36:e67
115. Marsollier L, Robert R, Aubry J et al (2002) Aquatic insects as a vector for *Mycobacterium ulcerans*. Appl Environ Microbiol 68:4623
116. Marsoiller L, Legras P, Manceau AL et al (2002) Role des punaises d'eau dans la transmission de *M. ulcerans*. Bull ALLF 10:23
117. Marsoiller L, Aubry J, Saint-Andre JP et al (2003) Ecology and transmission of *Mycobacterium ulcerans*. Pathol Biol 51:490
118. Marsoiller L, Aubry J, Cutanceau JP et al (2005) Colonization of the salivary glands of *Naucoris cimicoides* by *Mycobacterium ulcerans* requires host plasmocytes and a macrolide toxin, mycolactone. Cell Microbiol 7:935
119. Mosi L, Williamson H, Wallace JR et al (2008) Persistent association of *Mycobacterium ulcerans* with West African predaceous insects of the family Belostomatidae. Appl Environ Microbiol 74:7036
120. Marsollier L, André JP, Frigui W et al (2007) Early trafficking events of *Mycobacterium ulcerans* within *Naucoris cimicoides*. Cell Microbiol 9:347
121. Silva MT, Portaels F, Pedrosa J (2007) Aquatic insects and *Mycobacterium ulcerans*: an association relevant to Buruli ulcer control? PLoS Med 4:e63
122. Marsollier L, Sévérin T, Aubry J et al (2004) Aquatic snails, passive hosts of *Mycobacterium ulcerans*. Appl Environ Microbiol 70:6296
123. Veicht MGK, Johnson DPR, Flood P et al (1997) A large localized outbreak of *Mycobcaterium ulcerans* infection on a temperate southern Australian island. Epidemiol Infect 119:313
124. Johnson PD, Veitch MG, Flood PE et al (1995) *Mycobacterium ulcerans* infection on Phillip Island, Victoria. Med J Aust 162:221
125. Fyfe JA, Lavender CJ, Handasyde KA et al (2010) A major role for mammals in the ecology of *Mycobacterium ulcerans*. PLoS Negl Trop Dis 4:e791
126. Forbes BR, Wannan JS, Kirkland WB (1954) Indolent cutaneous ulceration due to infection with *Mycobacterium ulcerans*. Med J Aust 41:475
127. Connor DH, Washington CM, Fletcher LH (1966) Buruli ulceration. A clinicopathologic study of 38 Ugandans with *Mycobacterium ulcerans* ulceration. Arch Pathol 81:183
128. Goto M, Nakanaga K, Aung T et al (2006) Nerve damage in *Mycobacterium ulcerans*-infected mice: probable cause of painlessness in Buruli ulcer. Am J Pathol 168:805
129. Sarfo FS, Phillips R, Wansbrough-Jones M et al (2016) Recent advances: role of mycolactone in the pathogenesis and monitoring of *Mycobacterium ulcerans* infection/Buruli ulcer disease. Cell Microbiol 18:17
130. Mve-Obiang A, Lee RE, Portaels F et al (2003) Heterogeneity of mycolactones produced by clinical isolates of *Mycobacterium ulcerans*: implications for virulence. Infect Immunol 71:774

131. Pidot SJ, Hong H, Seemann T et al (2008) Deciphering the genetic basis for polyketide variation among mycobacteria producing mycolactones. BMC Genomics 9:462
132. Sarfo FS, Phillips RO, Rangers B et al (2010) Detection of mycolactone A/B in *Mycobacterium ulcerans*-infected human tissue. PLoS Negl Trop Dis 4:e577
133. Sarfo FS, Phillips RO, Zhang J et al (2014) Kinetics of mycolactone in human subcutaneous tissue during antibiotic therapy for *Mycobacterium ulcerans* disease. BMC Infect Dis 14:202
134. Hong H, Coutanceau E, Leclerc M et al (2008) Mycolactone diffuses from *Mycobacterium ulcerans*-infected tissues and targets mononuclear cells in peripheral blood and lymphoid organs. PLoS Negl Trop Dis 2:e325
135. Sarfo FS, Le Chevalier F, Aka N et al (2011) Mycolactone diffuses into the peripheral blood of Buruli ulcer patients—implications for diagnosis and disease monitoring. PLoS Negl Trop Dis 5:e1237
136. O'Brien DP, Comte E, Serafini M et al (2014) The urgent need for clinical, diagnostic, and operational research for management of Buruli ulcer in Africa. Lancet Infect Dis 14:435
137. Marion E, Song OR, Christophe T et al (2014) Mycobacterial toxin induces analgesia in Buruli ulcer by targeting the angiotensin pathways. Cell 157:1565
138. George KM, Pascopella L, Welty DM et al (2000) A *Mycobacterium ulcerans* toxin, mycolactone, causes apoptosis in guinea pig ulcers and tissue culture cells. Infect Immunol 68:877
139. Coutanceau E, Decalf J, Martino A et al (2007) Selective suppression of dendritic cell functions by *Mycobacterium ulcerans* toxin mycolactone. J Exp Med 204:1395
140. Simmonds RE, Lali FV, Smallie T et al (2009) Mycolactone inhibits monocyte cytokine production by a posttranscriptional mechanism. J Immunol 182:2194
141. Boulkroun S, Guenin-Macé L, Thoulouze MI et al (2010) Mycolactone suppresses T cell responsiveness by altering both early signaling and posttranslational events. J Immunol 184:1436
142. Adusumilli S, Mve-Obiang A, Sparer T et al (2005) *Mycobacterium ulcerans* toxic macrolide, mycolactone, modulates the host immune response and cellular location of *M. ulcerans in vitro* and *in vivo*. Cell Microbiol 7:1295
143. Schütte D, Um-Boock A, Mensah-Quainoo E et al (2007) Development of highly organized lymphoid structures in Buruli ulcer lesions after treatment with rifampicin and streptomycin. PLoS Negl Trop Dis 1:e2
144. Hall B, Simmonds R (2014) Pleiotropic molecular effects of the *Mycobacterium ulcerans* virulence factor mycolactone underlying the cell death and immunosuppression seen in Buruli ulcer. Biochem Soc Trans 42:177
145. Vincent QB, Ardant MF, Adeye A et al (2014) Clinical epidemiology of laboratory-confirmed Buruli ulcer in Benin: a cohort study. Lancet Glob Health 2:e422
146. Amofah G, Bonsu F, Tetteh C et al (2002) Buruli ulcer in Ghana: results of a national case search. Emerg Infect Dis 8:167
147. Boyd SC, Athan E, Friedman ND et al (2012) Epidemiology, clinical features and diagnosis of *Mycobacterium ulcerans* in an Australian population. Med J Aust 196:341
148. O'Brien DP, Friedman ND, Cowan R et al (2015) *Mycobacterium ulcerans* in the elderly: more severe disease and suboptimal outcomes. PLoS Negl Trop Dis 9:e0004253
149. Eddyani M, Debacker M, Martin A et al (2008) Primary culture of *Mycobacterium ulcerans* from human tissue specimens after storage in semisolid transport medium. J Clin Microbiol 46:69
150. Bratschi MW, Bolz M, Grize L et al (2014) Primary cultivation: factors affecting contamination and *Mycobacterium ulcerans* growth after long turnover time of clinical specimens. BMC Infect Dis 14:636
151. Converse PJ, Xing Y, Kim KH et al (2014) Accelerated detection of mycolactone production and response to antibiotic treatment in a mouse model of *Mycobacterium ulcerans* disease. PLoS Negl Trop Dis 8:e2618
152. Affolabi D, Bankole H, Ablordey A et al (2008) Effects of grinding surgical tissue specimens and smear staining methods on Buruli ulcer microscopic diagnosis. Tropical Med Int Health 13:187

153. Herbinger KH, Adjei O, Awua-Boateng NY et al (2009) Comparative study of the sensitivity of different diagnostic methods for the laboratory diagnosis of Buruli ulcer disease. Clin Infect Dis 48:1055
154. Phillips RO, Sarfo FS, Osei-Sarpong F et al (2009) Sensitivity of PCR targeting *Mycobacterium ulcerans* by use of fine-needle aspirates for diagnosis of Buruli ulcer. J Clin Microbiol 47:924
155. Portaels F (ed) (2014) Laboratory diagnosis of Buruli ulcer: a mammal for health care providers. World Health Organization, Geneva
156. Lavender CJ, Fyfe JA (2013) Direct detection of *Mycobacterium ulcerans* in clinical specimens and environmental samples. Methods Mol Biol 943:201
157. Mitjà O, Lukehart SA, Pokowas G et al (2014) *Haemophilus ducreyi* as a cause of skin ulcers in children from a yaws-endemic area of Papua New Guinea: a prospective cohort study. Lancet Glob Health 2:e235
158. Lindo SD, Daniels F Jr (1974) Buruli ulcer in New York City. JAMA 228:1138
159. Faber WR, de Jong B, de Vries HJ et al (2015) Buruli ulcer in traveler from Suriname, South America, to the Netherlands. Emerg Infect Dis 21:497
160. Phillips R, Horsfield C, Kujper S et al (2005) Sensitivity of PCR targeting the *IS2404* insertion sequence of *Mycobacterium ulcerans* in an assay using punch biopsy specimens for diagnosis of Buruli ulcer. J Clin Microbiol 43:3650
161. Johnson RC, Nackers F, Glynn JR et al (2008) Association of HIV infection and *Mycobacterium ulcerans* disease in Benin. AIDS 22:901
162. Portaels F, Zinson C, Aguiar J et al (2003) Les atteintes osseuses dans l'ulcère de Buruli: à propos de 73 cas. Bull Séanc Acad R Sci Outre-Mer 49:161
163. Phillips R, Sarfo FS, Guenin-Macé L et al (2009) Immunosuppressive signature of cutaneous *Mycobacterium ulcerans* infection in the peripheral blood of patients with Buruli ulcer disease. J Infect Dis 200:1675
164. Bahebeck J, Bedimo R, Eyenga V et al (2004) The management of musculoskeletal infection in HIV carriers. Acta Orthop Belg 70:355
165. Toll A, Gallardo F, Ferran M et al (2005) Aggressive multifocal Buruli ulcer with associated osteomyelitis in an HIV-positive patient. Clin Exp Dermatol 30:649
166. Christinet V, Comte E, Ciaffi L et al (2014) Impact of human immunodeficiency virus on the severity of Buruli ulcer disease: results of a retrospective study in Cameroon. Open Forum Infect Dis 1:ofu021
167. World Health Organization (2004) Provisional guidance on the role of specific antibiotics in the management of *Mycobacterium ulcerans* disease (Buruli ulcer). WHO.CDS/CPE&GB11.10
168. Klis S, Stienstra Y, Phillips RO et al (2014) Long term streptomycin toxicity in the treatment of Buruli ulcer: follow-up of participants in the BURULICO drug trial. PLoS Negl Trop Dis 8:e2739
169. O'Brien DP, Jenkin G, Buntine J et al (2014) Treatment and prevention of *Mycobacterium ulcerans* infection (Buruli ulcer) in Australia: guideline update. Med J Aust 200:267
170. Sugawara M, Ishii N, Nakanaga K et al (2015) Exploration of a standard treatment for Buruli ulcer through a comprehensive analysis of all cases diagnosed in Japan. J Dermatol 42:588
171. Phillips R, Kuijper S, Benjamin N et al (2004) *In vitro* killing of *Mycobacterium ulcerans* by acidified nitrite. Antimicrob Agents Chemother 48:3130
172. Phillips R, Adjei O, Lucas S et al (2004) Pilot randomized double-blind trial of treatment of *Mycobacterium ulcerans* disease (Buruli ulcer) with topical nitrogen oxides. Antimicrob Agents Chemother 48:2866
173. Adjei O, Evans MR, Asiedu A (1998) Phenytoin in the treatment of Buruli ulcer. Trans R Soc Trop Med Hyg 92:108
174. World Health Organization (2012) Treatment of *Mycobacterium ulcerans* disease (Buruli ulcer). World Health Organization, Geneva
175. Ruf MT, Chauty A, Adeye A et al (2011) Secondary Buruli ulcer skin lesions emerging several months after completion of chemotherapy: paradoxical reaction or evidence for immune protection? PLoS Negl Trop Dis 5:e1252

176. Nienhuis WA, Stienstra Y, Abass KM et al (2012) Paradoxical responses after start of antimicrobial treatment in *Mycobacterium ulcerans* infection. Clin Infect Dis 54:519
177. Sambourg E, Dufour J, Edouard S et al (2014) Paradoxical reactions and responses during antibiotic treatment for *Mycobacterium ulcerans* infection (Buruli ulcer). Four cases from French Guiana. Ann Dermatol Venereol 141:413
178. Asiedu K, Raviglione MC, Scherphier R (2000) World Health Organization. Global Buruli ulcer iniziative. Buruli ulcer: *Mycobacterium ulcerans* infection. World Health Organization, Geneva
179. Meyers WM, Shelly WM, Connor DH (1974) Heat treatment of *Mycobacterium ulcerans* infections without surgical excision. Am J Trop Med Hyg 23:924
180. Junghanss T, Um Boock A, Vogel M et al (2009) Phase change material for thermotherapy of Buruli ulcer: a prospective observational single centre proof-of-principle trial. PLoS Negl Trop Dis 3:e380
181. Braxmeier S, Hellmann M, Beck A et al (2009) Phase change material for thermotherapy of Buruli ulcer: modelling as an aid to implementation. J Med Eng Technol 33:559
182. Vogel M, Bayi PF, Ruf MT et al (2016) Local heat application for the treatment of Buruli ulcer: results of a phase II open label single center non comparative clinical trial. Clin Infect Dis 62:342
183. Smith PG, Revill WD, Lukwago E et al (1976) The protective effect of BCG against *Mycobacterium ulcerans* disease: a controlled trial in an endemic area of Uganda. Trans R Soc Trop Med Hyg 70:449
184. Portaels F, Aguiar J, Debacker M et al (2002) Prophylactic effect of *Mycobacterium bovis* BCG vaccination against osteomyelitis in children with *Mycobacterium ulcerans* disease (Buruli ulcer). Clin Diagn Lab Immunol 9:1389
185. Nackers F, Dramaix M, Johnson RC et al (2006) BCG vaccine effectiveness against Buruli ulcer: a case-control study in Benin. Am J Trop Med Hyg 75:768
186. Tanghe A, Adnet PY, Gartner T et al (2007) A booster vaccination with *Mycobacterium bovis* BCG does not increase the protective effect of the vaccine against experimental *Mycobacterium ulcerans* infection in mice. Infect Immunol 75:2642
187. Hart BE, Hale LP, Lee S (2015) Recombinant BCG expressing *Mycobacterium ulcerans* Ag85A imparts enhanced protection against experimental Buruli ulcer. PLoS Negl Trop Dis 9:e0004046
188. Phillips RO, Phanzu DM, Beissner M et al (2015) Effectiveness of routine BCG vaccination on Buruli ulcer disease: a case-control study in the Democratic Republic of Congo, Ghana and Togo. PLoS Negl Trop Dis 9:e3457
189. Pedrique B, Strub-Wourgaft N, Some C et al (2013) The drug and vaccine landscape for neglected diseases (2000–11): a systematic assessment. Lancet Glob Health 1:e371
190. O'Brien DP, Ford N, Vitoria M et al (2015) Generating evidence to improve the response to neglected diseases: how operational research in a Médecins Sans Frontières Buruli ulcer treatment programme informed international management guidance. PLoS Negl Trop Dis 9:e0004075
191. Wadagni A, Frimpong M, Phanzu DM et al (2015) Simple, rapid *Mycobacterium ulcerans* disease diagnosis from clinical samples by fluorescence of mycolactone on thin layer chromatography. PLoS Negl Trop Dis 9:e0004247

Other Nontuberculous Mycobacteria and Skin Infection

11

Domenico Bonamonte, Pietro Verni, and Gianni Angelini

Various other mycobacteria can be pathogenic for man [1–6]. Here, those that most often induce skin manifestations will be considered. These complaints, too, are to be considered non contagious, since person-to-person transmission has never yet been documented [4, 7].

11.1 *Mycobacterium avium* Complex

The *Mycobacterium avium* complex (MAC) includes two species, *M. avium* and *M. intracellulare* (MAI), that cannot be differentiated using traditional physical and biochemical tests but require specific DNA probes. *M. avium* is the major pathogen in disseminated diseases, while *M. intracellulare* is the most common pulmonary pathogen among the nontuberculous mycobacteria. It is not generally necessary to differentiate between the two species because there are no prognostic or therapeutic advantages [4].

MAC organisms inhabit a vast environmental habitat; they are present in water (indoor water systems, pools, hot tubes), soil, and in animals [8–12]. Aerosols of fresh- and saltwater may contain MAC; recirculating hot-water systems are the access route of MAC in subjects with AIDS [10, 12]. Nevertheless, infection sources are difficult to identify: only 15% of cases are linked to water, suggesting that there

D. Bonamonte, MD, PhD (✉)
Department of Biomedical Science and Human Oncology,
University of Bari "Aldo Moro", Bari, Italy
e-mail: domenico.bonamonte@uniba.it

P. Verni, MD
University of Bari "Aldo Moro", Bari, Italy

G. Angelini, MD
Professor of Dermatology, Former Professor and Chairman, University of Bari "Aldo Moro", Bari, Italy

D. Bonamonte, G. Angelini (eds.), *Mycobacterial Skin Infections*,
DOI 10.1007/978-3-319-48538-6_11

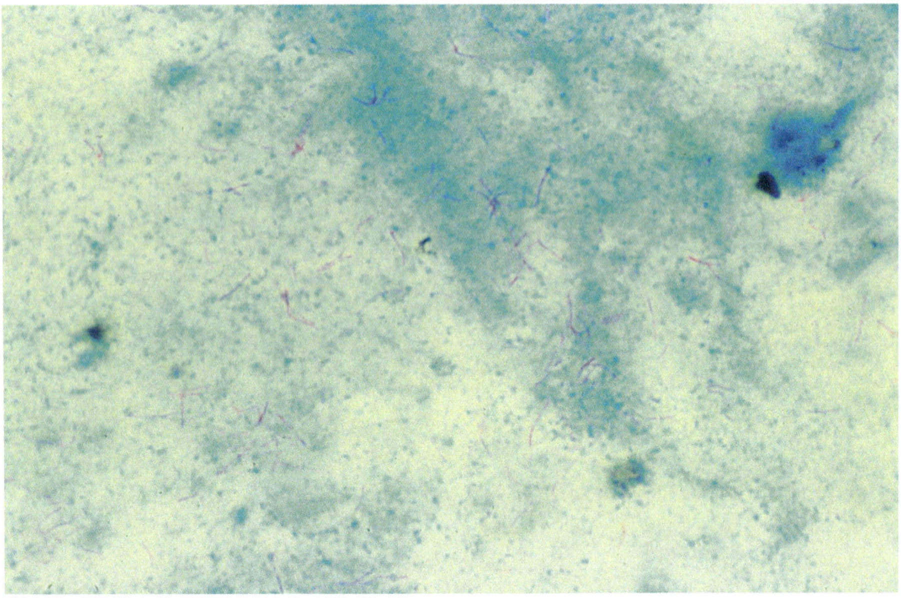

Fig. 11.1 *Mycobacterium avium* in sputum

are various other environmental sources. There does not seem to be any evidence of man-to-man or animal-to-animal transmission [6]. These organisms have also been isolated in the feces of 30% of healthy subjects [13].

Although classified as nonchromogens, some *M. avium* strains may produce a pale yellow pigment. The organism grows in 2–4 weeks in Löwenstein-Jensen medium, and rapidly in BACTEC 12B medium [1].

The *M. avium* complex most commonly causes pulmonary infection in patients with underlying lung disease (Fig. 11.1), but may also involve skin, soft tissue, tendons and joints and sometimes bone; it also is a cause of lymphadenitis in children [14]. Disseminated MAC infection is common in AIDS patients [15]. Cutaneous lesions may be primary after traumatic inoculation or secondary to disseminated infection.

Primary cutaneous infection is rare and presents with painful subcutaneous nodules, which ulcerate and discharge blood and serum; it may also appear as panniculitis or fasciitis [16, 17]. Five cases of primary cutaneous involvement were reported among Japanese patients aged between 2 and 10 years; there was no history of preceding trauma or underlying illness. The patients had multiple abscesses on the trunk or limbs [18].

In immunocompromised subjects, skin manifestations, that are frequently multiple, are secondary to dissemination [19–22]. They are generally observed in severely immunodepressed subjects undergoing antiretroviral therapy [21, 22]. MAC is one of the most common opportunistic bacteria producing disease in AIDS. Multiple purulent leg ulcers and papulo-pustules are sometimes observed [16]. A papulo-necrotic tuberculid-like eruption due to disseminated *M. avium* complex was also reported in patients with AIDS [23]. These forms are accompanied by fever, night sweats, weight loss, bone pain, hepatosplenomegaly, lymphadenopathy, and anemia. Because of the strong association with disseminated disease, in patients with MAC-induced cutaneous lesions, culture specimens should be obtained from blood, skin, sputum, urine, and lymph nodes [24].

Histopathology demonstrates a tuberculous granuloma with mononuclear cell infiltration, endothelial cell proliferation, giant cells, and extravasated erythrocytes [19]. There may also be histiocytic inflammation without granulomas. Acid-fast bacilli are seen in histiocytes [25].

Diagnosis is based on blood cultures or culture of bone marrow or liver biopsies, the predominant sites of the disseminated involvement. Matter obtained from the skin can also yield a positive culture. It is important to differentiate *M. avium* infection from lepromatous leprosy, other causes of panniculitis and ulcers, fungal infections and cutaneous tuberculosis.

MAC is nearly always resistant to single antitubercular treatment and must be treated with multidrug regimens. Some authors advise daily treatment with a four-drug regimen of isoniazid (300 mg), rifampicin (600 mg), ethambutol (25 mg/kg for the first 2 months, then 15 mg/kg), and streptomycin (optimal dose not established) for 3–6 months [16]. Instead, other authors believe that treatment should be prolonged to 12 months [4]. Among the newer macrolides, clarithromycin, combined with ethambutol, rifampicin, or both, has proven highly active, although in monotherapy, clarithromycin resistance often arises [26].

11.2 *Mycobacterium kansasii*

M. kansasii was first isolated in Kansas City in 1953 [27]. It produces yellow pigmented colonies after exposure to light and for this reason has been classified in group I of the Runyon classification [28, 29]. The organism is recognized as one of the most frequently isolated nontuberculous mycobacteria in Europe and the United States [30]. It is primarily a pulmonary pathogen, but cases of extrapulmonary and disseminated disease have also been observed [31]. Various authors have labeled *M. kansasii* as the most pathogenic nontuberculous mycobacterium [32, 33].

Unlike other common nontuberculous mycobacteria, *M. kansasii* is rarely isolated from natural water sources or soil; the major reservoir appears to be tap water [4]. Human-to-human transmission seems not to occur, although there have been two reports of familial clustering [34, 35].

M. kansasii is a slowly growing mycobacterium and grows in up to 6 weeks in various media, such as BACTEC broth, Middlebrook 7H10 agar, and Löwenstein-Jensen agar. Culture colonies are smooth or rough with a yellow pigment; they turn reddish-orange after prolonged incubation. *M. kansasii* is longer and broader than *M. tuberculosis*, and often shows a beaded or cross-barred appearance with Ziehl-Neelsen staining. It may be identified through routine tests and by means of a species-specific DNA probe [30]. Five subtypes have been identified [36].

Subspecies I is responsible for most human infections in the United States, Europe and Japan.

The incidence of *M. kansasii* infection varies by region, and has fluctuated over time. In Northern America, the highest rates are recorded in the central and southern States [37], whereas in Europe high rates are reported in England [38], Spain [39], and the Czech Republic [40]. Some studies have shown an urban predominance or an association with mining practices [39–42].

M. kansasii infection usually occurs in men with chronic obstructive pulmonary disease [4, 29]. Extrapulmonary disease can affect the lymph nodes, skin, musculoskeletal and genitourinary systems. Cutaneous disease manifests in various ways [43, 44] such as papulopustules [45], sporotrichoid verrucous nodules [46, 47], cellulitis [48], ulcers [18, 49], and granulomatous plaques [50]. It is often associated with immunosuppression or trauma [4]. Generally, immunocompetent patients present with localized lesions and a history of corticosteroid injection or skin trauma. Immunosuppressed patients, such as HIV-positive subjects, present with more diffuse lesions.

Histopathologically, the inflammation is present in the dermis and subcutaneous tissue, with acid-fast bacilli within histiocytes; chronic tuberculoid granulomas are generally devoid of bacilli [1].

There are few data to guide the treatment of extrapulmonary infection. A combination of isoniazid (300–600 mg), rifampicin (600 mg), and ethambutol (15 mg/kg) is usually recommended, given daily for 12–18 months [16, 31, 51]. Clarithromycin, shown to be highly active in vitro, may be clinically useful [26]. In patients with AIDS, streptomycin (1 g intramuscularly twice weekly) may be added to the regimen for the first 3 months [16]. Patients with acquired rifampicin resistance may be treated with daily isoniazid, ethambutol, trimethoprim-sulfamethoxazole, and initial streptomycin [52]. As an alternative to streptomycin, pyridoxine associated with an aminoglycoside, such as clarithromycin and/or moxifloxacin can be administered [31].

11.3 *Mycobacterium haemophilum*

Neither the reservoir for *M. haemophilum* nor the route of infection have yet been identified [53]. This organism has been found in patients in various areas worldwide [54–59], in particular from cities in close proximity to the ocean, Mediterranean Sea, and the Great Lakes region [60]. It was initially identified as a cause of cutaneous ulcers in an Israeli woman with Hodgkin's disease [61]. Many cases of infection have been reported in immunocompromised patients, associated with conditions such as organ or bone marrow transplantation, lymphoma or AIDS [62]. Recently, cases in immunocompetent children have also been reported [63, 64].

M. haemophilum is non pigmented and slow growing; optimal growth occurs between 28 and 30 °C in 2–4 weeks, in a atmosphere of 10% carbon dioxide with hemin (the addition of hemolyzed sheep erythrocytes is necessary, hence the name *M. haemophilum*) or ferric ammonium citrate-enriched media, or both [53, 61, 65].

Due to the low optimal growth temperature of the organism, the infection preferentially affects cooler sites of the body [53, 58, 62]. The disease may be focal or widespread. Cutaneous and subcutaneous lesions are the most common: they can be papulo-pustular, nodular, or plaques which often undergo abscess formation and ulceration. The lesions are usually multiple and located on the extremities, frequently overlying joints [53, 66]. *M. haemophilum* may also cause contagious septic arthritis and osteomyelitis, and rarely, pneumonia. More than 50% of cases have been reported in patients with AIDS [53, 58, 64, 65]. Immunocompetent children usually present with perihilar, cervical, or submandibular lymphadenitis alone [53, 64].

M. haemophilum lesions are characterized by granulomatous inflammation with suppuration, Langhans giant cells, necrosis, and acid-fast bacilli [61]. The organisms can be seen to aggregate in globi, as in lepromatous leprosy. Caseating granulomas as well as non granulomatous forms have also been reported [1].

Most *M. haemophilum* strains demonstrate in vitro susceptibility to amikacin, clarithromycin, ciprofloxacin, rifampicin and rifabutin [4, 53], but all isolated are resistant to ethambutol [4]. Optimal treatment for disseminated infection is unknown but good results have been obtained with regimens that included ciprofloxacin, clarithromycin and rifampicin [58, 67, 68]. The duration of therapy must usually be at least 6–9 months, while in immunocompromised patients the treatment duration may be indefinite [1]. Immunocompetent children with localized lymphadenitis usually respond well to surgical excision alone [59].

11.4 *Mycobacterium gordonae*

M. gordonae is a scotochromogen, slowly growing organism, generally isolated as yellow/orange colonies after incubation for 3 weeks or more at 37 °C. It is ubiquitous in the environment and is commonly isolated from soil and water sources, including tap water. This is why it was called *M. aquae* and is now known as the "tap water bacillus" [5]. Owing to its presence in water, it is associated with numerous nosocomial pseudoinfections and pseudoepidemics [69–72].

M. gordonae is the most frequently isolated mycobacterial contaminant, and is often considered non pathogenic [4]. As well as in freshwater, it is isolated from pipelines and laboratory faucets. A molecular DNA probe is available for species identification [4]. A literature review of 24 cases showed that 5 presented with disseminated disease and 19 with localized forms (8 at pulmonary, 7 soft tissue, 3 peritoneum and 1 at cornea level) [72]. Literature data demonstrate that *M. gordonae* can colonize and cause infection in patients with AIDS [73–75]. The skin manifestations consist of inflammatory nodules, most often on the limbs in immunodepressed subjects [76].

Optimal treatment in cases of infection due to *M. gordonae* has not been defined. Most of the isolates tested showed in vitro resistance to isoniazid and pyrazinamide, whereas many are susceptible to ethambutol, rifabutin, rifampicin, linezolid, erythromycin, and fluoroquinolones [4, 77].

11.5 *Mycobacterium malmoense*

M. malmoense, first described in 1977, is nonchromogenic and slow growing (at least 6 weeks) in primary isolation [78]. It is common worldwide and has been isolated from natural waters in Finland and soils in Zaire and Japan [79]. In many North Europe areas, *M. malmoense* is the second most common nontuberculous mycobacterium after MAC, and is isolated from sputum and cervical lymph nodes specimens in children [4].

Clinically, this organism has most often been associated with pulmonary disease [80, 81]. An association with coal workers' pneumoconiosis has been reported [82]. Cases of extrapulmonary disease have been described, with tenosynovitis and cervical lymphadenopathy in children [79, 83]. Disseminated infection with cutaneous lesions has also been reported, in particular in patients with AIDS or leukemia [83–85].

Most isolates are susceptible in vitro to ethambutol, ethionamide, and cycloserine, showing some resistance to streptomycin, rifampicin and capreomycin [78]. However, many authors have reported a lack of correlation between the clinical response and in vitro susceptibility among strains [81, 83, 86, 87]. Some patients were successfully treated with rifabutin, rifampicin, clofazimine, ethambutol, and clarithromycin [82, 83].

11.6 *Mycobacterium smegmatis*

As well as *M. smegmatis*, the *M. smegmatis* complex includes *M. wolinskyi* and *M. goodii*. Isolation of the three species is now possible using molecular techniques including RFLP analysis of the *hsp*65 gene [4]. This group is differentiated from the other group of rapid growing mycobacteria (*M. abscessus*, *M. chelonae*, and *M. fortuitum*) by its lack of in vitro susceptibility to clarithromycin [4].

M. smegmatis is a rapidly growing environmental saprophyte, that was isolated from smegma and syphilitic chancres in the 1880s, but has only recently been recognized as a human pathogen. *M. smegmatis* has also been isolated from soil samples, and so may have an etiological role in cases of soil-contaminated wounds. It is a rare cause of imported infections. As well as infecting the lungs and pleura, it can be associated with lymphadenitis, osteomyelitis, cellulitis, and soft tissue infection following injury or surgery [88, 89]. Disseminated infections have been reported [90].

Cutaneous infection usually needs surgical debridement.

M. smegmatis is resistant to isoniazid, rifampicin, and clarithromycin, whereas it may be susceptible to ethambutol, sulfamethoxazole, doxycycline, ciprofloxacin, ofloxacin, amikacin, and imipenem [4].

11.7 *Mycobacterium szulgai*

M. szulgai grows slowly and produces smooth or rough colonies after 2–4 weeks. It is scotochromogenic at 37 °C and photochromogenic at 25 °C. It is only rarely isolated in the environment, and only in one case has it been isolated from water [4, 91].

In most cases it affects the lungs, inducing a picture that is difficult to differentiate from those linked to *M. tuberculosis*. Other infection sites include the bursa, tendons, bones, lymph nodes, urinary tract, and skin [4]. Disseminated infection has been reported in immunocompromised patients [92].

M. szulgai is susceptible to most antitubercular drugs. Combination treatment, based on in vitro susceptibility and administered for at least 4–6 months, is recommended for extrapulmonary infection [4].

References

1. Weitzul S, Eichlrorn PJ, Pandya AG (2000) Nontuberculous mycobacterial infections of the skin. Dermatol Clin 18:359
2. Pradinaud R, Couppié P, Versapuech J (2003) Mycobactérioses cutanées enviromentales don't l'infection à *Mycobacterium ulcerans* (ulcère de Buruli). Encycl Med Chir, Editions Scientifiques et Médicales, Paris, Elsevier SAS, Maladies Infectieuses, 8-038-F-15
3. Ramos-e-Silva M, Ribeiro de Castro MC (2003) Mycobacterial infections. In: Bolognia JL, Jorizzo JL, Rapini RP et al (eds) Dermatology. Moby, London, p 1145
4. Griffith DE, Aksamit T, Brown-Elliott BA et al (2007) An official ATS/IDSA statement: diagnosis, treatment, and prevention of nontuberculous mycobacterial diseases. Am J Resp Crit Care Med 175:367
5. Bittner MJ, Preheim LC (2011) Other nontuberculous mycobacteria. In: Schlossberg D (ed) Tuberculosis and nontuberculous mycobacterial infections, 6th edn. ASM Press, Washington, DC, p 618
6. Sethi A (2012) Tuberculosis and infections with atypical mycobacteria. In: Goldsmith LA, Katz SI, Gilchrest BA et al (eds). Fitzpatrick's Dermatology in general medicine, vol 2, 8th edn. Mc Graw Hill, New York, p 2225
7. Piersimoni C, Scarparo C (2009) Extrapulmonary infections associated with nontuberculous mycobacteria in immunocompetent persons. Emerg Infect Dis 15:1351
8. du Moulin G, Stottmeier K, Pelletier P et al (1988) Concentration of *Mycobacterium avium* by hospital hot water systems. JAMA 260:1599
9. Kahana L, Kay M, Yakrus M et al (1997) *Mycobacterium avium* complex infection in an immunocompetent young adult related to hot tube exposure. Chest 111:242
10. von Reyn CF, Maslow JN, Barber TW et al (1994) Persistent colonization of potable water as a source of *Mycobacterium avium* infection in AIDS. Lancet 343:1137
11. Tobin-D'Angelo MJ, Blass MA, del Rio C et al (2004) Hospital water as a source of *Mycobacterium avium* complex (MAC) isolates in respiratory specimens. J Infect Dis 189:98
12. Sugita Y, Ishii N, Katsuno M et al (2000) Familial cluster of cutaneous *Mycobacterium avium* infection resulting from use of a circulating, constantly heated bath water system. Br J Dermatol 142:789
13. Portales F, Larsson L, Smeets P (1988) Isolation of mycobacteria from healthy persons' stools. Int J Lepr Other Mycobact Dis 56:468
14. Wolinsky E (1992) Mycobacterial diseases other than tuberculosis. Clin Infect Dis 15:1
15. Benson CA, Ellner JJ (1993) *Mycobacterium avium* complex infection and AIDS: advances in theory and practice. Clin Infect Dis 17:7
16. Hautmann G, Lotti T (1994) Atypical mycobacterial infections of the skin. Dermatol Clin 12:657
17. Sanderson TL, Moskowitz L, Hensley GT et al (1982) Disseminated *Mycobacterium avium-intracellulare* infection appearing as a panniculitis. Arch Pathol Lab Med 106:112
18. Ichiki Y, Hirose M, Akiyama T et al (1997) Skin infection caused by *Mycobacterium avium*. Br J Dermatol 136:260
19. Friedman BF, Dearborn E, Kirkpatrick CH (1988) *Mycobacterium avium-intracellulare*: cutaneous presentations of disseminate diseases. Am J Med 85:257

20. Wolinsky E (1979) Nontuberculous mycobacteria and associated diseases. Am Rev Respir Dis 119:107
21. Del Giudice P, Durant J, Counillon E et al (1999) Mycobacterial cutaneous manifestations: a new sign of immune restoration syndrome in patients with acquired immunodeficiency syndrome. Arch Dermatol 135:1129
22. Pelgrom J, Bastian I, van den Enden E et al (2000) Cutaneous ulcer caused by *Mycobacterium avium* and recurrent genital herpes after antiretroviral therapy. Arch Dermatol 139:129
23. Kullavanijaya P (1999) Atypical mycobacterial cutaneous infection. Clin Dermatol 17:153
24. Zakowiski P, Fligiel S, Berlin GW et al (1982) Disseminated *Mycobacterium avium-intracellulare* infection in homosexual men dying of acquired immunodeficiency. JAMA 248:2980
25. Sagerman PM, Relman DA, Niroomand F et al (1992) Localization of *Mycobacterium avium-intracellulare* within a skin lesion of bacillary angiomatosis in a patient with AIDS. Diagn Mol Pathol 1:212
26. Wallace RJ Jr, Glassroth J, Griffith DE et al (1997) Diagnosis and treatment of disease caused by nontuberculous mycobacteria. Am J Respir Crit Care Med 156:s1
27. Buhler VB, Pollack A (1953) Human infection with atypical acid fast organisms: report of two cases with pathologic findings. Am J Clin Pathol 23:363
28. Runyon EH (1959) Anonymous mycobacteria in pulmonary disease. Med Clin N Am 43:273
29. Hirsch FS, Saffold OE (1976) *Mycobacterium kansasii* infection with dermatologic manifestations. Arch Dermatol 112:706
30. Martin-Casabona N, Bahrmand AR, Bennedsen J et al (2004) Nontuberculous mycobacteria: patterns of isolation. A multicountry retrospective survey. Int J Tuberc Lung Dis 8:1186
31. Johnston JC, Elwood K (2011) *Mycobacterium kansasii*. In: Schlossberg D (ed) Tuberculosis and nontuberculous mycobacterial infections, 6th edn. ASM Press, Washington, DC, p 578
32. Marras TK, Daley CL (2002) Epidemiology of human pulmonary infection with nontuberculous mycobacteria. Clin Chest Med 23:553
33. Hernandez-Garduno E, Rodigues M, Elwood RK (2009) The incidence of pulmonary nontuberculous mycobacteria in British Columbia. Int J Tuberc Lung Dis 13:1086
34. Oustad GD (1969) Familial aggregations of group I atypical mycobacterial disease. Am Rev Respir Dis 99:426
35. Penny ME, Cole RB, Gray J (1982) Two cases of *Mycobacterium kansasii* infection occurring in the same household. Tubercle 63:129
36. Picardeau M, Prod'Hom G, Raskine L et al (1997) Genotypic characterization of five subspecies of *Mycobacterium kansasii*. J Clin Microbiol 35:25
37. Good RC (1979) Isolation of nontuberculous mycobacteria in the United States. J Infect Dis 142:779
38. Lambden K, Watson JM, Knerer G et al (1996) Opportunistic mycobacteria in England and Wales, 1982–1994. CDR Rev 11:147
39. Leal Arranz MV, Gaafar A, Unzaga Baranano MJ et al (2005) Clinical and epidemiological study of disease caused by *Mycobacterium kansasii* in the metropolitan area of Bilbao, Spain. Arch Broncopneumol 41:189
40. Kubin M, Svandova E, Medek B et al (1980) *Mycobacterium kansasii* infection in an endemic area of Czechoslovakia. Tubercle 51:207
41. Ahn CH, Lowell JR, Onstad GD et al (1979) A demographic study of disease due to *Mycobacterium kansasii* or *M. intracellulare–avium* in Texas. Chest 75:120
42. Isaac-Renton JL, Allen EA, Chao CW et al (1985) Isolation and geographic distribution of mycobacteria other than *M. tuberculosis* in British Columbia, 1972–1981. Can Med Assoc J 133:573
43. Breathnach A, Levell N, Munro C et al (1995) Cutaneous *Mycobacterium kansasii* infection: case report and review. Clin Infect Dis 20:812
44. Razavi B, Cleveland MG (2000) Cutaneous infection due to *Mycobacterium kansasii*. Diagn Microbiol Infect Dis 38:173
45. Bolivar R, Satterwhite TK, Floyd M (1980) Cutaneous lesions due to *Mycobacterium kansasii*. Arch Dermatol 116:207

46. Maberry JD, Mullins JF, Stone OJ (1965) Cutaneous infection due to *Mycobacterium kansasii*. JAMA 194:1135
47. Owens DW, Mc Bride ME (1969) Sporotrichoid cutaneous infections with *Mycobacterium kansasii*. Arch Dermatol 100:54
48. Fraser DW, Buxton AE, Naji A et al (1975) Disseminated *Mycobacterium kansasii* infection presenting as cellulitis in a recipient of a renal homograft. Am Rev Respir Dis 112:125
49. Drabik JJ, Hoover DL, Roth RE et al (1988) Ulcerative perianal lesions due to *Mycobacterium kansasii*. J Am Acad Dermatol 18:1146
50. Hauke CW, Temofeew RK, Slama SL (1987) *Mycobacterium kansasii* infection with multiple cutaneous lesions. J Am Acad Dermatol 16:1122
51. Davidson PT (1989) The diagnosis and management of disease caused by *M. avium* complex, *M. kansasii*, and other mycobacteria. Clin Chest Med 10:431
52. Wallace RJ Jr, Dunbar D, Brown BA et al (1994) Rifampicin-resistant *Mycobacterium kansasii*. Clin Infect Dis 18:736
53. Kiehn TE, White M (1994) *Mycobacterium haemophilum*: an emerging pathogen. Eur J Clin Microbiol Infect Dis 13:925
54. Lindeboom JA, Prins JM, Bruijnesteijn van Coppenraet ES et al (2005) Cervico-facial lymphadenitis in children caused by *Mycobacterium haemophilum*. Clin Infect Dis 41:1569
55. Lesla ES, Coppenraet BV, Kuijper EJ et al (2005) *Mycobacterium haemophilum* and lymphadenitis in children. Emerg Infect Dis 11:62
56. Artenstein AW, Fritzinger D, Gasser RA Jr et al. Infection due to *Mycobacterium haemophilum* identified by whole cell lipid analysis and nucleic acid sequencing. Clin Infect Dis 1994;19:1155
57. Bernard EM, Edwards FF, Kiehn TE et al (1993) Activities of antimicrobial agents against clinical isolates of *Mycobacterium haemophilum*. Antimicrob Agents Chemother 37:2323
58. Straus WL, Ostroff SM, Jernigan DB et al (1994) Clinical and epidemiologic characteristics of *Mycobacterium haemophilum*, an emerging pathogen in immunocompromised patients. Ann Intern Med 120:118
59. Saubolle MA, Kiehn TE, White MH et al (1996) *Mycobacterium haemophilum*: microbiology and expanding clinical and geografhic spectra of disease in humans. Clin Microbiol Rev 9:435
60. Becherer P, Hopper RL (1992) Infection with *Mycobacterium haemophilum*. Clin Infect Dis 14:793
61. Sompolinsky D, Lagziel A, Naveh D et al (1978) *Mycobacterium haemophilum* sp. nov., a new pathogen of humans. Int J Syst Bacteriol 28:67
62. Rogers PL, Walker RE, Lane HC et al (1988) Disseminated *Mycobacterium haemophilum* infection in two patients with the acquired immunodeficiency syndrome. Am J Med 84:640
63. Cohen YH, Amir J, Ashkenazi S et al (2008) *Mycobacterium haemophilum* and lymphadenitis in immunocompetent children, Israel. Emerg Infect Dis 14:1437
64. Armostrong KL, James RW, Dawson DJ et al (1992) *Mycobacterium haemophilum* causing perihilar or cervical lymphadenitis in healthy children. J Pediatr 121:202
65. Mezo A, Jennis F, McCarthy SW et al (1979) Unusual mycobacteria in 5 cases of opportunistic infections. Pathology 11:377
66. Dever LL, Martin JW, Seaworth B et al (1992) Varied presentations and responses to treatment of infections caused by *Mycobacterium haemophilum* in patients with AIDS. Clin Infect Dis 14:1195
67. Plemmous RM, McAllister CK, Garces MC et al (1997) Osteomyelitis due to *Mycobacterium haemophilum* in a cardiac transplant patient: case report and analysis of interactions among clarithromycin, rifampicin, and cyclosporine. Clin Infect Dis 24:995
68. White MH, Papadopoulos E, Small TN et al (1995) *Mycobacterium haemophilum* infection in bone marrow transplant recipients. Transplantation 60:957
69. Steere A, Corrales J, von Graevenitz A (1979) A cluster of *Mycobacterium gordonae* isolates from bronchoscopy specimens. Am Rev Respir Dis 120:214
70. Panwalker AP, Fuhse E (1986) Nosocomial *Mycobacterium gordonae* pseudoinfection from contamined ice machines. Infect Control 7:67

71. Stine TM, Harris AA, Levin S et al (1987) A pseudoepidemic due to atypical mycobacteria in a hospital water supply. JAMA 258:809
72. Weinberger M, Berg SL, Feuerstein IM et al (1992) Disseminated infection with *Mycobacterium gordonae*: report of a case and critical review of the literature. Clin Infect Dis 14:1229
73. Horsburgh C Jr, Selike R (1989) The epidemiology of disseminated nontuberculous mycobacterial infection in the acquire immunodeficiency syndrome (AIDS). Am Rev Respir Dis 139:4
74. Barber TW, Croven DE, Farber HW (1991) *Mycobacterium gordonae*: a possible opportunistic respiratory tract pathogen in patients with advanced human immunodeficiency virus, type 1 infection. Chest 100:716
75. Lessnau KD, Milanese S, Talavera W (1993) *Mycobacterium gordonae*: a treatable disease in HIV-positive patients. Chest 104:1779
76. Zala L, Hunziker T, Braathen LR (1993) Chronic cutaneous infection caused by *Mycobacterium gordonae*. Dermatology 187:301
77. Brown BA, Wallace RJ Jr, Onyi GO (1992) Activities of clarithromycin against eight slowly growing species of nontuberculous mycobacteria, determined by using a broth microdilution MIC system. Antimicrob Agents Chemother 36:1987
78. Schroder KH, Juhlin I (1977) *Mycobacterium malmoense* sp. nov. Int J Syst Bacteriol 27:241
79. Henriques B, Hoffner SE, Petrini B et al (1990) Infection with *Mycobacterium malmoense* in Sweden: report of 221 cases. Clin Infect Dis 29:149
80. Hoefsloot W, van Ingen J, de Lange WCM et al (2009) Clinical relevance of *Mycobacterium malmoense* isolation in the Netherlands. Eur Respir J 34:926
81. Research Committee of the British Thoracic Society (2003) Pulmonary disease caused by *M. malmoense* in HIV negative patients: 5-yr follow-up of patients receiving standardized treatment. Eur Respir J 21:478
82. Mc Grath EE, Bardsley P (2009) An association between *Mycobacterium malmoense* and coal workers' pneumoconiosis. Lung 87:51
83. Zaugg M, Salfinger M, Opravil M et al (1993) Extrapulmonary and disseminated infections due to *Mycobacterium malmoense*: case report and review. Clin Infect Dis 16:540
84. Chocarra A, Gonzales Lopez A, Breznes MF et al (1994) Disseminated infection due to *Mycobacterium malmoense* in a patient infected with human immunodeficiency virus. Clin Infect Dis 19:203
85. Shmoor P, Descamps V, Lebrun-Vignes B et al (2001) Infection cutanée à *Mycobacterium malmoense* chez un malade immunocompétent. Ann Dermatol Vénéréol 128:139
86. Bucholz UT, Mc Neill MM, Keyes LE et al (1998) *Mycobacterium malmoense* infections in the United States, January 1993 through June 1995. Clin Infect Dis 27:551
87. Hoffner SE, Henriques B, Petrini B et al (1991) *Mycobacterium malmoense*: an easily missed pathogen. J Clin Microbiol 29:2673
88. Wallace RJ Jr, Nash DR, Tsukamura M et al (1988) Human disease due to *Mycobacterium smegmatis*. J Infect Dis:52
89. Newton JA Jr, Weiss PJ, Bowler WA et al (1993) Soft-tissue infection due to *Mycobacterium smegmatis*: report of two cases. Clin Infect Dis 16:531
90. Pierre-Audigier C, Jouanguy E, Lamhamedi S et al (1997) Fatal disseminated *Mycobacterium smegmatis* infection in a child with inherited interferon-gamma receptor deficiency. Clin Infect Dis 24:982
91. Maloney JM, Gregg CR, Stephen DS et al (1987) Infections caused by *Mycobacterium szulgai* in humans. Rev Infect Dis 9:1120
92. Gur H, Porat S, Haas H et al (1984) Disseminated mycobacterial disease caused by *Mycobacterium szulgai*. Arch Intern Med 144:1861

Printed and bound by PG in the USA